Hutchison's Clinical Methods

Hutchison's Clinical Methods

Eighteenth Edition

Michael Swash MD, FRCP, MRCPath
Consultant Physician to The London Hospital

Stuart Mason MD, FRCP
Hon. Consulting Physician, The London Hospital

Baillière Tindall London Philadelphia Toronto
Mexico City Rio de Janeiro Sydney Tokyo Hong Kong

Baillière Tindall 1 St Anne's Road
Eastbourne, East Sussex BN21 3UN, England

West Washington Square
Philadelphia, PA 19105, U.S.A.

1 Goldthorne Avenue
Toronto, Ontaria M8Z 5T9, Canada

Apartado 26370–Cedro 512
Mexico 4, D.F., Mexico

Rua Evaristo da Veiga, 55–20° andar
Rio de Janeiro – RJ, Brazil

ABP Australia Ltd, 44 Waterloo Road
North Ryde, NSW 2064, Australia

Ichibancho Central Building, 22-1 Ichibancho
Chiyoda-ku, Tokyo 102, Japan

10/FL, Inter-Continental Plaza, 94 Granville Road
Tsim Sha Tsui East, Kowloon, Hong Kong

First published 1897
Seventeenth edition 1980
Eighteenth edition 1984

English Language Book Society Edition of Eighteenth Edition 1984
Greek edition (Gregory Parisianos) 1971
Spanish edition (Idepsa Principe de Vergara) in preparation

Typeset by Inforum Ltd, Portsmouth
Printed in Great Britain by Bemrose Printing - C.I.P., Derby

British Library Cataloguing in Publication Data
Hutchison, *Sir* Robert, *bart*
Hutchison's clinical methods.—18th ed.
1. Diagnosis
I. Title II. Swash, Michael
III. Mason, Stuart, *1919–*
616.07'5 RC71

ISBN 0 7020 1031 6

Contents

List of plates

Preface

This eighteenth edition is the fruit of much revision and some addition. Nevertheless the book continues the aims set out by Robert Hutchison, who prefaced the first edition in 1897 with these lines: 'The title *Clinical Methods* describes the scope of this book better than any other. It is not intended as a treatise upon medical diagnosis . . . It aims rather at describing those methods of clinical investigation by the proper application of which a correct diagnosis can alone be arrived at. To every student when he first begins work in a medical ward the question presents itself: How shall I investigate this case? To that question the present work is intended to provide an answer.'

We have emphasized the importance of considering the patient as a person, not a case, and to that end we have added a chapter on psychiatric assessment. The chapters on the cardiovascular system and the ear, nose and throat are new presentations. In them, as in other chapters, we have briefly introduced modern imaging techniques and physiological tests in order to show how these illustrate the nature of symptoms and physical signs. There is additional material in several of the other chapters.

We sadly record the death of Richard Bomford prior to the preparation of this edition. He was truly a patient's physician and his influence on this book is abiding.

Once again we are greatly indebted to our colleagues, listed overleaf, for their contributions. We also pay tribute to our publishers for their skill and forbearance. The responsibility for any errors is ours alone.

Michael Swash
Stuart Mason

Acknowledgements

We wish to thank the following for their help:

J. M. Pfeffer MB BS, BSc, MRCPsych	The psychiatric assessment
H. Baker MD, FRCP	The skin
A. D. W. Maclean MB BS, FRCS	The abdomen
F. P. Marsh MB BChir, FRCS	The urine, The faeces
D. T. D. Hughes BM BCh, FRCP	The respiratory system
P. G. Mills BM BCh, MRCP	The cardiovascular system
A. W. Morrison MB ChB, FRCS, DLO with G. S. Kenyon MB ChB, FRCS Ed	The ear, nose and throat
I. S. Levy BM BCh, FRCS	The eye
J. D. Perry MB BS, MRCP	The locomotor system
G. C. Jenkins MB BS, PhD, FRCPath with B. T. Colvin MB BChir, MRCP, MRCPath	The blood
A. D. M. Jackson MD, FRCP, DCH	Examination of children

1
Doctor and patient

It is easy to talk of the principles of medicine but difficult to provide accurate succinct definitions. One statement that gets near to the truth is that 'diagnosis should precede treatment whenever possible'. There are two steps in making a diagnosis. The first is observation by history taking, physical examination and ancillary investigations. The second is interpretation of the information obtained in terms of a disorder of function and structure, then in terms of pathology. This book is about observation rather than interpretation; pathology, the study of disease, is largely outside its scope. However, information and interpretation go hand in hand. The nature of further observation is determined by interpretation of information already obtained. In practice, of course, patients do not present with a diagnosis; they come with problems. The wise doctor does not think of himself as a diagnostician but rather as someone who elucidates human problems. He also realizes that labelling a disease process is but one step in the management of a problem.

THE HISTORY

The aim is to get from the person concerned an accurate account of his complaint and to see this against the background of his life as a whole. The findings should be recorded under the following headings:

1 Presenting complaint
2 History of present illness
3 Previous history of illness
4 Menstrual history
5 Treatment history

6 Family history
7 Social and occupational history

Some doctors prefer to record the patient's social and occupational history and the past and family histories before the history of the presenting complaint, since the patient's presenting illness is then viewed more clearly in the context of what has happened before. Further, it is often wise to find out about the patient's life, at least to some degree, before tackling the presenting illness itself. However, in taking the history it is neither possible nor desirable to tie a patient down to any particular sequence. He must be allowed to tell his story in his own way. Further, a good doctor begins the examination of a patient as the latter walks into the room—his general appearance, the way he walks, the way he answers questions and so on—and only finishes taking the history when the consultation is over. Occasionally a vital piece of information may come out just when the patient is leaving.

The list of headings may appear formidable and it does take some experience to know in a given case which part of the history is particularly worth pursuing. If, for instance, the patient's complaint is undue bleeding, a careful *family history* may virtually make the diagnosis. If he has chest symptoms, the fact that he worked with asbestos even twenty years earlier (*occupational history*) may be the vital clue. If his complaints are those of a severe anaemia, the fact that he has been treated with chloramphenicol (*treatment history*) may be all-important. If he has a fever, the fact that his plane put down in West Africa (*social history*) may be the clue. These are rare examples; more commonly it may be his *social circumstances*—his relations with his wife or his employer—that are at fault. When students start case taking they are wise to make at least some enquiry under all the headings listed. When they have had more experience, they may know on which they should concentrate; but in a difficult case even the most experienced doctor would be unwise to neglect any of the headings listed.

In a simple case—provided one can be sure that the case in point is simple—a few direct questions may obtain all the necessary information. As a rule it is best just to let the patient talk, even if the process seems time-consuming. One should 'listen to the patient telling one the diagnosis': the woman complaining of an itching skin rash may end her story with a remark that her husband irritates her.

History taking is a *special form of the art of communication*. It is necessarily a two-way business: two people studying each other. This is the beginning of the doctor–patient relationship on which will depend the value of the patient's history and his confidence in his doctor. For many patients consulting a doctor is an ordeal as bad as a *viva voce* for some students. However anxious the patient is to seek medical advice, he may feel, at the margins of consciousness, that the doctor is a threatening formidable figure. It is the doctor's job to put the patient at ease and encourage him to talk freely. To do this you need the right words emphasized by body language or non-verbal communication. Make it clear from your stance, gestures and expression that the patient has your whole attention and that you will not be shocked or angered by anything he says. Gazing out of the window or continually writing notes will put off the patient.

Common courtesy goes a long way towards good communication. So greet the patient, by name if possible. Whenever visiting a patient for the first time, tell him who you are and why you have come to see him. It is usually possible to start the interview with some non-committal remarks. The discovery of a common county of origin or a mutual interest in a hobby or a pet may work wonders. When the patient is telling his story always watch his body language to see if it matches his words. His eyes may give more information than his words. The clenched fist may betray tension when the words sound emotionless.

Never underestimate the power of communication inherent in touching your patient. Try holding the hand of a frightened old lady and see how it gives her more comfort than your words of reassurance. When it comes to physical examination does the patient feel your touch as an attack or caress? Gentleness is all important; indeed abdominal palpation, to be successful, must be like a caress. Patients are often greatly reassured by a thorough gentle examination. It is all part of gaining the patient's confidence.

In telling the history the patient may appear to be evasive; this is seldom, if ever, deliberate. It may be due to dementia, aphasia or sub-normal intelligence, but is commonly due to anxiety or even fright. Sometimes the symptoms cannot easily be put into words. 'I feel rotten' or 'I just don't feel myself' may be the presenting complaint of a whole spectrum of disorders. Psychological symptoms are often very difficult for the patient to express. Many people feel that such symptoms are not respectable ones to present to a doctor and substitute these symptoms by complaints of vaguely described physical discomfort, often implying polysymptomatic complaints. Later such a patient may be able to say that everything is flat and hopeless and there is nothing to live for; in other words he is depressed. An anxious patient may come with symptoms of indigestion, headache or palpitations; later he may be able to voice his ever-present feeling that something awful is about to happen. Indeed this feeling may have become so much a part of him that he is almost unaware of it.

Evasiveness is, of course, particularly common if the real problem is a sexual one or involves feelings of guilt. The spinster caring for a difficult elderly mother will not easily associate her headaches with her feelings of anger. It is important for the doctor to recognize the reasons that make a patient difficult to handle. Anger and exasperation are natural reactions if there is no determined attempt to tolerate the patient and discover why the interview is arousing mutual antipathy. We all have our own strengths and weaknesses in personal relationships. It is the doctor's job to know himself and attempt to eliminate his weaknesses while developing his strengths. This is an essential part of learning to take a history. If a patient does make one angry, it is best to recognize this and try a fresh start to the interview by saying: 'I am afraid I find what you are saying difficult to follow. Let's start again and I'll try to get it right.'

In spite of a huge proliferation of ancillary aids, *history taking and physical examination remain essential skills for the doctor*, if only for two simple reasons. Those who work in large modern hospitals are apt to forget that most of the world's population have to be treated either where there are no ancillary aids or where these are very restricted. Even where these aids are freely available, they are in varying degrees costly and are not without discomfort or risk to the patient. It was the original author of this book who wrote: 'From making the cure of the disease more grievous than the endurance thereof, good Lord deliver us.'

Special investigations should therefore be used with discretion; that is, they should be used selectively, when simpler clinical methods have indicated what further investigations are likely to be profitable. The answer to a question may aid diagnosis more than an expensive laboratory procedure. It is our view too that no doctor should request any special investigation unless he knows what information relevant to the problem it is likely to provide, and has some idea of its cost and of its possible dangers to the patient.

Thus case taking—the taking of histories and the performance of physical examinations under supervision during the period of medical clerking—remains an essential part of medical education. It is also the means of establishing the all-important relationship between patient and doctor. In this first chapter we deal with history taking and physical examination in general terms. In later chapters we shall elaborate by considering different systems individually, and the book ends with a short section about cooperation with the laboratory.

There is no one method of history taking applicable to all patients in all situations. The method will vary according to whether the history is being taken in the wards, the out-patient clinic, the surgery or the home, and according to the state of the patient and the time available. It is wise to open a non-urgent consultation with some general question such as 'What can I do for you?' or 'How can I help you?' This gives the patient an opportunity to say what he wants from the consultation. To know this at the outset may be valuable and may indeed save time. Here we attempt to describe the methods that we think should be used by students undertaking medical clerking in hospital. We shall consider these for convenience under the headings mentioned above, but must emphasize once more that patients cannot be tied down to an orderly sequence. They must be allowed as far as possible to tell their story in their own words and in their own way. Only when they have done this should they be asked to enlarge on what appear to be the more important aspects of the story and only after that should specific questions be asked.

Personal history taking must never become a stereotyped routine of asking standard questions and recording the answers, though questionnaires may be useful for special purposes.

The presenting complaint

Try to define the main complaint and its duration. The presenting complaint is simply the complaint which made the patient come to the doctor. The remarks above about apparent evasiveness may apply here, but most patients with physical disease have no difficulty. They have pain in the belly or headache or shortness of breath. In writing up the history students should avoid the temptation to include a mini-history under the presenting complaint. In most cases there is one symptom which made the patient come to the doctor and ideally this is all that should be included under this heading. One must admit, however, that some patients have more than one main complaint and a few have so many that it is impossible to identify a presenting complaint.

The question of duration may be difficult. First, many people, particularly the elderly, cannot remember the duration of their symptoms. One could indeed regard this as the normal state of affairs and suspect the patient who can remember every detail of his illness of being unduly introspective and hypochondriacal.

Most patients with long-standing symptoms tend to date them by events rather than by years, even though there is no causal relationship. The symptoms started 'after my husband died' or 'at the time of the last General Election'. With patience it is possible to get at the likely duration. After that it is wise to ask some such question as 'Did you ever have anything wrong before that?' or even 'When were you last perfectly well?' In this way earlier symptoms, which the patient regards as unimportant, may be revealed. One should remember too that patients often use the word 'chronic' to mean 'severe', rather than of prolonged duration.

The history of the present illness

Ask the patient to tell you the story of his illness from the beginning. Ideally you should allow him to do this without interruption, but this may be a counsel of perfection. It may require some tactful encouragement to make a dour or nervous patient tell you his story at all, while some talkative ones cannot keep anywhere near the point. A particular difficulty is the patient who will use pseudo-medical terms or terms of which he does not know the medical meaning. Patients who insist on talking about rheumatism, migraine, acidity, catarrh or disc should be gently discouraged and asked to describe what they actually feel to be wrong. Others will insist on talking about 'what my other doctors said'.

When the patient has told you all that he will spontaneously, ask him to enlarge on any points that you may think to be important or that you may have misunderstood. Also try to clear up any doubt about the time of onset and the duration of the main symptoms. Some patients have symptoms which come and go, and it is important to try to find out whether the relapses and remissions are related in any way to times, seasons or events in the patient's life.

When you think that you have the patient's story clearly, you should take each main symptom in turn and examine it in detail. The first step is to try to make sure that you and the patient are talking about the same thing. Ask the patient to rephrase any part of the story if his original words were unclear to you. Sometimes the history has to be elaborated before it can be understood. A patient may, for instance, complain of wind or flatulence. Since flatus is considered in our culture to be an indelicate subject, it may be assumed that he means bringing up wind, whereas he may well mean passing wind by the bowel; or he may mean that he has a feeling that he wants to get rid of wind but is unable to do so. Therefore enquire directly: 'Do you mean that you bring the wind up or that you pass it down or that you feel that you want to get rid of it but can't?' It should be unnecessary to point out that one should avoid leading questions, which themselves suggest the answer expected, as far as possible, but some questions, such as 'Have you ever spat blood?' may be essential.

Perhaps the commonest complaint which brings a patient to a doctor is a *pain* of some sort and this will serve to illustrate one way in which the nature of a symptom can be further explored.

Ask about the following points:

Site Where is it? Note whether the patient points to one spot or spreads his hands over a wide area.

Radiation Does it stay in one place or does it move or spread?

Severity Does it interfere with his activities and does it ever keep him awake at night? If it never interferes in any way with his activities and never keeps him awake at night, he is probably talking about what should properly be called discomfort. Patients who use such exaggerated terms as continual agony are usually seeking sympathy and one should try to discover the real reason for their distress, which is often social or psychological.

Timing When did it start? When does it come and when does it go?

Character What is it like? Most descriptions of the character of a pain, e.g. stabbing, burning, pricking or gnawing, are unhelpful. It is very difficult for anyone to describe a pain in words. On the other hand the distinction between a colic, which waxes and wanes and may cause a patient to roll about, and a steady pain like that of peritonitis, which causes the patient to try to avoid all movement, may be very important.

The following points are often particularly helpful in deducing what disturbance of normal function is responsible for the pain:

Occurrence or aggravation What brings it on? And what makes it worse? A pain in the centre of the chest which always comes on after a certain amount of exertion, or is made worse by exertion, is almost certainly due to ischaemia of the heart. A very similar pain which comes on a short time after eating is probably oesophageal.

Relief What makes it better? Pains may be relieved by simple measures. Pain arising in the musculoskeletal system, for instance, may be relieved by a change of position. Upper gastrointestinal pains, e.g. duodenal ulcer, are usually promptly relieved by eating. Lower gastrointestinal pains may be relieved by defaecation or the passage of wind. Cardiac pain, brought on by exertion, is relieved by rest. Any definite relief by simple things of this sort may be a valuable clue to the disturbance of function or structure involved.

The effect of drugs may also be of diagnostic value. Ischaemic cardiac pain is usually promptly relieved by trinitrites. Musculoskeletal pains are usually relieved by simple analgesics like aspirin, while discomforts associated with stress and tension are not. Most physical back pains are therefore relieved to some extent by aspirin, while tension pains usually are not so relieved. In the rare event of a back pain made worse by aspirin, one would have to think of an abdominal cause, e.g. a peptic ulcer adherent to the posterior abdominal wall.

Pain is a symptom which can usually only be further explored in clinical terms. It may, however, be possible to explore other symptoms, thirst for example, in more precise physiological terms.

Thirst must first be distinguished from the dry mouth of oral infections or of defective salivary secretion. Compulsive water drinkers complain of severe thirst but are seldom woken up by it. Thirst is, however, most commonly the prime symptom of loss of body water (with or without loss of salt). The principal causes of loss of body water are diminished intake, vomiting, diarrhoea, increased sweating (with fever or exposure to heat), increased output of urine and severe haemorrhage. Observation or simple questions will therefore uncover the immediate disorder of function or functions that are responsible for the symptom, but further questions and investigations may be necessary to explain it in terms of pathology.

If, for instance, the thirst appears to be due to loss of body water due to increased urinary output, one must recall that the huge output of urine of low specific gravity of diabetes insipidus and the similar output of urine of high specific gravity (due to glucose) of diabetes mellitus can both cause severe thirst. The passage of large amounts of urine with a specific gravity of 1010 (isotonic with plasma) in renal failure may be sufficient to cause thirst, persistent through day and night. Hypercalcaemia, by diminishing the action of antidiuretic hormone and so increasing water loss, may produce thirst and finally the administration of diuretics (or even excessive tea or coffee drinking) may promote salt and water loss with increased urine volume and so thirst.

These two examples—pain and thirst—thus serve to illustrate different ways in which all important symptoms should be explored, with the object of identifying, if possible, the disturbance of function and/or structure responsible for them.

While concerning oneself with the details of a patient's symptoms it is important not to lose sight of what may be called the shape of the illness. Is it something that began insidiously and has gradually got worse up to the present time? Or something intermittent? Or something which began acutely and is slowly getting better, but has not yet gone? Does it relate to some past illness or to a chronic disorder already diagnosed? Sometimes this shape of the illness may be more significant than individual symptoms.

Another valuable question in patients with long-standing symptoms (particularly psychological ones) is: 'What made you decide to come and see me at this particular time?' The answer is sometimes illuminating. It may well be: 'I wouldn't have dreamt of coming, but my wife made me', or it may be because an acquaintance has recently died with what appeared to the patient to be rather similar symptoms.

On pages 11–18 there is a scheme, arranged under systems, of the kinds of questions that doctors usually ask when taking a history. Such a scheme is of limited value. When the patient has told his story and the stage of examining individual symptoms is reached, the doctor should be asking himself first, 'Are we both talking about the same thing?' and then, 'What does this thing (i.e. symptom) mean in terms of disturbance of function and/or structure?' and should be framing his questions accordingly, rather than be repeating a list of standard questions. It is usual, however, to conclude the history of the present illness with a brief review of the other systems which do not appear to be implicated.

Previous history of illness

The previous history should include all important illnesses from infancy onwards. Beware of accepting ready-made diagnoses, particularly, as explained above, in the case of such terms as influenza, arthritis, rheumatism and so on. Even if more precise diagnostic terms are used, it is wise to ask a few questions about the nature of the illness to check whether the diagnosis seems likely. Questions about common infections should usually include a tactful enquiry about venereal disease and its treatment.

In some cases it may be necessary to communicate with doctors or hospitals that have treated the patient in the past to obtain information necessary for correct treatment. The name and, if possible, the address of the doctor or hospital concerned with the treatment of a previous illness should therefore be recorded, together with the name and address of the patient at the time of the previous illness, if this has changed in the interval, and in the case of a married woman her name before marriage.

The menstrual history

Women should be asked about menstruation. In the majority of cases menstruation occurs about every 28 days. Ask at what age menstruation began and, if menstruation has ceased, ask how long it has been absent. The menopause usually occurs about the age of 40 to 50 years. Enquire also whether the patient is losing more or less blood than usual. The menstrual flow is to be regarded as abnormal if it lasts for fewer than 2 or more than 8 days. Ask about premenstrual tension and about the presence or absence of pain at the periods; and ask whether the patient is or has been taking oral contraceptives.

The treatment history

The treatment history should include details of drugs taken, including psychotropic drugs, surgery, radiotherapy and psychotherapy. Adverse reactions to drugs, including hypersensitivities (especially to penicillin), are now a common cause of disease. It is essential to learn if the patient has had previous adverse effects from a drug so that its prescription can be avoided. Knowledge of current therapy is also necessary to avoid adverse drug interaction when other drugs are prescribed. A major difficulty is that patients may not be able to remember, nor may any record exist, about past treatments. Many of his remedies may in any case have been bought across the counter. In this case, and probably always, it helps to ask about remedies taken for particular complaints, e.g. 'What do you take when you have a headache?'; 'What do you take for the bowels?' Patients' memories can be aided by asking them to bring up the whole contents of their medicine store. It is often extensive and outdated. Relatives often remember more than the patient if he is very old, very young or mentally sick. It is important to discover not only whether someone was given a drug to take, but whether he took it and for the appropriate time. If the drugs were not taken as prescribed, the reasons for them not being taken must be discovered. Patients frequently do not comply with instructions. Vocabulary matters: medicines often mean something liquid or something sold in a pharmacy; drugs may mean doctors' prescriptions or illicit narcotics to a patient; and tablets may not be distinguished from capsules. It is often better to ask a patient what remedies he took for particular complaints and whether these ever disagreed with him, than to use technical terms. Hospital drug information units can help with the names of unusual drugs imported from overseas and with listing the adverse effects of any drug. Much difficulty would be avoided if all doctors used official rather than proprietary names.

The family history

Note the patient's position in the family and the ages of the children if any. Usually it is only necessary to record the state of health, the important illnesses and the cause of death of immediate relatives. If, however, there is a question of an hereditary disorder one should enquire about all known relations and attempt to construct a family tree showing those affected and those not affected.

The social and occupational history

Enquire about what may be grouped together as the patient's physical and emotional environment, his surroundings both at home and work, his habits and his own mental attitude to life and to his work. Try to visualize his life, sharing his emotions and viewing step by step his home, family, daily habits, diet and work. It may help to ask him to give an account of a typical day. Ask about:

1 The *exact nature of his occupation* (not just the name of his trade but what precisely his work involves) and whether it exposes him to injurious influences. Former occupations should also be noted. One should ask about his attitude to his work, his employers and his workmates. Sometimes one should enquire into a patient's business affairs and the possibility of financial worries.

2 His *domestic and marital relationships*, his feelings about other members of his family, his interests, hobbies, hopes, fears, the holidays he gets and whether he enjoys them, the amount of exercise he takes, the games he plays, and, in general, the sort of life he leads and the sort of person he is.

3 His *home surroundings*, their sanitary condition and the possible existence of overcrowding or of loneliness. What pets does he keep? Where did they come from and were they recently imported?

4 His *diet* and his *use of alcohol and tobacco*. It is important to ask about past habits in these respects. A man who says that he neither drinks nor smokes may have been a heavy drinker or smoker in the past. Remember too that many alcoholics will convincingly deny their dependence. Distinguish between cigarette smoking and pipe or cigar smoking. Cigarette smoking is a cause of bronchial carcinoma and vascular disease; therefore a detailed history of smoking is essential in many cases.

5 *Whether or not he has lived abroad* and if so whether he was ill there. Recent travel may be important; a patient may for instance suffer from malaria in the U.K. if he has recently travelled from or even through a malarious area.

There are two more points about history taking which should be mentioned. *First* it is sometimes as important to record that a symptom was not present as to record that it was present. Under each system therefore the absence of the most important symptoms, e.g. breathlessness and cough in the case of the respiratory system, breathlessness on exertion or cardiac pain in the case of the cardiovascular system, and paralysis, headaches or fits in the case of the nervous system, should be recorded.

Secondly the history does not end when the patient is first seen. Continuation notes should record the disappearance of symptoms or the appearance of new ones, or any other relevant fact which becomes apparent while the patient is under observation.

There follows a scheme of the kind of questions which most doctors ask in taking a history.

ROUTINE QUESTIONS

General

Weight Is it increasing, decreasing or stationary?

Sleep Has the sleeping pattern changed? Is there difficulty in getting to sleep or unusually early waking? Is the patient sleepy during the day? Are 'sleeping pills' taken?

Energy Tiredness is a universal complaint. Is it loss of energy or boredom? Is it part of general malaise?

Gastrointestinal system, abdomen and pelvis

Upper alimentary tract

If the symptoms point to disease of the upper alimentary tract, inquire about:

Pain What is its severity and site? Is it localized or diffuse? Does it radiate in any particular direction? For how long has the patient had it? Does he have intervals of freedom? If so, for how long? What is its relation to meals (if any)? Does it wake him at night? What things aggravate it? What affords relief (e.g. food, antacid powders, vomiting)? Distinguish especially between 'pain' and 'sense of discomfort' or 'fullness'.

Appetite Is it increased or reduced? If reduced, is his appetite really bad, or is the patient afraid to eat on account of pain?

Vomiting Frequency. Its relation to pain; does it relieve pain or not? Distinguish between vomiting (contraction of abdominal muscles and diaphragm) and regurgitation (contraction of stomach muscles against closed pylorus).

General characteristics of vomited matter Its amount and colour. Does it ever contain blood? Does it ever look like 'coffee-grounds'? Is it ever sour and frothy? Does it contain residues of food taken the day before?

Flatulence Does the wind tend to escape downwards or upwards? Does either form relieve the symptoms?

Water brash Does the patient ever experience excessive secretion of saliva into the mouth, with regurgitation of mouthfuls of clear, tasteless fluid?

Heartburn Does the patient suffer from pain behind the sternum? Does it come on especially when he is lying down?

Dysphagia Is there any difficulty in swallowing? If so, where does the food appear to 'stick'? Is it worse with liquids or with solids? Is swallowing painful?

Lower alimentary tract

If the symptoms point to a disorder of the lower alimentary tract, inquire about:

Diarrhoea Number and time of occurrence of motions during the day; their relation to meals or to special articles of food. Colour of the motions; are they formed, unformed, porridge-like, frothy, or frankly watery? Do they float in the lavatory pan or are they difficult to flush away? Has he ever passed any blood or slime? Is there pain during defaecation? Does the patient use purgatives or does he take anything else, e.g. beer, likely to produce loose motions?

Constipation What is the patient's usual bowel habit? Has there been any recent change in habit? If so, can this be explained by change in diet, medicines, etc.? Does the constipation alternate with diarrhoea? If so, can this be explained by the taking of purgatives? Has he any colicky pain? Has he passed blood? Has he had any vomiting? Does he take codeine in any form?

Pain Site, radiation and character? Persistent or intermittent? Where is it felt worst? Is it relieved by defaecation or by the passage of flatus?

Liver and gallbladder

If the symptoms point to disease of the liver or gallbladder, e.g. the patient is jaundiced or has pain in the region of the liver, inquire about:

Jaundice Has the patient noticed any change of colour of the urine or faeces? Does the skin itch? Have there been any other cases of jaundice among his family, friends or workmates? Has he had any kind of injection in the last three or four months?

Pain Its site. Has the patient ever had attacks of very severe pain, coming on suddenly and lasting for a few hours? If so did the pain radiate and in what direction? Was he yellow after it subsided? Has he ever had pain in the tip of the shoulder or in the middle of his back?

Inquire also regarding his digestion on the lines already laid down.

Genital system

If the symptoms point to an affection of the genital system:

Patients will usually talk spontaneously about structural things, such as a urethral discharge, swelling of the testicles or ulceration of the penis or scrotum in the male; and gynaecological abnormalities in the case of the female.

Often, however, their real complaint is of a disorder of function which is to them intensely personal and embarrassing. Tact and sympathetic listening may enable such patients to discuss disorders of coital function, such as impotence, premature ejaculation or frigidity, problems of infertility and possible anxieties about masturbation or homosexuality.

The cardiovascular system

If the symptoms point to disease of the circulatory system, inquire about:

Rheumatic fever or chorea A history of rheumatic fever or chorea is significant. If the patient is a child, also ask about sore throats and 'growing pains'.

Dyspnoea How short of breath is the patient? When does it come on? Is it present at rest or only on exertion? What degree of exertion is necessary to produce it? Does he have attacks of breathlessness at night (paroxysmal nocturnal dyspnoea)? Does he have to sit up or can he sleep lying down?

Pain or distress What is its exact site and character? If the patient has chest pain or tightness, does it radiate to the left arm, neck, shoulder or interscapular region? If so, in what direction? What precipitates it, and what, if anything, relieves it? Angina pectoris and cardiac pain are discussed on p. 233. A cramp-like pain and tiredness in the legs on exercise may be due to intermittent claudication; this is felt in the muscles of the legs, especially in the calves. Is it present only on exertion, or also at rest? Is it relieved by rest?

Palpitation What brings on palpitation and how long does it last? Does the heart give an occasional thump now and then? Is the pulse rate increased during an attack and is the pulse regular or irregular? Enquire also about cough, sputum and haemoptysis, as under respiratory system.

Do the feet swell?

Does he ever have pain in the calves when walking? Or is there undue coldness, redness or blueness of the extremities?

The blood

If the symptoms and appearances point to a blood disorder, inquire about:

Family history of bleeding. Has the patient had any loss of blood? Has he noticed any red spots in the skin? Does he bruise easily? Do his gums bleed? Has he been taking aspirin in any form? Are the stools ever black? Has he bleeding piles? (If a woman, is menstruation excessive or diminished?) What kind of diet does he eat? What drugs has he been taking and to what chemical substances is he exposed in his work or home?

Ask also about such subjective sensations as breathlessness on exertion, headache, giddiness or palpitation.

Do the feet swell?

The respiratory system

If the symptoms point to disease of the respiratory system, ask about:

Family history of tuberculosis or allergies; occupation (including past occupations) and possible exposure to animal, mineral or vegetable dusts. Ask particularly about smoking habits, past and present.

Cough Whether dry or productive. Worst at which time of day? Worsened by any particular conditions, such as cold, dust or pollen? Painful or not?

Sputum Quantity. Most produced at what time of day? Consistency, colour, and odour. Purulent or not? Ever blood-stained, and if so whether with streaks or clots, and on how many occasions?

Breathing Is the patient dyspnoeic? Does dyspnoea occur at rest, or after varying degrees of exertion? Various 'grades' of dyspnoea have been described, but for the student it is best to inquire from the patient what sort of activity (walking upstairs, running for a bus, etc.) produces dyspnoea. Patients with severe pulmonary disease may by dyspnoeic at rest.

Wheeze Wheezing may be associated with dyspnoea. The student should inquire when wheezing occurs. Is it constant or intermittent? Does anything provoke it? Is it worse at any particular time of day or night?

Chest pain Where is it? Is it aggravated by deep breathing or coughing? Was it associated with increase in cough, sputum or dyspnoea? Was the onset sudden, as in spontaneous pneumothorax?

The urinary system

If the symptoms point to disease of the *kidneys*, e.g. oedema, or *urinary system*, e.g. pain on micturition, ask about:

History of tonsillitis or previous renal disease. Family history of renal disease or high blood pressure. What analgesics has the patient taken?

Has he any pain in the lumbar region or any attacks of acute pain shooting down into the groin or testicles?

The following remote symptoms: headache, vomiting, drowsiness, fits, dimness of vision, dyspnoea.

Does the face ever look puffy in the morning? Are the ankles swollen?

What is the state of the bowels?

Inquire regarding micturition, as follows:

Urine Is the urine altered in amount? Does the patient have to get up at night to pass it?

Is it altered in colour? Is it clear or turbid when passed? Any blood in it? If so, at what period of micturition is it present? Is the urine frothy?

Is there any increased frequency of micturition? Is the increase by day or by night? Is there an increase in volume passed? Is frequency associated with undue thirst? Distinguish between *polyuria* as in diabetes and chronic renal failure and *frequency* as in cystitis.

Is there any pain during micturition? Is it before, during or after the act? What is its character, and where is it felt?

Skin diseases

Inquire carefully into the patient's personal habits as regards diet, clothing and washing. What is his occupation? Does he handle chemical substances or other irritants? Ask if he has been taking any drugs recently. It may be necessary to inquire carefully regarding syphilis. Does the eruption itch? If so, when is the itching worst? Did the eruption appear all at once or in crops? Does he suffer from asthma, hay fever or any other allergic conditions? What are his hobbies? Is he in contact with animals, with insects, with plants? What has he applied to his skin on his own initiative, or on the instructions of his doctor? What cosmetics does she use? Is there a *family* history of skin disease, asthma, hay fever, urticaria? Is there a family history of loss of hair or of excessive hair?

The nervous system

If symptoms point to a disorder of the nervous system, ask about:

A family history of mental illness, paralysis, or fits. The nature of the patient's work; is he exposed to any poisons, e.g. lead, mercury, manganese, carbon disulphide or other volatile substances? Syphilis and alcohol should be inquired about. Has he been exposed to tropical infestations?

It is always important to inquire about discharge from the ear and about recent or remote head injury.

If the patient complains of *fits* or *blackouts* the following questions should be asked in order to clarify the nature of the attacks:

Age at first attack? Describe the first attack. When did the second occur? What has been shortest and longest interval between attacks? Do they occur in sleep or not? Has he any premonition or *aura*? What is its character? Does the patient go rigid? Does he lose consciousness? Is the onset sudden or gradual? Are convulsions present? Are they general or local? Where do they begin and end? Does he fall? Has he ever hurt himself? Does he bite his tongue, micturate of defaecate during the fit? Are there any after-symptoms, such as sleep, headache, automatism or paralysis? Is there any subsequent mental disturbance? Because these patients are seldom clear as to the exact nature of their fits, it is important to obtain a description from a witness of the patient's attacks. The word 'fit' is often undesirable and 'attack' or 'seizure' is preferable.

If he complains of *paralysis* or *stroke* inquire regarding symptoms of heart disease, hypertension, or diabetes (see Cardiovascular and Urinary Systems). Had he any premonitory symptoms before the onset? How did the paralysis come on? Suddenly or gradually? Has he any headache or vomiting? Where is the headache situated? Describe the patient's disability in detail. Other subjective symptoms of nervous disease are considered in Chapter 10.

If the patient complains of *headache*, describe its site, the factors which improve, worsen or precipitate it, its quality, severity and timing, and the effect of recent treatment. What does the patient think has caused it? Are there family problems or other sources of personal or emotional conflict and tension? Does the patient fear brain tumour? Is there a history of recent head trauma and, if so, is litigation pending? Does the headache have the characteristics of raised intracranial pressure? Is it migrainous? Is there a family history of headache?

Dizziness is another common symptom. Is it intermittent? Does it relate to changes in head posture? Is there a history of deafness or ear problems? Is there a history of trauma? Is it getting better or worse? Are there any features to suggest brain stem disease, e.g. unsteadiness of gait, slurred speech, double vision or facial numbness?

The locomotor system

If the symptoms point to a disorder of the bones or joints:

Inquire for previous manifestations of rheumatoid arthritis, rheumatic fever or gout. Ask about possible associated conditions in the skin (e.g. dermatomyositis, psoriasis, disseminated lupus erythematosus, scleroderma and erythema nodosum), the bowels (ulcerative colitis) and the eyes (e.g. conjunctivitis, uveitis and Sjögren's disease). Ask about the presence of a urethral discharge in the male or of vaginal discharge in the female. Has the patient been exposed to rubella? Is there a family history of gout or other rheumatic disorder?

If there is pain referred to a bone, ask whether it is worse in the day or in the night. Bone pains are often described as being deep and boring.

If the pain is in a joint, ask whether it is present constantly or only when the joint is moved. Has the joint been visibly swollen? Does the pain move from one joint to another, as is characteristic of acute or subacute rheumatism?

Describe the patient's gait and other disabilities.

Children

If the patient is a young child, the following special questions should be put to the mother or other responsible person:

How many other children are there in the family? What are their sexes and ages? Have there been any miscarriages or stillbirths? If so, when? Is there a history of illness in the parents or siblings, or in the parents' near relatives?

Was the mother well during pregnancy and did she take any drugs? Was this a fullterm infant? What was the birth weight? Was the child born at home or in hospital, and was the labour normal? Were there any unusual symptoms, such as jaundice, cyanosis or fits, in the newborn period?

Was the baby breast-fed, and for how long? If bottle-fed, what type of milk was used? Were vitamin supplements given? When was mixed feeding introduced? Was there a satisfactory weight-gain in infancy? What immunizations were given, and when?

It is particularly important to inquire about the 'milestones of development' (p. 469). When did the baby first smile, sit up, walk and talk? When did he acquire control of bowels and bladder?

What are the child's present habits with regard to eating, sleeping, bowels and micturition? What is his general behaviour like in comparison with his siblings or other children of the same age? If the child is of school age, does he attend school regularly, does he get on well with his lessons, and does he like school?

Has the child ever been separated from his mother? If so, when and for how long? What is the social background? Are the living conditions satisfactory? Does the mother go out to work? If she does, who looks after the child while she is away? Is this an immigrant family? If so, where do they come from, and how long have they been in this country?

Finally, inquire about previous illnesses, their nature and severity, and the ages at which they occurred—infectious diseases, fits, bowel disturbances, upper respiratory infections, discharging ears. If there is a history of cough, was it spasmodic, associated with vomiting, particularly bad at night? And was there a whoop? What drugs has the child received? Has the child ever been in hospital? Have there ever been any accidents involving physical injury, burns or poisoning?

In taking the history try to discover what is really worrying the parents. It may be something deeper than is suggested by the child's symptoms, for example leukaemia or some other serious disease which affected another child in the family.

The occupational history

In clinical practice the occupational history is often valuable, and there are few surer and quicker means of gaining a patient's confidence than the display of an intelligent knowledge of his or her job. If there is any suspicion that the patient's symptoms are due to his occupation it is necessary to take the occupational history from the time the patient left school. Record the dates and items of all subsequent jobs. He may be exposed to a noxious substance responsible for his ill-health in his present occupation, but this should not be assumed. An ice-cream vendor may have a mesothelioma due to exposure to asbestos many years before. Cancer of the genito-urinary tract may be the result of exposure in the past to certain aromatic amines used as intermediates in the dye-stuffs industry, as an anti-oxidant in rubber and cable-making. Ask the patient the name of his trade, the processes employed, the tools used and the substances handled. The name of an occupation may be misleading, as different names are used for the same process in different places.

The man may be ignorant of the nature of a substance he uses and knows it only by a trade name. In such cases it is best to communicate with his works manager and ask about the substance in question.

Question him on the general conditions at his place of work. Is the job dusty, and if so what tools make the dust? Are there fumes or vapours, and if so what are the chemical substances involved? Most of the toxic substances encountered in the dangerous trades enter the body by inhalation. Ask whether a hood is installed over his bench, and whether it is connected to a suction system. Ask about the provision of protective clothing at his place of work. Does he wear a special suit, gloves or goggles, and why? Finally ask whether any similar illness has befallen a fellow workman.

Other aspects of the history are no less important. A particular illness may render a man temporarily or permanently unfit to do his work. The doctor should know that conditions peculiar to certain trades may cause disease which predisposes to infection. Thus, silicosis leads to an excessive mortality from pulmonary tuberculosis and also from pneumonia. Diseases other than infections may be involved. For example, a heavy mortality from cirrhosis of the liver as well as from tuberculosis exists among publicans, barmen, brewers' draymen and others who have ready access to alcohol.

The doctor should have regard for his patient's work even when he is suffering from a disease which is non-occupational. One must know whether a man does a job which makes him a danger to others. A dairyman with open tuberculosis can contaminate milk with tubercle bacilli by coughing into it, and those who handle food can initiate outbreaks of typhoid fever, dysentery and *Salmonella* infection by acting as carriers. Those who drive heavy goods or public transport vehicles come under stringent medical regulations. The possible effect of any drug on the patient's occupation must always be considered. Antihistamines may cure hay fever but make the patient so sleepy that he cannot work without danger to himself or others.

THE PHYSICAL EXAMINATION

The examination of the general state of the patient and of the different systems is described in Chapters 2 to 17. Though the findings should be recorded under systems, patients in medical wards are usually examined from above downwards, by the methods of inspection, palpation, percussion and auscultation, as may be appropriate to the different parts of the body. One should therefore develop a routine of physical examination which combines speed with thoroughness, but disturbs the patient no more than necessary. With practice a routine examination of the kind outlined here can be performed in 15 minutes or less. It need hardly be said that the examination must be carried out as gently as possible, without tiring or exposing the patient more than necessary. In the case of severely ill patients it may be necessary to postpone a routine examination and to perform only the minimum necessary for a provisional diagnosis and treatment. Ill patients must obviously be treated with special care and consideration.

Different doctors have different routines for examining patients in different circumstances, and for writing up their case notes.

The following is the kind of routine examination which students are expected to carry out on patients in medical wards in hospital. Such a routine may have to be modified according to the needs of the patient, e.g. minimum necessary examination in an acutely ill patient, complete examination of the nervous system in a patient with neurological symptoms (see Chapter 10) or according to the circumstances, e.g. in the doctor's surgery or in the patient's home.

During the taking of the history and the performance of the examination the following should be observed:

General

General appearance of illness (does the patient look healthy, unwell or ill?)
Intelligence (see p. 62)
Mental state (see pp. 59 and 277)
Expression

Build
State of nutrition, obesity, oedema
Skin colour, cyanosis, anaemia, jaundice, pigmentation
Skin eruptions, petechiae, spider naevi (see Chapter 4)
Body hair
Deformities, swellings
Temperature, pulse, respiration rate

Hair

Area of scalp covered
Texture

Eyes

Simple tests of visual acuity: compare one eye against the other
Exophthalmos or enophthalmos
Ptosis
Oedema of the lids
Conjunctivae: anaemia, jaundice or inflammation
Pupils: size, equality, regularity, reaction to light, accommodation
Eye movement, nystagmus, strabismus
Ophthalmoscopic examination of the fundi

Face

Facies
Function of motor part of trigeminal nerve
Function of facial nerve

Mouth and pharynx (a torch and tongue depressor should be used)

Breath odours
Lips: colour and eruptions
Tongue: protrusion and appearance
Teeth and gums (if patient has dentures, notice whether they fit and ask whether they are worn for meals or only for adornment)
Buccal mucous membrane: colour and pigmentation
Pharynx
Movement of soft palate
State of tonsils

Neck

Movements

Veins
Lymphatic glands
Thyroid
Carotid pulses

Upper limbs

General examination of arms and hands
Fingernails: clubbing or koilonychia
Pulse rate, rhythm, volume and character
State of arterial wall of radials and brachials
Axillae, lymph glands
Blood pressure
Test for power, tone, reflexes, coordination and sensation
Joints

Thorax

Anteriorly and laterally
- Type of chest, asymmetry if any, breasts
- Rate, depth and character of respiration
- Pulsations
- Dilated vessels
- Position of trachea by palpation
- Look for and palpate apex beat
- Palpate over praecordium for thrills
- Palpate respiratory movements
- Estimate tactile vocal fremitus
- Percuss the lungs
- Auscultate the hearts sounds
- Auscultate the breath sounds
- Estimate vocal resonance

Posteriorly (patient sitting)
- Inspect and palpate respiratory movement
- Estimate tactile vocal fremitus
- Percuss the lung resonance
- Auscultate the breath sounds
- Estimate vocal resonance
- Note movements and deformities of the spine
- Palpate from behind, cervical glands, thyroid
- Look for sacral oedema

Abdomen

Inspection: size, distension, symmetry

Abdominal wall: movement, scars, dilated vessels
Visible peristalsis or pulsation
Pubic hair
Hernial orifices
Palpation: tenderness, rigidity, hyperaesthesia, splashing, masses, liver, gall-bladder, spleen, kidneys, bladder
Percussion: masses, liver, spleen, bladder
Auscultation: bowel sounds, murmurs
Impulse on coughing at hernial orifices
Inguinal glands
Genitalia: penis, scrotum, spermatic cord
Abdominal reflexes
Rectal examination when indicated
Gynaecological examination when indicated

Lower limbs

General examination of legs and feet
Oedema
Varicose veins
Test for power, tone, reflexes (including plantar response), coordination and sensation
Joints
Peripheral pulses
Temperature of feet

Examination of excreta

Urine, sputum, stools, vomit: examine by naked eye and measure or estimate amount
Test urine for specific gravity, sugar, protein and blood

WRITING OUT THE HISTORY AND EXAMINATION

Different doctors record the history and examination in different ways. The aim is to write a complete yet concise record of a patient's illness. For easy reference this is best done in note form, with important facts starred or underlined. It is often helpful to record routine details of the patient's marital status, children, age, occupation, financial and racial status, and the family history and past medical history first. The patient's presenting complaint and the history of the presenting illness then fall naturally into context with this background information. This approach is particularly pertinent when taking and recording a history of symptoms likely to be psychogenic, or related to potentially serious or difficult problems, e.g. the consequences of head injury or of cancer and its treatment.

The physical examination, although performed from above downwards, should be written out under systems. A short statement of the findings under each system should be included, for the absence of signs, as well as of symptoms, can be as important as their presence. The minimum statement about a patient's cardiovascular system might for example read as follows:

pulse 76 regular
neck veins not distended
BP 130/80
apex beat not displaced
heart sounds I and II heard in all areas
no murmurs

Simple line drawings can often convey more information than much writing. It is usual for a student to conclude his writing-up of a case with a list of tentative diagnoses and a list of investigations required, followed by continuation notes. This part of the medical record in particular has been much criticized. A formal scheme of recording with the self-explanatory title, 'Problem-orientated medical records' or POMR, has been adopted by some institutions, and was well described in the *British Journal of Hospital Medicine* (1972) 7, 603. However, the decision to adopt POMR is really one for the department or unit rather than for the individual student, although tentative diagnoses, if not the records, can be problem-orientated with advantage.

PRESENTING A CASE

The value of a student's or doctor's notes on a case is much diminished if he is unable to communicate them in concise form to other students or doctors. Students should therefore practise making a short summary of their findings, emphasizing both important positive findings and relevant negative ones. The summary should always begin with the name, age, sex and occupation of the patient, and can with advantage end with a brief statement of the problems to which the findings have given rise.

INTERPRETATION

The object of history taking, physical examination and ancillary investigations is the *making of a diagnosis*. In the past this has often been taken simply to mean the detection of a disease process, e.g. 'This patient has Hodgkin's disease'. If no disease process was detected the complaints were described as functional. This was illogical since all disease involves some disorder of function. The majority of patients consult a doctor about bodily disorders that express mental distress. The detection and alleviation of these problems are as important as the diagnosis of an organic disease process. Furthermore, the patient's own concept of his disease and his reaction to it has to be assessed alongside the doctor's diagnosis. Ultimately, it is the patient's symptoms that must be relieved.

One should begin the process of making a diagnosis by asking oneself some such broad questions as 'What is this person's problem?' and 'Has he a disability?' If one decides that he has a disability, one should ask:

1 *How far* can this person's disability be explained by his environment, i.e. in geographical, socio-economic and cultural terms?
2 *How far* can this person's disability be explained by his own attitude and mental make-up, i.e. in psychological terms?
3 *How far* can this person's disability be explained by a disease process or processes, i.e. in pathological terms?

Such an approach is clearly more reasonable than to search for a disease process and then to label as functional any disability not so accounted for.

It used also to be axiomatic that one should try to account for all a patient's symptoms by one disease process. But a surprising number of patients have in fact more than one (e.g. coronary artery disease and an hiatus hernia, both of which may produce central chest pain) and still more have a disease process which either does not explain their symptoms at all or does not explain all their symptoms (e.g. weakness and tiredness in a patient with mild angina pectoris or mild anaemia). Moreover an apparently simple event may have a complex medical background. For instance, an old lady gets out of bed, trips and breaks her wrist. Very probably she was hurrying to the lavatory as she had cystitis, tripped because her vision was impaired by cataract, and the bones broke because they were weakened by osteoporosis.

In making a diagnosis one should try to account for a person's total disability and should not be dismayed if this involves mentioning more than one item. Thus the diagnosis in an old lady with multiple symptoms might well be:

1 Loneliness
2 Depression
3 Mild degenerative osteoarthritis

or in a young man with dyspepsia:

1 Impending marriage
2 Anxiety state
3 Duodenal ulcer

A diagnosis of this kind gives a true picture of the state of affairs as it lists the patient's problems and is not confined to labelling organic disease.

2 General considerations

A good physical examination requires a cooperative patient and a quiet, warm and well-lit room. Daylight is better than artificial light because the latter may mask changes in skin colour, for example the faint yellow tinge of slight jaundice. Although in practice the examination may have to be made under all sorts of circumstances, every attempt should be made to reassure and relax the patient. For a complete examination the patient should be asked to take off all his clothes and should then be covered by a blanket or dressing gown. Patients are often examined while wearing underpants, but it is essential to remember to examine the buttocks and genitalia. Ideally a chaperone should be present when a male doctor is examining a female patient and during rectal and vaginal examinations, both to reassure the patient and to protect the doctor from subsequent accusations of improper conduct.

Considering the general appearance, the most important step is to make a rapid assessment of the *degree of 'illness'*. This is not making a diagnosis. One has simply to answer the question: 'Does this patient look well, mildly ill, or severely ill and therefore in need of urgent attention?' Experienced nurses are often highly skilled in this kind of assessment and their opinion should never be ignored. Some severely ill patients complain little; occasionally one meets a patient whose appearance of excellent health belies his protestations of unbearable agony.

It has already been said that a good doctor begins his examination as soon as he meets the patient, and continues taking the history until the consultation ends. An abnormal finding on examination may indicate the need for further questioning. The examination may provide information about organs and functions, but in physical examination as well as in history taking it is important to try to view the patient as a whole person and to find his reaction to his illness.

The mental and emotional state

One should therefore make some assessment of the patient's intelligence and of his mental and emotional state. Simple tests of intelligence (p. 62) and mental state (pp. 59 and 277) may be necessary. Observation, as well as the history, may assist in the assessment of the emotional state. Thus an anxious person may be restless, with wide palpebral fissures and sweating palms. Is the anxiety reasonable in the circumstances or is the patient over-anxious? The lowered mood, inability to concentrate or make decisions, mental retardation, apathy or even obvious misery of a depressed patient my be clearly evident; but so-called 'masked depression', in which these features are less obvious, is an important cause of physical symptoms. Apparently severe disability, without appropriate concern or anxiety, should suggest malingering or hysteria (*la belle indifférence*).

The attitude

The attitude of a patient may give valuable information. Severely ill patients slip down into the most uncomfortable attitudes and are unable to correct their position for themselves. Patients with congestive heart failure may become dyspnoeic if they lie flat (*orthopnoea*). Patients with abdominal pain due to peritonitis lie still, while patients with colic are restless or even roll about in futile attempts to find relief. Patients with painful joint diseases often have an attitude of helplessness. Various neurological disorders produce characteristic postures (Chapter 10). In the severest cases of meningitis the neck may be bent backwards so that the head appears to bore into the pillow (*neck retraction*). In very severe cases, and in migraine, photophobia is prominent.

The gait

The gait should be observed in patients able to walk. Important abnormalities of the gait are described in Chapters 10 and 14, but note that simple things like a painful corn, an ill-fitting shoe or a strained muscle may produce a temporary limp.

Physique

Much can be learned from a general inspection of the patient's physique. Is his appearance consistent with his age? Is he tall, short, fat, thin, muscular or asthenic? Are there any obvious deformities and is the body proportionate? Height should be roughly equal to the finger-tip to finger-tip measurement of outstretched arms and twice the leg length from pubis to heel. Dwarfism with a stocky body and very short legs is characteristic of achondroplasia. Hypopituitarism arising in childhood produces a proportionate, but dwarfed, adult with an unusually youthful appearance.

'Ideal' weights, as used in life insurance assessment, are listed in Tables 2.1 and 2.2. Obesity is a problem of developed countries. In some parts of the world signs of malnutrition such as wasting, apathy, anaemia and skin changes may be encountered; they should also be looked for in neglected elderly patients in the U.K. A history of weight gain or loss can be checked by observation, remembering that fluid retention (*oedema*) will increase weight. Obvious weight loss, mainly from loss of adipose tissue, when food intake has increased is seen in thyrotoxicosis and diabetes mellitus. Psychogenic loss of appetite in girls (anorexia nervosa) causes extreme emaciation while physical activity remains unimpaired.

Table 2.1 Ideal weights for men aged 25 and over

Height ft in	cm	Small frame lb	Small frame kg	Medium frame lb	Medium frame kg	Large frame lb	Large frame kg
5 2	157.5	112–120	50.8–54.4	118–129	53.5–58.5	126–141	57.2–64.0
5 3	160.0	115–123	52.2–55.8	121–133	54.9–60.3	129–144	58.5–65.3
5 4	162.6	118–126	53.5–57.2	124–136	56.2–61.7	132–148	59.9–67.1
5 5	165.1	121–129	54.9–58.5	127–139	57.6–63.0	135–152	61.2–68.9
5 6	167.6	124–133	56.2–60.3	130–143	59.0–64.9	138–156	62.6–70.8
5 7	170.2	128–137	58.1–62.1	134–147	60.8–66.7	142–161	64.4–73.0
5 8	172.7	132–141	59.9–64.0	138–152	62.6–68.9	147–166	66.7–75.3
5 9	175.3	136–145	61.7–65.8	142–156	64.4–70.8	151–170	68.5–77.1
5 10	177.8	140–150	63.5–68.0	146–160	66.2–72.6	155–174	70.3–78.9
5 11	180.3	144–154	65.3–69.9	150–165	68.0–74.8	159–179	72.1–81.2
6 0	182.9	148–158	67.1–71.7	154–170	69.9–77.1	164–184	74.4–83.5
6 1	185.4	152–162	68.9–73.5	158–175	71.7–79.4	168–189	76.2–85.7
6 2	188.0	156–167	70.8–75.7	162–180	73.5–81.6	173–194	78.5–88.0
6 3	190.5	160–171	72.6–77.6	167–185	75.7–83.5	178–199	80.7–90.3
6 4	193.0	164–175	74.4–79.4	172–190	78.1–86.2	182–204	82.7–92.5

Heights are measured wearing ordinary shoes and weights in ordinary indoor clothing. Notice that tables of this kind make no allowance for 'middle-aged spread'.

Table 2.2 Ideal weights for women aged 25 and over

Height ft in	cm	Small frame lb	Small frame kg	Medium frame lb	Medium frame kg	Large frame lb	Large frame kg
4 10	147.3	92– 98	41.7–44.5	96–107	43.5–48.5	104–119	47.2–54.0
4 11	149.9	94–101	42.6–45.8	98–110	44.5–49.9	106–122	48.1–55.3
5 0	152.4	96–104	43.5–47.2	101–113	45.8–51.3	109–125	49.4–56.7
5 1	154.9	99–107	44.9–48.5	104–116	47.2–52.6	112–128	50.8–58.1
5 2	157.5	102–110	46.3–49.9	107–119	48.5–54.0	115–131	52.2–59.4
5 3	160.0	105–113	47.6–51.3	110–122	49.9–55.3	118–134	53.5–60.8
5 4	162.6	108–116	49.0–52.6	113–126	51.3–57.2	121–138	54.9–62.6
5 5	165.1	111–119	50.3–54.0	116–130	52.6–59.0	125–142	56.7–64.4
5 6	167.6	114–123	51.7–55.8	120–135	54.4–61.2	129–146	59.5–66.2
5 7	170.2	118–127	53.5–57.6	124–139	56.2–63.0	133–150	60.3–68.0
5 8	172.7	122–131	55.3–59.4	128–143	58.1–64.9	137–154	62.1–69.9
5 9	175.3	126–135	57.2–61.2	132–147	59.9–66.7	141–158	64.0–71.7
5 10	177.8	130–140	59.0–63.5	136–151	61.7–68.5	145–163	65.8–73.9
5 11	180.3	134–144	60.8–65.3	140–155	63.5–70.3	149–168	67.6–76.2
6 0	182.9	138–148	62.6–67.1	144–159	65.3–72.1	153–173	69.4–78.5

Heights are measured wearing ordinary shoes and weights in ordinary indoor clothing. Notice that tables of this kind make no allowance for 'middle-aged spread'.

The face

Observe the patient's face. His expression, and particularly his eyes, may indicate his real feelings better than do his words. The characteristic facies of various diseases, e.g. myxoedema, thyrotoxicosis, acromegaly, 3rd and 7th cranial nerve palsies (pp. 298, 310) and paralysis of the cervical sympathetic (Horner's syndrome) (p. 306), must be learnt in practice.

Parotid swellings are obvious on inspection of the face. The temporary tender bilateral parotid swelling of mumps or the unilateral swelling with reddening of the skin from acute parotitis can be contrasted with the non-tender bilateral persistent enlargement, accompanied by dry tearless eyes, of Sjögren's syndrome, or the more irregular unilateral lump of a mixed parotid tumour.

The *cheeks* give some information regarding the patient's health: in anaemia and hypopituitarism they are pale; in the nephrotic syndrome they are pale and puffy; in cases of mitral stenosis there is sometimes a bright circumscribed flush over the malar bones; in many persons who lead an open-air life they are red and high-coloured; in congestive heart failure they may also be high-coloured, but the colour is of a bluish tint which cannot be mistaken for the red cheeks of weather-beaten people. In some cases of disseminated lupus erythematosus there is a red raised eruption on the bridge of the nose extending on to the cheeks in a 'bat's-wing' distribution. *Telangiectases*, minute capillary tortuosities, or *naevi*, may be seen on the face in liver disease and, rarely, as a hereditary disorder (Fig. 2.1).

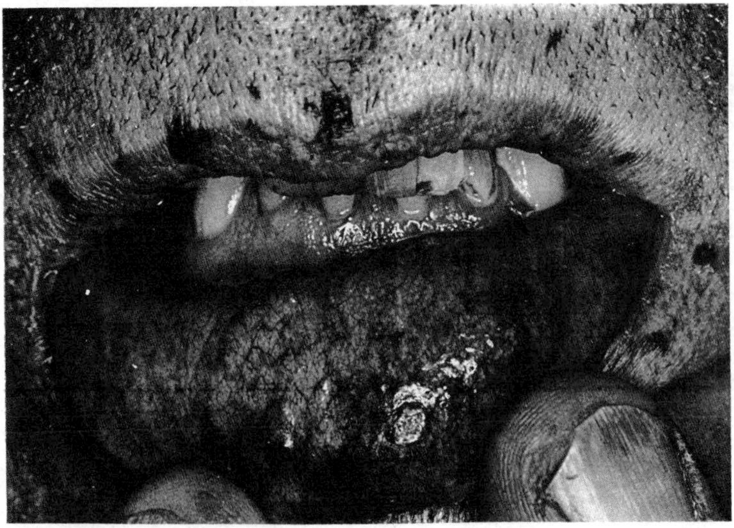

Fig.2.1 Hereditary telangiectasia. The telangiectasia can be seen at the margins of the lips and on the lower lip.

The skin

The detailed examination of the skin is described in Chapter 4.

The most important abnormalities in a general examination are pallor, yellowness, pigmentation, cyanosis and cutaneous eruptions. In dehydration the skin is dry and inelastic; it can be pinched up into a ridge. The skin is atrophied by age and sometimes after treatment with glucocorticoids. It is thickened, greasy and loose in acromegaly.

Pallor depends on the thickness and quality of the skin, and the amount and quality of the blood in the capillaries. It is thus seen in persons with thick or opaque skins, who are always pale; in hypopituitarism; in states where the blood flow in the capillaries is diminished, such as shock, syncope or left heart failure; locally in a limb deprived of its blood supply; or in the fingers or toes when arterial spasm occurs on exposure to cold, as in Raynaud's disease. Generalized pallor may also occur in severe anaemia. Anaemia, however, is to be judged 'by the colour of the blood rather than that of the patient' and the colour of the skin may be most misleading; that of the mucous membranes of the mouth and conjunctivae gives a better indication, and so does the colour of the creases in the palm of the hand.

Yellowness may be due to haemolytic jaundice, when the tint is pale lemon-yellow, or to obstructive jaundice, when it may be of a dark yellow or orange tint. In obstructive jaundice there may be scratch marks that result from the itching which the bile salts evoke. In rare cases yellowness may be due to carotenaemia.

Pigmentation is most commonly racial or actinic. The pigmentation of Addison's disease affects the buccal mucous membranes as well as the skin of exposed parts and parts subject to friction.

Cyanosis is a bluish colour of the skin and mucous membranes due to an increase in the amount of reduced haemoglobin in the blood. It may be divided into central and peripheral. Central cyanosis results from imperfect oxygenation of blood, as in heart failure and some lung diseases, or from the mixture of arterial and venous blood in the presence of right-to-left or venous–arterial shunts in the heart. In this case the cyanosis is general and the cyanosed extremities are warm. It characteristically affects the tongue. Peripheral cyanosis is due to excessive reduction of oxyhaemoglobin in the capillaries when the flow of blood is slowed. This may happen on exposure to cold, when there is venous obstruction or in heart failure. The cyanosed extremity or extremities are then cold and the tongue is unaffected. The cyanosis of heart failure is often of a mixed type, due to both central and peripheral causes. A similar bluish or leaden colour may in rare cases be produced by methaemoglobinaemia or sulphaemoglobinaemia, usually due to the taking of drugs such as phenacetin. This should be considered in any patient who is cyanosed but not breathless. Carbon monoxide poisoning produces a generalized cherry-red discoloration.

Cutaneous eruptions are described in Chapter 4.

An excess of fluid in the subcutaneous tissue causing swelling of the tissues is known as *oedema*. Thus in acute nephritis an early symptom is oedema of the face, which is most marked when the patient rises in the morning. In dependent oedema, however, which is typically present in congestive heart failure, and in conditions associated with a low plasma protein level, the swelling first appears at the ankles and over the dorsum of the foot, and only gradually mounts to the legs, thighs and trunk. In local venous obstruction, the oedema is confined to the parts from which the return of blood is impeded. In this way one finds oedema of an arm when malignant glands constrict the axillary vein or oedema of a leg in thrombosis of the popliteal or femoral vein. Oedema of the whole upper part of the body may result from intrathoracic tumours. Oedema may be recognized by the pallid and glossy appearance of the skin over the swollen part, by its doughy feel, and by the fact that it pits on finger pressure. In recumbent patients oedema often appears first over the sacrum. In eliciting pitting it is important to press firmly and for a sustained period, or slight oedema may be missed. The oedema of lymphatic obstruction does not pit on pressure.

Localized oedema may be due to local changes in capillary permeability, as in angioneurotic oedema and giant urticaria. Oedema is also a feature of cutaneous or subcutaneous inflammation.

Subcutaneous emphysema is uncommon, but if present can be readily recognized by the crackling sensation produced by pinching the part affected.

The hands

The hands of the patient should be examined. Notice the strength of grip as he shakes hands; this often indicates improvement or deterioration with considerable accuracy. Their general shape should be noted, along with the state of the joints, the character of the nails, the presence or absence of finger-clubbing and the presence of staining with nicotine.

In osteoarthrosis the finger joints are often implicated, and bony nodules, known as *Heberden's nodes* (Fig. 2.2), are formed at the bases of the terminal phalanges. In rheumatoid arthritis there is characteristically a spindle-shaped swelling of the interphalangeal joints and later an ulnar deviation of the fingers. *Trophic changes* in the skin may be present in neurological disease and in disorders of the peripheral circulation (e.g. Raynaud's disease). Characteristic movements or attitudes of the hand may also be seen in athetosis, tetany, and lead palsy. *Tremor* of the hands may occasionally be congenital. In other cases it is due to nervousness, senility, parkinsonism, thyrotoxicosis, alcoholism, disseminated sclerosis, uraemia, hepatic failure or mercurial poisoning. This and other abnormal movements are considered on p. 335. In ulnar paralysis the hand becomes deformed by over-extension of the first phalanges, combined with excessive flexion of the rest, so that a claw-like attitude is produced. This is known as the '*main en griffe*'. Wasting of the small muscles of the hand, due for example to median or ulnar nerve lesions, cervical root (C8) disease or loss of

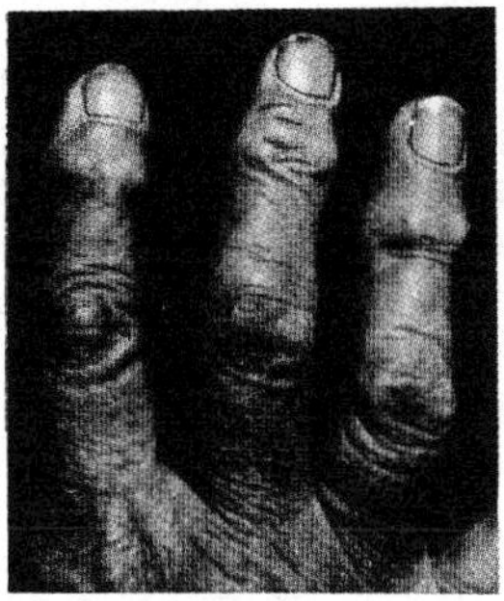

Fig.2.2 Heberden's nodes.

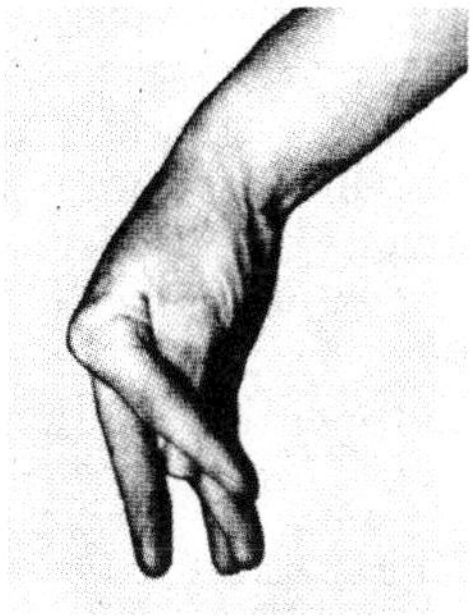

Fig.2.3 Tetany.

anterior horn cells at the same level, gives the hand a flattened appearance. The characteristic posture of the hand in tetany is shown in Fig. 2.3. In *Dupuytren's contracture* there is a thickening of the palmar fascia, which may lead to a flexion contracture of the ring and other fingers. In acromegaly the hands are massive, the fingers spatulate with square tips and the skin thickened.

In *clubbing of the fingers* (Fig. 2.4), the tissues at the base of the nail are thickened, and the angle between the nail base and the adjacent skin of the finger is obliterated. The nail itself loses its longitudinal ridges and becomes convex from above down as well as from side to side. In extreme cases the terminal segment of the finger is bulbous like the end of a drumstick. The condition may occasionally be congenital. Gross degrees of clubbing are found in association with severe chronic cyanosis, as in congenital heart disease, and in association with chronic suppuration within the chest, as in bronchiectasis and empyema. Lesser degrees may be found in carcinoma of the lung, pulmonary tuberculosis, and chronic abdominal conditions such as polyposis of the colon, Crohn's disease and ulcerative colitis. Clubbing is also an important

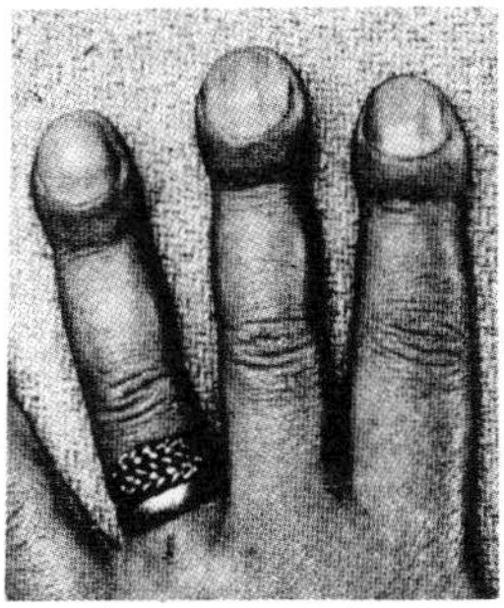

Fig.2.4 Clubbing.

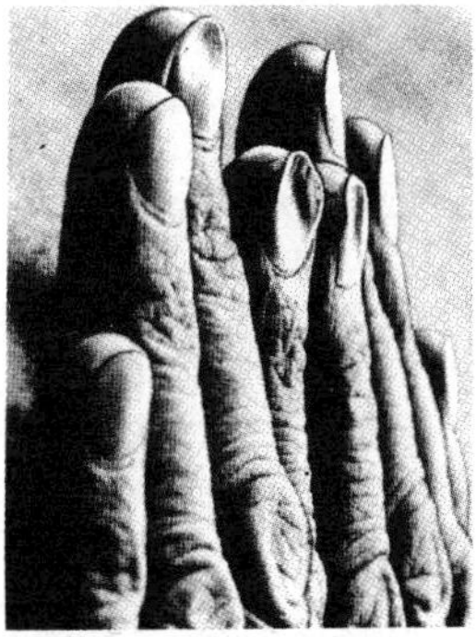

Fig.2.5 Koilonychia.

sign of subacute bacterial endocarditis, when it may be associated with Osler's nodes, tender transient swellings about the size of a pea in the pulp of the fingers and toes, and 'splinter' haemorrhages beneath the nails. In hypertrophic pulmonary osteoarthropathy there is, besides clubbing of the fingers, thickening of the periosteum of radius, ulna, tibia and fibula. This gives rise to swelling above the wrist and ankle. *Koilonychia* (Fig. 2.5) occurs in iron-deficiency anaemia. The nails are soft, thin, brittle and 'spoon-shaped'. The normal convexity is lost and replaced by a concavity.

The feet

The feet must not remain obscured under bedclothes or socks. Apart from looking for pitting oedema, the condition of the skin of the feet is of importance, especially in diabetics and the elderly. Peripheral vascular disease will make the skin shiny, and hair does not grow on ischaemic legs or feet. The dorsalis pedis and posterior tibial pulses may be reduced or absent. If the toes of an ischaemic foot are compressed their dull purple colour will blanch and only slowly return. Painless trophic lesions, often with deep ulceration, on the soles are seen frequently in diabetic peripheral neuropathy.

The neck

The neck should be inspected and palpated. Swellings in the neck are usually felt best from behind. Note:

The lymphatic and salivary glands In infected conditions of the tonsils the glands at the angles of the jaw are enlarged, as are those below the jaw in cases of malignant disease of the mouth. Glands draining an inflammatory focus are usually tender. Enlarged tuberculous glands may occur in groups or in long chains behind the sterno-mastoid, and scars may mark the points of past suppuration in severe untreated cases. In Hodgkin's disease and other reticuloses the glands are enlarged and discrete. In lymphatic leukaemia there may be great enlargement of the glands on both sides. In secondary syphilis the glands under the upper part of the trapezius are often palpable. If enlarged glands are found either in the neck or elsewhere, it is important to observe whether they are firm and distinct, or fused together, whether fluctuation can be elicited, and whether they are adherent to adjacent structures. The *submandibular salivary glands* should also be palpated when the neck is being examined from behind. If they are swollen and tender, the opening of their ducts into the mouth should be inspected with the tip of the patient's tongue rolled upwards; a salivary calculus may be seen.

The thyroid gland Inspect the neck for any general or local enlargement of the gland, and observe its movement with the larynx as the patient swallows.

Patients find this easier if they are given a glass of water. Then stand behind the patient and palpate the gland with one hand on each side of the neck. Determine if any swelling exists, and if so whether it is uniform or nodular, hard or soft. Sometimes such enlargements press on the trachea and occasionally extend into the thorax behind the sternum; at other times, particularly if the disease is malignant, the recurrent laryngeal nerves may become implicated. In cases where there is difficulty in determining whether a tumour is connected with the thyroid, it is helpful to remember that the gland and any tumour connected with it moves up and down on swallowing. Minor degrees of enlargement of the thyroid are often better seen than felt. A bruit heard over the thyroid shows that the gland is hyperactive.

Pulsations Pulsations in the vessels must be noted. Any arterial pulsation is both seen and felt as a distinct thrust, whereas venous pulsation is seen but is not felt as thrust, if it is felt at all. In aortic incompetence the carotid arteries are seen to pulsate forcibly. In aortic stenosis a systolic thrill is felt. Women patients with hypertension sometimes show kinking of the right common carotid artery which simulates aneurysm. The jugular veins may be distended and pulsatile in congestive heart failure (p. 206). In superior mediastinal obstruction due to retrosternal goitre or malignant neoplasm in the mediastinum, non-pulsatile distended veins may be seen over the neck and upper part of the body; cyanosis and oedema of the upper part of the body may accompany this sign. Distended neck veins may also be seen in large pericardial effusions.

The breasts

The chance of finding a treatable cancer should make a full examination of the breasts a necessary feature of every general examination of a woman. With the patient reclining, arms to the sides, inspect the development and symmetry of breasts and nipples. Look for any reddening of the skin, ulceration or dimpling (*peau d'orange*). Retraction (rather than inversion) of one nipple may signpost the cancer beneath. If there is a discharge from the nipple determine whether it is bloody, serous or milky.

Palpate each breast with the flat of the fingers, working over the whole breast as if it was mapped out in quadrants. Repeat this when the patient has her hands placed behind her head. If a lump is found the qualities to be observed hold good for any lump felt anywhere in the body. Determine the situation, size, shape, surface and edge; feel its consistency and mobility in relation to deep and superficial structures.

Axillae Then examine the axillae. It is difficult to feel enlarged lymph glands unless the patient's arm is raised to allow the examining fingers to be pushed high into the axilla. The arm is then lowered and palpation is continued downwards along the chest wall. Any swelling of the male breast is likely to be seen at a glance. The swelling can be distinguished as breast tissue rather than pectoral fat by palpation when the patient's hands are behind his head. At some stage of puberty the majority of normal boys will have a palpable disc of breast tissue beneath the areola.

Temperature

When taking the temperature, the following points must be remembered:

1 The thermometer must be accurate.

2 The thermometer must be kept in position long enough to allow the mercury to reach the body temperature. It is advisable to exceed the period which the instrument professes to require. The ordinary 'half-minute' thermometer should be left in position for one or two minutes. Collapsed, comatose and elderly patients should have the rectal temperature taken with a special 'low-reading' thermometer. Accidental hypothermia is not uncommon in the elderly.

3 In conscious adults the temperature is taken in the mouth or in the axilla. In young children the thermometer should be placed in the fold of the groin, and the thigh flexed on the abdomen; or it may be inserted into the rectum. The temperature of the mouth and rectum is generally at least half a degree higher than that of the groin or axilla. When the temperature is taken in the mouth, the patient must breathe through the nose and keep the lips firmly closed during the observation.

4 Before inserting the thermometer, make it an invariable rule to wash it in antiseptic or in cold water, and see that the mercury is well shaken down. Wash it again before replacing it in its case. The Centigrade (Celsius) scale is in general use, although in Great Britain many people are still more familiar with the Fahrenheit scale (for comparison of the two scales see p. 478).

Normal	36.6–37.2°C	(98–99°F)
Subnormal	below 36.6°C	(below 98°F)
Febrile	above 37.2°C	(above 99°F)
Hyperpyrexia	above 41.6°C	(above 107°F)
Hypothermia	below 35°C	(below 95°F)

In many conditions, notably acute fevers, there is a disturbance of heat regulation, which may be looked on as the setting of the 'thermostatic' mechanism controlling heat gain and loss at a level higher than normal. While the temperature is rising to this new level, heat is being conserved, the skin vessels are constricted so that the body feels cold, and the patient may even shiver violently. This shivering is referred to as a *rigor*. When the higher temperature is reached, heat loss again becomes apparent; the skin vessels dilate and the body feels warm. This is the state of affairs present in sustained fever or *pyrexia*.

There are three classical *types of fever*—the continued, the remittent and the

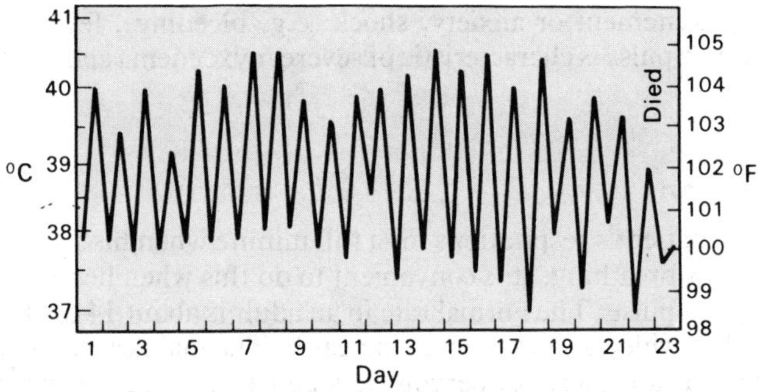

Fig.2.6 Remittent fever.

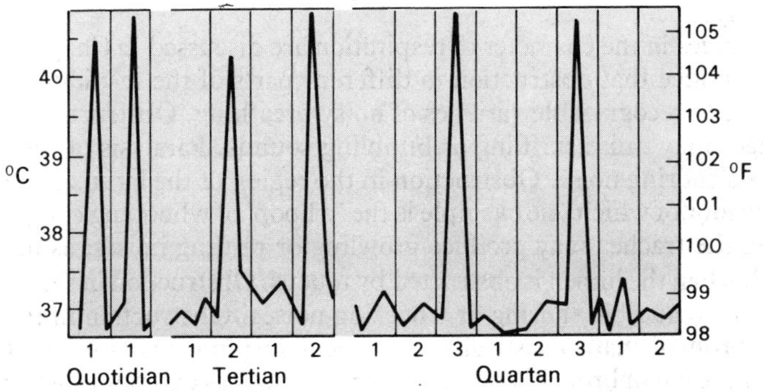

Fig.2.7 Intermittent fever.

intermittent. When fever does not fluctuate more than about 1°C (or 1.5°F) during the twenty-four hours, but at no time touches the normal, it is described as *continued*. When the daily fluctuations exceed 2°C, it is known as *remittent* (Fig. 2.6); and when fever is present only for several hours during the day it is called *intermittent*. When a paroxysm of intermittent fever occurs daily, the type is *quotidian*; when on alternate days, *tertian*; when two days intervene between consecutive attacks, *quartan* (Fig. 2.7). However, with the use of antibiotics and other specific drugs, these classical types of fever are not often seen.

Pulse

Count the pulse for a full minute when the patient is at rest and composed. Abnormalities due to cardiovascular causes are described in Chapter 9. The rate in health and under conditions of a medical examination varies from about 60 to 80 beats a minute. The common causes of a rapid pulse are recent exercise, excitement or anxiety, shock (e.g. bleeding), fever and thyrotoxicosis. A slow pulse is characteristic of severe myxoedema and of complete heart block.

Respiration

Count the patient's respirations for a full minute when his attention is distracted from his breathing. It is convenient to do this when he thinks you are still counting his pulse. The normal rate in an adult is about 14 to 18 respirations a minute, but wide variations occur in health. The main causes of fast breathing (tachypnoea) are exercise, nervousness and fever; pulmonary, pleuritic and cardiac conditions causing hypoxia; cerebral disturbance, metabolic acidosis and hysterical overbreathing, which later may give rise to alkalosis and attacks of tetany.

Changes in the character of respiration are discussed in Chapter 8, but one should notice that obstruction in different parts of the respiratory tract may give rise to recognizable varieties of noisy breathing. Obstruction in the nasal passages may cause sniffling or bubbling sounds. Paralysis of the soft palate causes a snoring noise. Obstruction in the region of the larynx causes inspiratory stridor of which one example is the 'whoop' of whooping cough. Obstruction in the trachea may produce growling or rattling noises, as in the 'death rattle', when the lumen is obstructed by mucus. Obstruction in the bronchi may give rise to audible snoring or wheezing noises. Obstruction in the larynx or larger bronchi characteristically gives rise to inspiratory noises, while obstruction in the small bronchi and bronchioles produces expiratory wheezing. The latter is heard in bronchitis and asthma (obstructive airways disease). Alternating periods of cessation of respiration and hyperventilation (*Cheyne–Stokes respiration*) occur in left heart failure and in various cerebral disturbances. The breathing may be characteristic of diseases quite distinct from those of the respiratory system. Examples of this are the stertorous breathing of apoplexy, the hissing expiration of uraemia, and the 'air-hunger' of diabetic keto-acidotic coma, which affects both inspiration and expiration.

Odours The odours of alcohol and paraldehyde are easily recognizable in the breath. That of alcohol does not necessarily mean the patient's condition is due to alcoholic intoxication. The odour of diabetic ketosis has been described as 'sweet and sickly'; that of uraemia as 'ammoniacal or fishy'; and that of hepatic failure as 'mousy', but one should not rely too far on such delicate distinctions.

The mental state

The examination of the mental state is the equivalent in psychiatry of the physical examination in general medicine. The patient's words should be recorded exactly. With mute or otherwise disturbed patients the 'mental state' examination may be merely a description of behaviour.

Special attention needs to be paid to the mental state of the *elderly*. The bright and smiling face of an old lady may well mask considerable defects of memory and orientation.

Detailed accounts of the examination of the mental state are given in relation to the psychiatric assessment in Chapter 3 and in relation to the neurological examination in Chapter 10.

3 The psychiatric assessment

The prevalence of psychiatric disorder in the community is of such magnitude that every doctor must be able to carry out a psychiatric assessment. The range of presenting problems in patients with psychiatric disorders is wide. Many patients with emotional disturbance may present, not with overt psychiatric symptoms, but with 'more respectable' physical symptoms. In some patients physical and psychiatric illness may co-exist. There may be a direct causal relationship between the two, as in the depressed patient who takes a drug overdose or the elderly man with a post-operative confusional state. On the other hand, physical and psychiatric illnesses may be unrelated, as in the chronic schizophrenic who developes a neoplastic lesion. In addition, every patient's reaction to his illness will be influenced by his emotional state and this will itself affect the course of the illness.

As in physical illness the approach to diagnosis and treatment depends on an adequate formulation of the problem. This necessitates following the basic steps of taking a history, examining the patient and, when necessary, arranging appropriate investigations. In psychiatry exact measurements are often not readily available. Emphasis is therefore placed on the history and examination and further investigations consist mainly of clarification of this information by interview and observation and by involvement of other sources of information. In addition specific psychological investigations including measures of the cognitive state and, less frequently, of personality and mood are also used. Laboratory tests and X-rays are used in some patients.

THE PSYCHIATRIC HISTORY

Interview technique

As in every medical interview it is important to put the patient at his ease and to establish a relationship with him in a warm and empathic way using words that the patient can understand. On the interview technique will depend not only the accuracy of the information gathered, and therefore the adequacy of the formulation, but also the patient's compliance in any treatment suggested. In no branch of medicine are interviewing skills so important as in psychiatry. The doctor's ability to communicate with the patient is doubly important as psychiatric patients, by the very nature of their disturbances, may be particularly difficult to interview. Even for the most well-adjusted person the interview itself may involve being asked searching and potentially embarrassing questions. Awareness of these difficulties is helpful to the interviewer. Aspects of the doctor–patient relationship in general are discussed in Chapter 1.

History taking scheme

The psychiatric history should be carried out systematically under the following headings; *reason for referral*; *presenting complaints*; *history of present illness*; *family history*; and *personal history*. The latter can be subdivided into *childhood*; *schooling*; *occupation*; *psychosexual and marital*; *forensic*; *past medical and past psychiatric history*; *drug and alcohol abuse*; *premorbid personality*; and *social circumstances*. Taking a psychiatric history often requires more than one interview. The number of interviews depends on many factors including the amount of information to be gathered and the rapport established between the patient and doctor. Obviously the above scheme must be adapted to meet the needs of the patient, different aspects receiving different degrees of emphasis in different patients.

History of present illness

The patient must be given the opportunity of telling the doctor what is worrying him. It is often useful to write down the patient's complaints verbatim since they may constitute a summary of the disorder.

Initially the patient should do most of the talking. The doctor can clarify the problem later if necessary by asking leading questions. For each symptom the following points should be elicited:

1 The date and circumstances of onset of the symptoms, including any precipitating factors or recent stresses. Since the illness may have been present for some time before the onset of the presenting symptoms it may only be by asking the patient when he was last well that the true date of onset of his illness can be decided.

2 Relieving and aggravating factors.

3 Consistency—variation from day to day and during the day. This includes searching for any periodicity such as diurnal mood variation; patients with a depressive illness often feel worse in the morning.
4 Severity—often best assessed by asking the patient how it interferes with his normal life.
5 Nature—it is important to clarify what the patient means by symptoms. Confusion may mean one thing to the layman and another to the doctor. Abnormal beliefs or experiences may not be clearly described but the doctor must be absolutely sure about them if he is to make the correct diagnosis.
6 Site and radiation—this is mostly relevant when the patient complains of physical symptoms but may be important when the patient is hearing voices; hearing them outside or inside the head may have a different significance.
7 Associated symptoms—it is important to ask in detail about any other symptoms associated with the major presenting complaint and at this time it is usual to ask about sleep, appetite and weight.

Sleep disturbance may be related to physical problems, such as pain or breathlessness, or to psychological problems. Examples of the latter include insomnia occurring in the presence of anxiety or drug withdrawal; early morning waking and nightmares with depression; excessive sleep with drugs or organic illness; reversed sleep pattern, i.e. increased during the day and decreased at night, in acute confusional states; and disturbed sleep with affective or organic illness. Sleep disturbance of recent onset is usually highly significant whereas chronic sleep impairment, although distressing to the patient, is usually of less importance in diagnosis.

Appetite is decreased in anorexia nervosa but may be increased in anxious patients who eat for comfort. In depression, appetite may decrease or increase. It is an alteration of pattern that is important. Associated with loss of appetite there may be a loss of weight as in depression, anorexia nervosa or self-neglect, and when appetite is increased there may be weight gain, which also occurs during treatment with some psychotropic drugs.
8 Previous history of similar symptoms and the type of treatment and the patient's response to it.
9 A family history of similar symptoms and the response of family members to treatment.

Family history

The patient's family background is important in many psychiatric disorders. For example, in schizophrenia and the affective psychoses genetic factors may be relevant. Environmental factors are often complex. The loss of a mother in early life predisposes to depression in later life; failure of bonding may lead to difficulties with relationships in adult life and over-protective parents may produce anxious children. This aspect of the history must be covered in some

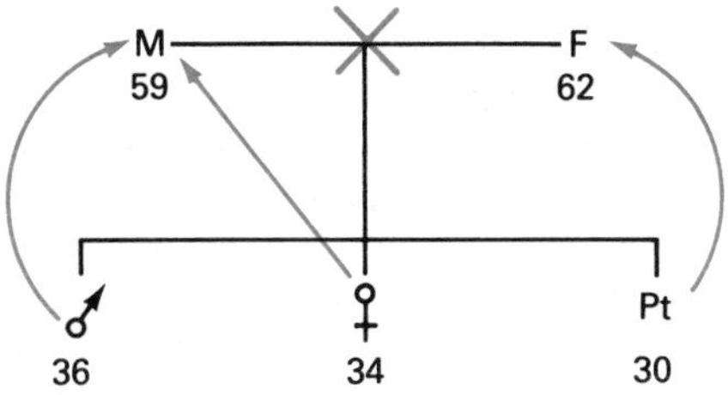

Fig. 3.1 X = broken relationship; → = direction of attachment.

detail including information mainly about parents and siblings, and also, when relevant, about members of the non-nuclear family.

For each parent, if alive, one should ask about age and physical and psychiatric health, both present and previous. If dead, then the age of the parent at the time of death, the cause of death and the patient's age and reaction to the bereavement need to be ascertained, as well as their parents' health while they were alive. The parents' occupation and personality, and their relationship with each other and with the patient, including any separations in childhood from the patient are all relevant. Children whose parents have had a bad marriage are themselves vulnerable to the development of pychosexual and marital difficulties. For each sibling similar details should be obtained including information about their marital status. By this stage, one will usually have acquired some idea of the family atmosphere and inter-family relationships and the position of the patient within the family, though one may have to ask directly about these areas. It is useful to draw a family tree to facilitate the assimilation and display of the information gathered. This can vary from a simple diagram of the family members with their ages to the use of symbols to denote the emotional relationships between the various family members (Fig. 3.1). As long as one is consistent and a reference key is provided it does not matter what symbols are used. For example, in the above family (Fig. 3.1) if the parents were divorced and the elder two siblings were closer to their mother, and the younger to his father, these relationships could be indicated by arrows. In some cases it may be relevant to ask about other members of the family, e.g. in instances in which the patient is brought up by or is particularly close to a grandparent, or in which a grandparent or parental sibling lives or has lived in the nuclear family home. Finally one should ask about the family psychiatric and medical history both in the nuclear and in the wider family. This inquiry should include psychiatric disturbance, alcoholism and suicide. An unexplained death in the family may hint at suicide. If any member of the family has had psychiatric treatment the date and place of this treatment should be ascertained.

Personal history

The question to be answered is why have *these* symptoms occurred in *this* patient at *this* time. This requires familiarity with the patient's earlier circumstances; for example, a severely anxious child with a fear of going to school and inability to separate from his parents may well develop symptoms of anxiety (such as agoraphobia) in later life, whereas a person with a long history of difficulty in coping with authority may present later with anti-social behaviour. A systematic scheme of enquiries such as that detailed below helps to ensure that important areas are not omitted, though the weight placed on different aspects of the personal history may differ from patient to patient. A visual display of the information by means of a life chart (Fig. 3.2) may help to clarify the relationship between different areas of the patient's life and illuminate the cause of the current symptoms.

Date	Age	Social history	Family history	Psychosexual history	Medical history	Psychiatric history
1952	0	↑				
1957	5					
1962	10	School	Parents' divorce		Pain in chest	Difficulties at school
1967	15	↓↑				
1972	20	Secretary ↓		Marries (leaves home)	Pain in back	Relieved by Valium
1977	25			First child born		Puerperal depression
1982	30			Second child born	Pain in back	Sleep and appetite impaired Lethargy

Fig. 3.2 This is the life chart of a 30-year-old married mother of two from a broken home referred to the Orthopaedic Department with backache. No cause for this could be found. Associated symptoms included sleep disturbance, poor appetite and lethargy. Given this patient's background, in particular the divorce of her parents, one would not be surprised if she were vulnerable in psychosexual areas, and this is shown clearly in the chart to be the case by the development of emotional disturbance at the time of her marriage and the birth of her first child. One would therefore anticipate that the birth of her second child would also be a traumatic time for her. The presentation with physical symptoms—pain in the back—as a manifestation of psychiatric disorder is consistent both with her symptomatology after her parents' divorce, and at the time of her marriage, and the presence of the associated symptoms of sleep and appetite disturbance and lethargy, all common manifestations of emotional upset. The life chart clearly displays the links described above.

Childhood

This is the logical place to start the personal history. Begin with questions about the patient's birth. Was it planned, what was the length of gestation? Find out about the mother's health during pregnancy and the nature of the delivery. Note the infantile and childhood milestones, and inquire about neonatal or feeding difficulties; most people are only aware of these if their parents have told them of any difficulties in these areas.

In later childhood, neurotic traits may become apparent such as particular fears, physical symptoms at times of stress, or periods of unhappiness. These and additional traits such as bed-wetting, temper tantrums, and periods of physical or emotional disorder must be considered in the light of relationships with peers, the atmosphere at home, separations from and relationships with family members, and any bereavement or other major life event.

Adolescence

Assessment of adolescence includes questions that usually arise when dealing with the psychosexual history. Relevant areas of enquiry are peer and family relationships, episodes of disturbance whether anti-social or emotional, and difficulties in growing up. Adolescence is interrelated with *schooling* and *occupation*.

Schooling

It is usual to ask about dates of starting, leaving and changing schools, academic achievement, relationships with peers and teachers, any difficulties in learning or behaviour and periods of non-attendance. The latter includes *truancy*, in which the child, usually without the parents' knowledge, indulges, often with others, in more enjoyable pastimes instead of going to school, and *school refusal*, in which the child stays at home with the knowledge of his parents because of a fear of leaving home or going to school. Enforced *absence* is usually due to illness, although it must be remembered that the latter may also be a manifestation of school refusal.

Similar details are required if the patient has gone on to higher education.

Occupation

A comprehensive work history entails asking about every job the patient has had since leaving school. Enquiry should concentrate on duration of job, level of achievement and promotion, attendance and ability, enjoyment or difficulties, relationship with peers and superiors, reasons for leaving and the duration of any periods of unemployment.

If the person has had numerous jobs this may become a repetitive and tedious process. In these cases one can use a shortened approach and ask about the number of jobs, the length of time unemployed in total and in the last 5 years, the longest job, the highest level of achievement, any difficulties at work including being dismissed from a job, general relationship with workmates and employers, and the general work record, while asking in more detail about the present job.

Where relevant, military service can be dealt with in much the same way as any other form of occupation.

Psychosexual history

This is usually the most difficult area to assess, relying as it does on asking highly personal questions which may be as embarrassing for the doctor as the patient. It is important not to allow this potential difficulty to harm the patient–doctor relationship. However, failure to ask these questions may result in the omission of a vital piece of information with serious effects on the overall assessment. In some cases it may be necessary to leave some of the questions to later interviews; sensitive and skilful interviewing usually enables adequate exploration of this area in the first interview. Shaping the enquiry so as to lead from easy to difficult questions, for example by taking a menstrual history before the sexual one, and asking questions in such a way as to make the patient feel his sexual behaviour is normal, for example 'How old were you when you first started to masturbate?' rather than 'Have you ever masturbated?' facilitates the acquisition of information. Try to use less emotionally laden wording, such as 'physical relationship' instead of 'sexual relationship'.

The sexual history should encompass the following points: puberty; menstrual history; sex education; masturbation and fantasies; relationships with members of the opposite sex, especially their duration, intensity and sexual contact and enjoyment; engagement; marriage (see below); any homosexual feelings and experiences; and, where appropriate, deviant sexual experiences and fantasies.

The *marital history* includes the relationship with the spouse from the time of meeting through the development of their relationship, engagement and marriage. The age and occupation of the spouse; the parents' attitude towards him or her; the quality of the marriage, including any areas of disagreement, overt disharmony or periods of separation; their current sexual relationship, both its frequency and enjoyment; and any extra-marital affairs should also be noted. One should enquire about pregnancies, terminations and miscarriages, stillbirths and livebirths with details of the ages and behaviour of the children and any difficulties with them. If there are no children and the couple have been together for a long time then it is important to know why. Is it out of choice because both husband and wife are career-orientated, or through a dislike or fear of children, suggesting possible psychosexual difficulties? Failure to conceive despite trying may have repercussions on the emotional state of the partners and their relationship. Similarly if there is only one child to a longstanding marriage or if there are large gaps between the birth of children it is worth asking the patient whether there is any reason for this.

When the patient is not married but is in a stable relationship the same questions should be asked as for the married patient, including future intentions as far as marriage or staying together are concerned. When the patient has been married before, the previous marriage and its ending by death or divorce should also be assessed. Finally, if the patient is neither married nor in a stable relationship it is worth asking about his desires for the future and whether he feels he has any difficulties in this area.

Forensic history

This encompasses any and all confrontations with the law and includes juvenile delinquency as well as anti-social behaviour later on in life. Details of offences committed and punishment received should be noted.

Past medical history

It is important to ask in chronological order about any illness or operations in childhood or during adult life, about periods of hospitalization or incapacity and any resulting disability and interference with the patient's life, the reaction of the patient and his family to these episodes and any remaining medical problems including current symptoms and medication. It is, for example, illuminating to find out that the patient who now presents with physical symptoms has had a number of previous episodes of similar symptoms at times of stress and has recovered when the stress was resolved, or that the anxious patient awaiting surgery has always reacted badly in the past to major illnesses or operations. It is useful here to ask about the frequency and nature of contact with the general practitioner.

Past psychiatric history

This includes any episodes of emotional upset, from that thought not severe enough to need medical attention through the minor neuroses treated by the general practitioner to severe psychiatric disorders needing expert psychiatric treatment, whether as outpatient, day-patient or inpatient on a voluntary or compulsory basis, Ask about circumstances, precipitating factors, place of treatment, duration and response to treatment and any continuing symptoms or medication. It is often worth asking whether the patient has ever taken psychotropic medication in the past, whether prescribed by his family doctor or obtained in other ways, not necessarily as any form of drug abuse but, perhaps, from other members of the family. Finally, it is also worth asking about contact with any voluntary organizations, such as the Samaritans, or with Social Services.

Alcohol abuse

Alcohol abuse may lead to physical, psychiatric and social sequelae and it affects an increasingly large number of people. Yet it is an area only too frequently neglected in the medical history. All patients should be asked whether they drink and, if so, roughly how much and in what circumstances, remembering that the answers frequently bear little resemblance to actual alcohol consumption.

Where there is any suspicion of alcohol-related problems a thorough and systematic drinking history must be obtained. One way of doing this is to construct a daily account of the patient's drinking habits including how he feels when he wakes up in the morning, how much sleep he has had, whether he remembers the night before, and, if he has withdrawal symptoms on getting up in the morning, such as shaking, nausea, retching, anxiety or craving for alcohol. Detailed questions about the content, time, place, type and circumstances of first and all subsequent drinks and whether he drinks alone or in company are often revealing. When dealing with the first drink of the day it is worth asking about the speed at which it is drunk as people with physical dependence often gulp rather than sip their first drink. Another helpful pointer to the current level of drinking is the amount of money the patient spends on drink, especially when related to his income.

Having dealt with the current drinking habit it is useful to take a more longitudinal perspective into the drinking history, covering such points as any family history of drinking, the age when the patient started drinking and when his alcohol consumption increased, the pattern of drinking, whether daily or in bouts, the type of alcohol consumed, and any precipitating factors, e.g. whether related to stress or mood. Personal difficulties caused by drinking—including its impact on the family, physical or psychiatric illness, loss of work or being drunk at work, or anti-social behaviour—and previous treatment or periods of abstinence or reduction in alcohol intake are important. A history of serious medical or social complications, such as delirium tremens, anti-social behaviour resulting in encounters with the police, or alcohol-related marital problems are especially important.

It is also important, for treatment, to ascertain whether the patient feels he is drinking too much and would like to cut down or even stop drinking, and what sort of help he feels he would require in order to do this.

Drug abuse

This term implies abuse not only of drugs of addiction, whether major, e.g. heroin, or minor, e.g. cannabis, but also prescribed drugs, commonly benzodiazepines, and non-prescribed drugs not normally considered addictive, such as cough linctus or analgesics. An assessment similar to that outlined above for alcohol should be used. Additional information concerning the route of drug intake and the source of the drugs may also be available.

Personality

Personality disorder is one of the commonest diagnoses used in psychiatry. Personality is defined as the sum of those characteristics that make a person into the individual he is. These characteristics include behaviour, both actions and reactions; attitude to self; ways of relating to others, both socially and sexually; attitude to authority; level of independence; mood; fantasy life; religious beliefs and moral attitudes; and interests and hobbies.

Personality may change with illness, e.g. the disinhibition that occurs with frontal lobe brain damage. However, to answer the question, in what sort of person has this illness developed, it is necessary to assess premorbid personality. This is most reliably assessed from an informant familiar with the patient before the onset of his illness. If such an objective opinion is unavailable it is worth asking the patient how others see him, for example: 'Would other people say you were a worrier?' Some features of personality, for example histrionic behaviour, will be obvious during the interview and others will already have been elicited in the history. Though many of the characteristics which make up the personality overlap (e.g. manipulative behaviour is a manifestation of behaviour itself and of a way of relating to others), they are best dealt with separately.

Actions includes level of achievement, histrionic or manipulative behaviour, deliberate self-harm or aggression towards others, disinhibition, obsessional behaviour (e.g. tidiness, being houseproud, perfectionist, conscientiousness or checking) and alcohol or drug abuse. Many of these will have been covered in the occupational, past psychiatric, forensic, and alcohol or drug abuse history.

Reactions to stressful events, e.g. illness, bereavement and other losses, examinations, promotion at work, failure and disappointment, and ability to cope with change. Types of reaction include being panicky, or unflappable and slow to react, short-tempered and easily angered, or placid (see 'Family, Occupational and Past Medical History').

Attitude to self Self-interested or thoughtful about others, level of self-esteem and self-criticism, self-consciousness and sensitivity, acceptance of abilities and achievements, self-confidence whether high, or low and constantly needing reassurance.

Relationship to others

Social ease of making and keeping social relationships, introverted or extraverted, suspiciousness, assertiveness, warm and affectionate or cold and undemonstrative, tolerant or authoritarian and intolerant. Include here relationships at work and with the family.

Psychosexual level of psychosexual development, especially capacity to make sexual relationships, direction of sexual attraction and areas of difficulty.

Attitudes to authority Well-adjusted and accepting, or anxious and uncertain? Is he generally tolerant or intolerant?

Level of independence Has the patient left home or is he still living with his parents? Can he accept responsibility and make decisions?

Usual mood Whether prone to anxiety, and if so about what, e.g. illness, work or family, pessimistic or optimistic, *cyclothymic*, i.e. swinging from elation to depression without reaching illness proportions, calm or irritable, bottles-up or shares feelings and emotions, calm or short-tempered and easily angered.

Religious beliefs and moral attitudes What religion, practising or not, whether tolerant of beliefs and attitudes of others, ability to show regret or remorse and limit actions according to conscience.

Interests or hobbies What types, time spent, passive spectator or active participant, social or solitary pastimes, energetic or sedentary.

Fantasy life Sexual and non-sexual fantasies, dreams and nightmares.

Social circumstances

Ask the patient about the place and type of his abode, his satisfaction with the accommodation and with other members of the household, his relationships with neighbours, current social contacts, financial problems and, if not already noted, any current or recent stresses including bereavement.

At the end of the history it is important to sum up to the patient what you have understood his problem to be. Ask him whether you have grasped it in its entirety, left out any important areas or perhaps even totally failed to understand what he has been trying to put over. Besides clarifying the history it also shows the patient that you have been listening to what he has been saying.

THE EXAMINATION

This can be subdivided into physical and psychiatric.

Physical examination

Physical examination of patients presenting with symptoms suggestive of psychiatric disorder is often necessary. The combination of psychiatric symptoms and physical disease is common. Acutely anxious patients may have signs of thyrotoxicosis. Evidence of liver disease may suggest alcoholism. Needle marks in the arms point to drug abuse; scars of slashed wrists or other signs of self-mutilation may point to psychiatric illness.

Psychiatric examination or mental state examination

This should be covered systematically under the following headings—appearance and behaviour; speech; mood; thought content; abnormal beliefs; abnormal experiences; cognitive state; insight and rapport. Where relevant, i.e. where organic brain disease is suspected, it is necessary to test further aspects of cerebral function.

Appearance and behaviour

The patient's appearance and behaviour often reveal the underlying psychiatric disorder. Important points to look for include dress, personal hygiene and general grooming. Note the shabbily dressed elderly man with food stains on his clothes, perhaps indicative of an underlying dementia or schizophrenic illness.

Facial expression is one of the outward signs of the patient's mood. For example, tearfulness or poverty of expression occur in depression, elation in mania, tenseness in anxiety, perplexity or blunting in schizophrenia. The *affect* may be inappropriate, such as the schizophrenic patient who laughs when relating upsetting material; it must be remembered, nonetheless, that anxious people may also laugh in similar circumstances. The emotional expression may be abnormally labile as in mania or organic brain disease.

The way the patient sits gives important hints to an underlying pathology; he may be relaxed and obviously at ease, or sit tensely and fidget restlessly, as in anxiety states. He may be so agitated that he gets up from the seat and paces up and down the room as in the agitated depressive or in the excited manic or the schizophrenic. He may leave the chair because he does not understand what is going on, as in the demented or confused patient, or because he feels threatened in the presence of delusions of persecution. He may appear to sit in a peculiar position as in catatonia or show no movement during the interview as in retarded depression or the anxious over-controlled patient who is holding himself rigidly. He may appear to drift off to sleep repeatedly, suggesting either a confusional state with fluctuating levels of consciousness or over-sedation.

His walking on the way to and from the interview room may show signs of ataxia due to organic brain disease, drug effect or excess alcohol consumption. In the latter his breath will smell of alcohol. There may be signs of *hysterical ataxia*, which may improve with suggestion or exhortation, or ataxia due to *malingering*, in which the limp varies from moment to moment and is most marked when the patient knows he is being watched.

There may be other abnormal movements, such as dystonia caused by major tranquillizers, choreiform movements in Huntington's chorea, or tic-like mannerisms, odd postures or other bizarre disorders of movement seen in patients with catatonia due to schizophrenia or organic brain disease. These include perseveration of posture so that the patient's limbs can be moved into an abnormal position which is maintained despite his being allowed to revert to his previous posture. When this movement is met by a waxy resistance it is termed *waxy flexibility*. The patient may keep on starting and stopping purposeful actions, for example when shaking hands with the interviewer, or show *negativism*, in which he opposes the examiner's intention. In *echopraxia* he copies the interviewer's actions; these abnormal postures and movements often occur in organic brain disease as well as in non-organic catatonia. There may be signs of slowing or retardation of movement even, at times, to the extent of stupor, which, in the case of catatonia, may be interspersed with periods of violent excitement. Stupor is commonly caused by organic disorders but functional psychosis, e.g. schizophrenia and depression, may also lead to stupor. Further, it may be hysterical in nature, or due to very high levels of anxiety following extreme stress; or it may be simulated by malingerers.

The patient's behaviour during the interview may be disinhibited, as in the manic patient who strips or the patient with organic brain disease who starts to urinate or masturbate during the interview. The patient may be manipulative or seductive and may threaten violence if his wishes are not met. There may be verbal aggression or physical violence, the latter against either the interviewer or objects in the room. On the other hand he may appear to be unduly submissive or self-critical, or may show little or no eye contact with the interviewer. He may appear to be suspicious of questions, which may be due to an underlying personality disorder or suggest a paranoid illness. The patient may also seem to be paying little attention to the interviewer or to be listening to someone else when there is no-one else in the room; this suggests that he is experiencing *auditory hallucinations*, i.e. hearing voices. He may even be talking to or arguing with these voices. The patient who appears unduly terrified without any obvious cause or to be touching or shooing away non-existent objects may be experiencing visual hallucinations.

It must, however, always be remembered that bizarre behaviour or inability to relate to the interviewer may be signs of subnormal intelligence.

Finally, obsessional patients may bring with them lists of their symptoms to present to the interviewer.

Speech

It is important to assess the form of speech as well as its content. Does the patient speak at all or is he mute and, if so, is this deliberate, organic, hysterical or part of a depressive or catatonic stupor? In the mute patient it is important to assess all aspects of speech production including the ability to produce sounds and communicate non-verbally. If he does speak, does he do so spontaneously or only in answer to questions, with monosyllabic or fuller and more elaborate replies? Is speech unduly slow as in depressive illness or so quick and continuous that it is impossible to interrupt as in hypomania and mania? Are there long pauses before the patient replies or does he stop in mid-sentence, e.g. in schizophrenia?

Are the words normal or are there neologisms as in some types of schizophrenia or organic brain disease? Is there evidence of dysphasia (see p. 283) or dysarthria (p. 282)? Where the words are normal, are the phrases and sentences normal and do they fit together, or does the patient seem to jump from topic to topic; if he does, is it possible to understand the link between topics, as in flight of ideas in mania, or is there no recognizable link as in *formal thought disorder*, e.g. schizophrenia? Is the link, if present, not one of content but of form as in rhyming or punning, usually features of mania? Is there evidence of echolalia, in which the patient repeats what the interviewer says, or perseveration, when he continues with the same theme when this is no longer appropriate? As an example of the latter, a 60-year-old man, replying to the question 'How old are you?', answers '60, 61, 62, 63, 64, 65, 66' and so on; when asked the subsequent question 'What year were you born?' he answers '1960' and to the next question 'What year is it?' now also answers '1960' (perseverence of a theme of 60). Both echolalia and perseveration are found in organic brain disease and in some types of schizophrenia.

When the speech is abnormal, samples of it should be written down verbatim, as this is the only reliable way of recording the abnormality for future assessment. Two doctors may differ in what they call formal thought disorder and therefore writing in the case notes 'There was evidence of formal thought disorder' is not very helpful. A recorded sample of the speech used gives much less room for disagreement.

Mood Mood has both a subjective component, which is reflected in the way the patient describes his emotional state, and an objective component, i.e. what the interviewer sees—for example, tears.

The subjective and objective components of mood are usually but not always congruent. Examples of incongruence are the inappropriate laughter of the schizophrenic or the smiling face of some severely depressed patients.

Subjective mood is assessed by asking the patient how he feels in himself, what his mood is, or what his spirits are like. If necessary leading questions such as 'Are you anxious or depressed?' may be used. Abnormal mood includes most commonly depression and anxiety but also elation, irritability, anger and perplexity. When the mood is abnormal it should be inquired into in the same way as any other presenting symptom.

Depression This may be mild and influenced by daily activities or severe. In severe depression symptoms may be worse in the morning, and associated with early morning waking, appetite and weight disturbance, lethargy, loss of concentration, and loss of interest and enjoyment in life. There may also be ideas of worthlessness, self-deprecation, poverty, guilt, persecution, bodily ill-health, nihilism and other morbid ideas. These may sometimes be delusional in intensity (see 'Abnormal experiences', below). The patient may be agitated or retarded, sometimes even to the point of stupor, and he may be mute or, in lesser cases, show retardation of speech.

The depressed patient may see no future, feel despairing and hopeless, and have thoughts of suicide. Suicidal ideation must *always* be sought for in depressed patients. Not only is it incorrect that discussing suicide with patients encourages them to do so, but failure to discuss it may lead to tragedies that could have been prevented. It can be asked for directly or led up to by a series of questions such as: 'How do you see the future?' 'Have you felt it would be nice to escape or be able to sleep and not wake up?' 'Do you feel at times that you would rather be dead or that you are such a burden to others that they would be better off if you were dead?' 'Have you had thoughts of suicide, however fleeting?' 'Have you made any plans?' Where it is felt that the patient is suicidal but he denies it, it is worth asking the questions 'What stops you killing yourself?' or 'What do you have to live for?' Some patients admit to having suicidal thoughts but deny that they would do anything because of the impact it would have on the family or because it is against their religion or they do not have the courage. Suicide, however, is not a respecter of family feelings, religious beliefs or personal bravery. Homicidal thoughts may also be present as in some mothers with puerperal depressive illnesses who kill their children because they are convinced they have passed on some terrible illness and death is better for them than a life of suffering.

Anxiety Patients with anxiety states may present with somatic symptoms related mainly to autonomic nervous system arousal or hyperventilation (Table 3.1), or with psychic symptoms (Table 3.2), or both. It may be free-floating or situation-dependent as in phobic disorders (e.g. agoraphobia), social phobias and other specific phobias.

The patient may complain of panic attacks with sudden surges of anxiety with physical symptoms and the desire to run away, sometimes coupled with an inability to move.

Table 3.1 Somatic symptoms of anxiety

Headaches and other muscular aches and pains
Palpitations
Tremor
Breathlessness
Chest pain
Urinary frequency
Faintness and lightheadedness
Fatigue
Pins and needles
Diarrhoea
Dry mouth
Abdominal discomfort
Flushes
Sweating

Table 3.2 Psychic symptoms of anxiety

Feelings of anxiety
Irritability
Inability to relax
Inability to concentrate
Initial insomnia—difficulty getting off to sleep
Feeling of impending doom
Depersonalization

Elation Elated patients usually describe themselves as being on top of the world, feeling happier than they have ever done before. This is a sign of hypomania and mania and is associated with over-activity, pressure of speech with flight of ideas, sleep impairment, irritability and grandiose ideas. Manic patients may also have moments of tearfulness or the mental state may show signs of both depression and elation, as in mixed affective states.

Other abnormal mood states Irritability may occur in many psychiatric disorders, especially anxiety states and hypomania, and in situational and relationship disturbances such as marital problems. It may also be part of the usual mood in some personalities, such as the intolerant person who does not suffer fools gladly. Anger may be related to a specific person or situation or may be part of an underlying psychiatric disturbance, in particular when ideas of persecution are present. Perplexity is usually found in schizophrenic patients who are suspicious that something is going on but cannot quite put their finger on what it is.

Thought content

The patient should be asked what his main worries are and whether he is preoccupied by any thoughts, e.g. morbid thoughts or *obsessional ruminations*. The latter are thoughts that the patient recognizes as his own, realizes are silly and tries to resist, but is unable to do so and feels compelled to have those thoughts. They occur in obsessive compulsive neurosis and may be associated with *obsessional rituals*. These are acts which the patient feels compelled to carry out, recognizes as coming from himself as opposed to being controlled by other sources (see 'Delusions of influence'), accepts as being absurd and tries to resist, but is unable to do so because of severe anxiety. An example of obsessional rumination is the patient who knows that his spouse is not unfaithful but has doubts about her which continuously run through his mind and which he is unable to suppress. Common obsessional rituals include hand washing; the patient may wash his hands forty or fifty times a day with disinfectant and strong detergents till they are raw. Obsessional checking is another common manifestation; for example, the patient who switches off his bedroom lights before leaving the house, gets to the bottom of the stairs and has to go back up again to check the lights are off, goes back down to the front door, has to go back again to check that the lights are off, gets to the bottom of the path and has to return, goes a few yards down the road and has to return and so on. In neither case is the patient able to stop his obsessional rituals without being consumed by extreme anxiety.

Abnormal beliefs

These vary from *delusions*, in which the patient has a false and unshakable belief out of keeping with the social milieu from which he comes, to *over-valued ideas*, in which the patient has false beliefs which, although of major concern to him, are not completely unshakable. These abnormal beliefs include misinterpretations, in which the patient concocts false explanations for various normal events which may or may not be delusional in extent. Abnormal ideas should be written down verbatim and asked about in detail.

Though abnormal beliefs usually denote the presence of a psychiatric illness, they may also occur in certain situations in normal people, as in the case of *ideas of reference*, in which the person feels that what others are saying refers to him or that they are laughing behind his back. This is commonly seen in sensitive people, especially in anxiety-provoking situations such as parties where they know no-one else.

Delusions may be primary, like sudden bolts from heaven, or secondary. In the latter their existence is understandable in terms of the rest of the patient's psychopathology, as in affective psychoses. Primary delusions may be *delusional ideas*. These are fully formed delusions that suddenly enter into the patient's mind, as in the person who for no reason suddenly believes that his food is being poisoned. This is often preceded by a *delusional mood*, in which the patient feels that there is something going on around him and that things are not quite right, but is unable to elaborate this feeling. In *delusional perceptions* the object is perceived normally but is interpreted in a delusional way, e.g. the patient who sees an ashtray on the table, recognizes it as an ashtray but believes that it has been put there to show people that he is a spy. This is not understandable in terms of the rest of the patient's psychopathology. If it were so understandable, it would be a *delusional misinterpretation*, which is a secondary delusion. Primary delusions should be diagnosed with extreme caution as, by the time the patient has presented, it may be very difficult to differentiate primary from secondary.

Delusions of persecution These are called *paranoid delusions*, although the term paranoid originally meant deluded. They are probably the most common delusions and may occur alone or with other abnormal mental signs. They occur in organic psychoses, such as confusional states, dementia, and alcohol and drug-induced psychoses, and associated with various organic illnesses such as some endocrine disorders and systemic lupus erythematosus. They also occur in functional psychoses such as paranoid schizophrenia, paraphrenia of the elderly, depressive illness and mania, in stress-induced, psychogenic psychoses or hysterical pseudopsychoses, and in some people with paranoid personality developments.

Delusions of grandeur These delusions occur in the now uncommon syphilitic general paralysis of the insane (GPI) and in mania and schizophrenia. Patients believe they are on a 'special mission' or are Napoleon or Christ.

Delusions of poverty and other depressive delusions Depressed patients may insist that they are destitute and have no clothes. Other common depressive delusions include *self-deprecation*, *worthlessness* and *guilt*; 'I have done something terrible and should be in prison and not in hospital.' Delusions of ill-health, often even potentially fatal, may occur and persist despite every assurance of the patient's physical health. These delusions occur in depression, schizophrenia, and abnormal personality development. Some people develop isolated abnormal ideas about their own appearance which may sometimes be delusional in intensity, e.g. their nose is too long or their hair is falling out.

These patients often have sensitive personalities, some of them may be depressed and some may become schizophrenic with time.

Nihilistic delusions occur in severe depressive illnesses. The patient with nihilistic delusions says that either he or part of his body is dead. This may have disastrous consequences since it may lead to self-harm. A rare delusion is of *infestation*, the patient believing that his house is infested by insects. Delusions of infestation occur in depression, in schizophrenia, or in organic illnesses.

Delusions of love Erotomania is another name for this symptom, in which the patient is convinced that someone is in love with him, despite the other person having shown no signs of this. He may act upon his misguided belief and pester the individual so that legal injunction may be necessary to restrain him. These delusions may occur in schizophrenia and occasionally in abnormal personality development.

Delusions of infidelity With these the patient is morbidly jealous of his wife, and is convinced that she is having an extra-marital affair. He may go to extreme lengths to confirm these abnormal beliefs. He often presses the unfortunate wife to admit her errant ways and these arguments may lead to violence that can end in murder. These delusions occur in people with suspicious personalities, especially when associated with alcohol abuse, and in schizophrenia and affective psychoses.

Delusions of influence (passivity or alienation phenomena) This is one of Schneider's first-rank symptoms, those symptoms which in the absence of organic brain disease are suggestive of schizophrenia (see Table 3.3).

Delusions of influence occur when the patient says that his mind or body is being controlled by outside forces such as laser beams transmitted by a neighbour. When the mind rather than the body is affected, the patient may complain that thoughts are either being forced into or out of his head. Another form of thought alienation is *thought broadcast*, in which the patient's thought

Table 3.3 Schneider's first-rank symptoms of schizophrenia

Hearing voices in the third person arguing or commenting on what the patient is doing
Hearing one's own thoughts spoken out loud
Thought alienation (insertion, withdrawal or broadcast)
Delusional perceptions
Somatic hallucinations (caused by others—experiences of bodily influence)
Everything in the spheres of feeling, drive, volition and actions which the patient experiences as imposed on him or influenced by others (passivity phenomena)

leaves his head, travels through the air and enters into other people's heads so that, when he thinks something, everyone else thinks the same. Alienation may also affect perception, as in patients who experience somatic hallucinations which they say are being caused by other people or by external forces. These are known as *'made' experiences* (see 'Tactile hallucinations', below).

Delusions of reference Some patients believe that the television, radio or newspaper contains special messages for them. This may occur as part of a paranoid illness.

Abnormal experiences

These may be divided into abnormal perceptions and abnormal experiences of the self or the environment.

Abnormal perceptions These may occur with any of the sensory modalities of hearing, vision, smell, taste and touch and vary in type. Objects may be distorted while remaining recognizable or they may be a new perception as in illusions or hallucinations. *Distortions* may occur in *intensity*, either increased or decreased, and due to functional or organic disorders in *quality*, e.g. colour, often due to toxic substances, or *form*, e.g. micropsia, when the object appears smaller or further away, or macropsia; these changes are due to organic lesions of the visual pathway (see Chapter 10). *Illusions* occur when the object is real but perception is disturbed. They are usually related, in the psychiatric sense, to disorders of the perceptual environment of the object, thereby leading to decrease in visual clarity coupled with a state of high emotion in the perceiver. A common example is the experience of walking through a lonely alley on a dark night when a tree in the distance may appear to be the figure of a man. Vision is impaired by the poor illumination and the lonely alley induces a feeling of fear thus leading to the illusion. Illusions occur not only in normal people, but also with psychiatric illness, particularly acute confusional states. They most commonly affect the visual and, to a lesser extent, the auditory modalities. An example of the latter is the woman with a puerperal depressive illness who hears the nurses talking outside her room without hearing clearly what they are saying but thinks thay are talking about her, saying how ill she is.

Hallucinations occur in the absence of an appropriate object yet the patient still insists that he has perceived something. The commonest hallucinations are auditory and visual but, as in any abnormal perception, they can occur in all sensory modalities. They may be due to organic disease of the nervous system or to extreme environmental disturbances as in sensory deprivation. In certain instances they may be non-pathological phenomena, as in hypnagogic and hypnopompic hallucinations experienced by a person going to sleep or waking up. Hypnagogic hallucinations also occur in narcolepsy.

In psychiatric illness, hallucinations occur in organic and functional psychoses, e.g. in schizophrenia and affective illnesses, severely raised levels of anxiety due to hyperventilation, grief reactions, and hysterical illnesses. They are occasionally displayed by malingerers. They may occur wherever the patient is or may only be present in certain places. Thus the paranoid patient who hears voices of his neighbours plotting against him while he is at home does not hear them while he is in hospital, yet they return when he is home again.

Auditory hallucinations The patient may complain of hearing noises, music, distant mumbling which he cannot identify, words, phrases or more elaborate speech. If the patient hears voices rather than sounds he may sometimes be able to recognize them as belonging to someone he knows. They may be talking to him, or talking about him (see below). The voices may be persecutory, neutral, or pleasing. The patient may talk back to the voices, or he may appear to be listening to them intently. In some cases the voices direct the patient to certain actions which he may feel duty-bound to follow.

Second-person voices with distressing content, 'You stink, you're horrible, go kill yourself' are found in severe depressive illnesses. Third-person voices, which discuss or argue about the patient or comment on what he is doing, are suggestive of schizophrenia in the absence of organic brain disease (see Table 3.3), as is hearing one's own thoughts spoken out loud (*echo de pensées*). In grief reactions, the bereaved person may hear the footsteps or other stigmata of the dead person.

Visual hallucinations Visual hallucinations may vary in complexity from simple flashes of light to sophisticated 'visions' of people or animals. They occur more commonly in organic psychoses, especially acute confusional states, than in functional psychoses, whereas the opposite is true with auditory hallucinations. They may be frightening, as in the case of hallucinations of spiders, insects and rats which occur in delirium tremens, or pleasing as with lilliputian hallucinations, in which the patient sees tiny people; these may also occur in delirium tremens. They may co-exist with auditory hallucinations as in temporal lobe epilepsy.

Olfactory hallucinations These may occur in temporal lobe epilepsy, when an unpleasant smell may be the initial symptom of the attack; in schizophrenia, as in the patient who said that people were making cars emit noxious smells at him; and in depressive illnesses, in which the patient insists that he emits a foul odour which he can smell.

Hallucinations of taste These are rare in psychiatric practice but characteristically occur in temporal lobe epilepsy.

Tactile and somatic hallucinations In cocaine psychosis patients may complain that insects are crawling over them (formication). Other patients insist that they are experiencing odd sensations in various parts of their body which are produced by others, as in the man who complained that his neighbour's laser gun was producing a cold feeling which travelled up his legs. This is another first-rank symptom of schizophrenia in the absence of organic brain disease (see Table 3.3). These hallucinations may have a sexual content, as in the patient who insisted that someone was having intercourse with her and she could feel it happening all the time.

Other hallucinations and illusions Some people complain that, when alone, they feel the presence of someone else beside them. This may occur in *grief reactions*, as illusions when the patient is frightened, as a manifestation of hysteria and in organic brain disease and schizophrenia. Finally vestibular hallucinations may occur, usually in acute organic brain disease, such as the patient with delirium tremens who has the sensation that he is flying through the air.

Abnormal experiences of self and environment

Déjà-vu This may occur in normal people but it is usually associated with temporal lobe epilepsy, and is characterized by the patient feeling that he has been in his current situation before.

Capgras' syndrome In this syndrome, which occurs most commonly in schizophrenia but may also occur in dementia, the patient asserts that people are not who they claim to be, but are their double.

Depersonalization This symptom is often a manifestation of heightened anxiety levels. The patient does not feel his normal self and may describe this unpleasant experience as if he is floating above his own body looking down on himself. He may also complain that he has lost the capacity to feel at an emotional level. This may be one of the most marked symptoms in depressed patients.

Derealization This often accompanies depersonalization. The patient says that his surroundings feel unreal or grey and colourless.

Cognitive state

All patients should have their cognitive state briefly tested, but in elderly people or where the presence of organic brain disease is suspected, e.g. acute confusional states, this assessment is extremely important.

Level of consciousness An assessment of the level of alertness of the patient or, if he is unconscious, of the level of unconsciousness must be made. Some patients appear to have fluctuating levels of consciousness; the mental state may then fluctuate between lucidity and gross abnormality. This is a manifestation of an acute confusional state. For a full account of the examination of the unconscious patient, see Chapter 11.

Orientation The patient's orientation in time, place and person should be formally assessed by direct questioning and the patient's answers written down verbatim. Disorientation is an important sign of organic brain disease, whether chronic or acute, but may also occur in chronic, disinterested, institutionalized schizophrenics and in hysterical dissociative states.

Time Ask about the day, date, month, year and time of day. If the patient does not know the month one should ask about the season. All patients should know the year and either the month or season and the approximate time of day, e.g. morning, afternoon, evening or night. Long stays in hospital, where one day is much like the next, however, are not conducive to an awareness of which particular day it is or the exact date of the month.

Place The patient should know where he is, e.g. home or hospital, and approximately where it is situated, e.g. what town or part of the town. Depending on how long he has been in the place where he is being interviewed, whether at home or in a hospital ward, he should know his way to such places as the bathroom or toilet. Some patients with acute confusional states may say they are in hospital but that the hospital is part of their own home.

Person If disorientation is suspected the patient should be asked if he knows his own name and his address.

Attention and concentration The patient's behaviour during the interview will have shown whether he is easily distractable or has been paying attention to and concentrating on the questions you have asked. This can be tested more formally by asking the patient to subtract serial sevens from a hundred or, as this may be difficult even for normal people, serial threes from twenty. Tasks such as recounting the months of the year and days of the week backwards or repeating a sequence of digits (digit span) forwards are also useful. Repetition of digits backwards, e.g. doctor says 165 to which the patient should reply 561, is dependent not only on attention and concentration but also on the ability to register the numbers 165 and remember them long enough to reverse them and is thus a test of immediate memory. Normal people should be able to manage seven digits forward and five backwards; telephone numbers in most large cities consist of seven digits.

Memory In chronic organic brain disease, memory for recent events is diminished, whereas early in the illness the patient often remains able to remember events which have happened in the past and is thus able to give a coherent account of the family and early personal history. Some patients with memory impairment as in Korsakoff's psychosis, which is usually due to vitamin B deficiency following poor nutrition and most commonly associated in the U.K. with heavy drinking, may attempt to cover their disability by confabulating. An example is the alcoholic with Korsakoff's psychosis seen after a six-week stay in hospital, who when asked how long he had been an inpatient stated that he had come in that day and been at work the day before, which he then described in great detail down to what he had had for his dessert in the staff canteen. Confabulation is not invention, but consists of the inappropriate recall of past, recent or distant, experiences. In the case of head injuries or in epileptic attacks, one should attempt to assess the presence of retrograde and anterograde amnesia, if any, in some detail. Memory impairment may be simulated for gain by some manipulative patients, some of whom may give approximate answers such as if the date is Monday, November 15th, 1984 they may say it is Tuesday, October 14th, 1983 and then correct themselves to Sunday, December 16th, 1985. Hysterical amnesia may occur in dissociative states in which there is a sudden total loss of memory. In contrast, in organic amnesia long-term memory and personal identity are usually spared until the later stages of the disorder. This is so even in dementing illnesses. Patients who are disinterested or depressed may appear to have memory impairment and in the latter case, called depressive pseudo-dementia, the aetiology may only become apparent when the depression lifts and the memory improves.

Past memory will already have been assessed while asking about the family and personal history, but recent memory will need more specific testing. A useful approach is to ask him whether he is interested in any sports. If this is so, concentrate on this; for example for football, ask about the fortunes of his favourite team, including past and present matches. Alternatively he can be asked about recent television programmes. Other recent events will include details about the hospital itself, and how the patient got there. Current affairs should also be asked about, e.g. the name of the monarch and her children and the Prime Minister and details of any recent happenings of major importance. A less direct question is to ask the patient what has been going on in the world or in this country recently. A more systematic approach to memory testing is to ask the patient to repeat a name and address immediately and again after five minutes or less, or to give him a sentence and see how many repetitions are necessary for accurate reproduction. One such sentence is: '*The one thing a nation needs in order to be rich and great is a large, secure supply of wood*.' Where relevant, visual as well as auditory memory should be tested. This can be done by giving the patient a picture depicting a series of objects and asking him a few minutes later to recall as many of the objects as he can.

The patient's answers to all specific questions about memory should be recorded verbatim.

Intelligence

An idea of the patient's level of intelligence is one of the most important pieces of information to be obtained from the interview. Not only will this help to determine suitable treatment (e.g. for psychotherapy the patient must be articulate and intelligent) but it will also affect the interpretation of the mental state examination itself. In the subnormal patient bizarre behaviour and abnormal ideas occurring as part of a *normal* fantasy life may be mistaken for psychiatric illness, when it represents only an attention-seeking device. An approximate assessment of intelligence can be obtained from the educational and occupational history and from an assessment of his general knowledge. Alternatively this can be tested more formally (see below). It is useful to enquire whether the patient can read and write, although this may correlate more with education than intelligence, and to see whether the patient is able to solve simple mathematical problems, especially where these are related to daily activities, e.g. shopping.

Further tests of cerebral function

In patients in whom organic brain disease is suspected, a more detailed assessment of cerebral function should be carried out. In addition to the above, this includes an assessment of speech both verbal and written, spatial, visual, motor and numerical abilities, awareness of body image and presence of released primitive reflexes. These fall into the rubric of the neurological examination (see Chapter 10).

FURTHER INVESTIGATIONS

In psychiatry this consists of information gathering, clarification and continuing assessment of the mental state, laboratory investigations, psychological testing, social enquiry and occupational therapy assessment.

Information gathering

Many patients will need more than one interview to take a full history. Other sources of information are needed to clarify and validate parts of the history. Spouse, family, friends and people at work or school may be able to help, but before they are contacted this should be discussed with the patient and his verbal or, in some cases, written consent obtained. In addition to separate interviews with the patient, spouse and family it is often necessary to bring them together in order to carry out diagnostic and therapeutic marital and family interviews. These interviews often provide information unavailable from either party on their own as well as affording an opportunity to see how the couple or family relate to each other. In addition, when feeding back your conclusions, it allows you to give all concerned parties the same information at the same time, thus avoiding potentially divisive miscommunication. If the other informant cannot be interviewed in person it may still be possible to do so over the telephone or by letter.

It is obviously important to obtain detailed medical records, from the general practitioner and from any hospital concerned; the grounds for previous diagnoses can be scrutinized and the response to past treatment assessed. Conditions in the patient's home may be assessed by a Social Worker, who may be able to see relatives who refuse to see a doctor. The patient's problems can be further assessed by asking him to write a diary of his symptoms, daily activities and emotional state. This often indicates links which may illuminate the aetiology of the current disorder. When one is dealing with a specific behavioural disorder, e.g. nervous diarrhoea, over-eating or aggressive behaviour, more systematic behavioural analysis may be necessary.

Mental state evaluation

The evaluation of the mental state is a continuous process and should be assessed at each interview. If the patient is admitted to hospital his behaviour on the ward should be observed and documented. This includes an account of the way he relates to other patients, to staff and visitors, and whether there are any signs of sleep or appetite disturbance or other abnormal behaviour.

Questionnaires and structured interview schedules may aid quantitative assessment of the mental state and be useful in evaluating progress.

Psychological testing

Psychological tests can be used to assess the patient's cognitive state, behaviour, personality and thinking process. Tests can be given to assess the level of intelligence, either briefly with the Mill Hill test and the Raven's Progressive Matrices test or in more detail with the WAIS (Wechsler Adult Intelligence Scale). In behaviour disorders it is useful to carry out a thorough behavioural analysis; this must be designed to be relevant to the individual problem. These investigations require specialized skills and they are best carried out by the clinical psychologist.

4
The skin, the nails and the hair

The skin is one organ; the whole of it should be examined to ensure that all physical signs are detected. Patients should be undressed as completely as possible and examined in good, preferably natural, light. The hair, nails and accessible mucosae should be included.

COLOUR AND PIGMENTATION

Before inspecting any rash, notice the colour of the skin. Normal skin is very variable in colour and depends on life style and light exposure as well as constitutional and ethnic factors. *Pallor* has many causes: temporary pallor occurs in shock, haemorrhage and intense emotion; persistent pallor occurs in anaemia or peripheral vasoconstriction. Although pallor is usual in anaemia, not all pale persons are anaemic. Conjunctival mucosal colour is a better indication of anaemia than skin colour. *Abnormal redness* is seen after overheating, extreme exertion, sunburn and in febrile, exanthematous and inflammatory skin diseases. Local redness may be due to telangiectasia, especially on the face. *Cyanosis* is a blue or purple–blue tint due to the presence of excessive reduced haemoglobin, either locally, as in impaired peripheral circulation, or generally, when oxygenation of the blood is defective. The tint of *methaemoglobinaemia* is more leaden than ordinary cyanosis; it is caused by drugs such as dapsone and certain poisons.

Jaundice varies from the 'subicteric', 'lemon-yellow', or 'daffodil' tints seen in pernicious anaemia and acholuric jaundice, to various shades of yellow, orange or dark olive-green in obstructive jaundice. Jaundice must be distinguished from the orange–yellow of carotenaemia, due to the presence of an excess of lipid-soluble yellow pigments in the plasma. Carotene does not stain the conjunctivae; jaundice does. Slight degrees of jaundice cannot be seen in artificial light.

Normal skin contains varying amounts of brown pigment (*melanin*). Brown pigmentation due to presence of haemosiderin is always pathological. A congenital absence of pigment in the skin which is generalized is known as *albinism*: if it is localized it is known as *piebaldism*. Patches of white and darkly pigmented skin are seen in *vitiligo*. Several autoimmune endocrine disorders are associated with vitiligo. A pale skin due to diminished pigment is also characteristic of *hypopituitarism* and *hypogonadism*. Increased pigmentation may be racial, due to sunburn or connected with various diseases. In *Addison's disease* there is a brown or dark-brown pigmentation, affecting exposed parts and parts not normally pigmented such as the axillae and the palmar creases; the lips and mouth may exhibit dark bluish-black areas. Note, however, that mucosal pigmentation is a normal finding in a substantial proportion of people of negro stock. More or less generalized pigmentation may also be seen in *haemochromatosis*, in which it has a peculiar greyish-bronze colour with a metallic sheen, due to excessive melanin and iron pigment; in *chronic arsenic poisoning*, in which it is finely dappled and affects covered more than exposed parts; in *argyria*, in which the deposition of silver in the skin produces a diffuse slatey-grey hue; and occasionally in the cachexia of advanced malignant disease. In *pregnancy* there may be pigmentation of the nipples and areolae, of the linea alba and, sometimes, a mask-like pigmentation of the face (chloasma). Chloasma may also be induced by steroid contraceptives. A similar condition, melasma, may be seen in Asian and African males. Localized pigmentation may be seen in *pellagra* and in scars of various kinds, particularly those due to X-irradiation therapy. Venous incompetence in the legs is often associated with chronic purpura, leading to haemosiderin pigmentation. The mixture of punctate, fresh purpura and haemosiderin may produce a golden hue. Pigmentation may also occur with chronic infestation by body lice. *Erythema ab igne*, a coarsely mottled pigmentation of the legs of women who habitually sit too near a fire, used to be common.

HAEMORRHAGE IN THE SKIN

Aggregations of extravasated red blood cells in the skin cause *purpura* (see Plate VII). Purpura may be punctate, from capillary haemorrhage, or may form larger macules according to the extent of haemorrhage and the size of vessels involved. The term *ecchymosis* implies a bruise, usually with cutaneous and subcutaneous haemorrhage causing a palpable lump. A frank fluctuant collection of blood is a *haematoma*.

Unlike erythema and telangiectasia, purpura cannot be blanched by pressure. It must not be confused with senile haemangioma (cherry angioma or Campbell de Morgan spot), which is common in later life and has no pathological significance.

DISTRIBUTION OF SKIN LESIONS

In the analysis of an eruption the two important points are its *distribution* and *morphology*.

Take distribution first and look at the whole eruption. Is it *symmetrical* or *asymmetrical*? Symmetry often implies internal causation whereas asymmetry may imply external factors. Is the eruption *centrifugal* or *centripetal*? Certain common diseases such as chickenpox and pityriasis rosea are characteristically centripetal whereas erythema multiforme is centrifugal. Smallpox, now probably eradicated, is also centrifugal. A disease may exhibit a *flexor* or *extensor bias*: atopic eczema in childhood is characteristically flexor whereas psoriasis in adults tends to be extensor. Are only *exposed areas* affected, implicating sunlight or some other external causative factor? If sunlight is suspected, are areas normally in shadow involved? Are the genitalia involved? *Localized distributions* may point immediately to an external contact as a cause, for example contact dermatitis from nickel in ear-rings, lipstick dermatitis, etc. Swelling of the eyelids is an important sign. Without redness and scaling, bilateral periorbital oedema may indicate acute nephritis, nephrosis or trichinosis. If there is *irritation*, insect bites or angio-oedema may be suspected; these are often unilateral. If there is *scaling* or *weeping and irritation*, contact dermatitis is the probable diagnosis. Dermatomyositis often produces swelling and heliotrope erythema of the eyelids.

MORPHOLOGY OF SKIN LESIONS

Assessment of morphology requires visual and tactile examination. Do not be afraid to feel the lesions. You will rarely be exposed to any danger in so doing, herpes simplex, herpes zoster and syphilis excepted. Proceed now to the *palpation* of the skin. Pass the hand gently over it, pinching it up between the forefinger and thumb, and note the following points: is it smooth or rough, thin or thick, dry or moist? Is there any visible sweating, either general or local? The *elasticity* of the skin should be investigated. If a fold of healthy skin is pinched up, it immediately flattens itself out again when released. Sometimes, however, it only does so very slowly, remaining for a considerable time in a creased condition. This is found frequently in healthy old people but may be an important sign of dehydration in conditions associated with prolonged vomiting and diarrhoea.

The condition of the subcutaneous tissue should be investigated. The presence of *oedema* is usually recognized by the fact that, if the skin is pressed firmly with the finger, a pit is left which persists for some little time. In some cases no pitting can be produced, especially when the oedema is of very long standing. The best place to look for slight degrees of oedema in cardiac disease is behind the malleoli at the ankles in patients who are ambulant, and over the sacrum in those who are confined to bed. The pressure of the finger should be maintained for 20–30 seconds, or small degrees of oedema will be overlooked. Pitting is minimal or absent in oedema due to lymphatic obstruction, where the skin is usually thickened and tough.

Subcutaneous emphysema gives rise to a characteristic crackling sensation on palpation. It starts in, and is usually confined to, the neighbourhood of the air passages. Rarely, it is due to clostridial infection of soft tissues after injury or gunshot wounds (gas gangrene).

A number of terms are used to describe the variety of lesions seen in the skin.

Macules Macules are areas of discoloration of the skin which are seen but not felt, being neither raised nor depressed nor thickened. They may be of any size. Macules may be erythematous, purpuric, pigmented or depigmented.

Papules Papules are palpable elevations of the skin of up to 5 mm diameter. Their surfaces may be pointed, rounded or flat. They are not deep-seated in the skin and are formed by proliferation of the skin's cells or by infiltration or exudation into the skin of cells and fluid. It may be possible to distinguish between predominantly dermal or epidermal papules. If the skin is stretched by applying tension on either side, a papule in the epidermis will retain its prominence, e.g. a wart, while a dermal papule will sink and become less prominent, e.g. a granuloma of tuberculosis, sarcoidosis or a lymphoma.

Nodules Nodules are larger than papules and may occasionally be enormous. They may be cutaneous or subcutaneous in origin. Nodules may be hard, for example the subcutaneous nodules of rheumatoid arthritis or the dermal nodules of metastatic carcinoma. Examples of soft nodules are lipoma (subcutaneous) or neurofibroma (very soft) as in von Recklinghausen's disease.

Vesicles Vesicles are small blisters of up to 5 mm diameter formed by the accumulation of fluid in the skin and associated with the disintegration of dermal cells in the affected areas. They are usually filled with serous fluid. If leucocytes are present, the fluid is opaque and yellow (*pustule*). Pustules are often follicular, as in coccal folliculitis. Non-follicular pustules may be a sequel to eczema or may be viral as in the later stages of herpes simplex or herpes zoster. Always note whether or not there is an area of redness around the base of a vesicle, for such redness indicates that the vesicle is planted upon an inflamed base—a fact which may be of diagnostic value, as in herpes simplex and herpes zoster (see Plate VI). Ruptured vesicles leave transient pits on the skin.

Bullae Bullae are larger blisters. They may be unilocular or multilocular and intra-epidermal or subepidermal. Bullae may contain serum, sero-purulent or haemorrhagic fluid.

Weals Weals are elevations of the skin caused by acute oedema of the dermis. They are caused by temporary increased permeability of the dermal capillaries due to local histamine release from mast cells. Often there is a surrounding erythematous macular flare. The lesions of urticaria (hives, nettle rash) are weals.

Scales Scaling of the skin surface indicates an abnormality of the process of epidermal keratinization and is found when imperfectly keratinized cells stick together in clumps. They may be small as in dandruff or large as in psoriasis. Scales must be distinguished from crusts (scabs), which are due to dried exudation. Crusts may be red from haemorrhage, yellow–green from pus, or honey-coloured from serum.

Burrows Burrows are short linear, straight or sinuous elevations of the outer epidermis, usually dark in colour. They are characteristic of infestation by scabies, and are made by the female scabies mite in the process of laying eggs.

Comedones (blackheads) Comedones are dark horny plugs of the pilo-sebaceous openings. They are the primary lesion of adolescent acne but may have an occupational cause in older men exposed to oils, e.g. ship's engineers. They are usually seen on the face.

Plaques Plaques are circumscribed flat areas of abnormal skin which are raised or sunk below the level of the surrounding skin, e.g. psoriasis or morphoea (the localized type of scleroderma). Plaques may also represent thickening of the skin by infiltration of inflammatory or neoplastic cells.

Fissures Fissures are small cracks in the epidermis, exposing the dermis, produced by the stretching of the skin after it has become inelastic owing to thickening of any kind. Fissures are often very painful.

Lichenification Skin which is continually rubbed, as in the chronic stage of atopic eczema, becomes thickened and the normal lines become more apparent. This is called lichenification because it resembles the lichen on trees.

Dyschromia Inflammation of the skin, especially in those of dark colour, often leads to hyperpigmentation or hypopigmentation.

Ulceration An ulcer is formed by destruction of the whole thickness of the skin by ischaemia, infection or neoplasia. In describing an ulcer, the nature of its floor, edge (flat, raised or undermined), and discharge should be noted. Any induration, inflammation or pigmentation of the surrounding skin should also be recorded. The draining lymph nodes should be examined.

Scar formation Scar formation represents an abnormal healing process in the skin. Describe the scar, noting especially whether it is atrophic or hypertrophic, freely movable or adherent to the deeper tissues, pale or livid, pitted, or surrounded by a zone of pigmentation.

Keloids are hypertrophic scars. They may be a sequel to burns but may also arise spontaneously or after chronic inflammation as in acne of the shoulders. Keloid formation is commoner in negro and Asiatic peoples than in Europeans. The skin over the sternum and shoulders is particularly prone to keloidal change.

THE HAIR

Hair colour and texture are racial characteristics, genetically determined. The yellow–brown mongol race has black straight hair, the negroids black, curly hair and the white caucasoids fair, brown, red or black hair. Secondary sexual hair begins to appear at puberty and has characteristic male and female patterns. Common baldness in men is genetically determined but requires adequate levels of circulating androgens for its expression. It occurs in women but only in old age.

Unlike other epithelial mitotic activity which is continuous throughout life, the growth of hair is cyclic, the hair follicle going through alternating phases of growth (anagen) and rest (telogen). Anagen in the scalp lasts 3 to 5 years; telogen is much shorter and constant at about 3 months.

Hair loss (alopecia) can have many causes. Any inflammatory or destructive disease of the scalp skin may destroy hair follicles in its wake. Thus, burns, heavy X-irradiation or zoster in the first division of the trigeminal nerve may cause a scarring alopecia. Alopecia in the presence of normal scalp skin may be patchy and localized as in traction alopecia in nervous children, ringworm infections (tinea capitis) or autoimmune alopecia areata. Secondary syphilis is a rare cause of a patchy 'moth-eaten' alopecia.

Diffuse scalp hair loss and growth of male-type body hair is characteristic of women with virilizing conditions. Metabolic causes include hypothyroidism and severe iron-deficiency anaemia. Anti-mitotic drugs may affect growing follicles, producing a diffuse anagen alopecia. Certain other drugs, such as anticoagulants, and dramatic metabolic upsets, such as childbirth, crash dieting and severe toxic illnesses, may precipitate follicles into the resting phase, producing an effluvium of telogen hairs three months later when anagen begins again.

THE NAILS

The nails should be carefully examined. Thimble pitting of the nails is characteristic of psoriasis but eczema and alopecia areata may also produce pitting. A severe illness may temporarily arrest nail growth; when growth starts again a transverse ridge develops. These are Beau's lines and can be used to date the time of onset of the illness. Inflammation of the cuticle (nail fold) may produce similar changes (chronic paronychia). The changes described above arise from disturbance of the nail matrix. The nail bed also makes a contribution to the nails. Disturbance of the nail bed may produce thick nails (pachyonychia) or separation of the nail from the bed (onycholysis). This may happen in psoriasis and other conditions. The nail may be destroyed in severe lichen planus or epidermolysis bullosa (a genetic abnormality in which the skin blisters in response to minor trauma). Some nails are missing in the genetic nail–patella syndrome. Splinter haemorrhages under the nails may result from trauma, psoriasis, rheumatoid arthritis or other 'collagen' diseases, bacterial endocarditis and trichinosis.

In iron-deficiency states, the fingernails and toenails lose their normal transverse convex curvature, becoming flattened or concave (see Figs. 2.4 and 2.5). Clubbing of the fingertips (see Chapters 2 and 8), in which the angle at the nail beds is lost and the fingertips expanded, is especially common in carcinoma of the lung and cyanotic heart disease but also occurs in other disorders (see p. 30).

CUTANEOUS MANIFESTATIONS OF INTERNAL DISEASE

White macules shaped like small ash leaves which are present at birth may be the first sign of tuberous sclerosis. Sometimes they are difficult to see by natural light but show up under the Wood's light. They should be looked for in infants suffering from fits. Pigmentation of the lips is a feature of *Peutz–Jegher syndrome*, genetically determined, in which multiple polyps of the stomach or colon appear which may undergo malignant transformation. Patchy depigmented macules which are hypoaesthetic and associated with enlargement of the peripheral nerves are features of certain types of *leprosy*. *Café au lait* patches are often the first sign of neurofibromatosis; they may be multiple. Another valuable sign of *von Recklinghausen's disease* is bilateral freckling of the axillary skin. The characteristic soft neurofibromata may be solitary or few or hundreds may be scattered over the body. *Paget's disease* of the nipple is a well defined red scaly condition which looks like eczema. It is associated in most instances with a duct carcinoma of the underlying breast. Several of the so-called collagen vascular diseases may have characteristic eruptions. *Systemic lupus erythematosus*, seen in females between puberty and the menopause, may show a symmetrical 'butterfly' erythema of the nose and cheeks. In *polyarteritis nodosa*, reticular livedo of the limbs, purpura, vasculitic papules and ulceration occur. In *scleroderma* (systemic sclerosis), acrosclerosis of the fingertips with scarring, ulceration and calcinosis follows a Raynaud's phenomenon of increasing severity. *Dermatomyositis* often presents with a heliotrope discoloration and oedema of the eyelids and fixed erythema over the dorsa of the knuckles and fingers and over the bony points. There is usually weakness of the proximal limb muscles. Dermatomyositis in the middle aged is associated in 30% of cases with internal malignancy.

Acanthosis nigricans is brownish thickening of the axillae and groins and the sides of the neck. Sometimes there is thickening of the palms, soles and gums. In the middle aged, acanthosis nigricans is associated with internal malignancy.

Icthyosis (fish skin) is usually present from childhood and is genetic but, if icthyosis is acquired in adult life, a search should be made for malignancy or other underlying disease. Generalized, severe *persistent pruritus* in the absence of obvious skin disease may be due to thyrotoxicosis, renal or hepatic failure, lymphoma or other malignancies. However, in old people with dry skin, it is common and of no systemic significance.

Diabetes mellitus has a number of skin manifestations: pruritus vulvae, boils, ulcers on the soles or toes due to neuropathy, and gangrene of the extremities from arteriosclerosis. *Necrobiosis lipoidica diabeticorum* produces reddish-brown plaques, usually on the shins, with central atrophy of the skin. Cutaneous or mucocutaneous candidosis and xanthomatous nodules in skin are also associated with diabetes. *Spider naevi* consist of a central arteriole feeding a cluster of surrounding vessels. Many young people have up to seven on the face, shoulders or arms. In older age groups pregnancy, the administration of oestrogens (as in oral contraceptives) and liver disease may cause multiple lesions. Pregnancy and liver disease may also produce erythema of the thenar and hypothenar eminences ('liver palms').

Xanthomata are yellow or orange deposits of lipid in the skin. They may be the effect of hyperlipoproteinaemia or of diabetes, liver disease, myxoedema or renal disease. White deposits of lipid (arcus senilis) in the cornea may have a similar explanation but may be a normal feature in those of 60 years or more. Flat lipid deposits around the eyes (xanthelasma) may be due to lipid disturbance but are also seen in the middle aged and elderly without any general metabolic upset.

Carotenaemia produces an orange yellow colour of the skin, especially of the palms and soles. It occurs in those who eat great quantities of carrots and other vegetables, in hypothyroid persons, in diabetics and also in those taking β-carotene for the treatment of erythropoietic porphyria.

Erythema nodosum is a condition in which tender, painful, red nodules appear, typically on the shins. They fade slowly over several weeks, leaving bruising, but never ulcerate. Sarcoidosis and drug sensitivity are the commonest causes but tuberculosis and streptococcal infection used to be common causes.

The skin is involved in various *venereal diseases*. Syphilis in all its stages, the pustules of chronic gonococcal septicaemia, type II genital herpes simplex and scabies are obvious examples.

Several of the commonest viral infections and illnesses of childhood are characterized by fever and a distinctive rash (*exanthem*), including measles, varicella and rubella. In measles, upper respiratory symptoms are quickly followed by a characteristic *maculopapular erythematous rash*. In rubella (German measles), the rash is more transient, *micropapular* and associated with occipital lymphodenopathy and less malaise. The exanthem of chickenpox (varicella) is *papulovesicular*, centripetal and there may be lesions in the mouth.

Other less common viral infections associated with a rash include hand, foot and mouth disease (due to Coxsackie A16 virus), whose name betrays the distribution of the *vesiculopustules*, and *erythema infectiosum*, where the exanthem on the face gives a 'slapped-cheeked' appearance. *Roseola infantum*, a disease of toddlers, mimics rubella.

DRUG ERUPTIONS

In the last quarter century, eruptions caused by drugs have become extremely common. Most, but not all, such rashes are due to allergic hypersensitivity.

Drug rashes can mimic almost every pattern of skin disease. Thus urticaria may be caused by penicillin; ampicillin may induce a measles-like (morbilliform) rash, especially when given in infectious mononucleosis; eczema-like rashes are seen from methyldopa and phenylbutazone, whereas gold and chloroquine rashes mimic lichen planus; generalized exfoliative dermatitis may be induced by sulphonylureas, indomethacin and allopurinol.

Drugs which may sensitize the skin to sunlight (phototoxic reaction) include tetracyclines, sulphonamides and nalidixic acid. Acne-like rashes may follow high-dose prednisolone therapy or use of isoniazid. Certain cytotoxic drugs cause hair loss. Both erythema nodosum and erythema multiforme may be induced by sulphonamides including co-trimoxazole.

Laboratory tests are of almost no value in the diagnosis of drug eruptions. Careful history taking and a knowledge of patterns of reactions usually allow accurate diagnosis.

SPECIAL TECHNIQUES IN EXAMINATION OF THE SKIN

Microscopical examination is useful in the diagnosis of scabies, pediculosis and fungal infection (tinea and candidosis).

Scabies

Scabies is due to the *Acarus* (*Sarcoptes*) *scabiei*. The female *Acarus* is larger than the male and burrows in the epidermis, depositing eggs. These burrows should be looked for between the fingers, on the hands or wrists and sides of the feet. They are recognized with the naked eye as little short dark lines terminating in a shining spot of skin. The eggs lie in the dark line, the insect in the shining spot. It may be picked out by means of a flat surgical needle passed along the black line to the clear spot. The use of a lens aids the operation—which is by no means invariably successful—and makes possible the recognition of the *Acarus*. The latter may be placed on a slide under the microscope for more detailed examination.

Pediculosis

Three varieties of pediculosis occur—*Pediculus capitis* on the head, *P. corporis* on the trunk, and *P. pubis* on the pubic and axillary hairs. The eggs or 'nits' of *P. capitis* are stuck on the hairs. From their position on the hairs one can judge roughly the duration of the condition, for they are fixed at first near the root of the hair, and are then carried up with the latter in its growth. The higher up the nits, the longer the pediculi have been present. *P. corporis* should be looked for in the seams of the clothes, especially where the latter come into close contact with the skin, e.g. over the shoulders. The bites of the parasite produce haemorrhagic spots, each with a dark centre and a paler areola. Marks of scratching should always be looked for on parts accessible to the patient's nails. *P. pubis* is venereally acquired and causes intense pubic itching. The nits are laid on the pubic hair.

Pediculosis corporis is seen only in the grossly deprived, vagabonds, down-and-out alcoholics, those living rough and in conditions of war and social upheaval. In contrast, pediculosis capitis is extremely common in schoolchildren, however clean, and is endemic in many schools.

Fungus infections

Fungus may grow in the skin, nails, or hair and cause disease (ringworm).

Skin Between the toes, the soles of the feet and the groins are the commonest sites of fungal infection. The lesions may be scaly or vesicular, tending to spread in a ring form with central healing; macerated, dead-white offensive-smelling epithelium is seen in the intertriginous areas such as the toe clefts.

Nails Discoloration, deformity, hypertrophy, and abnormal brittleness may result from fungus infection.

Hair Ringworm of the scalp is most common in children. It presents as round or oval areas of baldness covered with short, broken-off lustreless hair stumps. These hair stumps may fluoresce bright green under Wood's light. Some organisms are Wood's-light negative.

Microscopical examination for fungus infection Scales from the active edge of a lesion are scraped off lightly with a scalpel or the roofs of vesicles are snipped off with scissors. The material is placed in a drop of 10–20% aqueous potassium hydroxide solution on a microscope slide, covered with a cover slip and left for 30 minutes to clear. It is then examined with the 8 mm or 4 mm objective, using low illumination. The mycelia are recognized as branching refractile threads which boldly transgress the outlines of the squamous cells. Nails are examined in much the same way, but it is necessary to break up the snippings and shavings into small fragments. These are either heated in potassium hydroxide or are left to clear in it overnight before being examined. A scalp lesion is cleaned with 70% alcohol or with 1% cetrimide and infected stumps and scales are removed by scraping with a scalpel. The hairs are cleaned in potassium hydroxide in the same way as skin scales. Examination under the microscope reveals spores on the outside of the hair roots, and mycelia inside the hair substance. The species of fungus responsible may be established by culture on Sabouraud's glucose-agar.

5
The abdomen

THE MOUTH AND THROAT

The examination of the mouth and throat is conducted with the patient sitting up either in bed, with the head resting comfortably back on pillows, or in a chair. A bright torch, a tongue depressor (spatula) and fingercots are essential. The lips, teeth, gums, tongue, palate, fauces and oropharynx are then visualized systematically, and finally palpation of the sides of the tongue, floor of mouth and tonsillar regions are carried out.

Inspection

The lips

Look closely at the philtrum (the shallow depression running from nose to upper lip) for the tell-tale scar of a repaired cleft lip. When present, particularly if associated with 'nasal speech', inspect the palate carefully for signs of a cleft. Next, look at the corners of the mouth for cracks or fissures (angular stomatitis). The cracks are reddish brown, moist, superficial, linear ulcers radiating from the angles of the mouth. In children their origin is infective (perlèche); they are common in the elderly when ill-fitting or deficient dentures result in over-closure of the mouth. Cheilosis is also seen in severe iron-deficiency anaemia; it may provide a clue to the diagnosis of post-cricoid carcinoma in women with dysphagia; and also occurs in vitamin B_2 (riboflavine) deficiency.

Rhagades, white scars at the angles of the mouth indicating previous cheilosis due to congenital or tertiary syphilis, are now very rare. Here, however, the fissures extend into the mouth. A crack in the middle of the lower lip is common in cold weather; although difficult to heal because of constant movement of the lips and moistening by the tongue, such a fissure is of no sinister significance.

Observe any desquamation or inflammation of the lips (cheilitis). This is commonplace and self-limiting in cold weather. Grouped vesicles on the lips on a red base with crusted lesions are seen in herpes simplex labialis commonly associated with coryza. This infection is usually of short duration and the lack of induration and ulceration serve to distinguish it from other more serious conditions. Recurrent actinic cheilitis with small blisters and exfoliation, however, is a pre-malignant condition found in people constantly exposed to the sun and wind, such as farmers and fishermen.

Look for any ulcer on the lips. Carcinoma (epithelioma) usually occurs on the lower lip away from the midline; the ulcer is indolent, flat and shallow, although in time the edge may become heaped up and induration may be felt. Epithelioma has to be differentiated from a kerato-acanthoma, pyogenic granuloma and the chancre of primary syphilis. A kerato-acanthoma (molluscum sebaceum) is a lesion due to overgrowth of the stratum granulosum of the skin. It usually presents as a firm, rounded nodule sometimes with ulceration; it is more common on the upper lip and heals spontaneously without treatment. Pyogenic granuloma is a soft red raspberry-like nodule on the upper lip which often follows minor trauma. The upper lip is the commonest site of an extra-genital chancre, which appears as a small, round lesion that is firm and indurated. If it ulcerates it forms a serpiginous outline and exudes a stringy non-purulent exudate. In both epithelioma and chancre enlarged painless cervical nodes are commonly felt.

Very occasionally one sees multiple small brown or black spots on the skin around the mouth (circumoral pigmentation) which may also extend onto the lips and buccal mucosa. This pigmentation constitutes one of the triad of cardinal features of the Peutz–Jeghers syndrome and signifies underlying small bowel polyposis, a condition inherited as a mendelian dominant. On the buccal mucosa the pigmentation may look very like that seen in Addison's disease.

Now gently grasp the lower lip with the index finger and thumb of both hands and evert it fully, to display the mucous surface of the lip. Two lesions are commonly seen in this site: aphthous ulcers and retention cysts. Aphthous ulcers are small superficial painful ulcers with a white or yellow base and a narrow halo of hyperaemia. Such ulcers are also seen on the tongue, buccal mucosa and palate. Retention cysts of the mucous glands of the lips and buccal mucosa appear as round, translucent swellings, elevated from the surface with a characteristic white or bluish appearance. They are also found on the mucous surface of the lower lip.

The teeth

Ask the patient to grimace so as to show his teeth, or if he wears dentures to remove them and open the mouth widely. Using a tongue depressor to retract first the lips and then the cheeks, note the number of teeth present and look for decay (caries). The tooth most commonly 'missing' is an impacted unerupted third mandibular molar (wisdom). Inspect both the buccal and lingual aspects of the teeth. It is said that lack of teeth may cause indigestion, but many edentulous people suffer no indigestion whether they wear dentures or not. Look for any changes in:

Colour Tartar deposition occurs mainly on the lingual aspect of the lower incisor and canine teeth and consists of precipitated calcium salts of saliva which, in smokers, is stained brown. Children up to the age of eight treated with tetracycline (and children of expectant mothers so treated after the fourteenth week of pregnancy) are at risk of acquiring permanent staining of both the deciduous and permanent teeth. This takes the form of disfiguring horizontal bands, which may be yellow or grey and must not be mistaken for bands of hyperplasia on the enamel due to exanthematous fevers or any serious illness occurring during the development of the crowns. In endemic fluorosis, chalk-white patches appear on the teeth or the teeth present a dull, unglazed appearance, sometimes with pitting and brown staining (Maldon teeth).

Shape Ill-formed hypoplastic teeth have a broad, concave biting edge, whilst some notching of the incisors is seen in those who persistently bite cotton or hold hairclips between their teeth. They must not be mistaken for Hutchinson's teeth—a manifestation of congenital syphilis, but a very rare finding nowadays. In this condition the two central upper permanent incisors are rounded in section and notched at their biting edge. They may also be broader near the gum than at the crown, so as to be peg shaped. The first permanent molars may be dome shaped. The two central upper incisors are commonly lost in leprosy.

Ridging Transverse ridging is sometimes seen in the permanent teeth of those who had vitamin C and D deficiency in infancy.

Enlargement of the lower jaw in acromegaly leads to alteration of the bite, so that the lower teeth may close outside the upper ones.

The gums

Examine the gums at the same time as the teeth. Pink, healthy gums adhere closely to the necks of the teeth and have a sharp border. With increasing age gingival recession occurs, so making the teeth appear longer and exposing the cementum below the enamel. This makes it easier for infection to gain a hold.

In *chronic marginal gingivitis*, the gums are retracted, frequently bleed easily and lose their characteristic stippling. Sometimes pus can be squeezed from them (*pyorrhoea alveolaris*).

Acute herpetic gingivostomatitis due to the simplex virus occurs most commonly in infants and children. Many small vesicles appear on the gums, cheeks, palate, tongue and lips. The vesicles rupture to produce shallow ulcers with a yellowish floor and bright red margins. *Vincent's gingivostomatitis*, an infection due to fusiform spirochaetes, characteristically destroys the interdental papillae. A thick felted greenish grey slough is formed and halitosis is present. In patients exposed to lead compounds, a stippled blue line can often be observed running along the edge of the gum, especially opposite those teeth showing gingivitis. Similar lines may be produced by bismuth or mercury but these are uncommon signs. The gums in scurvy are swollen, irregular in outline, red, spongy and bleed easily. Hypertrophy of the gums may occur in pregnancy and in patients treated for long periods with phenytoin. Haemorrhages may be observed in the buccal mucous membrane in thrombocytopenic purpura and acute leukaemia.

Pus can form in a carious tooth to form an alveolar or dental abscess with throbbing pain, exacerbated by tapping the affected tooth. Localized swelling of the gum and swelling of the face (if pus has escaped through the lateral alveolar margin) are signs associated with this condition. Ill-fitting dentures can produce a granuloma or an ulcer on the gum at the point of pressure where the denture does not fit properly. Such a lesion has to be differentiated from a carcinomatous ulcer arising in the gum; the latter presents the same macroscopic features as malignant ulcers elsewhere in the mouth.

Epulis is a general term used to describe any swelling arising in the gum of the maxilla or mandible.

The tongue

Ask the patient to protrude the tongue. Inability to do so fully (*ankyloglossia*) is seen, very rarely, in infants due to tongue tie (a congenitally short frenulum linguae) or in advanced malignancy of the tongue involving the floor of the mouth. When carcinoma involves the side of the tongue (the commonest site) and the floor of the mouth, slight deviation towards the affected side may occur. Slight deviation is not uncommon and may be due to asymmetry of the jaws. In hemiplegia, deviation towards the paralysed side may be found. In lesions of the hypoglossal nerve or its nucleus there may be fasciculation of the affected side; later this side may be wasted and deeply grooved (lingual hemiatrophy). The tongue is large in acromegaly, cretinism, myxoedema and lymphangioma.

Tremor of the tongue may be due to nervousness, thyrotoxicosis, delirium tremens or parkinsonism.

Next examine the dorsum of the tongue.

Colour Is the tongue pale, red or discoloured? Pallor is seen in severe anaemia. Discoloration is most often due to the ingestion of coloured foods—e.g. red wine or coloured sweets.

Moistness The state of the tongue gives some indication of the state of hydration of the body, provided the patient is not a mouth breather. A dry, brown tongue may be found in the later stages of any severe illness, but is found particularly in advanced uraemia and acute intestinal obstruction.

Fur Furring of the tongue is of little value as an indication of disease. It is found in heavy smokers, mouth breathers, the edentulous and those on soft, milky or otherwise sloppy diets. A brown fur, the 'black hairy tongue', is due to a fungus infection and is of no special significance, though frequently a source of great alarm to its possessor. The tongue of scarlet fever at first shows bright red papillae standing out of a thick white fur. Later the white coat disappears leaving enlarged papillae on a bright red surface—'the strawberry tongue'.

The papillae Generalized atrophy of the papillae produces a smooth or bald tongue which is characteristic of pernicious anaemia, but may also sometimes be found in iron-deficiency anaemia, sprue, other gastrointestinal disorders and deficiency states, especially pellagra. In severe cases smoothness may be associated with wrinkling of the mucous membrane, which has then to be distinguished from fissuring of the tongue seen in chronic superficial glossitis due to syphilis, now rare in the United Kingdom, and congenital fissuring of the tongue or 'scrotal tongue', which is common and of no pathological significance. In chronic superficial glossitis, areas of leucoplakia (whitish opaque areas of thickened epithelium) are separated by intervening smooth and scarred areas; there are no normal papillae to be seen and the fissures run mainly in a longitudinal direction. In congenital fissuring the papillae are normal but the surface is interrupted by numerous irregular but more or less symmetrical folds which tend to run mainly horizontally. In median rhomboid glossitis a lozenge-shaped area of loss of papillae and fissuring is seen in the midline anterior to the foramen caecum. It feels nodular and may be mistaken for a carcinoma. It must also be distinguished from a lingual thyroid but this is situated posterior to the foramen caecum. 'Geographical tongue' is another harmless anomaly characterized by localized irregular red areas of desquamated epithelium and filiform papillae surrounded by a whitish-yellow border which change in distribution and give the appearance of a map. The 'false geographical tongue' with a similar appearance occurs chiefly in children with fever.

The sides and undersurface Ask the patient to open the mouth wide and protrude the tongue fully to one side. Then retract the cheek with a spatula. This displays the side and lateral undersurface well. Some patients find this impossible to do, so wrap a gauze swab around the tip of the tongue and with index finger and thumb gently pull the tongue out and to one side. Benign ulcers in this site are common and may be inflammatory or traumatic in origin, very often due to ill-fitting dentures or broken carious teeth; such ulcers tend to be painful, superficial and lack induration. However, in an elderly patient any ulcer at this site must be regarded as malignant until proved otherwise by biopsy; it is the most frequent site of carcinoma in the mouth and presents as a hard, indurated ulcer with everted raised edges.

Now ask the patient to retract the tongue fully and slightly elevate the tip with the mouth wide open. This displays the undersurface of the anterior tongue and floor of the mouth. Note the frenulum linguae and the orifice of the submandibular duct opening on either side of the base of the frenulum. The ampulla of each duct lies just proximal to the orifice and is a common site for calculi formed in the submandibular salivary gland to lodge. The calculus is seen as a white or yellow bleb distending an oedematous hyperaemic ampulla.

A small ulcer on the frenulum is sometimes seen in persistent coughing and particularly in whooping cough. Sublingual varicosities are common in the elderly. Two types of cyst may be found in the floor of the mouth: a ranula, which forms a bluish-white translucent swelling of variable size and is due to blockage of the duct of a mucous gland, and a sublingual dermoid cyst, a round opaque swelling lying beneath the mucosa either above or below the mylohyoid, which is due to sequestration of epidermal tissue beneath the skin along the embryological lines of fusion of the mouth.

The buccal mucosa

Inspect the buccal mucosa. Retract the cheek with a spatula. Note the opening of the parotid duct seen as a tiny swelling opposite the upper second molar tooth. In the catarrhal stage of measles, before the appearance of the rash, small bluish-white spots, surrounded by a red areola, may be seen opposite the molar teeth. These are known as Koplik's spots. In the same position irregular areas or dots of slatey-grey or blue pigmentation are seen in Addison's disease.

Aphthous ulcers, mucous retention cysts and papillomata present the same appearance on the buccal mucosa as elsewhere in the mouth. White opalescent patches (rather like white paint) of leucoplakia may also be seen on the inner aspect of the cheek; these should be differentiated from lichen planus, an oral manifestation of a skin disease, but in this case look elsewhere, especially on the arms and legs, for similar lesions. Thrush (monilial stomatitis), a fungal infection due to *Candida albicans*, presents as a different sort of white patch. It is seen as small white points raised somewhat above the surrounding surface, which is usually redder than normal. As the infection gains hold so the lesions coalesce and may form extensive sheets throughout the mouth. Patches of thrush are apt to be mistaken for small milk curds, but curds can be easily detached, while thrush patches can be removed only with difficulty and then tend to leave behind a raw surface. Thrush is common in debilitated children, beneath unclean dentures and in patients on cytotoxic or immunosuppressive drugs. It is also seen frequently on surgical wards, especially in ill patients with sepsis in the postoperative period and those treated with broad-spectrum antibiotics, which destroy the normal bacterial flora of the mouth and thus allow the fungi to flourish.

The palate, fauces, tonsils and pharynx

Ask the patient to put the head right back and keep the mouth wide open. Inspect the hard and soft palates and note the position of the uvula. Get the patient to say 'ah', which raises the soft palate and increases visibility of the fauces, tonsils and oropharynx. (For abnormalities of movement of the soft palate during phonation see p. 314.)

If a good view of these structures has not been obtained thus far, introduce a spatula to depress the base of the tongue and if necessary another spatula to retract the anterior pillar of the fauces to view the tonsils properly.

Again look for any ulcers, erythema or vesicles. Vesicles confined to one side of the hard palate which progress to painful oval ulcers are characteristic of herpes zoster of the maxillary division of the trigeminal nerve (5th cranial); this disorder usually occurs in older patients and is accompanied by a characteristic skin rash in the corresponding dermatome on the face. Herpes zoster infection of the glossopharyngeal nerve (9th cranial) produces similar lesions in the pharynx.

Malignant ulcers do occur on the hard palate but much less frequently than elsewhere in the mouth, and present the same appearances. Ectopic salivary gland tissue may be present in the mouth, the hard palate being the commonest site. Tumours of this tissue present as a smooth, hard swelling projecting from the surface of the hard palate, sometimes with central ulceration.

If a hole is seen in the hard palate it is usually due to one of the following causes:

1 Imperfect closure or breakdown after repair of a cleft palate.

2 Radionecrosis of bone following radiotherapy for treatment of local carcinoma.

3 Tertiary syphilis with formation of a gumma.

Petechiae on the palate are commonly seen in glandular fever, but they are also features of any form of thrombocytopenia, rubella and streptococcal tonsillitis. Oral lesions may be the presenting feature of glandular fever: enlarged tonsils are covered with a white exudate which tends to become confluent; there is oedema of the fauces and soft palate and erythema of the oropharynx. This contrasts with the yellow punctate folliculiar exudate seen in streptococcal tonsillitis. Whenever a membranous exudate is seen, diphtheria should spring to mind and, as in all cases of mouth infection, a swab should be taken for bacteriological examination. The membrane in diphtheria varies in colour from white to green and often starts on the tonsil before spreading to the fauces and pharynx.

Finally, look at the pharynx. The presence on its surface of a number of small round or oval swellings, somewhat like sago grains, is so common as to be almost normal in appearance. In pharyngitis these are much increased.

Notice any vesicles or ulcers. In chickenpox (herpes varicella) oral lesions may be apparent before the characteristic rash appears. There is erythema of the pharyngeal and buccal mucosae, followed by vesicles which progress to oval or round ulcers with a white slough. In herpangina (Coxsackie virus infection), which is also common in the young, similar lesions may be seen in the oropharynx, soft palate and uvula.

In the common cold (coryza), mucopus may be noticed on the posterior wall of the pharynx running down from the nasopharynx. Not very commonly seen nowadays are a peritonsillar abscess (quinsy) and retropharyngeal abscess. The latter forms a smooth, tense, tender swelling which bulges forwards from the posterior wall of the oropharynx.

The breath

Carious teeth, infection or ulceration of the gum, stomatitis, and retention and decomposition of secretion in the follicles of enlarged tonsils are the commonest sources of offensive breath. Characteristic odours may be recognized: in ketosis, the breath smells of acetone; in uraemia, there is a fishy or ammoniacal odour; and in hepatic failure, the odour is described as 'mousy'. In suppurative conditions of the lung the breath may have a putrid smell, whilst the odour of bronchiectasis has been compared to that of apple blossom with a hint of stale faeces. Paraldehyde and alcohol also impart their characteristic smell to the breath.

Palpation

Palpation forms an important, frequently neglected part of the examination of the mouth, particularly in patients who complain of oral symptoms or in whom unexplained cervical lymphadenopathy is found. Palpation is imperative in anyone with a solitary or suspected ulcer in the oral cavity, and bimanual palpation provides further information about such things as swellings in the floor of the mouth or cheek.

Impress on the patient that you will be as gentle as possible. Put on a disposable glove or fingercot, and ask the patient to remove any dentures and to open the mouth widely. With the tongue elevated and to one side, place the index finger of the right hand beneath the tongue on one side of the frenulum and run the finger back along the floor of the mouth. Even a small calculus can easily be felt in any part of the submandibular duct. Then come forwards, running the finger along the lingual side of the tongue to the midline and return on the buccal side of the gum towards the lower molar teeth. Now run the finger up the mucosa covering the ascending ramus of the mandible, and examine both palatal and buccal aspects of the gum of the upper jaw.

If an ulcer is present, try and decide whether any induration is present or not. To perform bimanual examination, with the index finger already inside the mouth, place the fingertips of the left hand flat beneath the mandible, or over the cheek, outside the mouth, and exert gentle pressure between your right index finger and the fingers of the left hand.

Now palpate the tongue and feel the dorsum and the lateral and under-surfaces with the index finger; it sometimes helps for the patient to protrude the tongue to one or other side to do this, and if necessary the tongue can be held in a gauze swab between finger and thumb of the other hand.

Palpation of the posterior third of the tongue, fauces and tonsils is the least pleasant part for the patient as it usually causes gagging, and it is thus left until last. As before, the index finger is used and run over these structures as rapidly as possible. One is concerned with detecting a small or hidden carcinoma in these sites, so feel for irregularity, ulceration and particularly induration.

Any abnormality felt in these sites in a patient with symptoms demands illuminated head lamp and laryngeal examination (p. 387).

THE ABDOMEN

It is helpful for recording in notes or when communicating information to colleagues to think of the abdomen as divided into regions (Fig. 5.1).

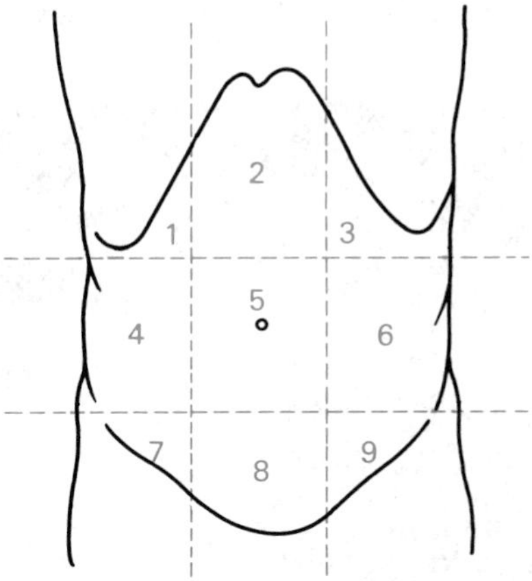

Fig. 5.1 Regions of the abdomen. 1 and 3: Right and left hypochondrium; 2: Epigastrium; 4 and 6: Right and left lumbar; 5: Umbilical; 7 and 9: Right and left iliac; 8: Hypogastrium or suprapubic.

The two *lateral vertical* planes pass from the femoral artery below to cross the costal margin close to the tip of the 9th costal cartilage.

The two *horizontal* planes, the sub-costal and inter-tubercular, pass across the abdomen to connect the lowest points on the costal margin, and the tubercles of the iliac crests respectively.

Remember that the area of each region will depend on the width of the sub-costal angle and the proximity of costal margin to iliac crest, in addition to other features of bodily habitus which naturally vary greatly from one patient to the next.

Inspection

The patient should be lying flat on his back, arms by his side, on a firm couch or mattress, the head and neck supported by enough pillows, normally one or two, to make him comfortable (Fig. 5.2). A sagging mattress makes examination, particularly palpation, difficult. Make sure there is a good light and the room is warm. Stand on the patient's right side and ensure your hands are warm. A shivering patient cannot relax and vital signs, especially on palpation, may be missed.

The abdomen is exposed by turning down all the bedclothes except the upper sheet. The clothing should then be drawn up to just above the xiphisternum and lastly the sheet folded down to expose the groins and genitalia across the upper thighs. This point is important because many is the patient who presents with intestinal obstruction due to a strangled femoral or inguinal hernia where the diagnosis is missed initially due to lack of proper exposure of the groins in an effort to save his embarrassment. However, once full inspection has taken place the sheet may be pulled up to the level of the symphysis pubis to allay anxiety.

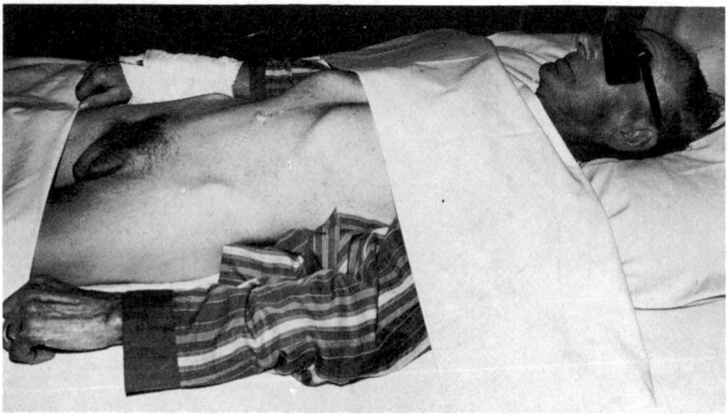

Fig. 5.2 Position of the patient and exposure for abdominal examination. Note that the genitalia must be exposed.

Inspection is an important and neglected part of abdominal examination. It is well worthwhile spending 30 seconds observing the abdomen from different positions to note the following features.

Shape Is the abdomen of normal contour and fullness, or distended? Is it scaphoid (sunken)?

Generalized fullness or distension may be due to fat, fluid, flatus, faeces, or fetus. *Localized distension* may be symmetrical and centred around the umbilicus, as in the case of the small bowel obstruction, or asymmetrical as in gross enlargement of the spleen, liver or ovary. Make a mental note of the site of any such *swelling* or distension; think of the anatomical structures in that region and note if there is any movement of the swelling, either with or independent of respiration.

A *scaphoid* abdomen is seen in advanced stages of starvation and malignant disease, particularly carcinoma of the oesophagus and stomach.

The umbilicus Normally the umbilicus is slightly retracted and inverted. Being at the centre of the abdomen one's eyes inevitably come to rest on it at the same time as noting the general shape of the abdomen. If it is everted then an umbilical hernia may be present and can be confirmed by feeling an expansile impulse on palpation of the swelling when the patient coughs. The hernial sac contains omentum, bowel or fluid. A frequent finding in the umbilicus of elderly obese women is a concentration of inspissated desquamated epithelium and other debris (omphalolith).

Movements of the abdominal wall Normally there is a gentle rise in the abdominal wall during inspiration and a fall during expiration; the movement should be free and equal on both sides. In generalized peritonitis this movement is absent or markedly diminished, which helps to limit further spread of infection within the peritoneal cavity and the pain of peritoneal irritation (the 'still, silent abdomen').

Visible pulsation of the abdominal aorta may be noticed in the epigastrium and is a frequent finding in nervous, thin patients. It must be distinguished from an aneurysm of the abdominal aorta, where pulsation is more obvious and a widened aorta is felt on palpation.

Visible peristalsis of the stomach or small intestine may be observed in three situations.

1. *Obstruction at the pylorus*. Visible peristalsis may occur where there is obstruction at the pylorus produced either by fibrosis following chronic duodenal ulceration or, less commonly, by carcinoma of the stomach in the pyloric antrum. Peristalsis will be seen as a slow wave either passing across the upper abdomen from left to right hypochondria or, if gross gastric dilatation is present, passing down to the suprapubic region and ascending to terminate in the right epigastrium. In pyloric obstruction, a diffuse swelling may be seen in

the left upper abdomen but, where obstruction is of long standing with severe gastric distension, this swelling may occupy the left mid and lower quadrants. Such a stomach may contain up to 2 litres of fluid and, on shaking the abdomen, a splashing noise is usually heard ('succussion splash'). This splash is frequently heard in healthy patients for up to three hours after a meal, so enquire when the patient last ate or drank. In congenital pyloric stenosis of infancy not only may visible peristalsis be apparent but the grossly hypertrophied circular muscle of the antrum and pylorus may be felt as a 'tumour' to the right of the midline in the epigastrium. Both these signs may be elicited more easily after the infant has been given a feed.

2. *Obstruction in the distal small bowel*. Peristalsis may be seen where there is intestinal obstruction in the distal small bowel, or coexisting large and small bowel hold-up produced by distal colonic obstruction, with an incompetent ileocaecal valve allowing reflux of gas and liquid faeces into the ileum. Not only is the abdomen distended and tympanitic (hyper-resonant) but the distended coils of small bowel may be visible in a thin patient and tend to stand out in the centre of the abdomen in a 'ladder pattern'.

3. *As a normal finding* in very thin, elderly patients with lax abdominal muscles or large wide-necked incisional herniae through an abdominal scar.

Skin and surface of the abdomen In marked distension the skin is smooth and shiny. *Striae atrophicae* or *gravidarum* are white or pink wrinkled linear marks on the abdominal skin. They are produced by gross stretching of the skin with rupture of the elastic fibres and indicate a recent change in size of the abdomen such as is found in pregnancy, ascites, wasting diseases, and severe

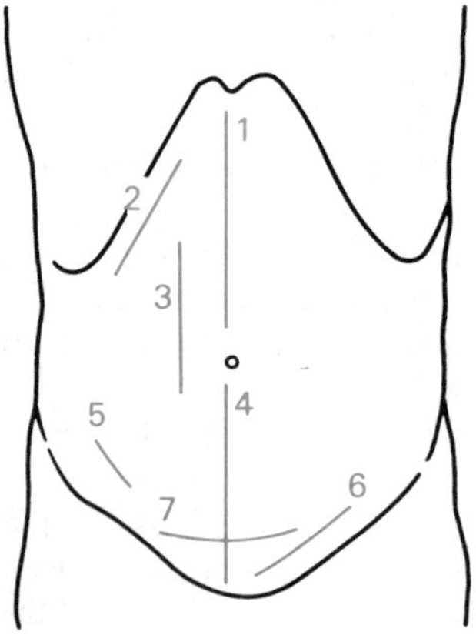

Fig. 5.3 Some commonly employed abdominal incisions. 1: Upper midline; 2: Right subcostal (Kocher's); 3: Right paramedian; 4: Lower midline; 5: Appendicectomy (Gridiron); 6: Left inguinal; 7: Suprapubic (Pfannenstiel).

dieting. Wide purple striae are characteristic of Cushing's syndrome and excessive steroid treatment.

Note any *scars* present, their site, whether they are old (white) or recent (red or pink), linear or stretched (and therefore likely to be weak and contain an incisional hernia). Common examples are given in Fig. 5.3.

Look for *prominent superficial veins*, which may be apparent in three situations (Fig. 5.4).

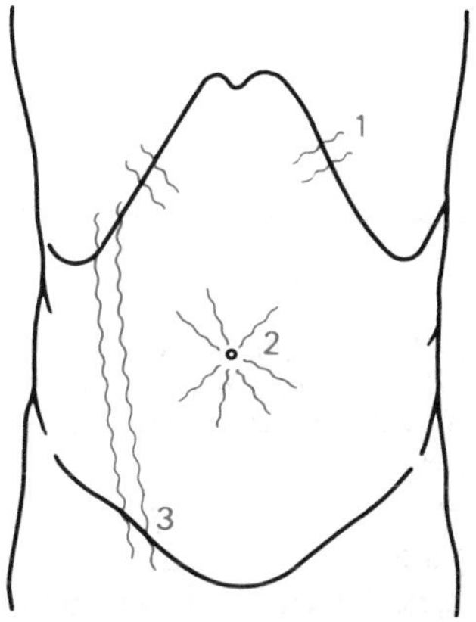

Fig. 5.4a Veins of the abdominal wall. 1: Thin veins over costal margin; 2: Caput medusae (see Fig. 5.4c); 3: Dilated veins in obstruction of inferior vena cava (see Fig. 5.4b).

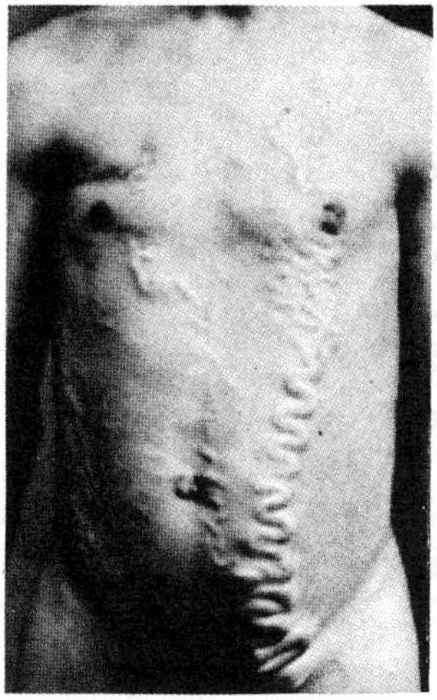

Fig. 5.4b Occlusion of inferior vena cava.

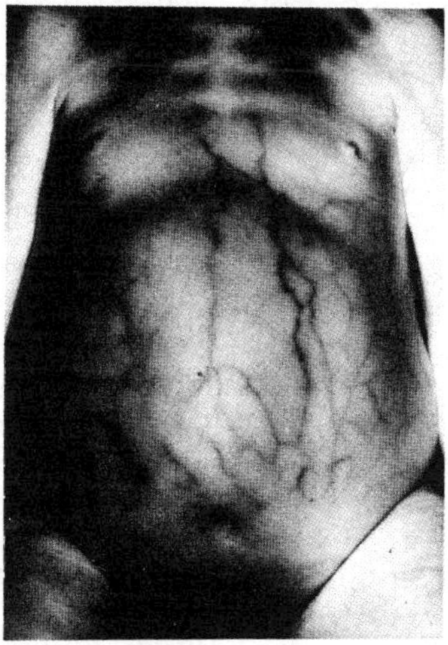

Fig. 5.4c Venous anastomosis in portal hypertension.

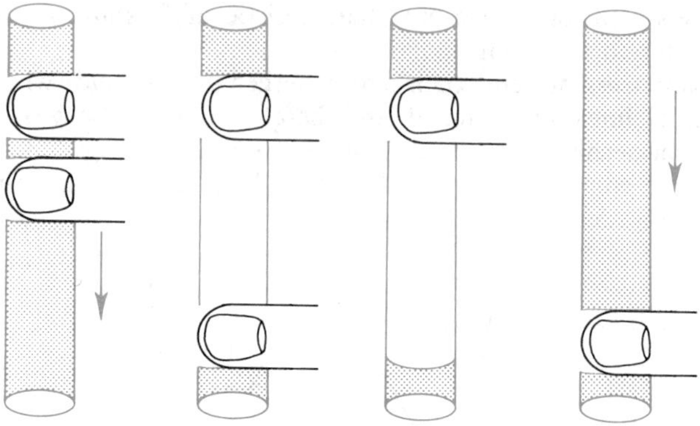

Fig. 5.5 A way of detecting the direction of blood flow in a vein. (a) Place 2 fingers side by side. (b) Move the lower finger away thus emptying part of the vein. (c) Remove the lower finger; in this example the vein remains empty. (d) Replace the lower finger and remove the upper finger; blood will be seen to run down from above.

Small, thin veins over the subcostal margins are common and usually of no significance. Distended veins around the umbilicus (caput medusae) are uncommon but, if present, signify portal hypertension, whose other signs include splenomegaly and ascites. Distended veins represent the opening up of anastomoses between portal and systemic veins and are seen in other sites, such as oesophageal varices and piles. In patients who have inferior vena caval obstruction, not only will there be oedema of the limbs, buttocks and groins, but in time distended veins on the abdominal wall and chest wall appear. These represent dilated anastomotic channels between the superficial epigastric and circumflex iliac veins below, and the lateral thoracic veins above, conveying the diverted blood from long saphenous vein to axillary vein; the direction of flow is therefore upwards. If the veins are prominent enough, try to detect the direction in which the blood is flowing (Fig. 5.5).

Pigmentation of the abdominal wall is seen in the midline below the umbilicus, where it forms the linea nigra and is a sign of pregnancy. Erythema ab igne is a brown mottled pigmentation produced by constant application of heat, usually a hot water bottle or heat pad, on the skin of the abdominal wall. It is a sign that the patient is experiencing severe pain.

Finally, inspect both groins, and the penis and scrotum in a male, for any swelling and to ensure that both testes are in their normal position. Then bring the sheet up just to cover the symphysis.

Palpation

Palpation forms the most important part of the abdominal examination. Tell the patient to relax as best he can, to breathe quietly and that you will be as gentle as possible. Enquire for the site of any pain and come to this region last. These points, together with unhurried palpation with a warm hand, will give the patient confidence and enable one to gain the maximum amount of information. It is helpful to have a logical sequence to follow and if this is done as a matter of routine then no important point will be omitted. The scheme below is suggested:

1 Start in the left iliac region palpating lightly and work anti-clockwise to end in the suprapubic region, repeat this using deeper palpation and with both hands if necessary

2 Next feel for left kidney

3 Feel for spleen

4 Feel for right kidney

5 Feel for liver

6 Feel for urinary bladder

7 Feel for aorta and para-aortic glands and common femoral vessels

8 If a swelling is palpable, spend time eliciting its features

9 Palpate both groins

10 Examine the external genitalia

Start by placing the right hand flat on the abdomen in the left iliac fossa with the wrist and forearm in the same horizontal plane where possible, even if this means the examiner is bending down or kneeling by the patient's side (Fig. 5.6).

The art is to 'mould' the relaxed right hand to the abdominal wall, not to hold it rigid. The best movement is gentle but with firm pressure with the fingers held almost straight with slight flexion at the metacarpophalangeal joints.

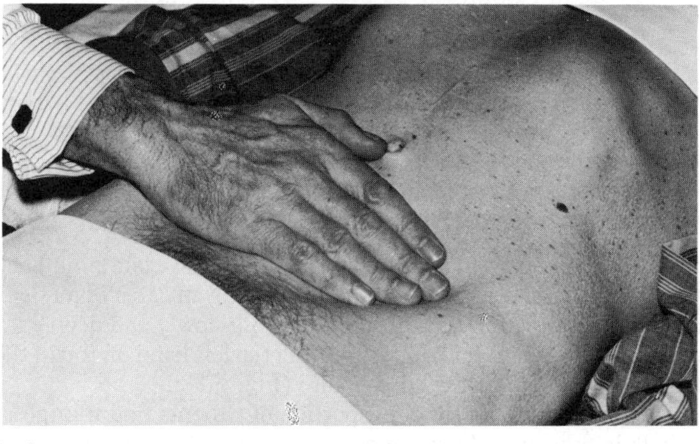

Fig. 5.6 Correct method of palpation. The hand is held flat and relaxed and 'moulded' to the abdominal wall.

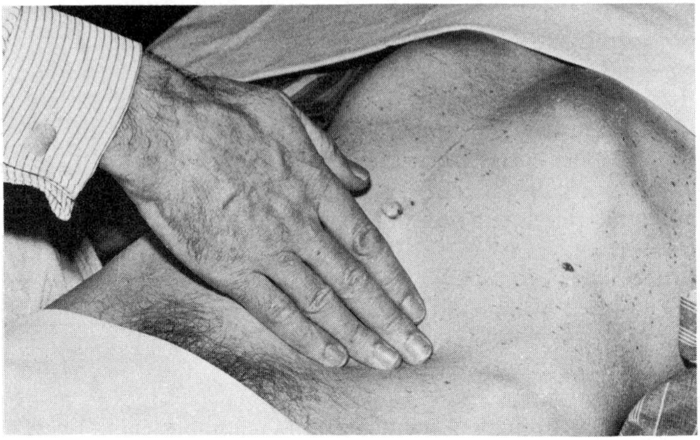

Fig. 5.7 Incorrect method of palpation. The hand is held rigid and mostly not in contact with the abdominal wall.

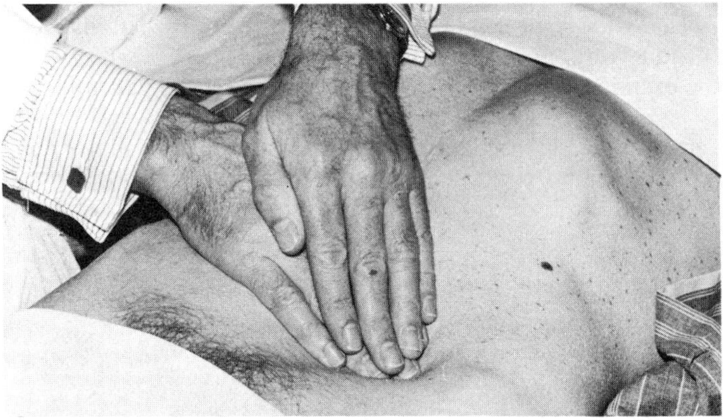

Fig. 5.8 Method of deep palpation in an obese, muscular or poorly relaxed patient.

At all costs avoid sudden poking with the fingertips (Fig. 5.7). Try and visualize the normal anatomical structures beneath the examining hand, and gently palpate each quadrant of the abdomen noting any area of tenderness or localized rigidity. Palpation is then repeated more slowly and deeply if necessary; in a fat or very muscular patient, putting the left hand on top of the right will enable you to exert increased pressure (Fig. 5.8).

There is no doubt that a small proportion of patients find it impossible to relax their abdominal muscles when being examined. In such cases it may help to ask them to breathe deeply, to bend their knees up or to distract their attention in other ways. No matter how experienced the examiner, he will gain little from palpation of a poorly relaxed abdomen.

Left kidney

The right hand is placed anteriorly in the left lumbar region whilst the left hand is placed posteriorly in the left loin (Fig. 5.9).

Ask the patient to take a deep breath in, press the left hand forwards, and the right hand backwards, upwards and inwards. The left kidney is not usually palpable unless either low in position or enlarged. Its lower pole, when palpable, is felt as a rounded firm swelling between both right and left hands (i.e. bimanually palpable) and it can be pushed from one hand to the other.

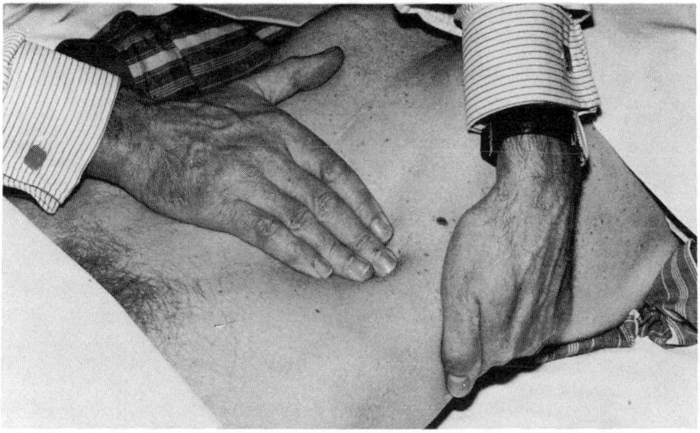

Fig. 5.9 Palpation of the left kidney.

Spleen

Like the left kidney the spleen is not normally palpable. It has to be enlarged to two or three times its usual size before it becomes so and then is felt beneath the left subcostal margin. It is not sufficiently appreciated that enlargement takes place in a superior and posterior direction before it becomes palpable subcostally. Once the spleen has appeared in this situation, the direction of further enlargement is downwards and towards the right iliac fossa (Fig. 5.10). Place the flat of the left hand over the lowermost rib cage posterolaterally, and the right hand beneath the costal margin way out to the left. Ask the patient to breathe in deeply, press in deeply with the fingers of the right hand beneath the costal margin, at the same time exerting considerable pressure medially and downwards with the left hand (Fig. 5.11). Repeat this manoeuvre with the

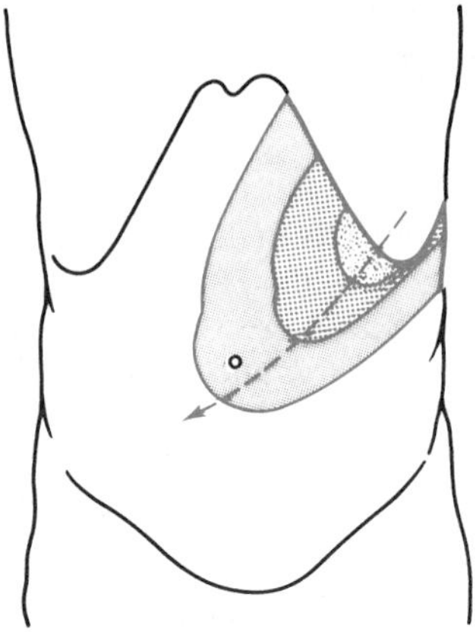

Fig. 5.10 The direction of enlargement of the spleen.

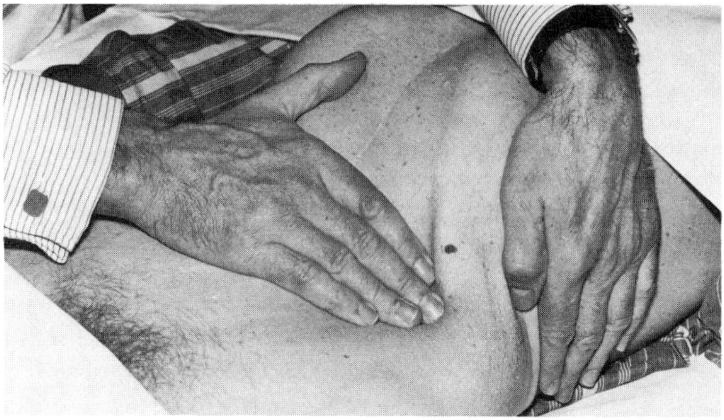

Fig. 5.11 Palpation of the spleen. Start well out to the left.

right hand being moved more medially beneath the costal margin on each occasion (Fig. 5.12). If enlargement of the spleen is suspected from the history and it is still not palpable, turn the patient half onto his right side and repeat the examination as above.

In minor degrees of enlargement, the spleen will be felt as a firm swelling with smooth rounded borders. Where considerable splenomegaly is present, its typical characteristics include a firm swelling appearing beneath the left subcostal margin in the left upper quadrant of the abdomen, which is dull to percussion, moves downwards on inspiration, is not bimanually palpable, whose upper border cannot be felt (i.e. one cannot 'get above it'), and in which a notch can often, though not invariably, be felt in the lower medial border.

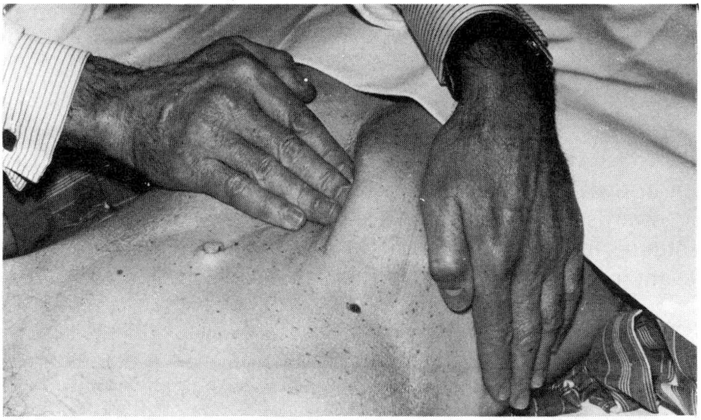

Fig. 5.12 Palpation of the spleen more medially than in Fig. 5.11.

The last three features distinguish the enlarged spleen from an enlarged left kidney; in addition there is usually a band of colonic resonance anterior to an enlarged kidney.

Right kidney

Feel for the right kidney in much the same way as for the left. Place the right hand horizontally in the right lumbar region anteriorly with the left hand placed posteriorly in the right loin. Push forwards with the left hand, ask the patient to take a deep breath in and press the right hand inwards and upwards (Fig. 5.13).

The lower pole of the right kidney, unlike the left, is commonly palpable in

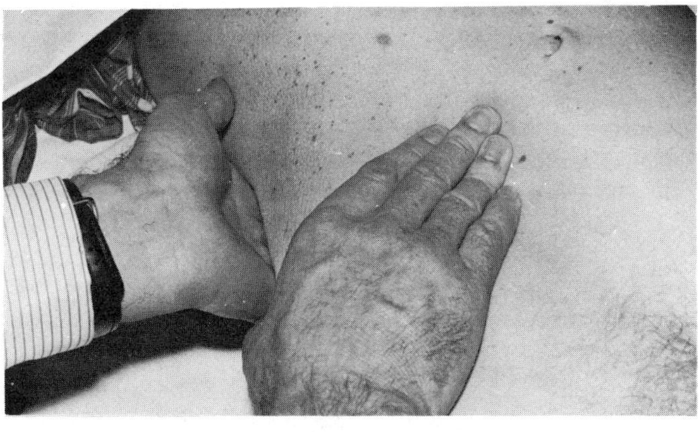

Fig. 5.13 Palpation of the right kidney.

thin patients and is felt as a smooth rounded swelling which descends on inspiration and is bimanually palpable.

Liver

Sit on the couch beside the patient. Place both hands side by side flat on the abdomen in the right subcostal region lateral to the rectus with the fingers pointing towards the ribs. If resistance is encountered move the hands further down until this resistance disappears. Ask the patient to breathe in deeply and at the height of inspiration press the fingers firmly inwards and upwards (Fig. 5.14).

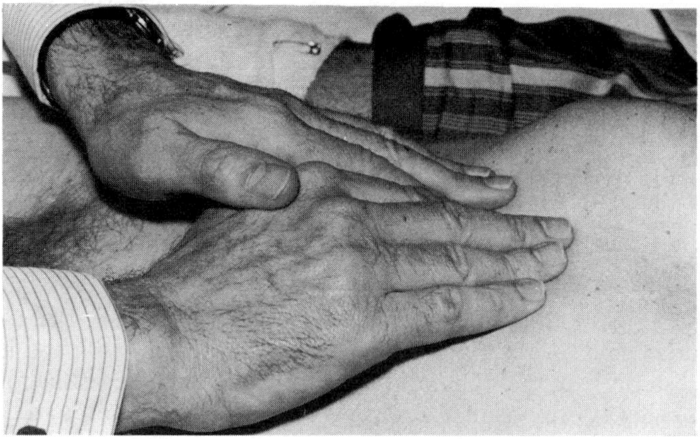

Fig. 5.14 Palpation of the liver: preferred method.

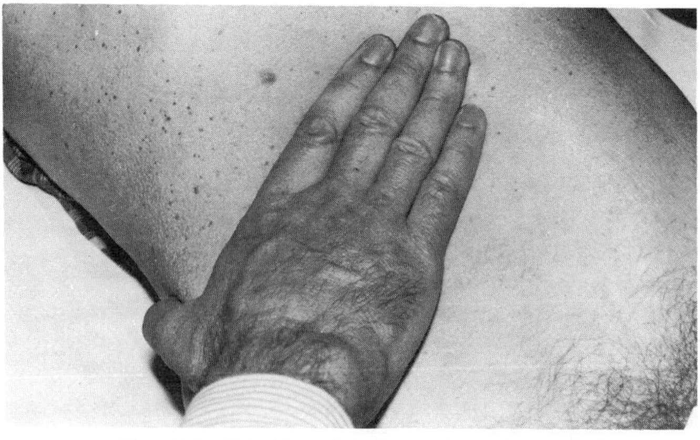

Fig. 5.15 Palpation of the liver: alternative method.

If the liver is palpable it will be felt as a sharp regular border which rides beneath the fingers. Repeat this manoeuvre working from lateral to medial regions to trace the liver edge as it passes upwards to cross from right hypochondrium to epigastrium. Another commonly employed, though less accurate, method of feeling for an enlarged liver is to place the right hand below and parallel to the right subcostal margin. The liver edge will then be felt against the radial border of the index finger (Fig. 5.15). The liver is often palpable in normal patients without being enlarged, whilst in patients with emphysema it is frequently felt. Considerable hepatomegaly is spoken of as being so many centimetres palpable below the right costal margin. Try and make out the character of its surface, i.e. whether it is soft, smooth and tender as in heart failure, very firm and regular as in obstructive jaundice and cirrhosis, or hard, irregular, painless and sometimes nodular as in advanced secondary carcinoma. In tricuspid regurgitation the liver may be felt to pulsate. Occasionally a congenital variant of the right lobe projects down lateral to the gallbladder as a tongue-shaped process, called Riedel's lobe. Though rare, it is important to be aware of this because it may be mistaken either for the gallbladder itself or the right kidney.

Gallbladder

The gallbladder is palpated in the same way as the liver. The normal gallbladder cannot be felt. When it is distended, however, it forms an important sign, and may be palpated as a firm, smooth, round or globular swelling with distinct borders, just lateral to the edge of the rectus abdominis near the tip of the 9th costal cartilage. It moves with respiration. Its upper border merges with the lower border of the right lobe of the liver, or disappears beneath the costal margin and therefore can never be felt (Fig. 5.16). When the liver is enlarged or the gallbladder grossly distended, the latter may be felt not in the hypochondrium, but in the right lumbar or even as low down as the right iliac region.

The ease of definition of the rounded borders of the gallbladder, its comparative mobility on respiration, the fact that it is not normally bimanually palpable and that it seems to lie just beneath the abdominal wall help to identify such a swelling as gallbladder rather than a palpable right kidney. This distinction may prove difficult, however, especially when the gallbladder lies in the mid or lower quadrants.

The gallbladder can usually be palpated in the following clinical situations. In *all* the swelling is painless.

1. In carcinoma of the head of the pancreas and other causes of malignant obstruction of the common bile duct, the ducts above become dilated as does the gallbladder. The patient is also deeply jaundiced.

2. In mucocele of the gallbladder, a gallstone becomes impacted in the neck of a collapsed empty uninfected gallbladder and mucus continues to be secreted

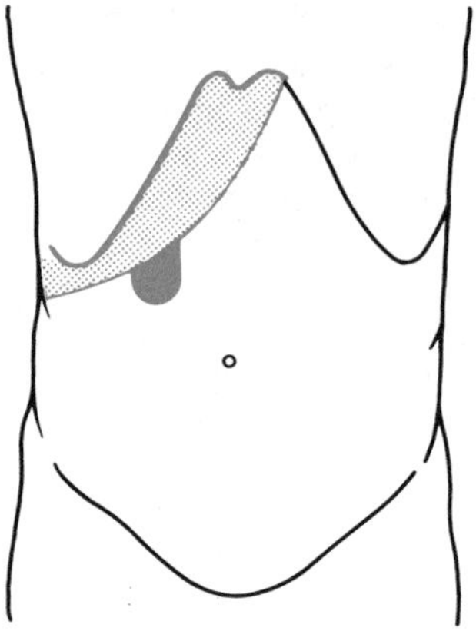

Fig. 5.16 Palpation of an enlarged gallbladder, showing how it merges with the inferior border of the liver so that only the fundus and part of the body can be palpated.

into its lumen. Finally the uninfected wall is so distended that it becomes palpable. In this case the bile ducts are normal and the patient is not jaundiced.

3. In carcinoma of the gallbladder, the gallbladder will be felt as a stony hard irregular swelling, whereas in 1 and 2 it is firm and regular.

Murphy's sign In acute inflammation of the gallbladder (acute cholecystitis) severe pain is present. Often an exquisitely tender but indefinite mass can be palpated which represents the underlying acutely inflamed gallbladder walled off by greater omentum. Ask the patient to breathe in deeply, and palpate for the gallbladder in the normal way; at the height of inspiration the breath is arrested with a gasp as the mass is felt. This represents Murphy's sign. The sign is *not* found in chronic cholecystitis or uncomplicated cases of gallstones.

The urinary bladder

Normally the urinary bladder is not palpable. When it is full and the patient cannot empty his bladder (retention of urine), a smooth firm regular oval-shaped swelling will be palpated in the suprapubic region and its dome (upper border) may reach as far as the umbilicus. The lateral and upper borders can be readily made out, but it is not possible to feel its lower border, i.e. the swelling is 'arising out of the pelvis'. The fact that this swelling is symmetrically placed in the suprapubic region beneath the umbilicus, that it is dull to percussion, and that pressure on it gives the patient a desire to micturate, together with the signs above, confirm such a swelling as the bladder (Fig. 5.17).

In women, however, the palpable bladder has to be differentiated from a gravid uterus (firmer, mobile side to side and vaginal signs different), a fibroid

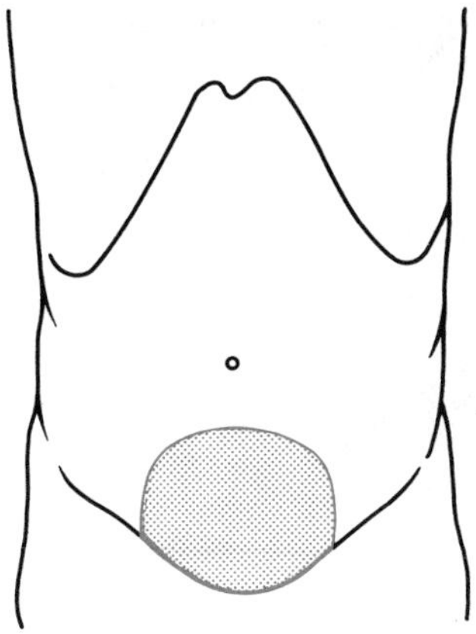

Fig. 5.17 Physical signs in retention of urine: smooth firm regular swelling arising out of the pelvis which one cannot 'get below' and which is dull to percussion.

uterus (may be bosselated, firmer and vaginal signs different) and an ovarian cyst (usually eccentrically placed to left or right side).

The aorta and common femoral vessels

The aorta is not readily felt but with practice it can usually be palpated a little above and to the left of the umbilicus; however, palpation has to be deep, so warn the patient of this. Palpation of the aorta is one of the few times that the fingertips are allowed as a means of palpation. Press the extended fingers of both hands, held side by side, deeply into the abdominal wall in the position shown in Fig. 5.18; make out the left wall of the aorta and note its pulsation. Remove both hands and repeat the manoeuvre an inch or so over to the right. In this way the pulsation and width of the aorta can be estimated. It is difficult to detect small aortic aneurysms; where a large one is present, its width may be assessed by placing a finger on either side of it and its expansile character noted by the fact that when pulsation occurs the width between each finger increases.

The common femoral vessels are found just below the inguinal ligament at the midpoint between the anterior superior iliac spine and symphysis pubis. Place the pulps of the right index, middle and ring fingers over this site in the right groin and palpate the wall of the vessel. Note the strength and character of its pulsation and then compare it with the opposite femoral pulse (Fig. 5.19).

Nodes lying along the aorta (para-aortic) are palpable only when considerably enlarged. They are felt as rounded, firm, often confluent, fixed masses in the umbilical region and epigastrium along the left border of the aorta.

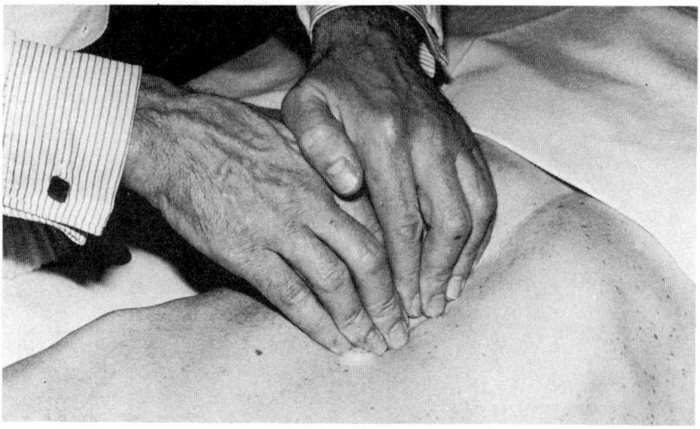

Fig. 5.18 Palpation of the abdominal aorta.

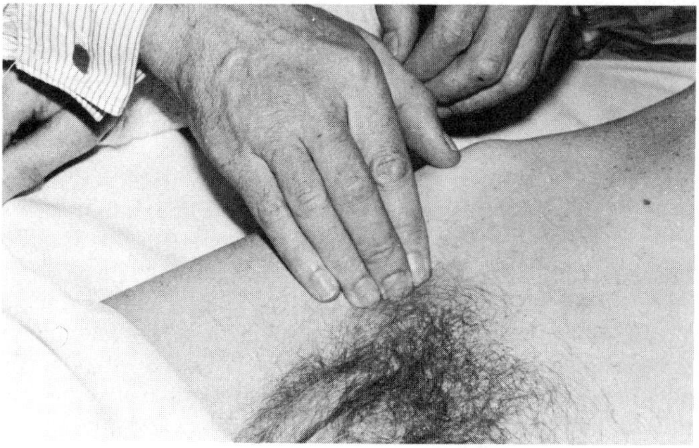

Fig. 5.19 Palpation of the right common femoral artery.

Causes of confusion on palpation

In many patients, especially those with a thin or lax abdominal wall, faeces in the colon may simulate an abdominal mass. The pelvic colon is frequently palpable, particularly when loaded with hard faeces. It is felt as a firm tubular structure some 12 cm in length situated low down in the left iliac fossa, parallel to the inguinal ligament. The caecum is often palpable in the right iliac fossa as a soft, rounded swelling with indistinct borders. The transverse colon is sometimes palpable in the epigastrium. It feels somewhat like the pelvic colon but rather larger and softer, with distinct upper and lower borders and a convex anterior surface.

In the epigastrium, the muscular bellies of rectus abdominis lying between its tendinous intersections can mimic an underlying mass and give rise to confusion. This can usually be resolved by asking the patient to tense the abdominal wall, when the 'mass' may be felt to contract.

What to do when an abdominal mass is palpable

When a swelling in the abdomen is palpable make sure first that it is not a *normal* structure, as described above. Next consider whether it could be due to enlargement of the liver, spleen, right or left kidney, gallbladder, urinary bladder, aorta or para-aortic nodes.

Now palpate the swelling again. The aim of examination is to decide the organ of origin and the pathological nature of the mass. In doing this it is helpful to bear in mind the following points:

Site First make sure that the swelling does indeed lie in the abdominal cavity and not in the anterior abdominal wall. Ask the patient to lift his head and shoulders off the pillow and press firmly against the forehead. Now feel the swelling again. If it disappears or becomes much less obvious then it lies within the peritoneal cavity, whereas if it remains the same size it must be within the layers of the abdominal wall.

Note the region which the swelling occupies. Think of the organs that normally lie in or near this region and consider whether the swelling could arise from one of these organs. For instance, a swelling in the right upper quadrant most probably arises from the liver, right kidney, hepatic flexure of colon, or gallbladder.

Now, if the swelling is in the upper abdomen, try and determine if it is possible to 'get above it' and, similarly, if it is in the lower abdomen, whether one can 'get below it'. By this is meant that one cannot feel the upper, or lower, border of the swelling as it disappears above the costal margin or into the pelvis respectively. If one cannot 'get above' an upper abdominal swelling, a hepatic, splenic, renal or gastric origin should be suspected. If one cannot 'get below' a lower abdominal mass the swelling probably arises in the bladder, uterus, ovary or occasionally upper rectum.

Size and shape As a general rule, gross enlargement of the liver, spleen, uterus, bladder or ovary presents no undue difficulty in diagnosis. On the other hand swellings arising from the stomach, small or large bowel, retroperitoneal structures such as pancreas, or the peritoneum (see under mobility), may be difficult to diagnose. The larger a swelling arising from one of these structures, the more it tends to distort the outline of the organ of origin. For example, the characteristic reniform outline of the kidney is retained early on, but when there is a large renal mass this outline is lost and recognition becomes difficult.

Surface, edge and consistency The pathological nature of a mass is suggested by a number of features. A swelling that is hard, irregular in outline and nodular is likely to be malignant, whilst a regular, round, smooth, tense swelling is likely to be cystic and benign, but remember degeneration and softening with cyst formation occurs in malignant tumours not infrequently. A solid, ill-defined and tender mass suggests an inflammatory lesion as in Crohn's disease of the ileocaecal region.

Mobility and attachments Considerable information can be gained from eliciting the mobility or fixity of an abdominal mass. Swellings arising in the liver, spleen, kidneys, gallbladder and distal stomach all show downward movement during inspiration, due to contraction of the diaphragm. One cannot, however, move such structures with the examining hand. In contrast, swellings originating in structures that have a mesenteric or other broad base of attachment are uninfluenced by respiratory movements but *can* be made to move freely by palpation, e.g. tumours of the small bowel and transverse colon, cysts in the mesentery, and large secondary deposits in the greater omentum.

When, on the other hand, the swelling is completely fixed it signifies usually one of three things: a mass of retroperitoneal origin, e.g. pancreas; part of an advanced tumour with extensive spread to the anterior or posterior abdominal walls or abdominal organs; or a swelling resulting from severe chronic inflammation involving other organs, e.g. diverticulitis of the sigmoid colon or a colovesical attachment or fistula.

In the lower abdomen, the side to side mobility of a fibroid or pregnant uterus rapidly establishes such a swelling as uterine in origin and as not arising from bladder or ovary.

Is it bimanually palpable or pulsatile? Bimanually palpable swellings in the lumbar region are usually renal in origin. Just occasionally, however, a posteriorly situated gallbladder or a mass in the postero-inferior part of the right lobe of the liver may give the impression of being bimanually palpable.

Finally, try to decide whether a swelling exhibits *pulsation*. It is often difficult to be certain whether a swelling in the upper abdomen that is pulsatile is merely transmitting pulsation from the underlying aorta or whether it is truly expansile in nature. The best way to determine this is to place two fingers on the swelling and observe what happens to them in systole. If the fingers remain parallel, then the pulsation is transmitted. If, however, the fingers tend to separate, then true expansile pulsation is present and the swelling is an aneurysm.

Percussion

Details of how to percuss correctly are given on page 179. In the abdomen only light percussion is necessary—a resonant (tympanitic) note is heard throughout except over the liver, where the note is dull. Whilst this technique is of limited value it can nevertheless provide important information.

Defining the boundaries of abdominal organs and masses

Liver The upper and lower borders of the right lobe of the liver can be mapped out accurately by percussion. Start anteriorly, at the 4th intercostal space, where the note will be resonant over the lungs, and work vertically downwards. In the normal liver the upper border is found at about the 5th intercostal space, where the note will become dull; this dullness extends down to the lower border found at or just below the right subcostal margin. The normal dullness over the upper part of the liver is reduced in severe emphysema, in the presence of a large right pneumothorax and when there is gas or air in the peritoneal cavity. The latter, occurring in a patient with severe abdominal pain, indicates perforation of a viscus (unless the patient has recently undergone laparotomy). This sign, however, is not one that should be relied on as there has to be a large volume of air or gas present to reduce the normal liver dullness, and this is not usually the case.

Spleen Percussion over an enlarged spleen provides rapid confirmation of the findings detected on palpation (p. 91 and Fig. 5.11). Dullness extends from the left lower ribs into the left hypochondrium and left lumbar region. The lower border of an enlarged spleen is readily mapped out; splenic dullness gives way to the resonance of surrounding bowel.

Bladder The findings in a patient with retention of urine are usually unmistakable on palpation alone (p. 91 and Fig. 5.17). The dullness on percussion provides reassurance that the swelling is cystic or solid and not gaseous; its superior and lateral borders can be readily defined from adjacent bowel, which is resonant.

Other masses The boundaries of any localized swelling in the abdominal cavity, or in the walls of the abdomen, can sometimes be defined more accurately by percussion than palpation. The dullness of a solid or cystic mass contrasts with the tympanitic note of surrounding loops of bowel.

Detection of ascites and its differentiation from ovarian cyst and intestinal obstruction

Three common causes of diffuse enlargement of the abdomen are:

1 The presence of free fluid in the peritoneum (ascites)
2 A massive ovarian cyst
3 Obstruction of the large bowel, distal small bowel, or both

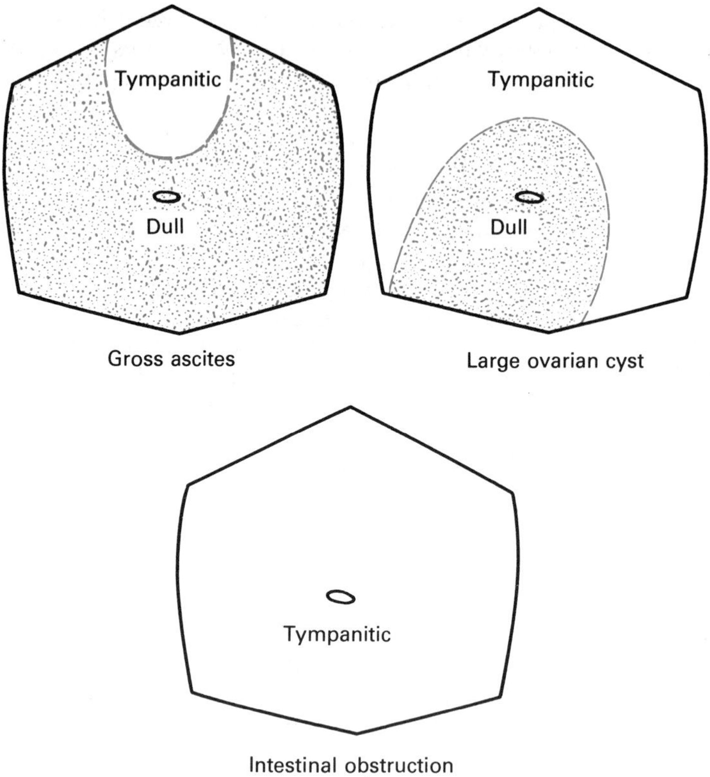

Fig. 5.20 Diffuse enlargement of the abdomen.
Gross ascites: dull in flanks; umbilicus is transverse and/or hernia present; shifting dullness positive; fluid thrill positive.
Large ovarian cysts: resonant in flanks; umbilicus is vertical and drawn up; large swelling felt arising out of pelvis which one cannot 'get below'.
Intestinal obstruction: resonant throughout; colicky pain, vomiting; constipation; increased and/or 'noisy' bowel sounds.

Percussion rapidly distinguishes between these three as can be seen in Fig. 5.20. Other helpful symptoms or signs that are usually present are also listed below.

It is unwise and difficult to diagnose *ascites* unless there is sufficient free fluid present to give generalized enlargement of the abdomen. Two signs, shifting dullness and a fluid thrill, present either singly or together, make the diagnosis of ascites certain. Useful as these two signs are, they can be elicited in only about half the cases of ascites. Absence of shifting dullness or of fluid thrill or both does *not* exclude a diagnosis of ascites.

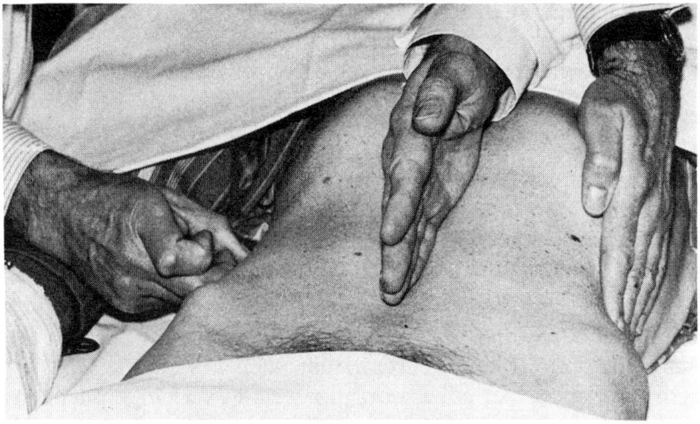

Fig. 5.21 Eliciting a fluid thrill.

To demonstrate *shifting dullness*, lie the patient supine and, on percussion, note dullness in the flanks and lower abdomen with a central area of resonance at and above the umbilicus. Now turn the patient on his right side. Allow time for the intestines to float upwards and the free fluid to gravitate down and percuss again. Note that whereas before the left flank was dull it is now resonant and that the height of the dullness on the lower side has risen. Now repeat this, turning the patient onto his left side.

To elicit a *fluid thrill* the patient is again laid on his back. Place one hand flat over the lumbar region of one side, get an assistant to put the side of his hand firmly in the midline of the abdomen, and then flick or tap the opposite lumbar region (Fig. 5.21). A fluid thrill or wave is felt as a definite and unmistakable impulse by the watching hand held flat in the lumbar region. The purpose of the assistant's hand is to dampen any impulse that may be transmitted through the fat of the abdominal wall. As a rule a fluid thrill is felt only when there is a large amount of ascites present which is under tension.

Auscultation

Auscultation is a useful way of listening for bowel sounds and deciding whether they are normal, increased or absent, and of detecting bruits in the aorta and main abdominal vessels.

The stethoscope should be placed on one site on the abdominal wall (just to the right of the umbilicus is best) and kept there until bowel sounds are heard. It should not be moved around from site to site. Normal bowel sounds are heard as intermittent low or medium pitched gurgles interspersed with an occasional high pitched noise or tinkle.

In *simple acute mechanical obstruction of the small bowel* the bowel sounds are excessive and exaggerated. Frequent loud low pitched gurgles (borborygmi) are heard, often rising to a crescendo of high pitched tinkles and occurring in a rhythmic pattern with peristaltic activity. The presence of such sounds occurring at the same time as the patient experiences bouts of colicky abdominal pain is pathognomonic of small bowel obstruction. In between the bouts of peristaltic activity and colicky pain, the bowel is quiet and no sounds are heard on auscultation.

In an obstructed loop of bowel, when strangulation and later gangrene supervene, however, peristalsis ceases, and the bowel sounds rapidly become less frequent and stop altogether. In *generalized peritonitis* bowel activity rapidly disappears and a state of *paralytic ileus* ensues, with gradually increasing abdominal distension. The abdomen is 'silent' but one must listen for several minutes before being certain that such a state exists. Frequently towards the end of this period, a short run of faint, very high pitched tinkling sounds is heard. This represents fluid spilling over from one distended gas- and fluid-filled loop to another and is characteristic of ileus.

A *succussion splash* may be elicited by palpation (p. 86) but also on auscultation. It may be heard in pyloric stenosis, advanced intestinal obstruction with grossly distended loops of bowel and in paralytic ileus. Place the stethoscope on the abdomen and with the free hand quickly depress the abdominal wall. A splashing noise is heard.

Bruits may also be heard in the abdomen. Press the bell of the stethoscope deeply into the abdominal wall over the abdominal aorta above and to the left of the umbilicus and listen for a bruit. Do likewise over each iliac artery in the corresponding iliac fossa, and over the common femoral arteries in each groin. If a bruit is heard it is a significant finding which indicates stenosis in the underlying vessel. Very occasionally bruits may be heard in the epigastrium when there is stenosis of the coeliac axis or superior mesenteric artery, or on either side of the midline in the mid-abdomen in patients with hypertension due to stenosis of the renal artery (see Chapter 15).

THE GROINS

Once the groins have been inspected (p. 84), ask the patient to turn his head to one side and cough. Look at both inguinal canals for any expansile impulse. If none is apparent, place the left hand in the left groin so that the fingers lie over and in line with the inguinal canal; place the right hand similarly in the right groin (Fig. 5.22). Now ask the patient to give a loud cough and feel for any expansile impulse with each hand. When a patient coughs, the muscles of the abdominal wall contract violently and this imparts a definite, though not expansile, impulse to the palpating hands which is a source of confusion to the inexperienced. Trying to differentiate this normal contraction from a small, fully reducible inguinal hernia is difficult, and the matter can usually be

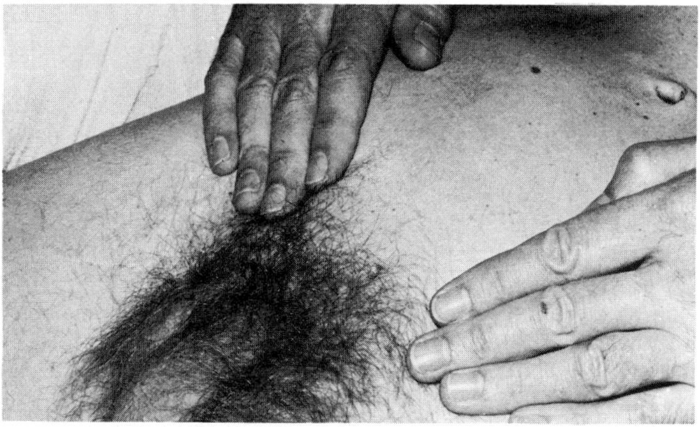

Fig. 5.22 Palpating the groins to detect an expansile impulse on coughing.

resolved only when the patient is standing up.

The femoral vessels have already been felt (p. 97 and Fig. 5.19) and auscultated (p. 104). Now palpate along the femoral artery for enlarged inguinal nodes, feeling with the fingers of the right hand, and carry this palpation medially beneath the inguinal ligament towards the perineum. Then repeat this on the left side. If the patient complains of a lump in the groin he should be examined lying down *and standing up*.

THE MALE GENITALIA

It is not always possible to avoid causing some discomfort, particularly in very sensitive patients, so always warn the patient what is about to happen. Tell him that the examination will be as gentle as possible and aim to make it so. Make sure the patient is warm; palpation is much more difficult, and therefore more likely to hurt, when the patient is cold.

Ask the patient to separate his legs slightly, which allows one to deliver the scrotum to an accessible position.

If there is any suspicion of venereal infection put on disposable gloves.

Inspection

Note the distribution of pubic hair, the appearance and size of the penis, the presence or absence of a prepuce, and the site of the external urethral orifice. Look at the scrotal skin for any redness, swelling, oedema or ulceration. If any swelling is present, observe whether it appears to extend into the groin, and note whether both testes are in the scrotum. Lift up the scrotum to inspect its posterior surface.

Palpation

The penis

Lift up the penis and palpate the corpora cavernosa, feeling for any induration, and the urethra, lying on the ventral aspect of the penis, from the glans to the perineum. If the patient is uncircumcised establish that the prepuce can be readily retracted by gently withdrawing it over the glans penis. This allows inspection of the inner lining of the prepuce, the glans penis, the coronal sulcus and the external urethral orifice (meatus). Always remember to draw the prepuce forwards, otherwise *paraphimosis*, painful oedema of the glans due to constriction by a retracted prepuce, may ensue. The internal male genitalia (prostate and seminal vesicles) are examined per rectum (p. 111).

Abrasions or small superficial sores on the outer surface of the prepuce or penile shaft are commonly due to trauma following intercourse. A *primary syphilitic chancre* is usually found on the inner aspect of the prepuce adjacent to or in the coronal sulcus. It commences as a small red papule which gradually hardens and erodes in the centre; a painless ulcer forms and typically the margins and base feel densely indurated. Retraction of the foreskin may reveal a *carcinoma*, which presents the characteristic features of a malignant ulcer with raised everted edges and an indurated base. It is almost unknown in those circumcised before puberty.

Phimosis is narrowing of the preputial orifice so preventing retraction of the foreskin. This commonly results in recurrent episodes of infection of the glans penis (balanitis) and of the prepuce (posthitis), which are termed *balanoposthitis*. *Hypospadias* is a congenital anomaly where the external urethral orifice opens not at the tip of the glans penis but on its ventral surface in the midline, anywhere from the glans to the shaft or even in the perineum. It is much more common than a similar opening situated on the dorsal surface of the penis, called *epispadias*.

In the skin of the scrotum, *sebaceous cysts* are common and often multiple, presenting as round, firm, whitish nodules. *Malignant ulcers* (epitheliomata) are still occasionally seen in those workers who constantly wear heavily oil-stained clothes. Ulceration can also occur as a result of fungation from an underlying tumour of the testis or from a gumma. Sinuses on the scrotal skin are uncommon now in the UK, but may occur as a result of tuberculous epididymo-orchitis in its advanced stages.

The testes

Now place the right hand below the scrotum and palpate the two testes. Arrange the hands and fingers as shown in Fig. 5.23; this 'fixes' the testis so that it cannot slip away from the examining fingers. The posterior aspect of the testis is supported by the middle, ring and little fingers of each hand, the right hand being inferior. This leaves the index fingers and thumb of each hand free

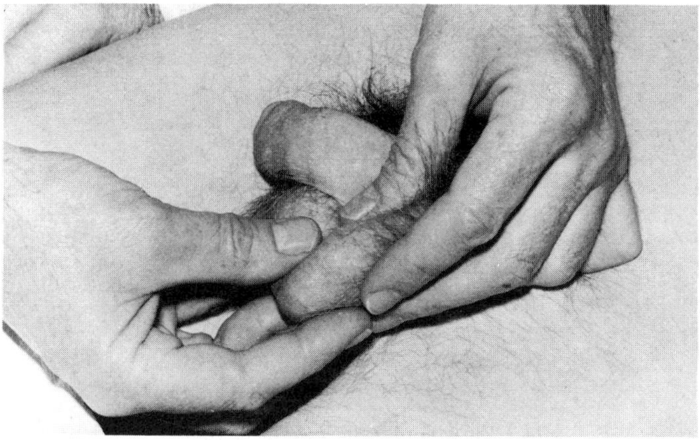

Fig. 5.23 Palpation of the left testis.

to palpate. Gently move the index finger and thumb over the anterior surface of the body of the testis, feel the lateral border with the index finger and the medial border with the pulp of each thumb. Note the size and consistency of the testis and any nodules or other irregularities. Now very gently approximate the fingers and thumb of the left hand (the effect of this is to move the testis inferiorly which is easily and painlessly done because of its great mobility inside the tunica vaginalis). In this way the upper pole of the testis can be readily felt between the approximated index finger and thumb of the left hand. Next move the testis upwards by reversing the movements of the hands and gently approximating the index finger and thumb of the right hand, so enabling the lower pole to be palpated.

The epididymis

Now palpate the epididymis. The head is found at the upper pole of the testis on its posterior aspect and is felt between the left thumb anteriorly and the index and middle fingers posteriorly. The epididymis is a soft nodular structure about 1 cm in length. The tail lies on the posterolateral aspect of the inferior pole of the testis and is felt between the thumb and fingers of the right hand. The tail too is soft but, unlike the head, its coiled tubular structure can usually be made out.

The spermatic cord

Finally palpate the spermatic cord (Fig. 5.24) with the left hand. Exert very gentle downward traction on the testis, place the fingers of the right hand behind the neck of the scrotum, and with the thumb placed anteriorly press

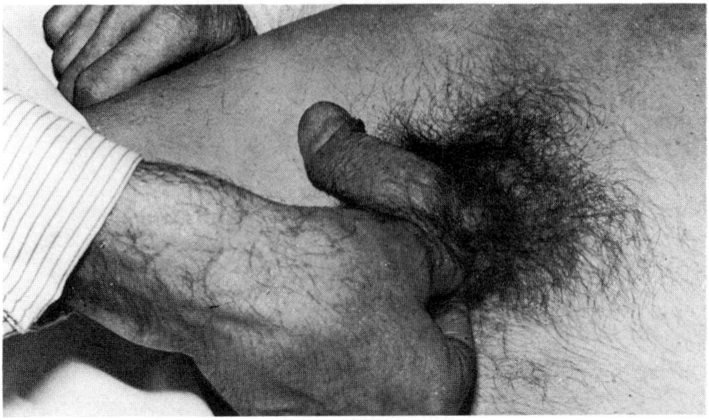

Fig. 5.24 Palpation of the left spermatic cord.

forward with the fingers of the right hand. The spermatic cord will be felt between the fingers and thumb; it is about 1 cm in width. The only structure that can be positively identified within it is the vas deferens, which feels like a thick piece of string. Having examined the testis, epididymis and cord on one side repeat the examination on the other side.

A *lump in the groin or scrotum* is a common clinical problem in all age groups. Most lumps in the groin are due either to herniae or enlarged inguinal nodes; inguinal herniae are considerably more common than femoral with an incidence ratio of 4:1. In the scrotum, hydrocele of the tunica vaginalis or a cyst of the epididymis are common causes of painless swelling; acute epididymo-orchitis is the most frequent cause of a painful swelling.

Examination of the groins and scrotum is only part of a general examination and must not be conducted in isolation. Generalized diseases such as lymphoma may present as a lump in the groin.

Usually the diagnosis of a lump in the groin or scrotum can be made simply and accurately. Remember that the patient should be examined not only lying down, but also standing up.

What to do if a patient complains of a lump in the groin

Ask the patient to stand in front of you, get him to point to the side and site of the swelling and note whether it extends into the scrotum. Get him to turn his head to one side and give a loud cough; look for an expansile impulse and try to decide whether it is above or below the crease of the inguinal ligament. If an expansile impulse is present on inspection, it is likely to be a hernia, so move to whichever side of the patient the lump in the groin is on. Stand beside and slightly behind the patient. If the right groin is being examined place the left hand over the right buttock to support the patient, the fingers of the right hand

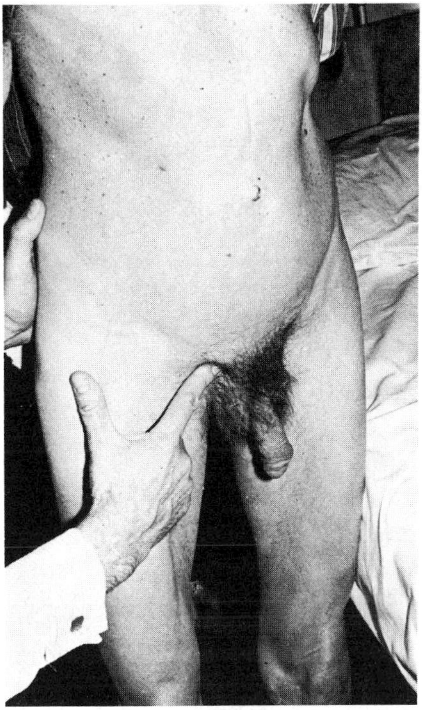

Fig. 5.25 Locating the pubic tubercle. *Note* the position of the examiner, at the side of the patient, with one hand supporting the buttock.

being placed obliquely over the inguinal canal. Now ask the patient to cough again. If an expansile impulse is felt then the lump must be a hernia.

Next decide whether the hernia is inguinal or femoral. The best way to do this is to determine the relationship of the sac to the pubic tubercle. To locate this structure push gently upwards from beneath the neck of the scrotum with the index finger (Fig. 5.25) but not invaginating the neck of the scrotum as this is painful. The tubercle will be felt as a small bony prominence 2 cm from the midline on the pubic crest. In thin patients the tubercle is easily felt but this is not so in the obese. If difficulty is found, follow up the tendon of adductor longus, which arises just below the tubercle.

If the hernial sac passes *medial to and above* the index finger placed on the pubic tubercle, then the hernia must be inguinal in site; if it is *lateral to and below*, then the hernia must be femoral in site.

If it has been decided that the hernia is inguinal then further points one needs to know are:

1 *What are the contents of the sac? Bowel* tends to gurgle, is soft and compres-

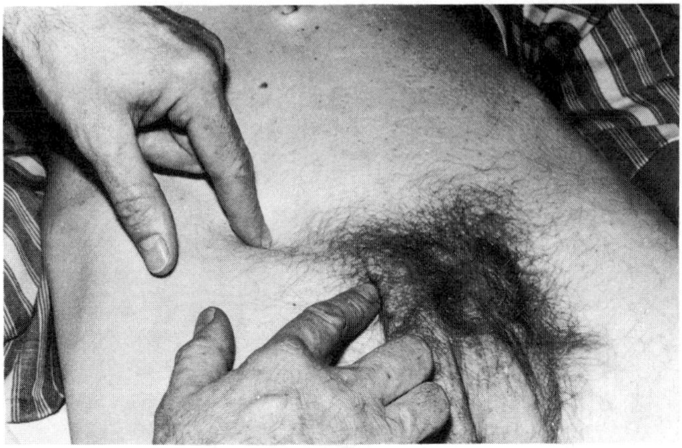

Fig. 5.26 *Left*: palpation of the pubic tubercle: index finger occluding the deep inguinal ring. *Right*: index finger on the pubic tubercle.

sible, whilst *omentum* feels firmer and is of a doughy consistency.
2 *Is the hernia fully reducible or not?* It is best to lay the patient down to decide this. Ask the patient whether the hernia is reducible and if so get him to reduce it himself to confirm this. It is more painful if the examiner reduces it.
3 *Is the hernia direct or indirect?* Again, it is best to lie the patient down to decide this. Inspection of the direction of the impulse is often diagnostic, especially in thin patients. A direct hernia tends to bulge straight out through the posterior wall of the inguinal canal, whilst in an indirect hernia the impulse can often be seen to travel obliquely down the inguinal canal. Another helpful point is to place one finger just above the mid-inguinal point over the deep inguinal ring (see Fig. 5.26). If a hernia is fully controlled by this finger then it must be an indirect inguinal hernia.

Apart from a femoral hernia, *the differential diagnosis of an inguinal hernia* includes a large hydrocele of the tunica vaginalis, a large cyst of the epididymis (one should be able to 'get above' and feel the upper border of both of these in the scrotum), an undescended or ectopic testis (there will be an empty scrotum on the affected side), a lipoma of the cord, and a hydrocele of the cord in a male, or a hydrocele of the canal of Nuck in a female.

In considering *the differential diagnosis of a femoral hernia*, one must think not only of an inguinal hernia but of a lipoma in the femoral triangle, an aneurysm of the femoral artery (expansile pulsation will be present), a sapheno-varix (the swelling disappears on lying down, has a bluish tinge to it, there are often varicose veins present and there may be a venous hum), a psoas abscess (the mass is fluctuant, and may be compressible beneath the inguinal ligament to appear above it in the iliac fossa), and an enlarged inguinal lymph node. Whenever the latter is found, the feet, legs, thighs, scrotum, perineum, and the pudendal and perianal areas must be carefully scrutinized for a source of infection or primary tumour.

The examination is completed by following the same scheme in the opposite groin.

What to do when the patient complains of a swelling in the scrotum

It is easier and better to examine the patient first lying down and afterwards standing up. Inspection, palpation and transillumination are the three keys to rapid, accurate diagnosis. After inspection of the scrotum and groins, try and answer the following questions.

1 *Can I 'get above' the swelling?* Palpate the neck of the scrotum between the fingers and thumb (see Fig. 5.24). If fingers and thumb cannot be approximated so that only the spermatic cord is palpable, then the swelling in question is not confined to the scrotum but is descending from the groin and is therefore an inguino-scrotal hernia, i.e. one 'cannot get above' it. (Very rarely an infantile hydrocele occurs which leads to the same signs though the testis is impalpable.) If fingers and thumb can be approximated so that one 'can get above' the swelling, that swelling can be arising only from the cord, the epididymis or the testis.

2 *Is the swelling cystic or solid? Is the testis palpable separate from the swelling?* Palpate the swelling in the same way as the testis and scrotal contents (p. 106), which will give a good indication whether the swelling is cystic or solid. *Now transilluminate the swelling*; tense the scrotal skin gently over the swelling and place a bright torch *behind* the swelling. If it transmits light then it must be a cystic swelling and is either a *cyst of the epididymis* (a spermatocele) or a *hydrocele of the tunica vaginalis*. The former lies above and a little behind the testis and the testis is palpable separate from the swelling. In the latter the testis is not palpable separate from the swelling, i.e. it is enclosed within the tunica vaginalis and therefore surrounded by fluid.

If the swelling is not translucent then its consistency is solid. Palpate the epididymis and testis again. Enlargement of the epididymis is found in inflammation (epididymitis): if it is tender it is acute; if it is painless, it is chronic (and usually tuberculous). Enlargement of the testis is found in orchitis (usually acute), when it is therefore tender, or, rarely, as a result of malignancy.

Finally stand the patient up. A swelling that is not apparent on lying down but appears on standing and which feels soft and rather like palpating a bag of worms is a *varicocele*, i.e. varicosity of the veins of the pampiniform and/or cremasteric plexi.

RECTAL EXAMINATION

Few other regions of the body reveal such a wealth of physical signs and

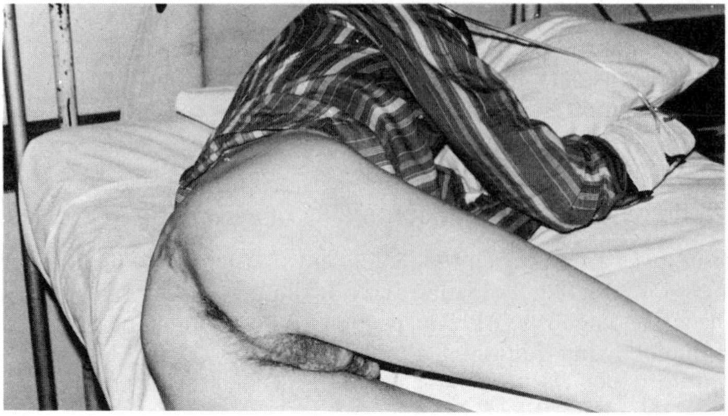

Fig. 5.27 Left lateral position for rectal examination.

diagnoses on inspection and digital examination as the perianal area, anus, and anal canal and rectum.

The left lateral position is best for routine examination of the rectum (Fig. 5.27). Make sure that the buttocks project over the side of the couch with the knees drawn well up, and that a good light is available. Put a disposable glove on the right hand and stand slightly behind the patient's buttocks, facing the patient's feet. Tell the patient what you are about to do and that you will be as gentle as possible.

Inspection

Separate the buttocks and carefully inspect the perianal area and anus. Note the presence of any *pruritus ani*, which may vary in appearance from mild erythema to a raw, red, moist, weeping dermatitis, or in chronic cases thickened white skin with exaggeration of the anal skin folds. The latter form *anal skin tags*, which may not only follow severe pruritus but also occur when prolapsing piles have been present over a period of time. Tags should not be confused with *anal warts* (condylomata acuminata), which are sessile or pedunculated papillomata with a red base and a white surface. Anal warts may be so numerous as to surround the anal verge, and even extend into the anal canal. Note any 'hole' or dimple near the anus with a telltale bead of pus or granulation tissue surrounding it, which represents the external opening of a *fistula-in-ano*. It is usually easy to distinguish fistula-in-ano from a *pilonidal sinus*, where the opening lies in the midline of the natal cleft but well posterior to the anus.

The following acutely painful anorectal conditions can usually be diagnosed readily on inspection. An *anal fissure* usually lies directly posterior in the midline. The outward pathognomonic sign of a chronic fissure is a tag of skin at the base (sentinel pile). The fissure can easily be demonstrated by gently drawing apart the anus to reveal the tear in the lining of the anal canal.

A *perianal haematoma* (thrombosed external pile) occurs as a result of rupture of a vein of the external haemorrhoidal plexus. It is seen as a small (1 cm), tense, bluish swelling on one aspect of the anal margin and is exquisitely tender to the touch. In *prolapsed strangulated piles*, there is gross swelling of the anal and perianal skin, which look like oedematous lips, with a deep red or purple strangulated pile appearing in between, and sometimes partly concealed by, the oedema of the swollen anus. In a *perianal abscess*, an acutely tender, red fluctuant swelling is visible which deforms the outline of the anus. It is usually easy to distinguish this from an *ischiorectal abscess* where the anal verge is not deformed, the signs of acute inflammation are often lacking and the point of maximum tenderness is located midway between the anus and ischial tuberosity.

Note the presence of any ulceration. Finally, if *prolapse* is suspected, ask the patient to bear down and note whether any pink rectal mucosa or bowel appears through the anus, or whether the perineum itself bulges downwards.

Palpation

Put a generous amount of lubricant on the gloved index finger of the right hand, place the *pulp* of the finger (not the tip) flat on the anus (Figs. 5.28 and 5.29) and press firmly and slowly in a slightly backwards direction. After initial resistance the anal sphincter relaxes and the finger can be passed into the anal canal. If severe pain is elicited attempting this manoeuvre then further examination should be abandoned as it is likely the patient has a fissure and unnecessary pain will be caused.

Rotate the finger through 360° in the anal canal and feel for any thickening or irregularity of the wall of the canal. Assess the tone of the anal musculature; it should normally grip the finger firmly. If there is any doubt ask the patient to contract the anus on the examining finger. In the normal patient the contraction will be readily appreciated, whilst in the old and infirm with anal incontinence or prolapse almost no appreciable contraction will be felt. With experience it is usually possible to feel a shallow groove just inside the anal canal which marks the dividing line between the external and internal sphincter. The anorectal ring may be felt as a stout band of muscle surrounding the junction between the anal canal and rectum.

Now pass the finger into the rectum. The examiner's left hand should be placed on the patient's right hip and later it can be placed in the suprapubic position to exert downward pressure on the sigmoid colon. Try to visualize the anatomy of the rectum, particularly in relation to its anterior wall. The rectal wall should be assessed with sweeping movements of the finger through 360°, 2, 5 and 8 cm inwards or until the finger cannot be pushed any higher into the rectum. Repeat these movements as the finger is being withdrawn. In this way

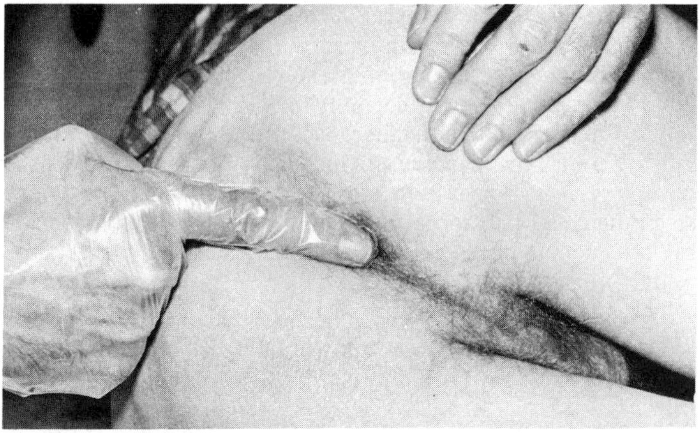

Fig. 5.28 Correct method for insertion of index finger in rectal examination. The pulp of the finger is placed flat against the anus.

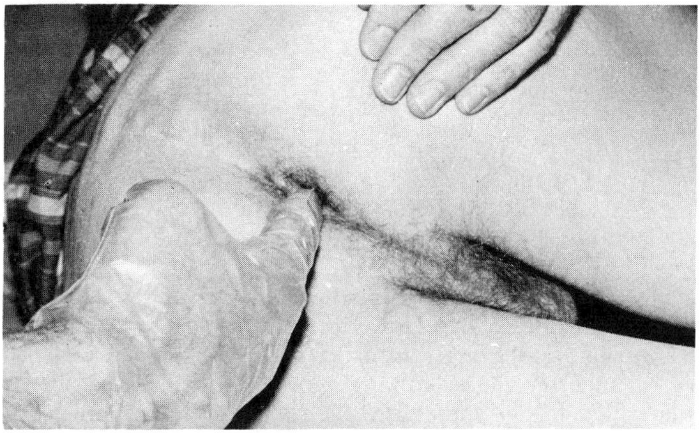

Fig. 5.29 Incorrect method of introduction of finger into anal canal.

it is possible to detect malignant ulcers, proliferative and stenosing carcinomas, polyps and villous adenomas. The hollow of the sacrum and coccyx can be felt posteriorly. Laterally, on either side, it is usually possible to reach the side walls of the pelvis. In men one should feel anteriorly for the *rectovesical* pouch, *seminal vesicles* and the *prostate*. Normally the rectovesical pouch and seminal vesicles are not palpable. In a patient with a pelvic abscess, however, pus gravitates to this pouch, which is then palpable as a boggy, tender swelling lying above the prostate. If the pouch contains malignant deposits, hard irregular nodules may be felt. In infection of the seminal vesicles, these structures become palpable as firm, almost tubular swellings deviating slightly from the midline just above the level of the prostate.

Assessment of the *prostate gland* is important. It forms a rubbery, firm swelling about the size of a large chestnut. Run the finger over each lateral lobe, which should be smooth and regular. Between the two lobes lies the median sulcus, which is palpable as a faint depression running vertically between each lateral lobe. Though one can say on rectal examination that a prostate is enlarged, accurate assessment of its true size is not possible. In carcinoma of the prostate, the gland loses its rubbery consistency and becomes hard, whilst the lateral lobes tend to be irregular and nodular and there is distortion or loss of the median sulcus.

In women, the cervix is felt as a firm rounded mass projecting back into the anterior wall of the rectum. This is often a disconcerting finding for the inexperienced. The body of a retroverted uterus, fibroid mass, ovarian cyst, malignant nodules or a pelvic abscess may all be palpated in the pouch of Douglas (recto-uterine pouch), which lies above the cervix. This aspect of rectal examination forms an essential part of pelvic assessment in female patients.

On withdrawing the finger after rectal examination look at it for evidence of mucus, pus and blood. If in doubt wipe the finger on a white swab. Finally make sure to wipe the patient clean before telling him or her that the examination is completed.

THE FEMALE GENITALIA

It goes without saying that any examination of the female genitalia must be performed with gentleness and consideration; otherwise the patient will not be relaxed and vital signs may be missed. A good light is essential and a chaperone should be present. Ask the patient to empty the bladder immediately prior to examination as this makes bimanual examination easier; little information can be gained with a full bladder.

Ask the patient to lie in the left lateral position (see p. 112). Put on a pair of disposable gloves.

Inspection

Look carefully at the external genitalia, perineum, anus and inner thigh regions. Using both hands, separate the inner thighs to display the labia majora adequately (in an obese patient this will be made easier by asking the patient to raise the right leg slightly). A swelling commonly seen in the posterior part of a labium majus is a Bartholin's cyst produced by blockage of the duct of Bartholin's gland; if infection supervenes an abscess develops. In *kraurosis vulvae* the labia are atrophic, the skin is white and rather thin and the introitus narrowed. In *leucoplakia of the vulva* white plaques, like white paint, are seen over the labia and perineum. Small wart-like papillary growths (condylomata acuminata) may be seen scattered over the vulva; these are due to a virus and not to syphilitic infection.

Hold the right buttock and thigh up slightly with the left hand, separate the labia minora with the index finger and thumb of the right hand and display the clitoris, urethral orifice and introitus of the vagina. The urethral orifice is seen as a small slit. In elderly women who complain of frequent painful micturition it is not uncommon to find an *urethral caruncle*, easily visible as a small, red polypoid lesion, rather like a tiny cherry, distorting the urethral orifice.

Note whether the hymen is intact. If it is, then digital examination per vaginam is not carried out; further information is gained by rectal examination and when necessary by vaginal examination under anaesthesia. Note any discharge at the introitus, its colour and amount. Inspection is completed by asking the patient to cough or bear down, at the same time observing the urethral orifice together with the anterior and posterior walls of the lower vagina. A small dribble or spout of urine issuing from the urethral orifice is apparent in *stress incontinence*. Bulging of the anterior vaginal wall backwards so that it appears to occlude the vaginal lumen is termed a *cystocele* and is due to prolapse of the urinary bladder. A large forward bulge in the posterior vaginal wall is a *rectocele*. Finally, the cervix may appear at the introitus in uterine prolapse (procidentia uteri). The common aetiology of these conditions is stretching and laxity of the pelvic muscles and ligaments following childbirth.

Palpation

Put lubricant jelly on the right index and middle fingers. Gently insert the index finger into the vagina, pressing towards the perineum. When the pelvic floor muscles are felt to relax, introduce the middle finger with the thumb raised forwards over the symphysis but held away from the urethral orifice and clitoris. Push up gently with both fingers extended and feel for the cervix. Note the direction in which the cervix points, its contour, size, mobility and any irregularity of its surface. Now place the tips of the fingers in each fornix— anterior, right lateral, left lateral and posterior (pouch of Douglas)— in turn, and feel for any induration, swelling or mass that may be present. By gentle pressure in each lateral fornix it is usually possible to reach the side walls of the pelvis.

Whilst bimanual palpation may be carried out in the left lateral position, more information will be gained if it is conducted with the patient lying supine, the knees drawn up and allowed to fall apart, and the heels together.

Uterus

The lubricated index and middle fingers are introduced into the vagina, and the cervix and fornices reassessed. Now place the fingers of the left hand in the

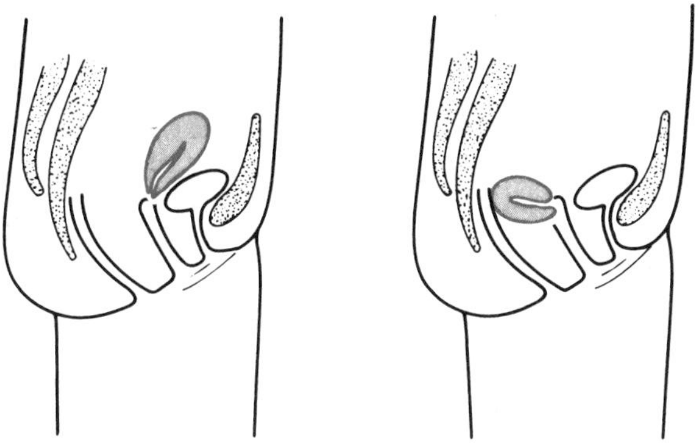

Normal anteverted uterus Retroverted uterus

Fig. 5.30 The uterus.

midline in the suprapubic region of the abdomen and press firmly downwards; the uterus will be pushed down towards the fingers of the right hand. Try to approximate the fingers of both hands; the fundus of the uterus will be felt and the position, size, contour and mobility of the uterus can be made out. Normally the uterus is palpable as a firm, non-tender, mobile swelling in the midline. In obese or poorly relaxed patients, however, this is not an easy thing to do.

Try to decide whether the uterus is *anteverted* or *retroverted* (Fig. 5.30). In the normal anteverted uterus, the cervix points backwards to make an angle of about 45° with the vagina, and the fundus and upper part of the body of the uterus are easily palpable. If the uterus is retroverted, the cervix will be felt either pointing in the long axis of the vagina or anteriorly, and the fundus will not be palpable suprapubically.

When the uterus is enlarged, symmetrical and soft, either pregnancy or carcinoma should be suspected. When it is enlarged, firm, mobile and nodular, such a finding is typical of fibroids. Fibroids may grow to a large size and may be palpable on abdominal examination as a swelling 'arising out of the pelvis'. When uterine mobility is reduced or the uterus is fixed and tender, there is usually an inflammatory cause. This is especially likely when there is associated induration in one of the vaginal fornices.

Adnexa

It is often not possible to feel the ovaries, fallopian tubes and parametrium unless they are enlarged or diseased. To palpate the adnexa, move the left hand to one side of the midline suprapubically and press down firmly whilst pushing gently upwards with the index and middle fingers of the right hand in the appropriate lateral fornix. Each fornix is palpated in this way and in the normal patient they should be soft and supple.

A normal ovary, if palpable, will be felt as a firm swelling about the size of a walnut, which is slightly mobile and tender.

An *ovarian cyst* is a common abnormality and often attains great size. It distorts the vaginal vault and is palpable as a swelling in the fornices, which has to be differentiated from fibroids or other uterine swelling. If sufficiently large, the cyst will be palpable through the abdomen as a swelling 'arising out of the pelvis', when it should be differentiated from a distended bladder, a fibroid uterus or ascites (p. 96).

As the normal fallopian tube is not palpable, any thickening or induration that is palpable in the lateral fornix is abnormal. Such thickening is usually indicative of local inflammation or malignant spread from carcinoma of the cervix. Firm, painless, discrete or confluent nodules felt in the posterior fornix (pouch of Douglas) are usually an indication of widespread secondary malignant deposits in the peritoneum (carcinomatosis peritonei).

Finally, another satisfactory and often helpful method of deep pelvic assessment is simultaneous palpation of the vagina and rectum with the index finger in the vagina and middle finger in the rectum. It is especially useful for assessment of swellings in the pouch of Douglas.

THE ACUTE ABDOMEN

Diagnosis and management of acute abdominal disorders depends on information derived both from the history and from the examination.

History

The patient usually presents with acute abdominal pain. In considering this symptom, its site, severity, radiation, character, time and circumstances of onset, and any relieving features are all important.

Site Ask the patient to point to the site of maximal pain with one finger. If pain is experienced mostly in the *upper abdomen* think of perforation of a gastric or duodenal ulcer, cholecystitis or pancreatitis. If pain is located in the *mid-abdomen*, disease of the small bowel is likely. Pain in the *right iliac fossa* is commonly due to appendicitis and pain in the *left iliac fossa* to diverticulitis. In women *low abdominal pain* of acute onset is often due to salpingitis, but rupture of an ectopic pregnancy should also be considered; the menstrual history is thus important. The coexistence of *severe back and abdominal pain* indicates a ruptured abdominal aneurysm or a dissecting aneurysm. When the parietal peritoneum is irritated, pain is felt at the site of the affected organ, but when the visceral peritoneum is predominantly involved pain is often referred in a somatic distribution. For example, in acute appendicitis pain is felt near the umbilicus at first but later, with parietal peritoneal involvement, the pain moves towards the site of the appendix, usually in the right iliac fossa.

Severity Try to assess how severe the pain is. Ask the patient whether it keeps him awake. In women, compare the severity with labour pains. Sometimes comparison to the pain of a fractured bone is useful.

Radiation If pain radiates from the right subcostal region to the shoulder or to the interscapular region, inflammation of the gallbladder (cholecystitis) is a likely diagnosis. If pain begins in the loin but then is felt in the lumbar region a renal stone or renal infection should be considered. Pain beginning in the loin and radiating to the groin is likely to be due to a ureteric calculus and umbilical pain radiating to the right iliac fossa is usually due to appendicitis. Central upper abdominal pain, later radiating through to the back, is common in pancreatitis.

Character and constancy Constant severe pain, felt over many hours, is likely to be due to infection. For example, diverticulitis or pyelonephritis can present in this manner. *Colicky pain* on the other hand, i.e. *pain lasting a few seconds or minutes and then passing off, leaving the patient free of pain for a further few minutes*, is pathognomonic of small bowel obstruction. If such pain is suddenly relieved after a period of several hours of severe pain, perforation of a viscus should be considered. Large bowel obstruction produces a more constant pain than small bowel obstruction, but colic is usually prominent.

Mode of onset In obstruction from mechanical disorders such as that due to biliary or ureteric stone, or obstruction of the bowel from adhesions or volvulus, the onset of colicky pain is usually sudden. It is often related to activity or movement in the previous few hours. In infective and inflammatory disorders the pain usually has a slower onset, sometimes over several days, and there is no relation to activity. Recent ingestion of a rich heavy meal often precedes pancreatitis. Alcohol excess or the ingestion of aspirin or steroid therapy are often observed as precipitating features in patients presenting with perforated peptic ulcer or with haematemesis.

Relieving features Abdominal pain relieved by rest suggests an infective or inflammatory disorder. If the patient cannot keep still and rolls around in agony then ureteric or biliary colic are likely diagnoses.

Vomiting A history of vomiting is not in itself very helpful because vomiting occurs as a response to pain of any type. However, effortless projectile vomiting often denotes pyloric stenosis or high small bowel obstruction. In peritonitis the vomitus is usually small in amount but vomiting is persistent. There may be a faeculent smell to the vomitus when there is low small bowel obstruction. Persistent vomiting with associated diarrhoea strongly suggests gastroenteritis. (See 'Examination of Vomit', p. 121.)

Bowels Constipation is the rule in the great majority of abdominal emergencies, whether inflammatory or obstructive. Absolute constipation occurs where there is complete intestinal obstruction. Absence of faecal matter occurs first and then the patient observes that the passage of flatus ceases and that abdominal distension has occurred. Diarrhoea occurring in the natural history of an acute abdominal disorder is evidence against a surgical cause. Alternating diarrhoea and constipation is seen in patients with diverticulitis or subacute intestinal obstruction. Sometimes a patient will be aware that the bowel sounds have become very noisy and frequent, which is evidence of chronic incomplete intestinal obstruction, probably in the colon.

The examination of the faeces is discussed in Chapter 7.

Micturition Increased frequency of micturition occurs both in urinary tract infections and in other pelvic inflammatory disorders as well as in patients with renal infections or ureteric stones. In the latter, haematuria commonly occurs.

Appetite and weight In patients with a chronic underlying disorder, such as abdominal cancer, there may be a history of anorexia and weight loss, although weight loss also occurs in a variety of other disorders. Sudden loss of appetite clearly indicates a disorder of sudden onset.

Other features It is important to note whether there have been previous episodes of abdominal pain and whether or not they have been severe. A tendency to improvement or worsening of the patient's symptoms after the onset is also important in deciding on management. The patient may have noticed swellings at the site of a hernial orifice indicating the likelihood of an obstructed hernia or there may be a history of blunt or penetrating abdominal trauma. Sometimes the patient may be aware of increasing abdominal distension, a phenomenon indicating intestinal obstruction or paralytic ileus probably associated with an inflammatory or infective underlying bowel disorder. Food poisoning may be suggested by a history of ingestion of unusual foods such as shell fish or a meal in unfamiliar surroundings. The menstrual history should never be forgotten, particularly in relation to the possibility of an ectopic pregnancy. Enquiry should always be made as to a purulent vaginal discharge, indicating salpingitis, or of discharge of mucus, pus or blood from the rectum, suggesting ulcerative colitis.

Examination

A detailed explanation of the findings in the very large number of causes of an acute abdomen is out of place in this book. The student should consult an appropriate textbook of surgery. What is intended here is a very brief explanation of the terms used and of the findings on palpation in acute inflammatory conditions of the peritoneum. The physical signs found on inspection (p. 85) and on auscultation (p. 103) have already been discussed.

Guarding Guarding is an involuntary reflex contraction of the muscles of the abdominal wall overlying an inflamed viscus and peritoneum, producing localized rigidity. It indicates localized peritonitis. What is felt on examination is spasm of the muscle, which prevents palpation of the underlying viscus. Guarding is seen classically in uncomplicated acute appendicitis. It is very important to distinguish this sign from voluntary contraction of muscle.

Rigidity Generalized or 'board-like' rigidity is an indication of diffuse peritonitis. It can be looked upon as an extension of guarding, with involuntary reflex rigidity of the muscles of the anterior abdominal wall. It is quite unmistakable on palpation, as the whole abdominal wall feels hard and 'board-like', precluding palpation of any underlying viscus. The least downward pressure with a palpating hand in a patient with generalized rigidity produces severe pain. It may be differentiated from voluntary spasm by getting the patient to breathe: in voluntary spasm the abdominal wall will be felt to relax during expiration.

Rebound tenderness Rebound tenderness is elicited by palpating slowly and deeply over a viscus and then suddenly releasing the palpating hand. If rebound tenderness is positive, then the patient experiences pain. This sign is explained by the fact that gradual stretching of the abdominal wall by deep palpation followed by sudden release of this pressure stimulates the parietal peritoneum which, if inflamed, produces pain. Rebound tenderness is not always a reliable sign and should be interpreted with caution, particularly in those patients with a low pain threshold.

EXAMINATION OF VOMIT

The character of the vomit varies with the nature of the food ingested and the absence or presence of bile, blood or intestinal obstruction. In pyloric stenosis the vomit is apt to be copious and sour smelling, contains recognizable food eaten many hours before and exhibits froth on the surface after standing. The presence of much mucus gives vomit a viscid consistency. The appearance of the vomit in haematemesis varies in relation to the site and severity of the bleeding. If bleeding is copious the vomit may present the appearance of pure blood, or it may be dark red and contain clots. Such bleeding may come from a gastric ulcer or from the oesophageal varices of portal hypertension. More commonly the blood is altered to a blackish or dark brown colour by being in contact with gastric juice. The dark brown colour is due to the conversion of haemoglobin into haematin. The altered blood gives to the vomit an appearance often compared to that of 'coffee grounds'. The taking of preparations of iron or red wine may produce a similar appearance in the vomit. Vomit which contains dark green bile may resemble vomit which contains blood; however, on diluting with water the green colour of the bile becomes more apparent while blood remains dark. Remember that blood in vomit may have come from the nose or lungs and been swallowed; bright red blood that is 'vomited' nearly always originates from the naso- or oropharynx and not from the stomach. Faeculent vomit, characteristic of advanced intestinal obstruction, is brown in colour, rather like vomited tea. Its main hallmark, however, is its typically faecal odour. Vomit containing formed faeces is rare but indicates a communication between the stomach and transverse colon, i.e. gastrocolic fistula.

ASPIRATION OF PERITONEAL FLUID

Aspiration of peritoneal fluid (paracentesis abdominis) is undertaken for diagnostic and therapeutic purposes. It is essential first to make sure that the bladder is empty; if there is any doubt a catheter should be passed before paracentesis is attempted.

The patient should be lying flat or propped up at a slight angle. An abdominal binder or many-tailed bandage should be placed in position around the patient's back before paracentesis is begun. The aspiration is usually performed in the right iliac fossa, a little outside the midpoint of a line drawn from the umbilicus to the anterior superior iliac spine.

With suitable sterile precautions, the skin at the point chosen should be infiltrated with local anaesthetic and the anaesthetic then injected down to the parietal peritoneum. If the puncture is made simply for diagnostic purposes, a 10 ml syringe and a suitable needle can be used. If it is intended to drain the peritoneum, a trocar and flanged cannula (which can be fixed to the skin with adhesive tape) should be employed. A tiny incision should be made in the anaesthetized area of the skin and then the trocar and cannula inserted. A resistance is felt as the trocar perforates the parietal peritoneum. The trocar is then withdrawn from the cannula and the fluid drained into a bottle via a tube connecting the cannula to the bottle. The binder is then secured over the abdomen, which helps to promote drainage. The rate of flow, which should not be too fast, can be controlled by means of a clip on the tubing. When aspiration is complete, the cannula should be withdrawn. The puncture wound is sealed with a plastic dressing and a dry dressing applied. Therapeutic drainage should, however, be avoided if possible as diuretics are preferable.

The fluid withdrawn is sent for bacteriological and cytological examination and chemical analysis. Transudates, such as occur in heart failure, cirrhosis and nephrosis, normally have a specific gravity less than 1·018 and a protein content under 25 g/litre. Exudates occurring in tuberculous peritonitis or in the presence of secondary deposits usually have a specific gravity above 1·018 and more than 23 g/litre of protein. The distinction, however, is somewhat unreliable. Tubercle bacilli may be demonstrated in the fluid in tuberculous peritonitis; blood-stained fluid strongly suggests metastases. Malignant cells may also be demonstrated in the latter condition, and in malignant ascites the fluid recurs rapidly after paracentesis.

THE GASTROINTESTINAL TRACT

Under this heading common and important methods of examining the *stomach* and *duodenum*, *small* and *large intestine*, the *liver*, *gallbladder* and *pancreas* will be described.

Stomach and duodenum

Intubation Intubation is used more for therapeutic than diagnostic purposes. In the former case it aids: (a) gastric decompression in intestinal obstruction and following abdominal surgery; (b) tube feeding in patients unable to swallow, or unconscious; and (c) gastric washouts prior to surgery in patients with pyloric holdup. Intubation is, however, a necessary preliminary to studies of gastric acid production.

The nasogastric tubes are now made of soft plastic (Portex). The blind gastric end is round and weighted with metal to render it radiopaque. The lubricated tube is passed via a nostril and then swallowed. For gastric acid studies it should lie in the most dependent part of the stomach and this should be confirmed by screening. If required, the tip can usually be passed into the duodenum by lying the patient on his right side and tilted forwards.

Gastric acid studies The patient should neither eat, drink nor smoke for eight hours before the study. After the tip's position has been confirmed by screening, all resting fluid should be removed by gentle manual suction with a syringe. The patient should then either sit up or lie on his left side, whichever is more comfortable. Constant manual suction is performed gently with a 20 ml syringe. It is usual to measure the basal acid output (BAO) and the maximum acid output (MAO), though the second is the more informative.

The *basal acid output* is measured after all resting fluid in the stomach has been removed. The basal secretion is then collected over the next one hour by continuous aspiration. In normal persons it is no more than a few millilitres per hour, containing up to 10 mmol/l of hydrogen ions.

The *maximum acid output* is measured after the administration of the synthetic peptide (pentagastrin) of the hormone gastrin.

After the basal secretion has been measured for one hour, a dose of 6.0 μg/kg body weight of pentagastrin is given by subcutaneous injection. This causes a maximal acid secretion. After the injection, the juice is collected for one hour. The total acid secreted in this hour is the MAO. In normal subjects this may reach a maximum of 27 mmol/l/hour in males and 25 mmol/l/hour in females. Patients with duodenal ulcer have normal or raised values (up to 50 mmol/l/hour), whilst those with gastric ulcer and carcinoma have normal or low values.

The insulin test This test consists of the injection of insulin, which produces hypoglycaemia and thus stimulates the nucleus of the vagus in the brain stem. Impulses then run down an intact vagal nerve and stimulate the production of a small amount of acid in the stomach. This does not happen after a complete vagotomy. Measurement of gastric acid production after an injection of insulin thus tests the completeness of a vagotomy. This investigation is particularly helpful when a patient develops a recurrent ulcer following vagotomy for duodenal ulceration. The blood sugar has to fall below 45 mg/100 ml for the test to be valid and it is measured before and after insulin is injected by slow i.v. infusion 0.04 units/kg/hour. Aspiration is then carried out for 120 minutes. The patient should be watched carefully and given intravenous glucose if severe hypoglycaemia occurs. A rise of acid secretion to 20 mmol/l/hour or more above basal unstimulated values probably indicates incomplete vagotomy.

Plain radiographs Plain radiographs of the abdomen with the patient supine and in the erect position are of great value in cases of suspected peritonitis due to perforation of a gastric or duodenal ulcer, when gas may be seen under the diaphragm, usually on the right side.

Barium meal The barium meal is a radiographic investigation in which the patient swallows a suspension of radiopaque barium sulphate, while the radiologist observes its passage on a fluorescent screen or on the TV monitor of an image intensifier. Films are taken to provide a permanent record of any abnormality discovered, but, as in all barium examinations of the alimentary tract, screening is important. The barium meal is principally used in the diagnosis of gastric and duodenal ulcer and of gastric carcinoma.

The barium-filled crater of a chronic gastric ulcer may be seen in the stomach as a projection from the wall ('profile view') or as a rounded deposit ('en face' view) with in either case mucosal folds radiating towards the crater. A duodenal ulcer is usually seen en face with a stellate appearance of the mucosal folds. Often no definite crater is seen, but the cap is deformed as a result of scarring, characteristically producing a trefoil deformity, sometimes with pseudo-diverticula. In cases of pyloric stenosis there is an increased amount of resting juice present and a grossly enlarged stomach which empties extremely slowly. Polypoid gastric carcinomas cause filling defects in the barium-filled organ. Malignant ulcers may be difficult to differentiate from simple ulcers, and the radiologist therefore pays particular attention to the mucosal folds and mobility of the wall in the region of the ulcer. Infiltrating tumours produce a rigid conical shape to the stomach with absence of peristalsis and no ulceration. Carcinomas involving the cardia and pylorus cause obstruction and, if small, may be difficult to differentiate from simple lesions.

Endoscopy and biopsy Flexible fibreoptic gastroscopes allow rapid and safe examination under outpatient conditions with the aid of local anaesthesia and light sedation (diazepam). By the use of suitable forward-viewing and side-viewing instruments it is possible to see the whole of the oesophagus, stomach and duodenum. The instruments carry a channel through which biopsy forceps or a brush can be introduced to obtain specimens for histological and cytological examination. Such instruments are of great value in differentiating benign from malignant lesions, assessing the response to treatment of benign gastric and duodenal ulcers, and in the rapid diagnosis of upper gastrointestinal bleeding.

Small intestine

Estimation of faecal fats Faecal fat analysis is useful in the demonstration of steatorrhoea (see Chapter 7).

Barium meal follow-through X-rays The small intestine may be studied by taking films of the abdomen at intervals after a barium meal. Abnormalities in the transit time to the colon and in small bowel pattern, e.g. dilatation, narrowing, increase in transverse barring or flocculation, may be demonstrated in malabsorption states. Areas of narrowing with proximal dilatation, fistulae and mucosal abnormalities may be produced by Crohn's disease. Small bowel diverticula or neoplasms may also be demonstrated.

The *small bowel enema* is an alternative to the barium meal and follow-through examination. This involves intubating the duodenum and passing small quantities of a non-flocculating barium suspension down the tube. This method is particularly valuable for detecting isolated focal lesions.

Biopsy Biopsy of the small intestinal mucosa can be performed using a spring-loaded capsule (the Crosby capsule). This capsule, about 1·5 cm long and 7 mm in diameter, contains a cutting blade which excises a small piece of intestinal mucosa when negative suction is applied to the thin polythene tube to which it is attached. The capsule is swallowed, and a small amount of radiopaque dye is injected, to check that it has passed through the pylorus. Its position in the small intestine can then be checked radiologically. After the biopsy has been taken the capsule is pulled up and the specimen placed on a small piece of card in a preservative solution. It should be examined immediately by the pathologist under a low-power microscope to assess the general appearance of the intestinal villi.

Biopsy must always be preceded by a barium meal and follow-through examination, as the technique might be dangerous if the capsule were to lodge in a duodenal or jejunal diverticulum.

The small intestinal biopsy is of particular importance in diagnosis of the malabsorption syndrome, where a flat mucosa is seen in place of the usual multiple villi. For further tests of intestinal function, such as the xylose and lactose absorption tests, special textbooks should be consulted.

Colon, rectum and anus

Proctoscopy The anal canal and lower rectum can be readily visualized with a proctoscope. Place the patient in the position described for rectal examination and gently pass the lubricated instrument to its full depth. Remove the obturator and inspect the mucosa as the instrument is slowly withdrawn. Piles are seen as reddish/blue swellings which bulge into the lumen of the instrument. The internal opening of an anal fistula, an anal or low rectal polyp and a chronic anal fissure are other abnormalities that may be seen.

Sigmoidoscopy It is often necessary to examine the rectum and colon more fully than is possible by proctoscopy, and in such cases the sigmoidoscope is employed. Sigmoidoscopy requires skill and experience. In accomplished hands the instrument can be passed for 30 cm. The procedure causes little discomfort and anaesthesia is unnecessary.

Proctitis, polyps and carcinomas may be seen and biopsies taken. Sigmoidoscopy is particularly useful in the differential diagnosis of diarrhoea of colonic origin.

In suspected amoebic dysentery, the mucous membrane may be inspected and portions of mucus and scrapings from the ulcer may be removed using a flexible sigmoidoscope and examined microscopically for amoebic cysts.

Barium enema Barium suspension is introduced via a tube into the rectum as an enema and manipulated around the rest of the colon to fill it. Screening is performed by a radiologist and films taken. The barium is then evacuated and further films taken. By this means, obstruction to the colon, tumours, diverticular disease, fistulae and other abnormalities can be recognized.

If, following evacuation, air is introduced into the colon, detailed study of the mucosa is facilitated. This method is especially valuable for detecting small lesions such as polyps and early tumours (Figs. 5.31 and 5.32).

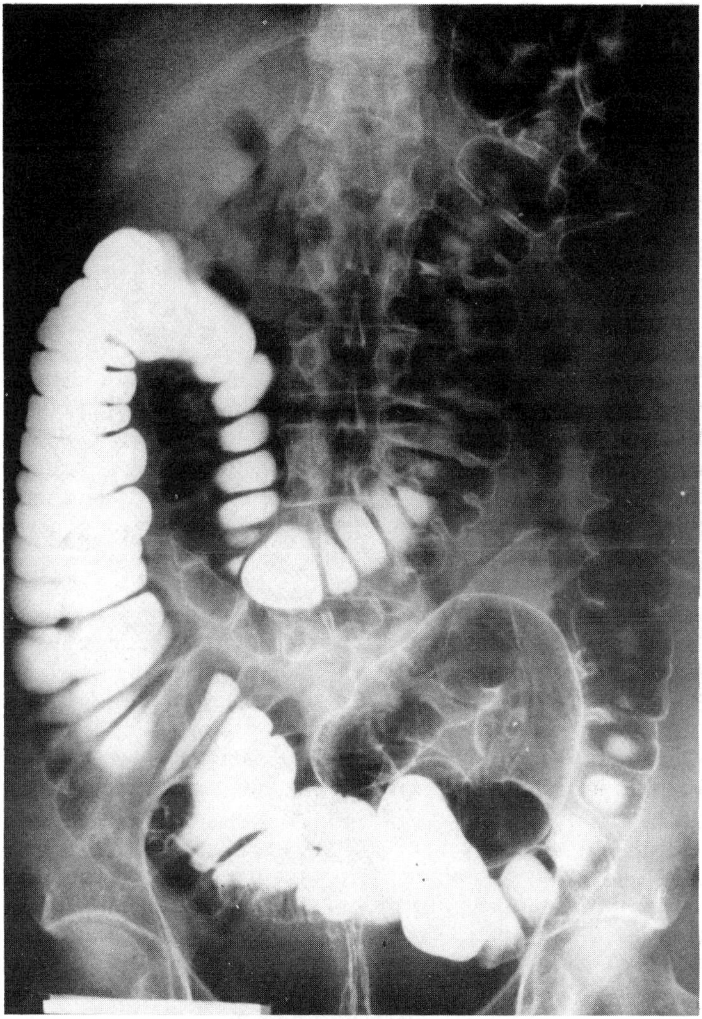

Fig. 5.31 Barium enema with air contrast. The right colon is outlined by barium sulphate, and the rectum, left colon and part of the transverse colon are outlined by air with a thin mucosal layer of barium sulphate. The patient is lying on his right side, thus allowing the air to fill the left side of the large bowel. Note the normal haustral pattern in the colon and the smooth appearance of the rectum. The anal canal can also be seen.

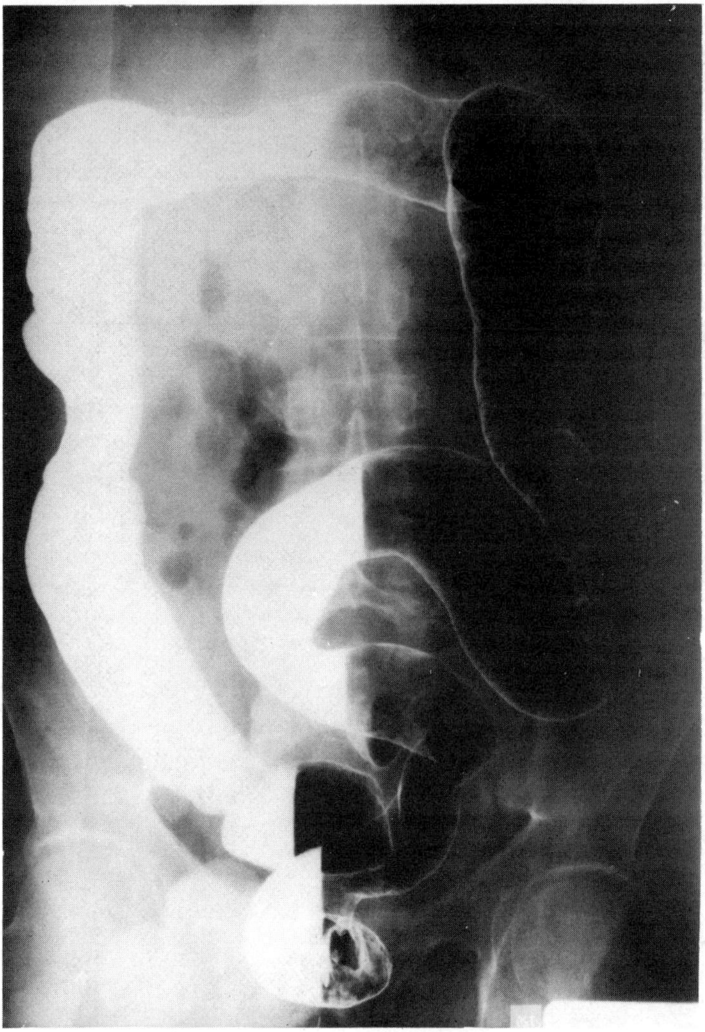

Fig. 5.32 Barium enema with air contrast. In this patient, with ulcerative colitis, the normal mucosal pattern, and the haustra themselves, have been obliterated. The patient is lying on his right side so that there are clear fluid levels in the barium sulphate suspension in the bowel.

Colonoscopy The use of flexible fibreoptic colonoscopes requires considerable skill and should be restricted to experts. It is frequently possible to inspect the whole of the colonic mucosa round to the caecum. Biopsies can be taken and pedunculated polyps removed by the use of diathermy snare loops, which thus do away with the need for laparotomy to excise such polyps.

The liver

Biochemical tests of liver function are used in the differential diagnosis of jaundice, to detect liver cell damage in other disorders and to monitor the results of surgery of the biliary system and pancreas. These include urinary urobilin, plasma bilirubin, alkaline phosphatase, serum aminotransferases, plasma proteins, plasma prothrombin and the sulphobromophthalein excretion test.

Isotope scan A radioisotope of technetium or colloidal gold is injected i.v. and is taken up by the reticuloendothelial system. A gamma camera is used to show the size and shape of the liver. Abnormal areas take up more, or less, isotope than normal; examples are primary or secondary hepatic tumours, abscesses and cysts.

Ultrasound scan A probe, emitting ultrasonic pulses, is passed across the liver and surrounding areas. Echoes detected from within the patient are received with a transducer, amplified and suitably displayed. The technique is of particular value in the diagnosis of fluid-filled lesions such as cysts and abscesses and in detecting intrahepatic bile ducts.

CT scanning Computerized axial tomography can be used to produce cross-sectional images of the liver and other intra-abdominal and retroperitoneal organs (pp. 159–160). This technique is of great value in the investigation of patients with disease of these organs.

Exploration of liver for liver abscess Liver abscesses due to *Entamoeba histolytica* are nearly always found in the right lobe. When suspected clinically, their presence and position may be demonstrated and localized radiologically or by isotope or ultrasound scanning. Metronidazole (Flagyl) 800 mg three times a day for ten days is now the first line of treatment and cures the great majority of cases. Where there is a lack of response to treatment after five days, exploration by needle aspiration for diagnostic and therapeutic purposes may be performed.

The procedure is conducted under local anaesthesia and strict asepsis. A needle of wide enough bore to admit a thick pus (a stout, old fashioned lumbar puncture needle is suitable) is selected and a piece of adhesive tape is wound around it 9 cm from its point. The needle is entered either at the site of maximum tenderness or in the right 8th, 9th or 10th intercostal space in the midaxillary line, and passed medially in a horizontal plane to a maximum depth of 9 cm. By this means the whole of the right lobe of the liver may be explored. When pus is encountered, strong suction has to be employed to remove as much of the pus as possible and this is done with the aid of a two-way syringe. As the pus is removed, it may be replaced by a suitable volume of air (about half the volume of pus removed). The patient is then X-rayed in several positions to determine the exact site and size of the abscess, and to allow the effect of treatment to be followed.

Needle biopsy of liver For many years needle biopsy was the standard method used in the diagnosis of liver abscess. In the last few decades it has been used to obtain material for histological study. Whilst needle biopsy can be conducted under mild sedation and local anaesthesia, it should be carried out only in hospital under supervision and blood should be available for transfusion if necessary. Generally the method is safe and reliable, but there is a tiny but definite mortality from the procedure due to leakage of bile and/or blood into the peritoneal cavity from the puncture site. The procedure should therefore always be regarded as a potentially dangerous investigation and should be performed only by those well trained in the technique. Contraindications include patients with a bleeding diathesis, deep obstructive jaundice or ascites.

Selective angiography of coeliac axis and hepatic artery Angiography is not commonly employed in the investigation of hepatic disease, since it is an invasive technique that demands considerable skill on the part of the radiologist. A catheter is passed retrogradely up the aorta from a femoral puncture; its tip is manipulated into the coeliac axis and thus into the hepatic artery. Radiopaque contrast material may then be injected to demonstrate the hepatic vasculature. The technique is occasionally valuable in demonstrating abnormal vascular patterns in isolated lesions, particularly in malignant disease, when other methods have failed.

Gallbladder and bile ducts

The main functions of the gallbladder are to concentrate and store hepatic bile, and to empty this bile into the duodenum after appropriate stimuli. The organ is investigated by performing *oral cholecystography*. This procedure depends on the fact that certain iodine-containing compounds, when absorbed from the gastrointestinal tract, are excreted by the liver and concentrated in the gallbladder, thus rendering it opaque.

Apart from a non-functioning gallbladder, radiolucent stones, abnormalities of the wall of the gallbladder, anatomical variations, and failure to contract in response to a fatty meal may also be demonstrated.

Intravenous cholangiography Intravenous cholangiography is used to demonstrate the bile ducts. The technique depends on the fact that an intravenously administered iodine-containing compound is excreted by the liver in the bile in such a concentration that it is radiopaque, and therefore does not depend on the concentrating power of the gallbladder as in cholecystography. As with cholecystography it cannot be performed in the jaundiced patient.

Of particular interest are the width of the common bile duct (usually less than 10 mm), the presence of stones seen as radiolucent filling defects, and the entry of dye into the duodenum. A dilated duct nearly always signifies an abnormality.

Percutaneous transhepatic cholangiography Percutaneous transhepatic cholangiography is a very useful investigation in patients with jaundice due to obstruction of the main bile ducts. The site of the obstruction due to tumours of the head of the pancreas, or iatrogenic and malignant bile duct strictures can be accurately localized and differentiated. The information gained prior to laparotomy is of great value to the surgeon.

ERCP (endoscopic retrograde cholangiopancreatography) The development of a side-viewing fibreoptic duodenoscope meant that the duodenal papilla could be readily identified. Biopsy and brushings of the papilla can be taken for histological and cytological examination. The papilla may be cannulated and then injected with dye to display the common bile ducts and pancreatic duct and thus demonstrate abnormalities in their outline or lumen. The technique is particularly useful in the rapid diagnosis and localization of the different causes of jaundice due to obstruction of the main bile ducts, in demonstrating the bile ducts where intravenous cholangiography has failed, and in the speed with which obstruction may be eliminated as a cause of jaundice in those patients with cholestasis.

Ultrasonic scan (see p. 129). This technique is being used increasingly in the diagnosis of gallbladder disease and the detection of gallstones in both the gallbladder and bile ducts.

The pancreas

Lundh test The Lundh test relies on an assessment of tryptic activity in pancreatic juice collected following duodenal intubation and indirect stimulation of the pancreas by prior ingestion of a meal. Where the mean tryptic activity is less than 6 IU/litre, exocrine insufficiency is present. The test is reliable in experienced hands and is cheap and simple to perform.

Triple test The triple test is so called becuse it consists of three parts. A special double lumen tube is swallowed and then screened into position in the duodenal loop. It has a weighted bulbous end and contains two sets of holes, one for duodenal and the other for gastric aspiration. The latter set of holes prevents contamination of the duodenal aspirate.

1 *Exocrine function*. After a short period allowed for stabilization, secretin is injected and duodenal aspirate collected continuously over the next 30 minutes. Pancreozymin (cholecystokinin) is then injected and the process repeated. The volume of aspirate and concentration and output of bicarbonate, amylase, lipase and trypsin are then measured and calculated. Patients with carcinoma of the pancreas, particularly of its head, produce low volumes of low enzyme levels. Patients with chronic pancreatitis secrete low volumes, the juice containing low levels of bicarbonate and normal or low enzyme levels.

2 *Cytology*. Fresh aspirate is examined for malignant cells stained by the Papanicoloau method. Interpretation, however, is difficult and requires an experienced cytologist.

3 *Hypotonic duodenography*. When the first two parts of the test are completed, an anti-spasmodic drug (Buscopan) is injected which paralyses the duodenum. A small amount of barium is injected down the duodenal lumen of the tube followed by 100 ml of air. This delineates the wall of the distended duodenum; ampullary carcinomas, and irregularity and distortion of the medial wall due to infiltration by a carcinoma of the head of the pancreas, may be visualized.

The triple test is more complex, and more unpleasant for the patient, than the Lundh test. In experienced hands the procedures should be regarded as valuable screening methods for pancreatic disease, especially where the following more sophisticated investigations are not available.

ERCP The ERCP procedure (p. 131) can display the entire pancreatic duct system. It is therefore valuable not only in the diagnosis of chronic pancreatitis but also in defining those cases which surgery could benefit.

After stimulation with secretin, pure pancreatic juice uncontaminated with duodenal content may be collected from the duct and cytological examination performed. This provides a better success rate (about 50%) in the diagnosis of pancreatic carcinoma than the similar examination in the triple test. The procedure should not be performed in patients with acute pancreatitis or those with suspected pseudopancreatic cysts.

Ultrasound and CT scans These are both useful methods in the diagnosis of pancreatic disease. Each method can differentiate solid from cystic lesions greater than 2.5 cm in size and the success rate in diagnosis is around 70%. Ultrasound is particularly useful in the diagnosis of true and pseudopancreatic cysts.

6
The urine

Sir Robert Hutchison used to say that the ghosts of dead patients do not ask why we did not employ the latest fad of clinical investigation; they ask 'Why did you not test my urine?' or 'Why did you not put a finger in my rectum?'

To the risk that the urine may not be tested at all, new dangers have been added, in that urine testing is increasingly delegated to non-medical persons, who may be inadequately trained in the performance and interpretation of the tests they use and unaware of their importance. All doctors and students should be thoroughly conversant with urine testing, which is an essential part of any medical examination.

Urine passed into a clean vessel is suitable for routine urine testing. Special methods of collection, designed to reduce contamination from urethra and vestibule, are desirable for microscopic examination (p. 145) and essential for bacteriological examination (p. 150).

The urine should be examined physically, chemically, microscopically and bacteriologically.

PHYSICAL EXAMINATION

Attention should be paid to the following points: quantity; colour and transparency; specific gravity; and naked-eye characteristics of the deposit.

Quantity

The normal quantity of urine passed daily varies widely, from 700 to 2500 ml, depending on the fluid intake. Normally, very much more urine is excreted during the day than during the night. An *increased excretion* of urine occurs *physiologically* after food or drink, and after exposure to cold. Conversely, *diminished excretion* occurs when little food or drink has been taken, and after heat-induced sweating.

A *pathological increase (polyuria)* occurs in diabetes mellitus and insipidus, during the elimination of oedema fluid and sometimes in renal failure. *Nocturnal polyuria*, usually shortened to the term *nocturia*, is often the first clinical indication of failure of the concentrating power of the kidney, and therefore is often the first symptom of chronic renal failure.

Abnormal reduction of urine output may be due to salt and water depletion from such factors as diarrhoea, vomiting, fever, excessive sweating and extensive burns; the sudden lowering of blood pressure; severe heart failure; or acute diffuse disease of the kidney tissue such as occurs in acute glomerulonephritis.

Complete cessation of urine output (*anuria*) is uncommon and most often results from an obstruction in the urinary tract itself.

Colour and transparency

Urochrome and *uroerythrin* are pigments which give normal urine its characteristic colour. The exact tint varies widely, and it darkens on standing due to the oxidation of colourless urobilinogen to coloured urobilin. The concentration of urine cannot be reliably estimated from its appearance.

Small quantities of *blood* give urine a smoky appearance; larger quantities make it brownish or red. Haemoglobin in large amounts, as in blackwater fever, gives it a colour varying from dark red (when it may be confused with the colour resulting from excessive consumption of beetroot) to brownish black or even almost black.

Bile pigment causes the urine to appear brown, with a green tint at the surface when viewed in the specimen glass against the light; it produces a yellow froth when the urine is shaken in a test tube.

The urine is abnormally pale when it is very dilute, i.e. with specific gravity of about 1.002, and in *renal failure*, when the normal colouring matter is greatly diminished or absent.

The taking of *drugs* may also lead to discoloration of the urine. Some examples are tetracyclines (yellow); anthracene purgatives (orange); desferrioxamine (reddish brown); phenindione (pink); nitrofurantoin, furazolidone and niridazole (brown); rifampicin and pyridium (red); methylene blue, present in some proprietary pills (green); and methyldopa and iron sorbitol (grey or black).

Normal urine is quite transparent when freshly passed but it may be *opalescent* from the presence of various substances in suspension, of which the most important are pus, bacteria, phosphates and urates. Phosphates dissolve on adding acid. If the opalescence persists after filtration, it is due to the presence of bacteria. Clear urine may become cloudy when cooled to room temperature; this is probably due to the precipitation of urates, which dissolve when the urine is re-warmed to body temperature.

Specific gravity

The concentration of urine is best expressed as its *osmolality*, which depends on the number of osmotically active solute particles per unit of solvent, and this may be determined by measuring its freezing point.

Although less accurate, it is often helpful, and usually more practicable, to measure the *specific gravity* with a *urinometer*. The specific gravity depends on the type as well as on the number of solute particles. To obtain satisfactory results certain precautions must be taken. The glassware used should be clean and free from detergents, and the urinometer should float freely in the measuring cylinder. The reading at the bottom of the meniscus is the relevant one. As the instrument is calibrated at 16°C, a falsely low reading will be obtained if urine is tested whilst warm, so it should be allowed to cool to room temperature. Otherwise 0.001 should be added to the specific gravity recorded for every 3°C by which the urine temperature exceeds 16°C. If there is insufficient urine for the urinometer to float freely, the urine should be diluted with an equal volume of distilled water and the last two figures of the urinometer reading doubled. Unfortunately, measurements of specific gravity using a urinometer are usually done with insufficient care, giving inaccurate results. Recently a commercial test strip (Multistix SG) has been introduced, which enables fairly accurate results to be obtained from a small quantity of urine within a few seconds. Randomly measured, the normal specific gravity varies from 1.002 to 1.025, depending on the state of hydration of the patient and the time of day—often being greatest on arising in the morning. It may occasionally rise to 1.035 even in health.

In normal urine the specific gravity is proportional to the urinary concentration of urea and sodium.

Approximate correlations between specific gravity and osmolality are as follows:

Specific gravity	*Osmolality* (mosmol/kg)
1.002	100
1.010	285
1.020	750
1.030	1200
1.035	1400

However, unusually high specific gravities compared with osmolalities may be found in urine containing a lot of heavy particles, e.g. radiographic contrast medium, glucose (as in diabetes mellitus) or protein. 15 mmol (2.7 g) per litre of glucose, or 4 g per litre of protein, cause the specific gravity to rise by 0.001.

In diabetes insipidus, on the other hand, the specific gravity may fall almost to that of distilled water, and this may also happen in compulsive water drinking.

Normally, the concentration of the urine, as reflected by its specific gravity, varies considerably from time to time. As renal failure develops, the kidneys progressively lose their ability to concentrate and dilute urine, whose specific gravity approximates more and more to 1.010 (the specific gravity of the glomerular filtrate) until eventually the urine is isotonic with plasma water. This is a simple and useful test of renal function which does not need laboratory facilities. The specimen passed on rising is usually tested for this purpose, as it is often the most concentrated that is passed in the day; however, this is not invariably so, and it may be helpful to test all specimens passed during a 24-hour period. If the specific gravity of this, or any other sample of urine, exceeds 1.018 it can be assumed that renal concentrating power is normal. Failure to achieve this does not mean that concentrating power is defective, because a period of fluid deprivation longer than overnight is required to achieve maximum concentration, but care must be taken that the patient does not become too dehydrated.

Naked-eye characteristics of the deposit

Normal urine is perfectly clear and transparent when voided. After it has stood for some time a deposit of 'mucus' appears in it. This forms a woolly cloud, which usually settles to the bottom of the glass, but if the urine is of high specific gravity it may be in the middle or at the top. If traces of blood are present in the urine, the cloud of 'mucus' may have a brownish tint.

Phosphates, urates and uric acid may precipitate in normal urine. Phosphates produce a white deposit when the urine is alkaline; warming increases their deposition because the urine becomes more alkaline due to the loss of carbon dioxide. They dissolve after acidification with acetic acid. Urates and uric acid form faintly pink deposits, particularly if the urine is concentrated or highly acidic; they disappear on warming or adding sodium hydroxide. Although usually of no significance, they may appear when purine breakdown is increased, as in myeloproliferative disorders, especially after treatment, when they may obstruct renal tubules acutely, or may form stones which themselves can obstruct the calyx, renal pelvis or ureter and cause colic.

Abundant leucocytes and bacteria may give the urine a turbid appearance; a gross deposit of yellow–white pus may rarely be formed. Gross haematuria may produce a red deposit.

CHEMICAL EXAMINATION

Many of the traditional chemical tests for urinary constituents have been replaced for routine purposes by commercial tablet or reagent 'stick' or 'strip' tests. Some of these will be described briefly, but for full details the manufacturers' literature should be consulted. This is especially necessary when a 'combination' indicator strip, e.g. Multistix, which tests for several different constituents of urine, is used because it is easy to confuse the colour bands, or to read the individual indicator areas at the wrong time.

In general the reagent strip is dipped briefly into the urine, its edge then being run against the rim of the urine container to remove excess moisture. The strip is held horizontally (to prevent the mixing of chemicals from adjacent bands) and the colour changes are noted at the times specified. Different bands are read at different times. *Failure to follow the manufacturer's instructions exactly, or failure to keep the reagents in a satisfactory condition, will result in incorrect deductions*. The indicator ends of reagent strips should not be handled, and urine for testing should be collected in clean containers, free from antiseptics or detergents.

pH

It is customary to test the reaction of the urine with pH indicator papers or commercial reagent test strips, but the result is rarely important except when a drug has been given with the intention of altering the pH for therapeutic purposes. Normal urine is nearly always acid. Rarely is it repeatedly neutral or alkaline when the patient is not taking alkalis, and this may indicate impairment of the ability of the tubules to eliminate acid. This can be confirmed by accurate measurement of the pH of the urine after giving ammonium chloride to the patient (p. 154).

Proteins

Before doing the 'traditional' tests for protein, it is essential that the urine should be absolutely clear and it may therefore be necessary to filter it. If the urine remains turbid after it has been filtered more than once, bacteria are probably present and the protein concentration is then best tested with commercial reagent strips. If the turbidity is due to urates, it will disappear when the urine is heated; if due to phosphates it will disappear after acidification.

Tests for protein

Commercial reagent strips The band for testing protein on commercial reagent strips (e.g. Multistix) is impregnated with buffered tetrabromophenol blue and changes from yellow to various shades of green depending on the concentration of protein in the urine. The colour of the indicator area on the strip is compared with the colours on the manufacturer's chart after the strip has been transiently dipped in the urine; the colour change is immediate, but the time of reading is not critical. The test is most sensitive for albumin, and the amount of albumin present in normal urine (up to 150 mg/l) may be indicated on the strip as a trace. Fluorescent light may make appreciation of the colour change difficult. The test is sensitive, semi-quantitative, quick and convenient, and is therefore widely used. It is less sensitive for globulin than albumin, and may give a negative result with urine containing Bence Jones protein; false positive results may occur if the urine is very alkaline, contaminated with certain detergents, and during treatment with phenothiazines.

The salicylsulphonic acid test The salicylsulphonic acid test for protein is simple, very reliable, semi-quantitative and does not require heat. However, it is less convenient than the commercial buffered strips, and is no longer in general use in the United Kingdom.

Filter the urine if cloudy. To 5 ml in a test tube add 20% salicylsulphonic acid, drop by drop. The presence of protein is indicated by a cloudy precipitate, best seen against a black background, but up to 25 drops may be required before it forms. Continue to add salicylsulphonic acid until no more precipitate occurs. For ordinary purposes it is sufficient to express the amount present as a haze, cloud or granular precipitate, a haze of protein representing about 20 mg per 100 ml; a heavier deposit may be allowed to settle (which may take an hour or so) and the quantity expressed as the proportion of the total urine volume occupied by the deposit. If this proportion is one half, the urine contains about 10 g protein/1. False positive results may be due to the presence of radiographic contrast medium; they may also occur with the urine of patients treated with sulphonamides, tolbutamide, para-aminosalicylic acid or large doses of penicillin, or if the urine contains a lot of uric acid.

The boiling test The boiling test is a satisfactory test for protein but is rather messy and less convenient than the salicylsulphonic acid test.

Fill a small test tube two-thirds full of urine which, if cloudy, has been filtered. If the urine is alkaline, add a small piece of indicator paper to the urine, then add 10% acetic acid, drop by drop, mixing thoroughly after each drop until pH 5 is reached. Incline the tube at an angle, boil the top 2 cm over a flame while holding the bottom of the tube and examine against a dark background. A cloudiness indicates the presence either of protein or of phosphates, which have precipitated because loss of carbon dioxide on boiling has made the urine more alkaline. If the precipitate disappears on adding acid it was due to phosphates; if it persists protein is present. If more than a light cloud persists boil all the urine, acidifying until no more protein is precipitated. Allow to settle and express semiquantitatively as described for the salicylsulphonic acid test. The boiling test is comparable in sensitivity to the latter test.

Treatment with tolbutamide or large doses of penicillin or the presence of radiographic contrast medium may result in false positive results.

If proteinuria is detected by either the salicylsulphonic acid or boiling test, but not by Multistix, the presence of Bence Jones protein should be suspected. This is confirmed if a precipitate forms as the urine is heated to about 45°C, only to disappear on boiling and re-precipitate during cooling; however, more sophisticated laboratory tests may be needed to detect it.

Esbach's albuminometer Urine protein concentration can be measured more accurately, but simply, using Esbach's albuminometer. The method is not often used. In it, picric and citric acids are added to the urine but, because the amount of coagulum depends on the type as well as on the amount of protein, the result is only approximate, and the method is perhaps best used for the serial assessment of protein concentration in an individual patient.

The instrument consists of a thick graduated glass tube. Make up Esbach's reagent by dissolving 10 g picric acid and 20 g citric acid in about 900 ml boiling water; allow to cool and make up to 1 litre with water. Filter the urine if not clear, and if alkaline render slightly acid with acetic acid. If the specific gravity is 1.010 or more it should be reduced to about 1.008 with water, the dilution factor being noted so that subsequent correction of the measured protein concentration can be made. Fill the tube with urine up to the mark 'U'. Pour in the reagent up to the mark 'R'. Close the tube with the rubber stopper and gently invert it several times to mix. Leave for 24 hours, then read off the upper level of the coagulum against the scale, whose figures represent grams of protein per litre of urine.

If the protein concentration exceeds 4 g per litre, greater accuracy can be obtained by repeating the test after dilution of the urine. However, protein concentrations of less than 1 g per litre cannot be properly measured.

Significance of proteinuria

Normally less than 150 mg protein is excreted in the urine over a 24-hour period, and random samples contain less than 20 mg/1. This rarely produces more than a trace reaction with commercial reagent sticks. It should be remembered that all these tests estimate protein concentration, not excretion rate, and as it is the latter which is of interest, consideration should be given to the amount of urine passed on the day of the test. One-third of protein in normal urine is albumin, identical with plasma albumin and apparently filtered through the glomerulus. Two-thirds consists of globulins, some of which are derived from plasma globulins, some originating in the renal tubules, and others from the lower urinary tract, e.g. prostatic and urethral secretions and semen; Tamm–Horsfall protein, a high molecular weight protein thought to be formed in the tubules, is the major proteinaceous non-cellular constituent of casts.

Fever and exercise may transiently increase urinary protein excretion in otherwise healthy people. Orthostatic proteinuria denotes the finding of protein in urine collected during the day, but not in the first urine passed after rising; it is usually of no importance save that it may lead to the mistaken belief that the kidneys are damaged. Persistent proteinuria usually indicates the presence of renal disease, but the amount does not indicate the severity of the disease. Proteinuria may also be due to extrarenal disease, such as congestive heart failure. Diseases affecting the lower urinary tract usually cause only slight proteinuria.

Blood and its derivatives

Whole blood may appear in the urine (*haematuria*) or blood pigment may appear without corpuscles (*haemoglobinuria*). Both conditions give positive chemical tests for haemoglobin, but can be differentiated by microscopy of the urine deposit for red cells.

Very small numbers of red cells, such as may be found for several days after an attack of renal colic, and in bacterial endocarditis, cause no discoloration of the urine. Larger numbers give it a peculiar opaque appearance to which the term 'smoky' is applied, and more still produce a brown or red colour, the cells often settling to form a similarly coloured deposit.

Tests for blood

Reagent strips A commercial reagent strip, e.g. Multistix, is momentarily dipped in a fresh uncentrifuged well-mixed sample of urine and the test area of the strip examined 25 seconds later. An even colour change from cream to green or blue indicates the presence of haemoglobin or myoglobin; a patchy discoloration suggests that blood is present. The test depends on the oxidation of orthotoluidine to a blue pigment, the reaction being catalysed by the globin. Therefore the use of stale or infected urine (containing peroxides produced by proliferating bacteria) or the presence of other oxidants (e.g. sodium hypochlorite antiseptic solution) may give a false positive reaction, and reducing agents (as in patients taking ascorbic acid) a false negative one.

Significance of blood and blood pigments in urine

Menstrual contamination is the most common cause of blood in the urine. Otherwise this is usually due to disease of kidney, ureter, bladder or urethra, although exercise may occasionally cause haematuria in healthy persons. The site of bleeding cannot be determined by examination of the urine unless the red cells form casts, which implies that there is bleeding into the renal tubules.

Haemoglobinuria may occasionally follow strenuous exertion in normal people but in disease may be due to haemolysis within blood vessels (as after mismatched blood transfusion) or in urine (as when blood cells lyse in dilute urine). Myoglobinuria is uncommon; it too can be produced by hard exercise and by muscle damage, such as found in crush injuries or in certain metabolic myopathies.

Urine which contains blood or haemoglobin must contain some protein, and it is often difficult to say whether the blood is sufficient to account for all the protein present or whether proteinuria exists in addition. If human blood is added to normal urine in an amount sufficient to produce distinct smokiness, the quantity of protein amounts to merely a trace. Even when the quantity added is sufficient to render the urine distinctly red, the amount of protein is only about 0.5 g/l.

Sugars

Several reducing sugars may be found in the urine. Glucose is by far the most important of these. In normal people it occurs in amounts too small to be detected by the usual methods employed, but if it is so detected its presence may be regarded as pathological. Glycosuria may be secondary to excessive blood glucose levels, as in diabetes mellitus, or to defective renal tubular reabsorption—'renal' glycosuria. If the glycosuria is accompanied by undoubted symptoms of diabetes mellitus the diagnosis is not in doubt. If no symptoms are present a random estimation of blood glucose concentration may confirm the diagnosis, although a formal glucose tolerance test is sometimes required.

The other reducing sugars which may be found in urine include lactose, fructose, pentose and galactose. Lactosuria occurs in late pregnancy and during lactation. Pentosuria, like galactosuria and fructosuria, is usually due to a rare inborn error of metabolism, but may follow the eating of large quantities of certain fruits, such as plums, cherries and grapes. It should be noted that sucrose is a sugar, but not a reducing one and, as unenlightened examiners have found to their embarrassment, artificially loading the urine with this substance does not produce a positive Clinitest.

Reducing substances which are not sugars may occasionally be found in the urine. Thus homogentisic acid (present in alcaptonuria, a rare inborn error of metabolism) and treatment with ascorbic acid, cephalosporins, nalidixic acid or aspirin may give a positive result with tests for reducing sugars. Similarly, Clinitest is used to ensure that formaldehyde, which also gives a positive reaction, has been thoroughly washed out of artificial kidneys sterilized with this substance, before they are used.

Tests for reducing substances

The presence of a *reducing substance* (glucose or otherwise) in the urine may be detected using Benedict's test or Clinitest tablets. Commercial strip tests are specific for glucose, so non-glucose reducing substances do not affect them.

Benedict's test To 5 ml of Benedict's reagent add 8 drops of the urine, boil for 2 minutes and allow to cool. If a reducing substance is present, a precipitate will appear, varying from a light green turbidity to a red precipitate. If the reduction is due to glucose, the test gives approximately quantitative results:

Light green turbidity	0.1–0.5 g/dl sugar
Green precipitate	0.5–1.0 g/dl sugar
Yellow precipitate	1.0–2.0 g/dl sugar
Red precipitate	2.0 g/dl sugar or over

Clinitest This is a convenient modification of Benedict's test, in which the ingredients are present in a tablet and the necessary heat is provided by the interaction of sodium hydroxide and citric acid. Five drops of urine are placed in the test tube using the dropper provided. The dropper is rinsed and 10 drops of water are added. One Clinitest tablet is dropped into the tube and the resulting reaction observed. Effervescence occurs, followed by boiling. Fifteen seconds after the boiling has ceased, the tube should be shaken gently and the colour of the contents compared with the colour scale provided. If the solution turns blue, the result is negative. When a reducing substance is present, the copper sulphate in the solution is converted to cuprous oxide, causing the colour change through green (0.5%) to orange (2%). If a transient orange 'flash' is seen during effervescence it indicates that the urine contains at least 2 g/dl reducing substance irrespective of the final colour.

Reagent strips These tests, e.g. Multistix, Diastix, are specific for glucose, but less easy to quantify than Clinitest. The reagent strip is dipped transiently in the urine and the colour of the test area is compared with the maker's colour chart several seconds later. A change from brown or blue through green indicates that the urine contains an abnormal amount of glucose. The test is semi-quantitative.

The tests are based on glucose oxidase or hexokinase enzyme reactions. The manufacturer's instructions should be followed carefully, because the time at which the colour change occurs should be recorded. The nature of the colour changes themselves varies with the type of strip used. The tests are highly sensitive unless inhibited by a high concentration of ascorbic acid in the urine, such as may occur with the oral administration of some tetracycline preparations. False positive reactions may be given by strong oxidizing agents, such as certain antiseptics, bleaches and detergents.

Ketones

Aceto-acetic acid and acetone (as well as hydroxybutyric acid, which is not a ketone) may appear in the urine of patients with severe diabetes mellitus, and after starvation or prolonged vomiting. The ketones may be detected using Rothera's nitroprusside test or one of its modifications such as Ketostix or Acetest, all of which are very sensitive. Severe degrees of ketonuria may be tested for using the ferric chloride (Gerhardt) test.

Tests for ketones

Rothera's test The urine must be fresh and unboiled because aceto-acetic acid is easily decomposed. 10 ml of urine is saturated with ammonium sulphate by adding an excess of the crystals; 3 drops of a strong freshly prepared solution of sodium nitroprusside and 2 ml of strong ammonia solution are then added. A deep permanganate colour is produced. This test is given both by acetone and aceto-acetic acid but by no other substances that may occur in fresh urine. If Rothera's test is negative, ketones are absent.

Acetest This is a modification of Rothera's test in tablet form. One drop of fresh urine is allowed to fall on an Acetest tablet on a clean white surface. A purple discoloration of the tablet 30 seconds later indicates the presence of aceto-acetic acid or acetone, and the amount can be estimated roughly by comparison with the maker's colour chart.

Reagent strips A reagent strip is dipped momentarily in the fresh urine. A mauve colour of the test end of the strip after 15 seconds constitutes a positive result. The test is semi-quantitative. False positive results may occur if the urine contains sulphobromophthalein, phenylketones or metabolites of L-dopa.

Gerhardt's test 10% ferric chloride solution is added drop by drop to 5 ml of urine in a test tube. A precipitate of ferric phosphate usually forms, but disappears again when more ferric chloride is added. The solution becomes brownish-red if aceto-acetic acid is present.

Aspirin and other salicylates, phenothiazines, phenol and some other drugs give a similar colour with ferric chloride. Boiling for about 5 minutes (before adding the ferric chloride) destroys aceto-acetic acid, but the other substances which react similarly with ferric chloride are unaffected. If, therefore, urine which has been boiled still gives the ferric chloride reaction, it may be inferred that the reaction was not due to aceto-acetic acid. Boiling after adding ferric chloride destroys the colour, whether this is due to aceto-acetic acid or to other substances.

A positive ferric chloride reaction is obtained only if aceto-acetic acid is present in considerable amount. If the urine reacts to Rothera's test but not to ferric chloride, it may be inferred that only small quantities of ketone bodies are present. If both are positive, the patient has a ketosis of considerable severity, demanding urgent treatment.

Bile pigments

Bilirubin

Bilirubin is the end product of metabolism of haem, contained in proteins such as haemoglobin and myoglobin, and formed mainly in reticuloendothelial cells. Normally bilirubin is transported in plasma in an unconjugated form, which is lipid soluble and strongly bound to protein, and therefore not excreted in the urine. Bilirubin is conjugated to form diglucuronide during its secretion into bile. This compound is water-soluble and less tightly bound to albumin, and can potentially pass across the glomerulus. In health bilirubin is not found in urine because it does not normally circulate in this form.

The finding of bilirubinuria in a jaundiced patient suggests that the jaundice is due to the appearance of conjugated bilirubin in the plasma, resulting from hepatocellular damage or hepatic obstruction. Jaundice due solely to unconjugated bilirubin, as in intravascular haemolysis, is not associated with bilirubinuria.

Urobilinogen and urobilin

Bilirubin secreted by the liver into bile is reduced by intestinal bacteria to urobilinogen, some of which is reabsorbed into the portal circulation to be excreted into bile by the liver again (enterohepatic circulation). A small amount reaches the systemic circulation and is excreted into urine. The colourless urobilinogen oxidises to the pigmented urobilin on standing, and, if present in quantity, colours the urine orange. Estimation of the urinary urobilinogen may be useful in several circumstances. Absence of urinary urobilinogen in a patient with obstructive jaundice indicates that the obstruction is so complete that no bile pigment is reaching the intestine. In a patient without jaundice, urobilinogenuria may imply that a normal liver is unable to cope with an unduly large load of urobilinogen or that a damaged liver is unable to excrete the normal amount of urobilinogen coming to it via the enterohepatic circulation. The first circumstance is found during haemolysis of red cells which may be insufficient to cause clinical jaundice and which does not produce bilirubinuria. The second occurs in the pre-icteric stage of infective hepatitis and in diffuse diseases of the liver such as severe cirrhosis when it may be accompanied by bilirubinuria.

Tests for bile pigment

Bile pigment makes the urine yellow or brownish in colour but this is not specific for bile. A crude test for its presence is to shake the urine in a test tube: a positive result is given by the formation of a stable yellow froth, the stability of which is due to the presence of bile salts and the colour to bilirubin. Ictotest is a more sensitive and reliable test for bilirubin.

Ictotest Five drops of urine are placed on the test mat provided. One Ictotest tablet is placed in the centre of the moistened area. Two drops of water are placed on the tablet and allowed to flow onto the mat and the colour change on the *mat* (not the tablet) is observed 30 seconds later. If bilirubin is present the mat turns bluish purple. A pink or red colour should be ignored as should any discoloration of the tablet. Chorpromazine in large quantities may produce a false positive result.

Ehrlich's aldehyde test and reagent strip tests An excess of urobilinogen in the urine can be detected by Ehrlich's aldehyde test or by the commercial strip test modification of this reaction. Colourless urobilinogen condenses with Ehrlich's aldehyde reagent in acid solution to form red dyes which can be extracted by a mixture of amyl and benzyl alcohols. The test must be performed on fresh urine because on standing urobilinogen undergoes spontaneous oxidation to urobilin, which does not give the reaction. Porphobilinogen (which is excreted in the urine in certain types of porphyria and condenses to porphyrins on standing, giving stale porphyric urine a port wine colour) also produces a red colour in the test, but the colour is not extracted into the alcohol phase.

1 ml of fresh urine at room temperature is mixed with 1 ml of Ehrlich's aldehyde reagent (2 g paradimethylaminobenzaldehyde, dissolved in 100 ml of 5% hydrochloric acid). After 1.5 minutes 2 ml saturated aqueous sodium acetate are added and mixed, followed by 2 ml of a 3:1 (v/v) mixture of amyl alcohol and benzyl alcohol. The test tube is stoppered and its contents are shaken gently for one minute. After the phases have separated a red colour of the upper (organic) phase indicates that urobilinogen is present, whilst a similar colour in the lower (aqueous) phase denotes porphobilinogen. Chloroform may be used in the test as an alternative to amyl and benzyl alcohols. It separates more quickly, into the *lower* layer, and therefore it is in this layer that the red colour due to urobilinogen may be seen. Fresh urine normally contains a little urobilinogen which may be sufficient to produce a slight pink discoloration in the test. Urine diluted 10 times with water will not do so.

In the commercial version, the reagent strip is dipped momentarily into fresh urine and the colour change in the test area compared with the makers' chart 45 seconds later. Positive reactions may also be produced by porphobilinogen and para-aminosalicylic acid.

MICROSCOPICAL EXAMINATION

It is customary to examine with a microscope the deposit from urine which has been centrifuged at 1000–1500 rpm for about three minutes; a cover slip should be used. This is useful for qualitative examination, and mid-stream urine (see 'Bacteriological Examination') is generally suitable for the purpose. However, it should be remembered that fragile items, such as casts, may be disrupted by prolonged or rapid centrifugation. Cells and casts disintegrate rapidly if urine is allowed to stand, and it is essential to examine fresh urine if red, white and epithelial cells are to be distinguished. Unstained cellular elements, especially casts, are not very refractile. They are best seen if the microscope diaphragm is partially closed and the condenser racked down.

Quantitative examination of the cellular deposit is best done on uncentrifuged urine in a haemocytometer chamber. Figs. 6.1, 6.2, 6.3 and 6.4 illustrate the urinary sediment as seen by phase contrast microscopy. Readers using ordinary microscopy must not expect to see casts and cells so clearly defined.

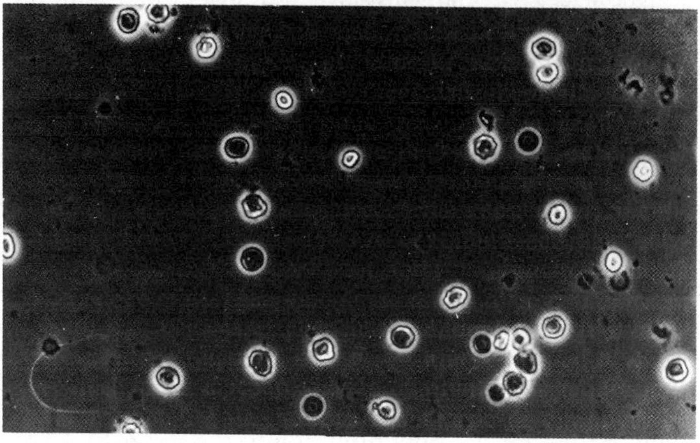

Fig. 6.1 Erythrocytes in urinary sediment.

Red blood corpuscles (Fig. 6.1)

Typically erythrocytes appear as roughly circular elements of about 7 μm diameter with clear yellowish centres. If the urine is concentrated they are shrunken and crenated, but in dilute urine they become larger and their biconcave shape changes to a more spherical one. Normal urine contains no more than 3 red cells/mm^3 of uncentrifuged urine or less than 1 per high power field (hpf) of centrifuged urine. Red cells may be confused with droplets of oil from fingers or catheter lubricant. However, oil droplets are easily differentiated by their variable size, their higher refractive index and the fact that they are more circular.

The detection of microscopic haematuria may be very important in diagnosis, particularly in patients with systemic diseases which may affect the kidney, e.g. subacute bacterial endocarditis. Small numbers of red cells do not discolour the urine, and may not give a positive chemical test for haemoglobin, especially if the urine is fresh.

Leucocytes (Fig. 6.2)

Leucocytes are slightly larger than red cells and can usually be recognized by their round shape, lobed nuclei and refractile granular cytoplasm. Their

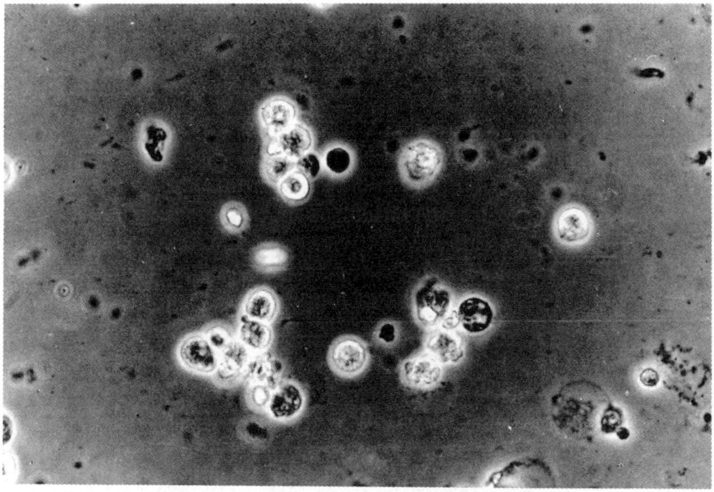

Fig. 6.2 Leucocytes in urinary sediment.

structure is more easily seen if the urine is acidified with a few drops of glacial acetic acid (which will cause the red cells to disintegrate) but, without the use of phase contrast microscopy or special stains, they cannot be differentiated reliably from renal tubular epithelial cells. When numerous, they tend to form clumps. They degenerate in a matter of hours and must be sought in fresh urine. More than 10 leucocytes/mm^3 of uncentrifuged mid-stream urine is abnormal in adult women, between 3 and 10 being of doubtful significance; more than 3 leucocytes/mm^3 is abnormal in men. This difference between men and women is a result of contamination of the urine by vaginal secretions. Centrifuged urine should not contain more than 5 leucocytes per high power field.

An increase in the number of leucocytes suggests that the urine is infected with bacteria, although it may occur without detectable infection, e.g. in patients with renal calculi. If pus cells are repeatedly found in apparently sterile urine, tuberculosis of the urinary tract must be considered. The diagnosis of bacterial urinary infection ultimately rests on culture, not microscopy, for infection can be present without any increase in urinary leucocytes.

Epithelial cells

Transitional epithelial cells from bladder or ureters appear as large oval cells with single nuclei. Polygonal squamous cells, sometimes in sheets, come from urethral or vaginal secretions; if present in quantity in urine collected from women, such sheets suggest that the specimen is contaminated and probably unsuitable for culture.

Spermatozoa

Spermatozoa occur at times in urine from males and females where their characteristic appearance makes is easy to recognize them. They have no pathological significance.

Prostatic threads

Prostatic threads are found when there is chronic inflammation of the prostate, especially after gonorrhoea. They are much larger than casts, being visible readily enough to the naked eye as they float in the urine or on its surface.

Casts

The precipitation of mucoprotein in renal tubules is thought to result in the formation of hyaline casts (Fig. 6.3). On this basic material erythrocytes (forming red cell casts), leucocytes (forming white cell casts), or tubular epithelial cells (forming epithelial casts or, if they contain fats, fatty casts) may be deposited. Disintegration of the cellular elements of a cast changes its appearance to that of a granular or waxy cast (Fig. 6.4). Very broad casts (called 'renal failure' casts) are so shaped because they are formed in tubules which are large and dilated through severe parenchymal disorganization.

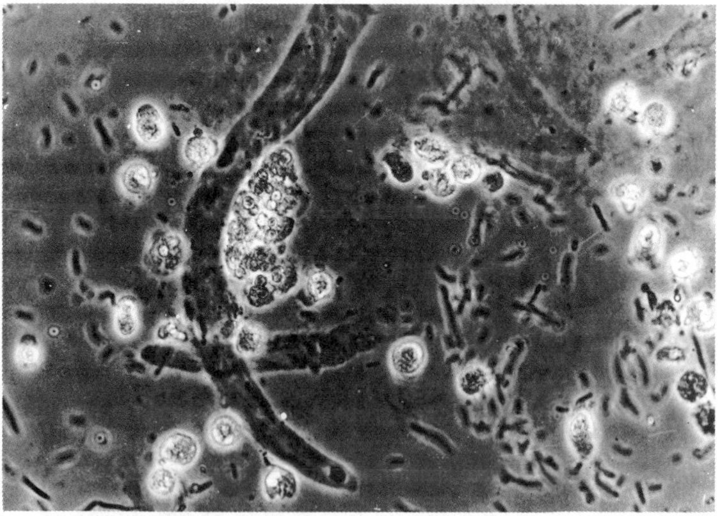

Fig. 6.3 Hyaline casts, leucocytes and bacteria in urinary sediment. Figs. 6.2. and 6.3 are reproduced from *Hand Atlas of the Urinary Sediment* (1971) by E.S. Spencer and I. Petersen, with kind permission of the authors and publisher (Munksgaard, Copenhagen).

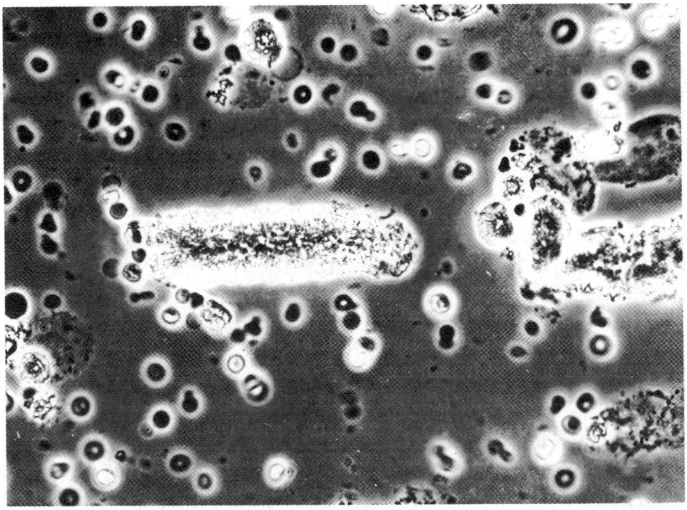

Fig. 6.4 Granular casts in urinary sediment.

The finding of an occasional hyaline cast is normal. Many such casts, or the presence of more complex casts, indicates that the kidneys are diseased.

Casts are easily missed if the microscopic illumination is too bright and disintegrate if the urine has been centrifuged too rapidly or for too long. They should be looked for towards the edges of the cover slip. They are distinguished from other objects which may be mistaken for them—such as hairs, wool, cotton, masses of urates, prostatic threads, and rolled-up epithelial cells—by their shape and characteristic outline. They are always cylindrical, and may have rounded ends, or one end may be ragged as if fractured. Hyaline casts are pale, transparent and homogeneous, and may be difficult to distinguish from the background unless phase contrast microscopy is used; they may be long and narrow with tapering ends and then are sometimes called cylindroids. Cellular casts are recognized by their constituent cells. Granular casts contain fine or coarse granules.

Crystals

Alkaline urine often contains crystals of ammonium magnesium phosphate (triple phosphate). Calcium oxalate crystals are normal in acid urine.

Amorphous or urate debris frequently obscures interesting cellular material, and dissolves on acidification or gentle warming respectively. Crystals are usually of no pathological significance, but occasionally are of diagnostic importance, e.g. cystine crystals, indicative of cystinuria.

Micro-organisms

Bacteria, especially if motile, may be seen during high power microscopy of unstained, uncentrifuged urine (Fig. 6.3), but they are more easily seen by Gram-staining the centrifuged deposit. Their finding on microscopy indicates that they are present in very large numbers and, if the urine is fresh and uncontaminated, strongly suggests a urinary infection. Urine from women may contain *Trichomonas vaginalis* or yeasts, which usually result from contamination with vaginal secretion. The former are pear-shaped or round parasites about twice the size of leucocytes and with unipolar flagellae that may be seen with difficulty. Yeasts are slightly smaller than red cells, and may be confused with them, with air bubbles, or with oil droplets.

Bilharzia

Schistosoma haematobium is best looked for in the last few millilitres of a stream of urine passed in mid-morning. The ova (Plate I) measure about 0.12 mm by 0.44 mm. A spine projects at one pole. The ova of *Schistosoma mansoni* are less often found in urine and have a lateral spine.

BACTERIOLOGICAL EXAMINATION

Collection of samples

It is rarely necessary to catheterize a patient for the purpose of obtaining urine for culture. A mid-stream urine specimen, collected after the vulva or glans penis has been cleaned with tap water, is suitable for most bacteriological purposes. Antiseptic solutions should not be used for cleaning, because enough antiseptic to interfere with the growth of bacteria during culture may get into the urine.

In women the labia are separated by patient or nurse and the vulva is cleaned twice in an anteroposterior direction with swabs soaked in tap water and then finally with a dry swab. Whilst the labia are still held apart some urine, perhaps 20–50 ml, is passed into a toilet or bowl, but the next portion ('mid-stream urine') is collected into a clean wide-mouthed jar. Urine collected in this way is unsuitable for culture if the patient is menstruating heavily, but reasonably satisfactory specimens can be collected after insertion of a vaginal tampon if menstruation is light.

Sometimes it is important to obtain a specimen free from urethral contaminants. This can be done by suprapubic aspiration of urine. The patient is asked not to micturate for several hours before attending the clinic, so that her bladder is full; if necessary she can be given water to drink on arrival. After bladder distension has been confirmed by percussion, the suprapubic area is shaved and cleaned with antiseptic. An 'intramuscular' needle is inserted at right angles to the skin surface immediately above the symphysis pubis and urine aspirated; it may be necessary to use a longer needle if the patient is fat. The technique is safe and, with slight modification, may be used in pregnant women and infants.

The most satisfactory specimen for culture is the one collected first after arising from sleep, for any bacteria in the bladder have been able to multiply undisturbed for several hours. This should be cultured as soon as possible (and certainly within two hours of collection) or refrigerated at 4°C immediately, in order to prevent contaminant bacteria from multiplying so much that they may be misinterpreted as pathogens. Mid-stream urines, and those obtained by catheterization, should be cultured quantitatively. The most accurate quantitative culture techniques, in which known volumes of serial dilutions of urine are mixed with molten agar or spread over solid agar, and the colonies of bacteria which grow are counted, are time-consuming and expensive. There are several simpler techniques which are less accurate but satisfactory for routine use. In the dipslide method a plastic graticule coated with agar on both sides is dipped momentarily into the urine, which because of surface tension leaves a thin film of approximately constant volume on the agar surface. The slide is incubated and the individual bacterial colonies counted in the normal way: the concentration of bacteria in the original urine can be estimated from the slide count. The technique is especially useful in that the patient can inoculate the slide herself at home, as instructed by a doctor, and post it to a laboratory for incubation.

An ingenious commercial dip-strip (Microstix 3) has three test areas. One, read at 30 seconds, provides a colorimetric estimation of the concentration in the urine of nitrite, which is produced from nitrate by certain bacteria. This is a quick, but insensitive method of estimating the concentration of bacteria in the urine. The other test pads are incubated according to the manufacturer's instructions for 18–24 hours, after which the density of coloured spots enables the concentration of Gram-negative bacteria, and that of all the bacteria in the urine, to be estimated separately. Subculture of the bacterial colonies cannot be made, and therefore the bacteria cannot be further identified nor their sensitivities to antibiotics determined.

Significance of bacteriuria

In general the finding of over 100 000 bacteria/ml (10^8/l) of mid-stream urine indicates the presence of urinary infection. However, contamination without infection may sometimes produce counts above this figure and urinary infection may sometimes be present with lower counts. It is therefore advisable to culture several mid-stream specimens if the patient's symptoms do not require early treatment and to discuss the results in doubtful cases with a bacteriologist. In such cases culture of a suprapubic aspirate may be helpful; any growth in such a specimen, other than a few skin contaminants, indicates that there is infection within the urinary tract. In patients with symptomatic infection the urinary leucocyte concentration is usually increased, but this is often not so when the patient has few or no symptoms.

ESTIMATION OF RENAL FUNCTION

One of the main functions of the kidneys is to rid the body of the waste products of metabolism which are presented to them in the blood stream. This they do by the excretion of waste products into the urine and by the retention of those substances which are not waste. The former is carried out primarily by the glomeruli, which filter off the contents of the plasma except those of high molecular weight or which are tightly bound to plasma protein. The tubules then reabsorb certain solutes, excrete others and reabsorb most of the filtered water. Progressive damage to the kidney by chronic renal disease is usually associated with destruction of, or cessation of function in, a large number of glomeruli. This leads to a reduction in the overall glomerular filtration rate which, if marked, causes a rise in the plasma urea concentration. At the same time there is a much greater flow of urine through the remaining tubules, which overloads the diluting and concentrating mechanisms at the distal ends of the tubules. The result is a progressive diminution in the ability of the kidneys to concentrate and dilute urine as renal destruction progresses, until finally the specific gravity becomes fixed at 1.010.

Plasma concentration of urea and creatinine

The plasma concentration of *urea* depends on a balance between its production from exogenous and endogenous protein and its excretion by the kidneys. Its level thus varies with protein intake and may also be raised in conditions such as fever and haemorrhage into the gastrointestinal tract, which increase endogenous production but where there is no renal involvement. In spite of these objections the plasma concentration of urea is widely used by clinicians as a crude indicator of renal function, and high levels correlate fairly well with the clinical picture of 'uraemia'. The normal range is usually given as 2.5–6.6 mmol/l (15–40 mg/dl). Raised levels may indicate renal failure due to disease of the kidneys themselves, their obstruction or their disturbance in conditions such as hypotension, saline depletion or heart failure which affect blood flow to or within the kidneys. The height of the urea is no guide to the cause of the renal failure and levels of 50 or 70 mmol/l (300 or 400 mg/dl), occasionally more, may be found.

Creatinine (normally 62–124 μmol/l or 0.7–1.4 mg/dl) is derived almost entirely from endogenous sources, but is more difficult to measure accurately than urea. Its plasma concentration correlates with the glomerular filtration rate better than does that of urea. Levels as high as 1500 μmol/l (20 mg/dl) may be reached in advanced renal failure.

The relationship between the plasma urea and creatinine concentrations on the one hand and the glomerular filtration rate on the other is hyperbolic not linear, and glomerular filtration must fall considerably before urea and creatinine concentrations become abnormal. For both clinical and research purposes it may be necessary to measure impairment of renal function short of that which produces a rise in their levels and to measure individual renal functions. Numerous methods are available and the subject is a complicated one. We shall describe here the estimation of the glomerular filtration rate (GFR) and tests of the renal concentrating and acidifying abilities.

Estimation of glomerular filtration rate

The reference method of estimating the glomerular filtration rate (GFR) is that of inulin clearance. The renal clearance of a substance is the smallest volume of plasma from which the amount of that substance excreted in the urine each minute could have been obtained at the time of the test. It is calculated from the expression UV/P, where U is the concentration of the substance in the urine (in μmol/litre), V is the volume of urine produced (in ml/min) and P is the plasma concentration of the substance (in μmol/litre).

If a substance is excreted by glomerular filtration, and is neither secreted nor reabsorbed by the tubules, its clearance is equal to the glomerular filtration rate. Although inulin clearance is considered to be an accurate measure of GFR there are practical difficulties in performing the test and other methods are preferred for routine use.

The clearance of endogenous creatinine is popular as a reasonably good index of GFR, but it over-estimates GFR at low filtration rates and in patients with the nephrotic syndrome. In order to minimize inaccuracies due to errors in the timing and measurement of urine collections, such collections should be made over 24 hours. It is not necessary to catheterize patients for the test. Urea clearance does not correlate well with GFR and should no longer be used for its measurement.

GFR can also be estimated by methods which do not require urine collections. It can be derived mathematically from the plasma creatinine concentration. The rate of disappearance of ^{51}Cr–EDTA or certain other isotopes from the circulation may be used to measure GFR accurately. The normal figure of about 120 ml/minute may be reduced by up to two-thirds before the plasma urea and creatinine concentrations become elevated.

Renal concentrating ability

The concentration of the urine, best measured as its osmolality, may be as low as 50 mosmol/kg after water loading, or as high as 1300 mosmol/kg after fluid deprivation. Specific gravity, as discussed earlier, is affected by the nature as well as by the number of osmotically active particles in solution. However, if a random specimen of urine has a specific gravity greater than 1.018 it can be assumed that concentrating ability is normal. Fluid deprivation for prolonged periods, or injection of vasopressin or an analogue of it, may be used to provide more accurate tests of concentrating ability; a urine osmolality of at least 750 mosmol/kg or a specific gravity of 1.020 should be attained if concentrating power is normal. In order to produce maximum concentration, fluid depletion for 24–36 hours may be necessary. This is unpleasant and may result in excessive dehydration if concentrating power is poor; it is a slightly more effective stimulus to concentration than vasopressin.

Renal acidifying ability

If the pH of a random specimen of urine is below 5.5, it can be assumed that renal acidifying ability is normal. In chronic glomerular disease the kidneys usually retain their ability to reduce urine pH below 5.5 until renal failure is advanced. In certain diseases affecting predominantly the renal tubules the urine cannot be adequately acidified, even when glomerular filtration rate is normal. In order to test for this, ammonium chloride capsules (0.1 g/kg body weight) are given orally; normally the urine pH is reduced to less than 5.4. The test should not be carried out if the patient is already acidotic. Renal tubular acidosis is a cause of renal calculi and nephrocalcinosis, the investigation of which is the most frequent reason for the test being performed.

Radiological investigations

Excretion urography

This depends on the excretion by the kidney of certain radiopaque organic compounds of iodine (Fig. 6.5). After a plain film of the whole abdomen has been taken, the contrast medium is injected intravenously and X-ray films of the kidneys, ureters and bladder are taken after various time intervals, the last being after the patient has emptied the bladder. This investigation provides evidence on the anatomy and function of the kidneys and their outflow tracts. It is important in the investigation of renal failure and of suspected urinary obstruction or other structural abnormalities, and is often performed in the investigation of hypertension. When renal function is poor the kidneys are more easily seen if tomographs and large doses of contrast medium are used.

Figure 6.6a shows the kidneys, pelvicalyceal systems and upper ureters 5 minutes after injection of contrast medium for intravenous urography. Figure 6.6b shows how important the plain film is: the pelvicalyceal system looks as if it is filled with contrast medium, but this has not yet been injected! A large calculus (so-called *staghorn calculus*) has formed a radiopaque cast of the outflow tract of each kidney. Figure 6.7 demonstrates a non-functioning left kidney with hydronephrosis on the right.

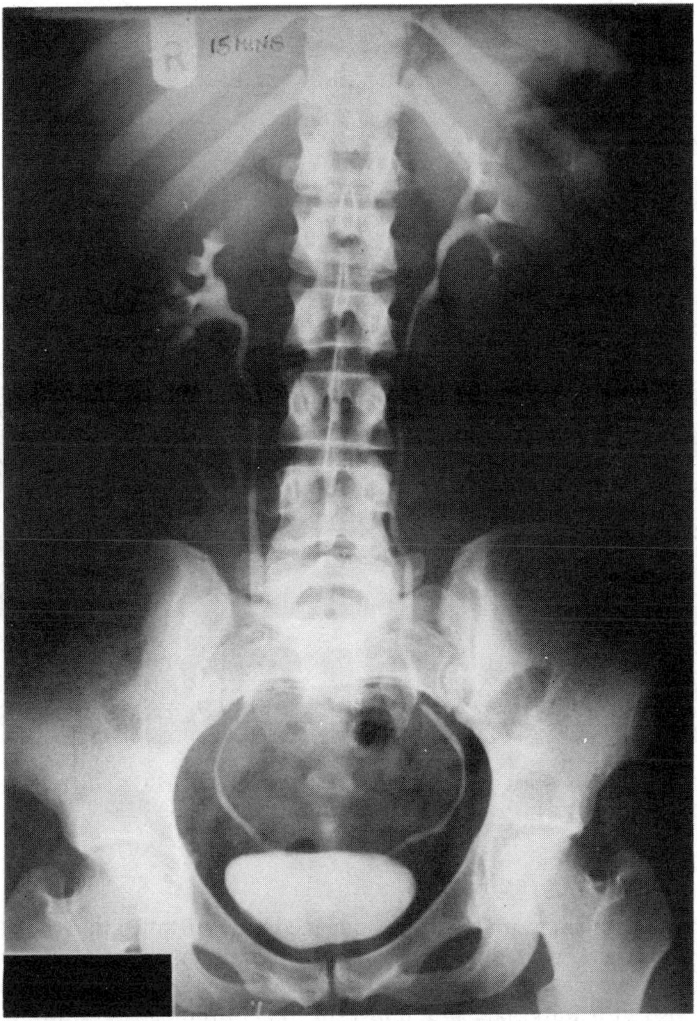

Fig. 6.5 Normal excretion urogram. In this film, taken 15 minutes after intravenous injection of the iodine-based contrast medium, the calyces of both kidneys, the ureters, and the bladder can be seen.

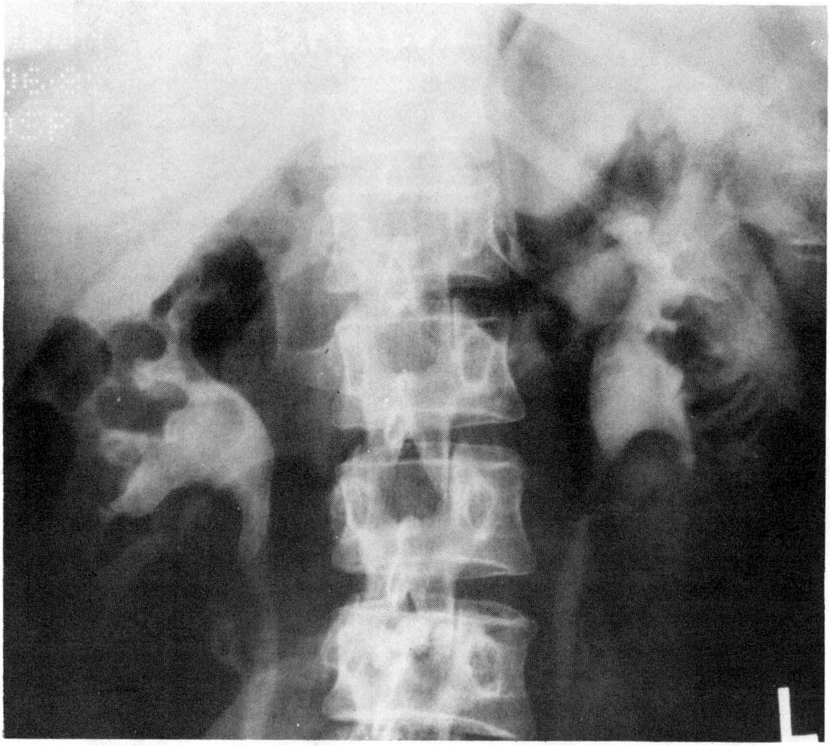

Fig. 6.6 Excretion urogram. (a) 5 minutes after injection of contrast. The ureters are opacified and the calyces also appear to be outlined by contrast (see b).

Micturating cystography

In this investigation a similar radiopaque medium is instilled into the bladder through a catheter passed with strict aseptic precautions. Cineradiograms are taken of the bladder, its outflow tract and the ureters, as the patient voids the dye. This test is important in the investigation of the bladder outflow tract, especially if vesico-ureteric reflex is suspected.

Computed tomography

The kidneys are easily examined in radiographic 'slices' of the body produced by computed X-ray tomography (CT). This technique is particularly useful for demonstrating collections of fluid (including cysts) and tumours (Figs. 6.8 and 6.9). Unlike ultrasound examination, CT scanning is helped rather than hindered by the presence of a lot of fat.

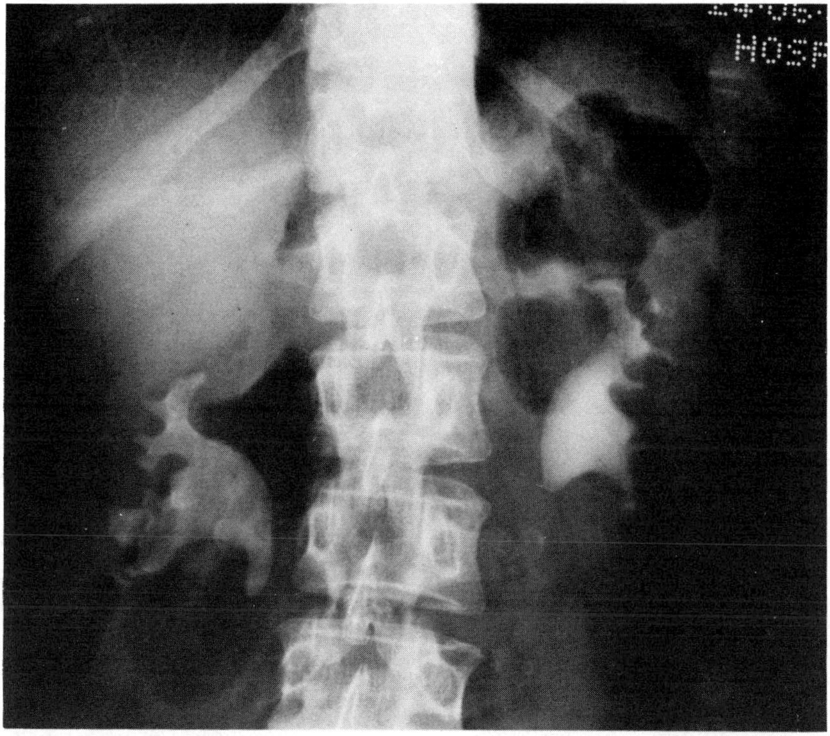

Fig. 6.6b Preliminary film, before contrast injection. The calyces are opacified by large staghorn calculi.

Ultrasound examination

The kidneys and their gross structure are relatively easily demonstrated, except in fat people, by ultrasound examination, in which the strength of echoes reflected from internal structures is used to build up an image. The technique is particularly useful for identifying collections of fluid (including cysts) and diagnosing outflow obstruction.

Interpretation of ultrasonic examinations is often difficult and the clinician is much more dependent on the doctor performing the test than he is for radiological investigations.

Radioisotope investigations

Radiographic and ultrasound techniques define the structure of organs well, but give comparatively little information about their function. The converse is true of radioisotope investigations. Their use is complex and the subject is rapidly developing. In studies of the urinary tract, radioisotopes (Figs. 6.10

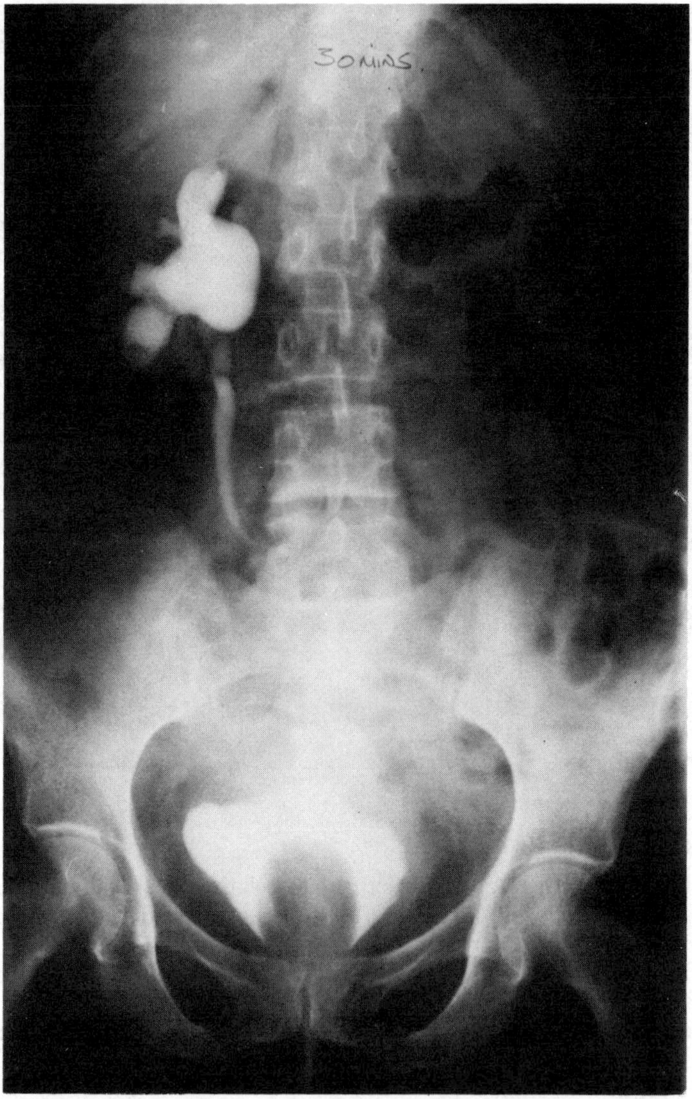

Fig. 6.7 Exretion urogram. In this film, made 30 minutes after injection of contrast, the left kidney fails to excrete a detectable concentration of contrast (non-functioning left kidney) and the right kidney shows dilated, hydronephrotic calyces. The right ureter is partially obstructed at the level of the body of the fifth lumbar vertebra. The circular lucency in the bladder is the dilated balloon of a Foley catheter.

(a)

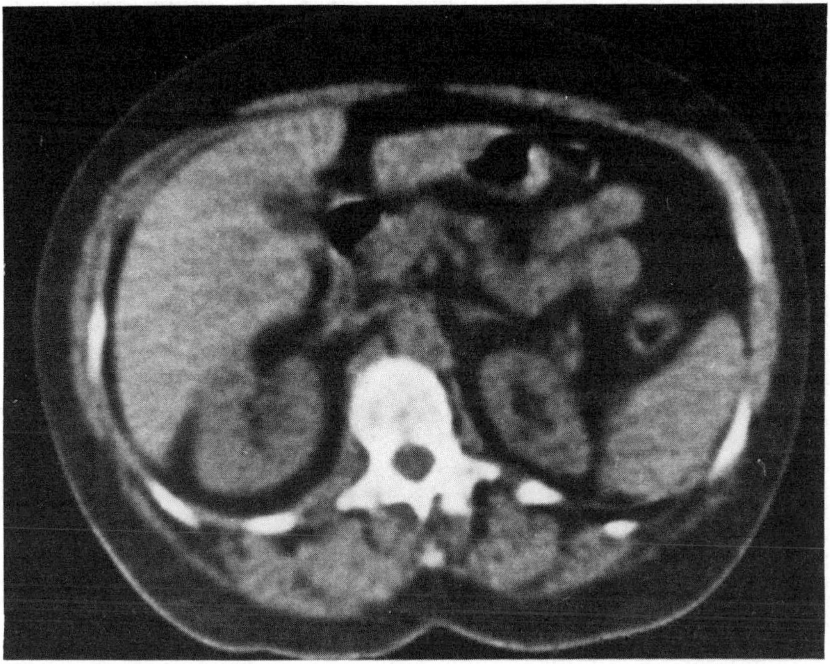

Fig. 6.8 (a) Computed tomographic scan (with drawing—b) showing normal kidneys. K = kidney; H = hilum; P = pelvis of kidney; A = aorta; I = intestine.

(b)

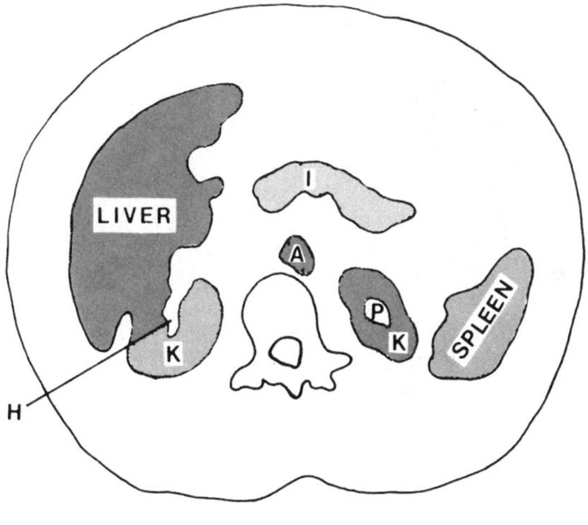

(a)

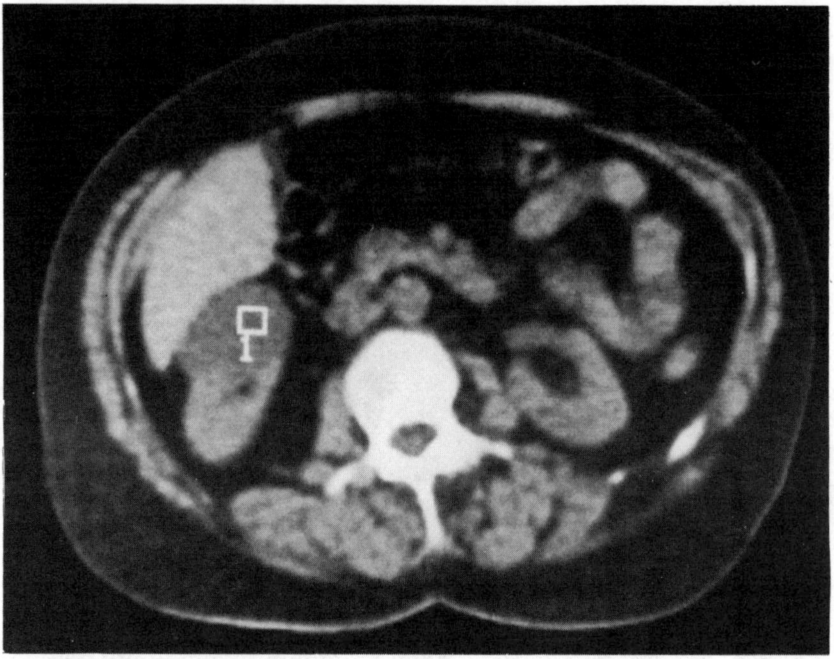

Fig. 6.9 (a) Computed tomographic scan (with drawing—b) showing cyst in right kidney. K = kidney; C = cyst in kidney; F = fat; M = muscle; IVC = inferior vena cava; I = intestine. ♀ denotes a region of interest (the cyst), in which measurements of tissue density can be made.

(b)

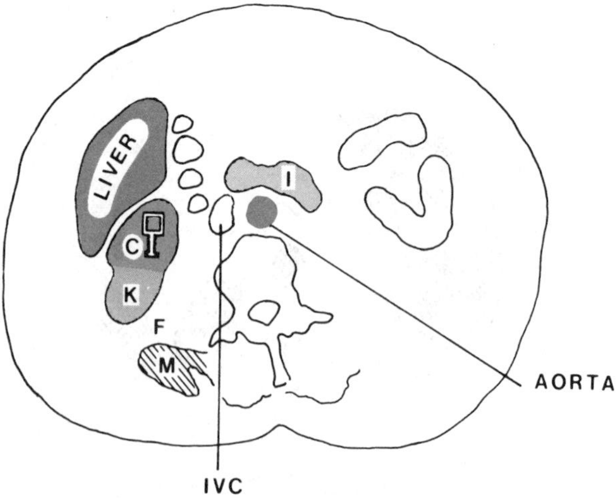

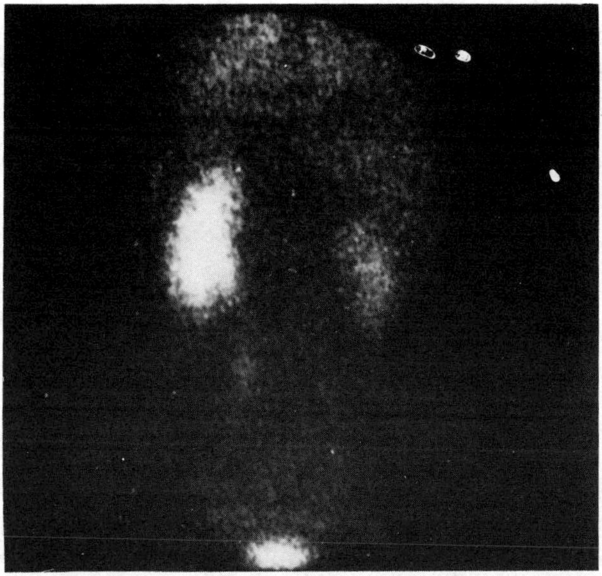

Fig. 6.10 Radioisotope gamma-camera scan of kidneys and bladder. The left kidney excretes more isotope than the right. The left ureter and the bladder can be seen (see also Fig. 6.11).

and 6.11) are most often used to measure glomerular filtration rate and similar aspects of renal function, to indicate the relative contribution of each kidney to overall renal function, to diagnose obstruction, and to assess bladder emptying and the retrograde passage of urine from bladder towards the kidney (vesico-ureteric reflux).

Cystoscopy and urethroscopy

The interiors of the bladder and urethra may be inspected through a cystoscope and urethroscope respectively. The main value of these procedures is in the diagnosis and treatment of tumours of the lining epithelium of the bladder and in assessment of the effects of disease of the prostate. It is possible to insert fine catheters through the cystoscope into the ureters, enabling urine from each kidney to be collected separately; by instilling contrast medium, radiographs of ureters, pelves and calyces can be taken.

Renal biopsy

By means of a special needle inserted into the back, biopsy specimens of the kidney may be obtained. Considerable skill is required and there is a small but definite risk to the patient. The method is of most clinical value in predicting

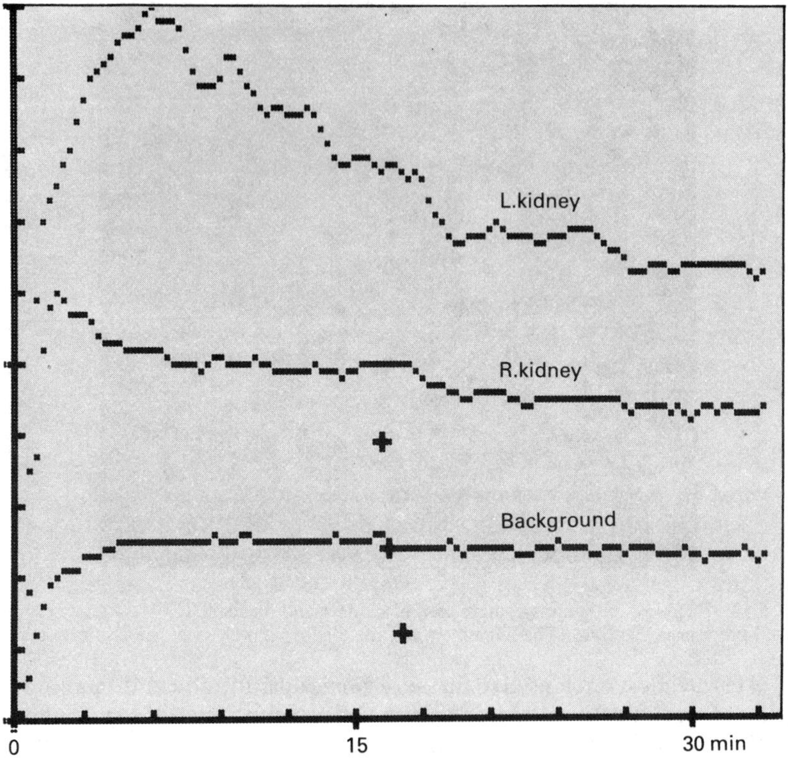

Fig. 6.11 Radioisotope excretion (ordinate) during the 30 minutes after intravenous injection in a patient with right renal artery stenosis and hypertension. The left kidney achieves more rapid excretion of isotope. The malfunctioning right kidney was the cause of the patient's hypertension.

the likely response to steroid therapy of certain patients with the nephrotic syndrome. It may also be valuable in the investigation of acute renal failure and in the diagnosis and assessment of systemic disorders such as amyloidosis and systemic lupus erythematosus.

7
The faeces

Examination of the faeces is an investigation of great importance all too easily omitted. No patient with bowel disturbance has been properly examined until the stools have been inspected. The white surface of a bedpan makes an ideal background for the detection of blood, pus and mucus.

NAKED-EYE INSPECTION

The following points should be noted:

The amount

It is sufficient to state whether the stools are copious or scanty.

Colour

Black stools may be produced by the ingestion of iron or bismuth. In haemorrhage occurring high up in the intestine the altered blood makes the stools dark, tarry-looking and very offensive, and all chemical tests for blood are strongly positive. *Pallor* of the stools may be due to lack of entrance of bile into the intestine, as in obstructive jaundice; to dilution and rapid passage of the stool through the intestine as in diarrhoea; or to an abnormally high fat content as in malabsorption.

Odour

The stools in jaundice are often very offensive. Cholera stools, on the other hand, contain very little organic matter, and are almost free from odour. The stools of acute bacillary dysentery are almost odourless, while those of amoebic dysentery have a characteristic odour, something like that of semen.

Form and consistency

In constipation the stools may be drier and harder than normal, and sometimes resemble sheep's stools. In all forms of diarrhoea they are more fluid than normal, and may be watery. Slimy stools are due to presence of an excess of mucus.

Abnormal ingredients

Abnormal ingredients can be detected by placing the stool on a fine sieve and adding a large quantity of water. The whole is shaken and stirred up till the soluble parts are all washed away. The residue is then examined. The head of a tapeworm can best be seen if this residue is strained through black muslin. The head is about as large as that of a large pin, and the neck about as thick as a stout thread.

Watery stools are found in all cases of profuse diarrhoea and after the administration of purgatives. To the stools of cholera the special name of *rice-water* stools is applied. Such a stool is colourless, almost devoid of odour, alkaline in reaction and contains a number of small flocculi consisting of shreds of epithelium and particles of mucus. Purulent or pus-containing stools are found in severe dysentery or ulcerative colitis, or in cases where an abscess has found its way into the intestines. Slimy stools are due to the presence of an excess of mucus, and point to an affection of the large bowel. The mucus may envelop the faecal masses or may be intimately mixed with them. Bloody stools vary in appearance according to the site of the haemorrhage. If the bleeding takes place high up, the stools look like tar. In an intussusception they may look like redcurrant jelly. If the haemorrhage is from the large intestine, the blood is less intimately mixed with the faecal matter, and may even be of a bright colour. In haemorrhage from the rectum or anus it may merely streak the faecal masses. The stools of bacillary dysentery consist at first of faecal material mixed with blood and pus, later of blood and pus without faecal material. Those of amoebic dysentery characteristically consist of fluid faecal material, mucus and small amounts of blood. The stools of steatorrhoea are very large, pale and putty-like or porridge-like and sometimes frothy. They are apt to stick to the sides of the lavatory pan and are difficult to flush away. If formed, they usually float.

CHEMICAL EXAMINATION

Tests for occult haemorrhage

Since benzidine ceased to be available, on account of a high incidence of carcinoma of the bladder in those who made it, orthotolidine has taken its place.

Orthotolidine test A portion of faeces the size of a pea is suspended in 5 ml of distilled water and boiled for 5 minutes. A 4% stock solution of orthotolidine in 95% ethyl alcohol is prepared. A 1 in 5 solution is made in glacial acetic acid. 1 ml of this reagent, 0.25 ml of the faecal suspension and 0.25 ml of hydrogen peroxide (20 vol. strength) are mixed in a test tube, and the result read in three minutes. A strong positive is indicated by a dark green colour and a weak positive by a pale green. This is a moderately sensitive test, and to avoid false positives the patient should have been on a meat-free diet for three days before the test and should not have been taking aspirin.

Hema-Chek slide test This test paper contains orthotolidine and strontium peroxide. A blue colour is produced when the test paper and developer are in contact with faeces containing blood.

A thin smear of faeces is made on the paper test 'slide' provided. The flap is closed and the paper 'slide' turned over. The flap is opened at the back and one or two drops of Hema-Chek developer are placed on the test area. A blue colour develops within 30 seconds if blood is present.

This test can be used on patients on a normal diet, but may not detect small amounts of gastrointestinal bleeding.

Both tests are of value in indicating the presence of gastrointestinal bleeding, but both may be negative in the presence of lesions which bleed intermittently or slightly, particularly those situated in the upper gastrointestinal tract. Spectroscopic methods and isotopic methods using radioactive chromium-labelled red cells are also available.

Fats in faeces

Fat is present in food as neutral fat or triglyceride. It is split to greater or lesser degree by lipases, mainly of the pancreas into glycerol and fatty acids. Some of the fatty acids, if unabsorbed, combine with bases to form soaps. Fat may, therefore, be found in the faeces as neutral fat, fatty acids and soaps.

The estimation of the proportion of split and unsplit fats present has been found unreliable as a method of distinguishing pancreatic from non-pancreatic steatorrhoea because of the effects of bacterial activity on neutral fats.

For the estimation of the fat in the stools, the patient may be placed on a diet containing 50 g of fat per day. The fat present in the stools collected over three or better five days is then estimated and should not exceed 6 g/day (or 12 g in three days). It has been found that equally reliable results are obtained if the patient eats a normal diet provided a three to five day collection is made.

MICROSCOPICAL EXAMINATION

See Protozoa (p. 169).

INTESTINAL PARASITES

The parasites which occur in the intestinal tract include worms and protozoa. Some of the nematode and cestode worms will be described.

Nematoda

The commonest of all internal parasites is the threadworm, *Enterobius vermicularis*, whose presence is associated with considerable itching about the anus. It inhabits the large intestines, caecum and appendix, and female specimens can often be seen wriggling about in the recently passed motion of their host. To the naked eye they look like small white threads, 0.5 to 1 cm in length. Under the microscope the female may be distinguished by her much larger size, by the large uterus filled with ova, and the pointed posterior end. For appearance of ovum, see Plate I.

Ascaris lumbricoides, the roundworm, has a general resemblance to an earthworm. It usually measures up to 25 cm but may be up to 33 cm long. The ova, which can occasionally be found in the faeces, have brownish-yellow granular contents, and in many cases the shell is surrounded by an irregular sheath (Plate I).

Ankylostoma duodenale, the hookworm, is an important cause of anaemia and debility in the tropics, where heavy infestations may occur. It is no longer indigenous in Great Britain, but may be found in immigrants. It lives for the most part in the upper part of the jejunum, and its presence there is probable when, in an infested district, severe anaemia, otherwise inexplicable, sets in. The diagnosis is confirmed by the discovery of ova in the motions (Plate I). They exhibit a segmented yolk enclosed in a thin shell, and are sufficiently numerous to be readily detected. The adult worm, which is rarely seen before therapeutic agents have been employed, is about 1 cm long, and the mouth is provided with four claw-like teeth.

Trichinella spiralis gains access to the body as the result of eating infested pork. Trichiniasis is rare when pork is eaten cooked, but small outbreaks and sporadic cases have been reported in Great Britain and in the USA. When man ingests the muscle trichinellae of the pig, larvae are set free in the small intestine, giving rise to the symptoms of the first stage of the illness—abdominal pain, vomiting and diarrhoea. The adult female, 3 mm long, penetrates the intestinal wall and discharges embryos into lymph spaces, whence they migrate into muscles. In this second stage of the illness the patient has fever and high eosinophilia and the muscles swell and become hard and tender. Rarely death may occur at the height of the myositis. Otherwise the embryo undergoes no further development, and its capsule becomes calcified. Unlike cysticerci, described below, calcified trichinellae are not visible in X-rays.

Cestoda

Many different kinds of tapeworm have been found as parasites in man, but the most important are *Taenia saginata*, *T. solium* and *Echinococcus granulosus*. Besides its occurrence in the fully developed state, *T. solium* may be present in the tissues in the form of a cysticercus; *T. saginata* is never found in this condition in man, whilst *E. granulosus* always occurs in the cystic stage, and has never been found in the mature condition in the human intestinal tract.

The presence of an adult tapeworm in the bowel is generally revealed by the passage of ripe proglottides in the stools, and, after the administration of antihelmintics, the head may be detected by the method previously described (p. 164).

Taenia saginata (mediocanellata) is the beef tapeworm. Infestation occurs as a result of consuming insufficiently cooked beef infested with the embryo of the worm. The adult parasite reaches a length of 4–8 m and consists of about 2000 segments. The ripe proglottides measure 13 by 6 mm. The head is quadrate, measures 2 mm in diameter, has 4 suckers, but is devoid of hooklets. The terminal gravid segments of the worm become separated from time to time and the ova may be then ingested by the bullock or cow, in the muscles of which the larva develops. It becomes a bladder worm, *Cysticercus bovis*, measuring 10 by 16 mm and containing an invaginated head which possesses in miniature the characteristics of the adult scolex. *Cysticercus bovis* is never found in human muscle tissue or brain. For appearance of ovum, see Plate I.

Taenia solium, the pork tapeworm, is not encountered in Britain but is endemic wherever infested pork is eaten raw or insufficiently cooked. It measures 2 to 4 m in length; a ripe proglottis is 10 by 5 mm. The head measures

1 mm in diameter and in addition to 4 suckers has a rostellum with 32 hooklets. The ova in the terminal proglottides may be ingested by the pig, in the muscles of which the bladder worm *Cysticercus cellulosae* develops. Occasionally persons in infected areas become infected with *Cysticercus cellulosae* from eating food contaminated with the ova of the parasite. The muscles of the human host are then infested by cysticerci, which are palpable through the skin as tense ovoid swellings 10 by 5 mm and of almost cartilaginous hardness. About four years after infestation they have become calcified and may then be demonstrated radiologically. The thigh muscles are those in which cysticerci are most easily demonstrated. Cysticerci may also occur in the brain and are a cause of epilepsy.

The adult stage of *Echinococcus granulosus*, which consists of a head and three segments, and whose length is only 3 to 8 mm, need not be fully described, since it is not found in man. The *cystic stage* is very important, as it gives rise to serious disease in man in many of the viscera and especially in the liver. The cysts of this are not simple, but produce from their inner surface one or two generations of secondary vesicles, on which the brood capsules, containing the cestode heads, are formed. During the period in which this process is going on, the primary vesicle dilates to accommodate its increasing contents, and may eventually reach the size of a coconut. The vesicles may rupture spontaneously, and their contents may escape by the lungs, the bowel or the urinary passages. Specimens may be obtained by aspiration or after surgical interference.

The diagnosis of suspected hydatid disease may rest upon the recognition of the nature of the fluid withdrawn, of hooklets or scolices, or the appearance of parts of the ectocyst, which are sometimes coughed up from the lungs. The Casoni intradermal test may be of some assistance, though cross reactions may occur in infestation with other cestodes.

The *fluid* is clear, alkaline, devoid of protein, and contains abundance of sodium chloride and traces of glucose. Its density is low, being generally under 1010. The *scolex*, if it is obtained in a perfect condition, is about 0.3 mm in diameter, and a number of them often spring in a group from one brood capsule. They have 4 suckers and a crown of hooklets. Portions of the *ectocyst* appear as whitish-yellow shreds, which can be recognized under the microscope by their lamination and by their pectinate markings on the laminae.

Diphyllobothrium latum (Dibothriocephalus latus), the fish tapeworm, is encountered in Sweden, Finland and Michigan. The adult worm measures from 3 to 10 m or more and has a total of 3000 segments. The scolex is small, spatula-shaped and possesses 2 deep suctorial grooves. The first larval host is a water flea and the second the pike, perch or salmon trout. Human infestation takes place from eating raw or undercooked fish. In a tiny proportion of cases, a vitamin B_{12} deficiency anaemia may be produced.

Trematodes

Schistosomes or blood flukes are the most important trematode parasites of man. They are found in three varieties, and produce the disease known as schistosomiasis or bilharziasis. *Schistosoma japonicum* and *Schistosoma mansoni* inhabit the portal blood stream, and the ova (Plate I) are passed in the faeces. *Schistosoma haematobium* characteristically inhabits the vesical plexus, so that the ova (Plate I) are passed in the urine (p. 150). They may occasionally also be found in the faeces. *Schistosoma mansoni* is found in Africa and South America; *Schistosoma haematobium* in Africa and the Near East, particularly in Egypt; and *Schistosoma japonicum* in the Orient.

Protozoa

A number of protozoa, many of them non-pathogenic, have been found in the faeces. Of these the most important clinically is *Entamoeba histolytica* (Plate I), which causes amoebic dysentery (as opposed to bacillary dysentery) and sometimes tropical abscess of the liver. *Entamoeba coli* (Plate I) is non-pathogenic.

Entamoeba histolytica is found in the stools in two forms. In acute attacks vegetative amoebae can generally be found, whilst in the more quiescent stage cysts are passed. So-called 'small' and 'large' races of *Entamoeba histolytica* have been described. It is likely that both are pathogenic.

If amoebic dysentery is suspected, a stool should be passed into a clean bedpan; this must be free from antiseptics, and the stool must not be mixed with urine. It should be taken immediately to the laboratory so that is is examined whilst warm.

With a platinum loop, select a piece of blood-stained mucus or, failing this, a small particle of faeces; emulsify it with a drop of warmed (37°C) normal saline and apply a cover-slip.

The diagnosis of vegetative *Entamoeba histolytica* depends for practical purposes on the demonstration of actively motile amoebae, which contain red cells. The slide must be examined on a heated stage, or, if this is not available, it may be kept warm by applying coins pre-heated in a Bunsen flame on each side of the cover-slip. Care must be taken not to overheat it. Motile amoebae are readily seen under the low power, and can be studied further under the 16 mm objective. Iodine will kill the amoebae, and must not be used.

Cysts can be seen under the low power as small round refractile bodies. They are seen even better if the stool is emulsified in 1% aqueous eosin, when, provided the stool is fresh, they show as white bodies against a pink background. The characteristic chromatoid bodies of *E. histolytica* are well shown by this method. Globules of oil or fat, which may be present in the faeces of patients who have been given oil as an aperient, may resemble them, and, if numerous, may make any attempt at further examination useless. Oil droplets vary in size, are structureless, and their edges cannot be sharply focused. If cysts are present, iodine should be used for their further identification. Make a further preparation using 1% Lugol's iodine. Find a suspected cyst under the low power. Apply the 16 mm objective and centre the cyst in the middle of the field. Rack up the microscope tube, apply a small drop of oil to the cover-slip without moving it, and carefully lower the oil-immersion objective into the drop. The main differences between *E. histolytica* and *E. coli* and their cysts are shown in Tables 7.1 and 7.2.

Table 7.1 *Entamoeba histolytica* and *Entamoeba coli*: vegetative forms

	Entamoeba histolytica	*Entamoeba coli*
Occurrence	Fairly abundant; when present, in amoebic dysenteric stools	Never abundant. Occasionally seen in dysenteric stools
Size	Variable, average 20 to 30 μm	Less variable. Generally larger than *E. histolytica*
Motility	Active. Large pseudopodia. These become larger as activity diminishes before death	Sluggish. Small cone-shaped pseudopodia
Cytoplasm	Homogeneous and 'ground-glass like'. Differentiation of ectoplasm and endoplasm clearly seen. Red blood corpuscles often seen	Appearance porcellanous. Ectoplasm less plentiful; line of demarcation between it and endoplasm inconspicuous. Endoplasm granular. Abundant food vacuoles with usually bacterial inclusions. Red blood corpuscles never present
Nucleus	Karyosome, not seen in unstained preparations, small and *central*. Periphery marked by ring-like layer of regular sized chromatin granules	Distinct. Karyosome usually large, irregular and *nearly always eccentric*. Ring-like layers of peripheral granules more pronounced and irregular in size and shape

Table 7.2 *Entamoeba histolytica* and *Entamoeba coli*: cysts

Entamoeba histolytica	*Entamoeba coli*
When mature, 4 nuclei, with nuclear karyosomes central. Peripheral chromatin often semilunar	When mature, 8 nuclei, with nuclear karyosomes usually eccentric
Size slightly smaller on average, varying from 10 to 20μm	Size slightly larger, varying from 10 to 20 μm
Glycogen less abundant	Glycogen more abundant
Refractility moderate	Refractility considerable
Rod-shaped 'chromidial bodies' usually seen in fresh specimen	'Chromatoid bodies' not often present: thread-like or in bundles when seen
Cyst wall rather thinner	Cyst wall rather thicker

Besides *E. coli*, there are three other non-pathogenic amoebae, which must not be mistaken for *E. histolytica*. They are *Endolimax nana*, *Iodamoeba bütschlii* and *Dientamoeba fragilis*. In the diagnosis of the vegetative forms this mistake will be avoided if it is remembered that *E. histolytica* alone is actively motile and contains red cells. The cysts of *Iodamoeba bütschlii* (Plate I) contain a single small nucleus, an eccentric karyosome and a very large compact mass of glycogen.

Giardia lamblia is a flagellete protozoon, which inhabits the duodenum and may be found in the stools of patients with diarrhoea in both cystic and vegetative form (Plate I). There is some doubt whether it is pathogenic. The fact that a course of metronidazole will eradicate it, with relief of the diarrhoea, suggests that it is.

Trichomonas hominis (Plate I) is another flagellate protozoon which may be seen in the stools in diarrhoea. It is probably non-pathogenic. Similar if not identical trichomonads may be found in the vagina in leucorrhoea and in the mouth in oral sepsis.

Isospora belli (I. hominis) (Plate I), one of a group of parasites which may produce coccidiosis in man, animals and birds, has occasionally been described as the cause of acute diarrhoea in man, particularly in the eastern Mediterranean.

Balantidium coli (Plate I) is a large ciliate protozoon found in the intestine of pigs. It occasionally infects man, and may rarely cause severe diarrhoea or frank dysentery.

8
The respiratory system

ANATOMICAL LANDMARKS

Lobes of the lungs

It is important to know the limits of the individual lobes. A line from the second thoracic spine to the sixth rib in the mammary line corresponds to the upper border of the lower lobe (the major interlobar fissure). A horizontal line on the right side from the sternum at the level of the fourth costal cartilage, drawn to meet the first, marks the boundary between the upper and middle lobes (the minor interlobar fissure). The greater part of each lung, as seen from behind, is composed of the lower lobe, only the apex belonging to the upper lobe; while the middle and upper lobes on the right side, and the upper lobe on the left, occupy most of the area in front. In the axillary regions, parts of all the lobes are accessible.

The bifurcation of the trachea corresponds in front with the lower border of the manubrium sterni, that is with the angle of Louis, and behind with the disc between the fourth and fifth thoracic vertebrae.

The ribs are best counted downwards from the second costal cartilage. This cartilage articulates with the sternum at the extremities of the angle of Louis, a transverse bony ridge at the junction of the body and the manubrium which is easily felt beneath the skin.

Anatomy of the bronchi

The two main bronchi each give off four main branches; on the right, one to the upper lobe, one to the middle lobe, one to the dorsal lobe (the upper and posterior part of the lower lobe), and one to the remainder of the lower lobe; and on the left, one to the upper lobe proper, one to the lingular process of the upper lobe (which represents the middle lobe on the left side), and a dorsal and a lower lobe bronchus as on the right side. These main bronchi then divide into segmental bronchi, which supply individual segments of lung. It is useful to know about these segments, because it is often possible from the signs and X-ray appearance to determine which segment and which segmental bronchus

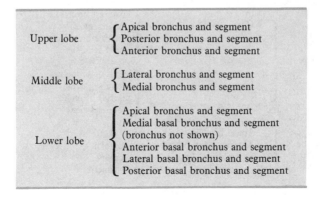

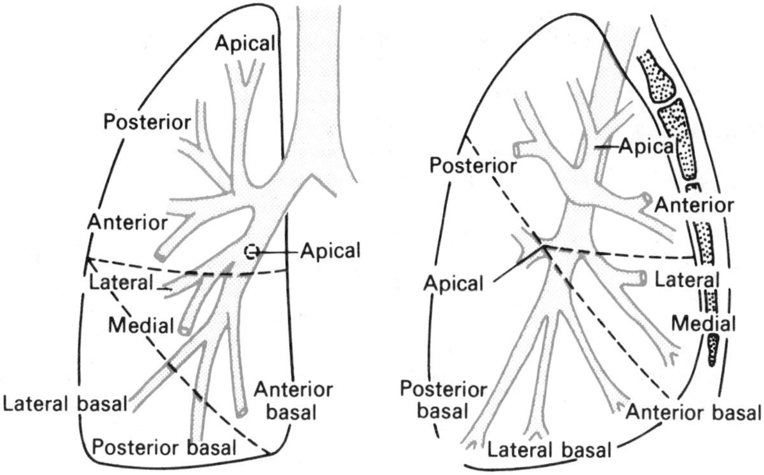

Fig. 8.1 The right lung (anterior and lateral aspects) showing the segmental bronchi. The dotted lines represent interlobar fissures.

Upper lobe	Apical bronchus and segment Posterior bronchus and segment Anterior bronchus and segment
Middle lobe	Lateral bronchus and segment Medial bronchus and segment
Lower lobe	Apical bronchus and segment Medial basal bronchus and segment (bronchus not shown) Anterior basal bronchus and segment Lateral basal bronchus and segment Posterior basal bronchus and segment

is affected by disease. The accompanying diagrams (Figs. 8.1–8.3) give a simplified scheme of the anatomy of the segmental bronchi and indicate the 'respiratory districts' or bronchopulmonary segments supplied by them.

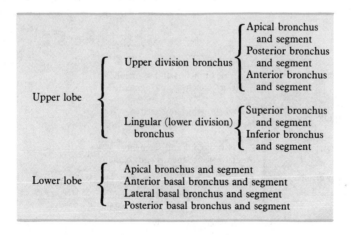

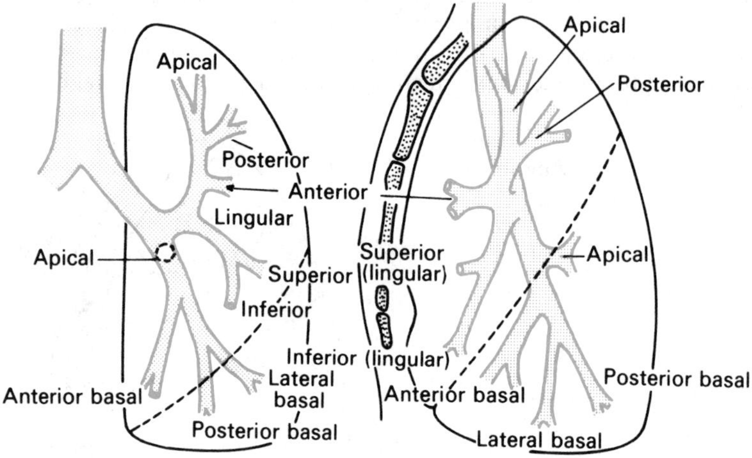

Fig. 8.2 The left lung (anterior and lateral aspects) showing the segmental bronchi. The dotted lines represent the interlobar fissure.

Upper lobe	Upper division bronchus	Apical bronchus and segment Posterior bronchus and segment Anterior bronchus and segment
	Lingular (lower division) bronchus	Superior bronchus and segment Inferior bronchus and segment
Lower lobe	Apical bronchus and segment Anterior basal bronchus and segment Lateral basal bronchus and segment Posterior basal bronchus and segment	

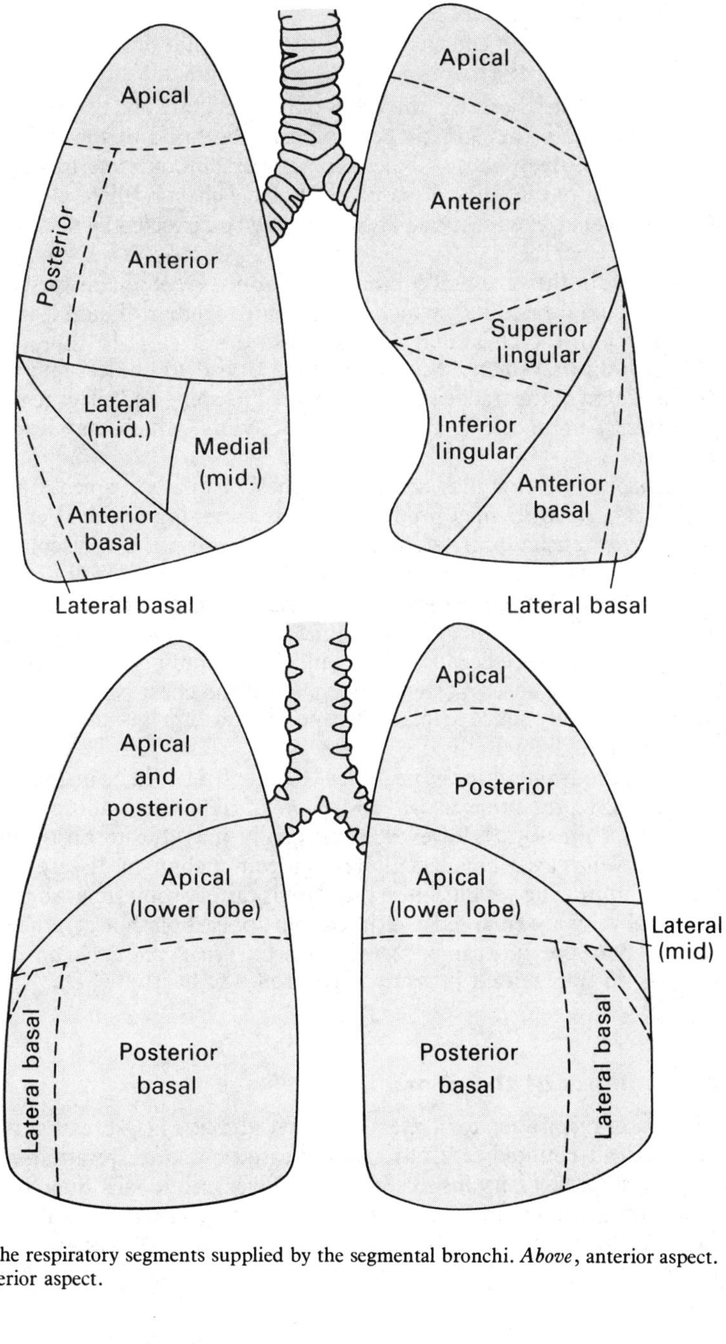

Fig. 8.3 The respiratory segments supplied by the segmental bronchi. *Above*, anterior aspect. *Below*, posterior aspect.

INSPECTION

Form of the chest

The shape of the chest, the thickness of its subcutaneous tissues and the slope of the shoulders vary greatly according to the build of the individual. The short, broad, deep chest of the thickset person contrasts to the long, flat, narrow chest of the tall and spare. The normal chest is bilaterally symmetrical and elliptical in cross section. The chest may be distorted by disease of the ribs or spinal vertebrae.

Disease of the vertebral column can produce *kyphosis* (forward bending) or *scoliosis* (lateral bending), which often occur together. These lead to obvious asymmetry of the chest and may decrease the size of the thoracic cage and restrict lung movement. Scoliosis may also lead to clinical and radiological displacement of the trachea and apex beat. The spine and rib cage may become particularly immobile in ankylosing spondylitis, which may lead to a fixed kyphosis.

Pulmonary disease may deform the chest. Unilateral apical fibrosis, often due to tuberculosis, may produce obvious flattening of the affected apex; in children, extensive unilateral fibrosis or collapse can cause scoliosis. Severe *obstructive airways disease* leads to a barrel-shaped chest. Expiration is obstructed so that the lungs are over-inflated and the chest is relatively fixed in full inspiration. The ribs are set less obliquely than normal and tend to move upwards in one piece because of the pull of the prominent accessory muscles of respiration. The anteroposterior diameter of the chest is increased, the spine becoming unduly concave forwards, and the sternum is arched forwards with a prominent angle of Louis.

The venous pulses in the neck (see Chapter 9) should be inspected. A raised venous pulse pressure is usually indicative of right heart failure, i.e. increased right atrial pressure. However, occasionally it is due to obstruction of the superior vena cava. This usually results from malignant disease in the upper mediastinum. The venous pulse pressure is raised, sometimes so much so that the facial veins are enlarged and the patient appears plethoric; if the upper level of the venous pressure can be seen in the neck, *venous pulsations are absent*, since there is no transmitted pressure wave from the heart.

Movements of the chest

The rate of respiration for a relaxed normal adult is 14–18 breaths/minute. The rate must be counted carefully. An increased rate of respiration, *tachypnoea*, may be caused by nervousness, exertion, fever or hypoxia. Such hypoxia may be due to cardiac, pulmonary, bronchial or laryngeal causes, to altered oxygen-carrying capacity of the blood or to interference with the reflex control of respiration. When breathing is painful, as in pleurisy or peritonitis, it is shallow and rapid to compensate for the reduced expansion.

The respiratory rhythm varies in health, particularly if the breathing is performed consciously, so the rhythm has to be noted when the patient is off his guard. Laryngeal and tracheal diseases may prolong inspiration; bronchial and pulmonary diseases tend to prolong expiration. Irregular breathing is usually not due to organic disease, but occurs terminally in patients with brain stem disease. A characteristic type of disturbed ventilatory rhythm, in which successive respirations gradually get deeper and deeper till a maximum is attained, and then fall off again until a pause of complete apnoea occurs, to be followed by another wave of gradually deepening and then diminishing respiration, is known as *Cheyne–Stokes breathing*. The pause may last for half a minute, though it is often shorter, and the whole cycle is usually completed in less than two minutes. It is most conspicuous when the patient who exhibits it is asleep or unconscious, but may be overlooked if the patient is awake, and particularly if he is talking. Cheyne–Stokes breathing occurs most commonly in cardiac and renal failure, severe pneumonia, increased intracranial pressure and other bilateral brain lesions, and narcotic drug poisoning. A spontaneous and sustained increased depth and rate of ventilation occurs in patients with cardiopulmonary disease, in whom gas exchange is disturbed and the amount of carbon dioxide in the blood is increased, in metabolic acidosis and in certain pontine brain stem lesions (*central pontine hyperventilation*).

Note the movement of the chest and whether it is expansile and symmetrical. Movement and expansion are not interchangeable terms; in emphysema the chest may move considerably, but there is little expansion. Chest expansion in men can be measured with a tape measure round the chest just below the nipples. In a fit young man it may be 5–8 cm; in emphysema it may be 1 cm or less.

Diminished or absent expansion may be due to pleural effusion, pneumothorax, consolidation, collapse, fibrosis or the presence of a neoplasm. It is also found in tuberculosis and lobar pneumonia, the former especially at the apices, the latter at the apex or base according to the situation of the disease.

PALPATION

Before making a systematic examination, it is useful to palpate any part of the chest which presents an obvious swelling or where the patient complains of pain.

Feel gently, as pressure may increase the pain, as in the case of pleurisy. Pain and tenderness may be due to recent injury to the chest wall, or to inflammatory conditions; to intercostal muscular pain, where, as a rule, especially painful spots can be discovered on pressure; to a painful costochondral junction; to secondary malignant deposits in the ribs; to herpes zoster, before the appearance of the eruption; or to pleurisy. Pain may also be due to cardiac causes, such as coronary thrombosis and pericarditis. The nature of any swelling should be investigated. Fluctuation occurs when an abscess has formed in the chest wall.

The positions of the cardiac impulse and trachea should then be determined. Feel for the trachea in the suprasternal notch and decide whether it is central or deviated to one side by its relation to the suprasternal notch and the insertion of the sternomastoids. Slight deviation of the trachea to the right may be found in healthy people. Displacement of the cardiac impulse alone may be due to scoliosis (the commoner form with its convexity to the right causing a displacement of the cardiac impulse to the left and vice versa), to funnel depression of the sternum or to enlargement of the left ventricle. In the absence of these conditions, a significant displacement of the cardiac impulse or trachea, or of both together, suggests that the position of the mediastinum has been altered by disease of the lungs or pleura. The mediastinum is 'pushed' away from the affected side by pleural effusion and pneumothorax; fibrosis or collapse of the lung will draw the mediastinum towards the affected side. In fibrosis or collapse of the upper lobe of a lung, the trachea only is displaced.

The *nature of the respiratory movements* must next be studied. Make certain that the two sides of the chest move to approximately the same extent. This is done by fixing the fingertips of either hand at the patient's sides and making the tips of the thumbs just meet in the middle line in front of the chest. As the patient takes a deep breath the increasing distance between the thumbs indicates the degree of expansion. The causes of diminished expansion have been mentioned under 'Inspection'.

Vibrations may be detected by palpation with the palm of the hand placed flat on the chest. The patient is then asked to repeat 'one, one, one', or 'ninety-nine', in a clear voice. The examining hand detects distinct vibration whilst this is done and one must determine whether the vibrations in corresponding areas on the two sides of the chest are approximately equal in intensity; do not, however, forget that where the heart encroaches on the left lung the fremitus is much diminished. *Vocal fremitus is increased* when the lung is consolidated, or contains a large cavity near the surface. *Vocal fremitus is diminished* when the corresponding bronchi are obstructed, or totally absent when the lung is separated from the chest wall by a pleural effusion. In this case the collapsed lung fails to convey the vibrations to the fluid; fluid itself is a good conductor of sound. In young persons and women, the vocal resonance is different both in character and intensity from that in male adults.

PERCUSSION

Method of percussion The middle finger of the left hand is placed firmly on the part which is to be percussed. The back of its middle phalanx is then struck with the tip of the middle finger of the right hand. The stroke should be delivered from the wrist and finger joints, not from the elbow, and the percussing finger should be so bent that when the blow is delivered its terminal phalanx is at right angles to the metacarpal bones and strikes the pleximeter finger perpendicularly. As soon as the blow has been given, the striking finger must be raised, just as the hammers of a piano fall back from the wires as soon as these have been struck. The blow should be no heavier than is necessary to elicit the resonance of the part being examined, and the wrist joint must move loosely. Repeated heavy blows cause much discomfort to patients. The *character of the sound produced* varies quantitatively and qualitatively. When the air in a cavity of sufficient size and appropriate shape is set into vibrations which are not modified by excessive tension of the containing walls of the space, the sound heard has a tympanitic character, as heard on percussion over an air-containing viscus, such as the stomach; but when the cavity is subdivided into a number of small loculi by numerous septa, more or less tense, a characteristic resonance, no longer tympanitic, is produced. The sound and feel of resonance over the healthy lung has to be learnt by practice. In general terms, this pulmonary resonance is low in pitch and clear in character.

Beginning in front, the examiner should tap lightly and directly (i.e. without pleximeter finger) on the most prominent point of each clavicle—being sure that the points examined correspond exactly with each other—and should observe the quality of the sound, and particularly whether the effects on the two sides are identical. Thereafter the other corresponding areas on either side should be carefully percussed in the manner already described. The presence of the heart will interfere, in parts of the left side, with the development of a sound resembling that from the corresponding point on the right. The back and axillary regions should then be examined in the same manner.

It is essential in all parts of the examination that the patient's attitude is a comfortable one and that his arms and shoulders are placed symmetrically, whether he is sitting up or lying down. When a very ill patient can only be examined at the back by rolling him on to his side, only gross differences in the note on the two sides are significant. If possible the patient should be examined lying first on one side and then on the other. Should the patient's chest be asymmetrical, from scoliosis or other cause, equal resonance on the two sides is not to be expected and again only gross differences between the two sides are significant.

The observer should have two objects in mind; first, to make a comparison of the percussion note in comparable areas on the two sides; and second, to map out the limits of lung resonance particularly at the apices, the bases and the area of cardiac dullness.

The *normal degree of resonance* varies from individual to individual and in different parts of the chest in the same individual, being most resonant below the clavicles and scapulae where the muscles are relatively thin, and least resonant over the scapulae.

The lower limits of lung resonance should be determined by percussing from above downwards. The *lower border of the right lung* lies over the liver and is thin; therefore its exact situation is best made out by light percussion. Posteriorly, however, the muffling due to the thick muscles and fat of the back makes it necessary to percuss more firmly. When the patient is obese, very heavy percussion may be necessary. In quiet respiration and on light percussion the lower border is found to lie in the mammary line at the sixth rib, in the mid-axillary line at the eighth rib, in the scapular line at the tenth rib. On heavier percussion some loss of resonance, due to the underlying liver and diaphragm, is found at higher levels and in the mammary line can be detected from the fourth interspace downwards.

On the left side the lower border overlaps the stomach and so the transition is not from lung resonance to dullness, but to tympanitic stomach resonance. Posteriorly, however, the splenic dullness and the dullness of the various solid structures which lie below the lung near the spine are interposed, so that the conditions resemble those found on the right. The position of the lower border corresponds pretty closely with that on the right side; it may, however, be found a trifle further down.

Resonance is increased when the pleural cavity contains air and the lung is more or less collapsed towards the hilum. The note varies from one that is hyper-resonant to one that is distinctly tympanitic, according to the amount of air in the pleural cavity.

A characteristic form of high-pitched tympanitic bell-like resonance may sometimes be heard in pneumothorax by percussion over the front of the chest with a couple of coins (one used as a plexor and the other as a pleximeter) whilst the observer listens with the stethoscope at the back of the patient. This sign is, however, absent in many cases of pneumothorax.

Although a definite tympanitic sound is found in pneumothorax, some observers have difficulty in recognizing this as definite '*hyper*-resonance' though recognizing it as being distinctly resonant. Such a sound may be found over some large cavities. In the diagnosis of emphysema it is more important to note the increased limits of resonance with loss of liver and cardiac dullness than the quality of the resonance.

Resonance is diminished when the pleura is thickened, when the underlying lung is more solid than usual for any reason, and when the pleural cavity contains fluid. Thus there may be slight impairment of resonance at one apex in a case of pulmonary tuberculosis due to local infiltration and fibrosis. Considerable impairment may be found over areas of lung affected by fibrosis or collapse. Percussion over a completely consolidated lobe produces a definitely dull note, whilst absolute dullness along with a peculiar sensation of resistance in the percussing finger, so-called 'stony dullness', is the characteristic finding over a pleural effusion of any size. In heart failure, impaired resonance or dullness may be found at the bases of both lungs, indicating oedema of the bases or bilateral effusions.

Myotatic irritability In certain conditions the muscles on the front of the thorax are unduly irritable, and a light tap over the sternum produces contractions, at some distance off, in the pectoral muscles. This phenomenon occurs in any wasting disease, and is known as myotatic irritability or myoidema. It is also found occasionally in healthy subjects.

AUSCULTATION

Three observations must be made at each point auscultated: first, the character of the breath sounds; second, the character of the vocal resonance; and third, the presence or absence of other sounds.

For good auscultation, a patient in bed should lean back against pillows, or lie on his back, and be completely relaxed. To examine the back, the patient should sit up, but if he is unable to do this he should be rolled round first to one side then to the other. In very ill patients the minimum necessary examination should be done. Take care that the chest-piece is accurately applied, that it is not allowed to move on the surface of the skin, and that no undue pressure is exerted. The patient should breathe with his mouth open, regularly and fairly deeply, but not noisily.

Breath sounds

There are two main types of breath sound (see Fig. 8.4). *Vesicular* breath sounds are produced by the passage of air in and out of normal lung tissue. Vesicular breathing is heard all over the healthy chest and, most typically, in the axillary and infrascapular regions. Throughout inspiration the sound is fairly intense and of low pitch with a characteristic rustle. There is no distinct pause before the expiratory sound, which is heard only in the early part of expiration. Normally the inspiratory sound is heard for at least twice as long as the expiratory sound. *Bronchial breath sounds* are produced by the passage of air through the trachea and large bronchi. Bronchial breathing is heard normally over the trachea, where it is very intense. The bronchial breathing heard over a diseased lung is far less intense but of the same quality. The inspiratory sound of bronchial breathing is harsh and aspirate, becoming inaudible shortly before the end of inspiration. The expiratory sound has the same character but

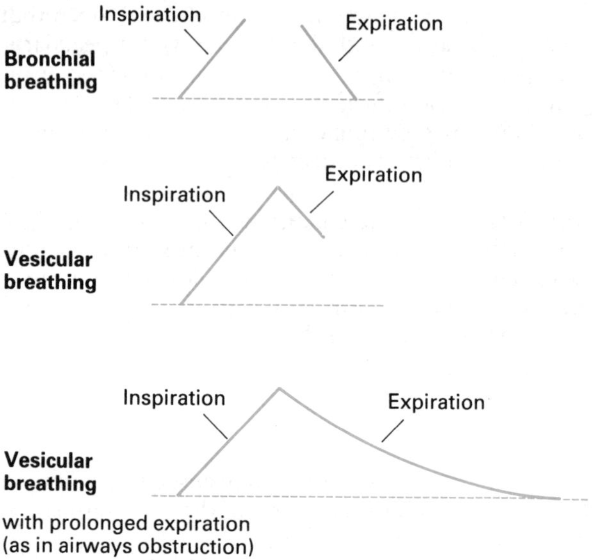

Fig. 8.4 Respiratory sounds.

is more intense and of higher pitch than the inspiratory; the sound lasts through most of expiration. Bronchial breathing is recognized best by the quality of the expiratory sound and the silent gap between inspiration and expiration. The slow expiration so characteristic of asthma and emphysema prolongs the normal expiratory sound but this is not to be confused with bronchial breathing.

The sound of breathing heard over a superficial bronchus combines bronchial and vesicular elements. This is *bronchovesicular breathing* with the expiratory sound having the more bronchial character. This type of breathing is heard normally near the root of the lungs behind and in the apical portions near the midline in front. It is more obvious over the right apex where the trachea is in immediate contact with the lung; at the left apex the aorta, internal carotid artery and oesophagus separate the trachea from the lung.

The intensity and quality of the breath sounds must be listened for in the regions already examined by percussion and the two sides of the chest accurately compared.

Breath sounds of any kind will be diminished or absent if their conduction is prevented by pleural thickening or effusion or by pneumothorax. They may also be absent if the nearest bronchus is occluded and no air is entering or leaving the alveoli; this may be found in collapse or fibrosis of the lung. Vesicular breath sounds will be diminished over any part of the lung where air is entering some but not all alveoli, as in bronchopneumonia. Bronchial breathing will be heard wherever the bronchus is patent and air is not entering the alveoli. This occurs classically over consolidated lung, occasionally over a large cavity and very rarely over a pleural effusion.

Vocal resonance

Palpation for vocal fremitus is closely allied to listening to *the intensity and character of the vocal resonance*. When the patient repeats the words 'one, one, one', or 'ninety-nine', the ear perceives, not the distinct syllables, but a resonant sound, the intensity of which depends on the loudness and depth of the patient's voice and on the conductivity of his lungs; the nearer the stethoscope is to a large bronchus, the more intense the sound.

Each point examined on one side of the chest should be at once compared with the corresponding point on the other side. Vocal resonance of normal intensity generally conveys the impression of being produced just at the chest-piece of the stethoscope. If it seems to be nearer the ear than this, the resonance is increased. When it appears to be near the earpiece of the stethoscope the increase is marked and the condition is often described as *bronchophony*.

If the words become clear and seem to be spoken right into the auscultator's ear, it will generally be found that whispered words are distinctly heard. This condition is called *whispering pectoriloquy*. Increased resonance occurs when the lung substance conducts the sound waves set up by the voice more clearly than usual from the bronchi. Consolidation is the commonest cause. Bronchophony and whispering pectoriloquy occur when a moderately large bronchus is surrounded by layer of solid lung reaching to the chest wall, as in lobar pneumonia. Whispering pectoriloquy is also fairly characteristic of a cavity of some size communicating with a bronchus and may be heard above the level of a pleural effusion. In some cases a certain degree of pectoriloquy is heard in health in the proximity of the trachea and large bronchi and particularly at the right apex.

Vocal resonance is either abolished or much diminished where a layer of fluid separates the lung from the chest wall (except when bronchial breathing is heard, see above) and in pneumothorax. It is also diminished in cases of thickened pleura and of emphysema.

Above the level of a pleural effusion or in some cases over an area of consolidation, the voice may sound nasal or bleating; this is known as *aegophony*.

Added sounds

Added sounds may arise in the lung or in the pleura. Sounds resembling pleural friction may be produced by movement of the stethoscope on the patient's skin, or of the observer's hands or clothes against the stethoscope. Sounds arising in the patient's muscles may resemble adventitious sounds and in particular the shivering of a cold patient makes any attempt at auscultation useless. The stethoscope rubbing over hairy skin may produce sounds indistinguishable from crepitations. Sounds resembling coarse crepitations may also be heard over a broken rib.

The nomenclature of the added sounds arising in the lung has been confused since their original description by Laennec. He introduced the French word *râle* to describe any added sound heard in the chest and also used the Latin word *rhonchus* in the same connotation. The least confusing classification of added sounds is to divide them into continuous wheezing sounds, or *rhonchi*, and interrupted bubbling or crackling sounds, or *crepitations*. Many British doctors merely use the terms 'wheezes' and 'crackles'.

Rhonchi, which are prolonged uninterrupted noises, arise in the bronchi and are due to partial obstruction of their lumen, by swelling of the mucosa, by viscid secretion or by constriction of bronchial smooth muscle often associated with turbulent air flow within the lumen. They may be high or low pitched, depending on whether they arise in small or large bronchial tubes. High-pitched rhonchi are called *sibilant* and have a squeaky quality; low-pitched rhonchi are called *sonorous* and have a snoring quality. They may also be palpable. Rhonchi are characteristic of bronchitis and asthma, and in the latter are high-pitched and expiratory. When they are localized to one side of the chest, the possibility of a localized obstruction of a bronchial tube should be considered, as for example in bronchial carcinoma. The word 'bronchospasm' as a description of a physical sign should be avoided.

Crepitations are discontinuous crackling or bubbling sounds. They may be produced in the alveoli, bronchi or, occasionally, in cavities. There are several types of crepitation produced by different mechanisms. They may be heard at any time in the respiratory cycle but are most commonly heard at the beginning of inspiration.

Fine crepitations are thought to be due to the presence of fluid in the alveoli as occurs in heart failure or the early stages of pneumonia when there is exudate in the alveoli.

Coarse crepitations can be produced by two distinct mechanisms. First, they can occur as bubbling or clicking sounds due to secretion in the bronchi in bronchitis and bronchiectasis. Second, in fibrosing alveolitis a more crackling sound is characteristically heard, especially in early inspiration. This is thought to be due to the sudden 'snapping open' of the relatively stiff alveoli that are associated with fibrosis. Such crepitations are usually only present at the lung bases.

A few crepitations may be heard in health, particularly at the lower borders of the lungs. These are abolished if the patient is asked to cough and are of no significance. In other cases crepitations are intensified after a cough or may only then make their appearance; these are known as *post-tussive crepitations*. They are an important sign of tuberculous infiltration, and may also be heard over cavities.

A *friction sound* or *pleural rub* is characteristic of pleurisy at the stage when exudation is not abundant enough to separate the inflamed and roughened pleural surfaces. It has a creaking or rubbing character, often quite characteristic, but sometimes rather hard to distinguish from a crepitation. The friction sound may be fine or coarse. In some instances it is palpable, but, since coarse crepitations may also be palpated sometimes, this does not distinguish them. The chief differences are that pleural friction sounds occur during that part of inspiration when the roughened surfaces are rubbing against each other, and reappear at a corresponding period of expiration. They are, moreover, unchanged after the patient has coughed, whereas crepitations may alter under these conditions because of changes in disposition of the secretion which causes them.

Finally there are certain manifestations of pulmonary disease which should be looked for outside the chest itself. These include clubbing of the fingers and cyanosis (both mentioned in previous chapters), and enlargement of cervical or axillary lymph nodes or of the liver from secondary carcinoma. Respiratory failure with carbon dioxide retention (p. 192) may be associated with certain neurological signs. These include a coarse flapping tremor of the hands (*asterixis*), generalized twitching movements and even convulsions. Such patients may become drowsy or stuporose and this is aggravated by sedatives or injudicious oxygen therapy. In some cases there is papilloedema.

THE SPUTUM

Sputum may be mucoid, purulent or frothy. Any of these varieties may contain blood, or the sputum may consist entirely of blood.

Mucoid sputum occurs characteristically in chronic bronchitis when secondary infection is not present. It is clear, tough and sticky and usually scanty. Particularly tenacious sputum may be found in asthma. This may block the bronchi by forming plugs, or else be coughed up as 'casts' of the bronchial tree—during or after an attack; alternatively, sticky particles like sago may be expectorated after an attack.

Mucopurulent sputum is seen in bronchitis (or other upper respiratory infections) when secondary bacterial infection has occurred: the sputum in bronchitis may also be frankly purulent.

Purulent sputum is thick and yellow (or green) and not sticky. It may occur in any condition in which infection is present and is characteristic of bronchiectasis, bronchopneumonia and lung abscess. In bronchiectasis and lung abscess it may be copious and its expectoration may be readily influenced by change of posture.

Frothy sputum, characteristic of pulmonary oedema, may be white or pink and is often copious.

Blood may be coughed up alone, or the sputum may be more or less blood-stained. It must be distinguished from blood brought into the mouth from epistaxis or haematemesis. Its brighter colour and its frothy appearance usually makes its origins obvious. Further, patients who have had a haemoptysis commonly bring up blood-stained sputum for a day or two, while bleeding from the upper intestinal tract is characteristically followed by melaena. Haemoptysis may be due to pulmonary causes, including tuberculosis, bronchiectasis, pulmonary embolus and carcinoma, and to cardiac causes, including mitral stenosis.

Several diseases cause a characteristic coloration of the sputum. In lobar pneumonia it may be rusty and so viscid that it will often not fall out of an inverted spittoon; it is bright yellow or green when a liver abscess has ruptured into the lung, and the latter colour also appears in some cases of pneumonia. When an amoebic hepatic abscess has discharged into the lung, the sputum has the appearance of anchovy sauce.

The quantity of sputum coughed up in 24 hours is important, especially whether change of position produces a large quantity. Bronchitic patients bring up most sputum during the first two hours after waking in the mornings.

The odour of the sputum is also important; it may be putrid in bronchiectasis or lung abscess.

Microscopical examination of sputum

The principal value of microscopical examination of the sputum is in the detection of bacteria and in the recognition of malignant cells. Eosinophils may be found in the sputum in allergic conditions, e.g. some cases of asthma, and in pneumonia due to parasitic worms and in aspergillosis.

Malignant cells may be seen in the sputum, particularly in patients with squamous carcinomas of the main bronchi. Skill is required to differentiate them from epithelium and other cellular debris, but their appearance is often unmistakable (Plate XIV).

Less common constituents of the sputum include fungi, yeasts and golden yellow asbestos bodies in asbestosis.

X-RAY EXAMINATION

Radiological examination of the chest is most important, because many localized and even some widespread infiltrative lesions (e.g. sarcoidosis) may produce no abnormal physical signs. It is paramount in the early diagnosis of tuberculosis and carcinoma. Serial X-rays form an integral part of the estimation of progress in many chest diseases. A brief outline of the standard methods will be given here.

Radiography

Posterior–anterior view

The ordinary standard X-ray film of the chest is a postero-anterior view, that is to say one taken with the film against the front of the patient's chest and the X-ray tube 2 metres behind the patient (Fig. 8.5). It is examined systematically on a viewing box. The following is a simple plan of examination:

1 *The bony skeleton*. Is the chest symmetrical? Is any scoliosis present? Are the ribs unduly crowded or widely spaced in any area? Are cervical ribs present? Are the ribs eroded or do they appear the site of malignant deposits?

2 *The position of the patient*. Is the patient straight or rotated? If straight, the

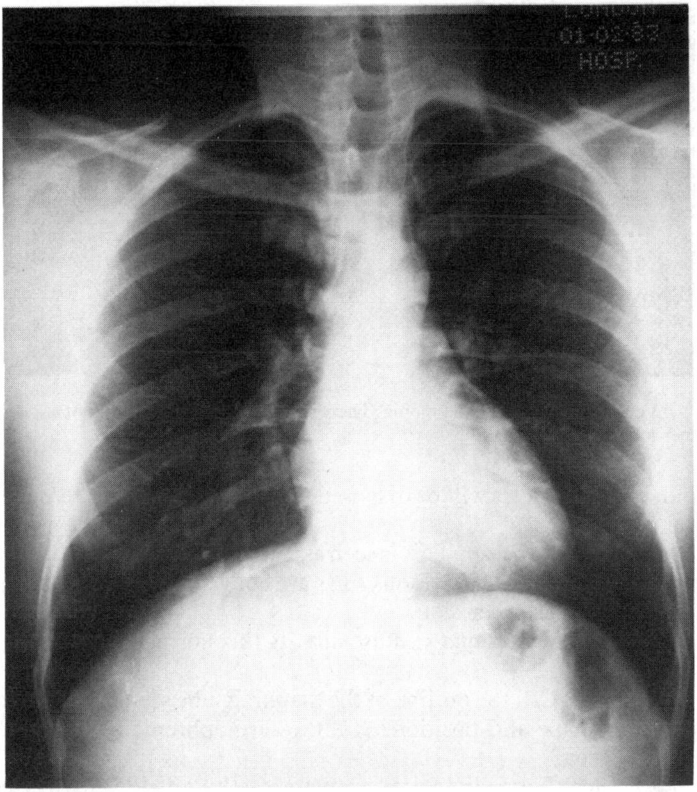

Fig. 8.5 Postero-anterior (PA) chest X-ray in a normal person. Note the position of the trachea, the size and shape of the heart and the relatively uniform appearance of the lung fields. The bony skeleton and diaphragm can clearly be seen. There is a little air in the stomach.

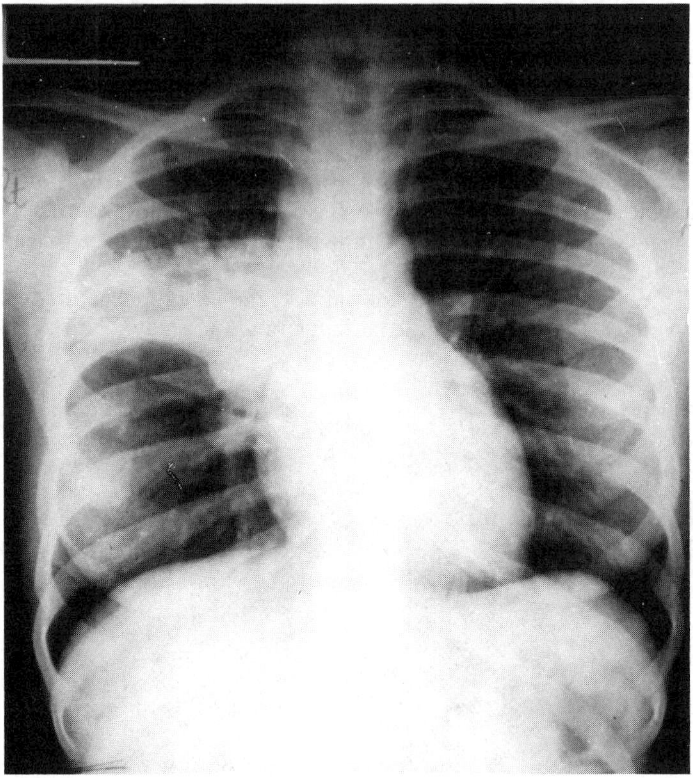

Fig. 8.6 PA chest X-ray. Lobar pneumonia. There is consolidation in the anterior segment of the right upper lobe.

inner ends of the clavicles will be disposed symmetrically with reference to the vertebral column.

3 *The position of the trachea*. This is seen as a dark column representing the air within the trachea. The cartilaginous rings are not visible. Is it centrally placed or deviated to one or other side?

4 *The outline of the heart and mediastinum*. Is this normal in size, shape and position?

5 *The diaphragm*. Can the outline of the diaphragm be seen on each side, and is it normal in shape and position? Are the cardiophrenic and costophrenic angles clearly seen?

6 *The lung fields*. For radiological purposes the lung fields are divided into three zones:

Zone 1 (upper zone) extends from the apex to a line drawn through the lower borders of the anterior ends of the second costal cartilages.

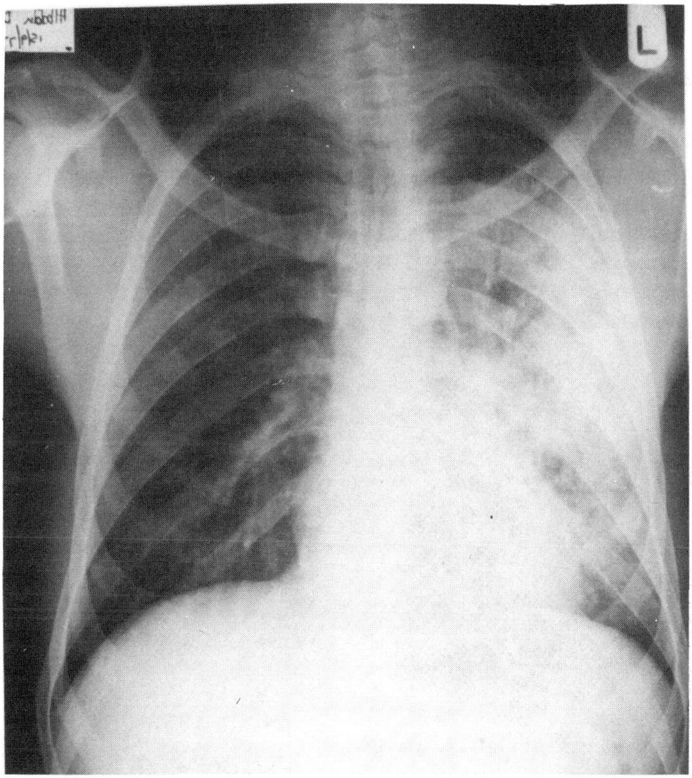

Fig. 8.7 PA chest X-ray. Bronchopneumonia. There is patchy consolidation in the mid and lower zones of the left lung. In this patient, this was due to tuberculosis. Note that the left lung is less well expanded than the right, as shown by the more acute angulation of the rib cage on the left side.

Zone 2 (mid zone) extends from this line to one drawn through the lower borders of the fourth costal cartilages and contains the hila of the lungs.

Zone 3 (lower zone) extends from this line to the bases of the lungs.

Each zone is systematically examined on the two sides and any area which appears abnormal is carefully compared with the corresponding area on the opposite side. The minor interlobar fissure, which separates the right upper and middle lobes, may sometimes be seen running horizontally in the third and fourth interspace on the right side. The major interlobar fissure, which separates the lower lobes from the remainder of the lungs, is not seen in a normal postero-anterior film. The typical radiographic features of lobar pneumonia, bronchopneumonia and obstructive airways disease are shown in Figs. 8.6, 8.7 and 8.8.

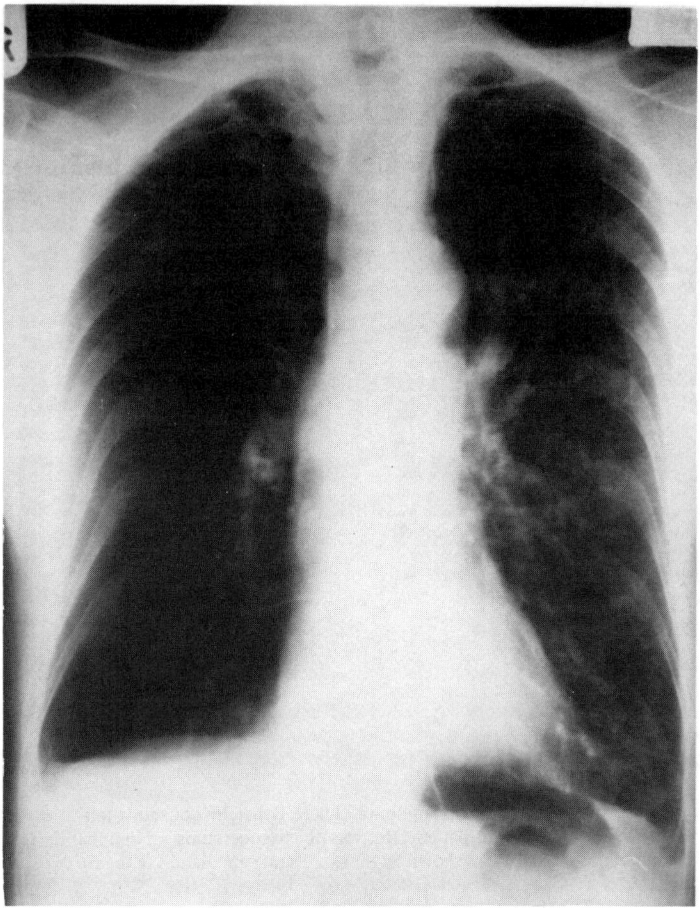

Fig. 8.8 PA chest X-ray. Obstructive airways disease. The lung fluids are darker, i.e. less radiopaque, than normal (compare with Fig. 8.5). The rib cage is deformed and the diaphragms are flattened and depressed. The heart shadow is long and narrow. The patient smoked heavily.

Lateral views

Lateral views are indispensable in the localization of lung lesions, for the postero-anterior view does not show whether a shadow is situated in the anterior or posterior part of the chest, or (if in the mid zone) whether in the upper or lower lobe. The following is a simple plan of examination.

1 *The bony skeleton*

2 *The position of the trachea*

3 *The diaphragm*. As the level of the diaphragm differs on the two sides, a

double outline may be seen, that of the side nearer the film being the clearer.
4 *The lung fields* are obscured by two relatively opaque areas, one above and behind, due to the shoulder joint, and one below and in front, due to the heart, which rests on the anterior part of the diaphragm. There are thus left two relatively clear areas—one above and in front, behind the upper part of the sternum, and one below and behind, including the angle between the diaphragm and the spine.

In the lateral views, the interlobar fissures are more often seen. Their normal positions have already been described (p. 173). Their recognition is useful both in localizing lesions and in detecting shrinkage of a lobe from fibrosis or collapse.

Screening

Screening is used mainly to detect abnormalities of the heart and paralysis of the diaphragm. By standing the patient in different positions, it is possible to see enlargement of the various chambers of the heart and main vessels and paradoxical pulsation of the left atrium. Enlargement of the left atrium is detected by noting displacement of the barium-filled oesophagus. When a diaphragmatic paralysis is present *paradoxical* movement is seen when the patient coughs or sniffs, the diaphragm ascending when it should descend, and vice versa.

Bronchography

After local anaesthesia, a radiopaque iodized oil is introduced into the trachea and allowed to run into the bronchi. X-ray pictures are taken and the corresponding bronchi are clearly outlined. With suitable manipulation, the whole of the bronchial tree can be outlined. Bronchography is rarely performed nowadays; its main use was to demonstrate bronchiectasis, now an uncommon disease.

Tomography

An ordinary X-ray picture consists of shadows at all depths in the chest, superimposed on one another. It has the disadvantage that not more than some 40% of the lung tissue is shown without its being obscured by shadows of the bony thorax or of mediastinal contents. The tomograph (Fig. 8.9) is a device whereby a picture is obtained of a section of the thorax at any given depth. The tube and plate are moved in the arc of a circle as the exposure is made, in such a manner that the structures in one section only remain in focus and anything out of the plane of this section is blurred out. Sections can be taken at different depths in the chest, as desired, and so the appearances in chest X-rays can often be greatly simplified. It is mainly used to detect cavitation in apparently opaque shadows in the lung fields, and to give a clearer picture of hilar

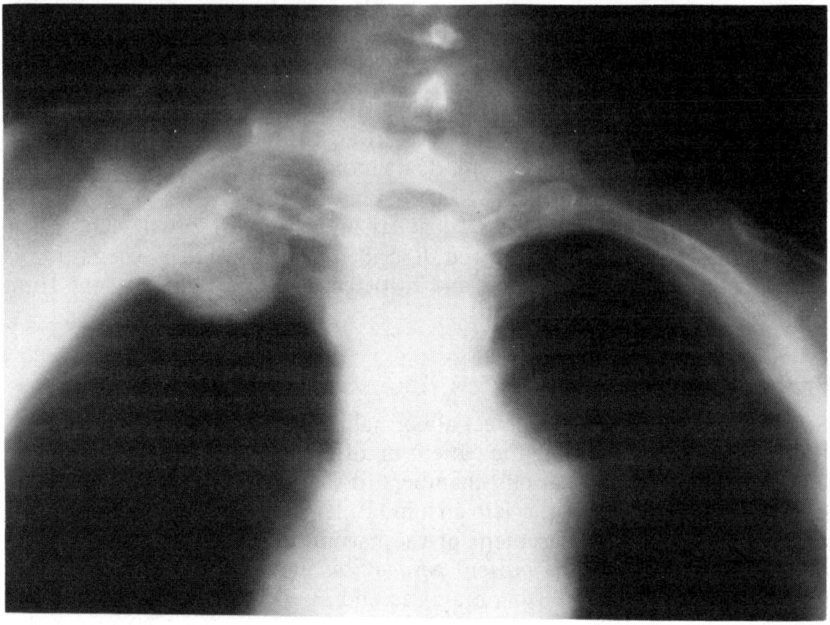

Fig. 8.9 PA tomogram of the chest. There is a radiopaque mass at the right apex. This proved to be tuberculosis, although radiographically bronchogenic carcinoma (Pancoast tumour) was considered more likely.

shadows. It may also indicate narrowing of a bronchus due to lesions such as carcinoma.

A complete tomographic picture of the lungs can be obtained by using computerized axial tomography (CT) scans. In this technique serial cuts in an axial plane are taken through the thorax. This technique may be especially sensitive in revealing:

1 Small secondary deposits
2 Enlarged glands (and other structures) in the mediastinum
3 Pleural involvement by fibrosis or mesothelioma.

BRONCHOSCOPY AND THORACOSCOPY

By means of the bronchoscope, the main bronchi and their branches can be inspected directly, small portions of tissue can be removed for biopsy, and therapeutic procedures carried out. The main value of bronchoscopy is in the diagnosis of carcinoma of the bronchus and in deciding whether this is operable. With the aid of flexible fibreoptic bronchoscopes, very small bronchi can be visualized and washings for cytological examination taken from separate lung segments. The flexible bronchoscope enables examination of patients with severe cervical or skeletal deformities, and affords a good view of the upper lobe bronchi and also permits transbronchial biopsy (see below). After an artificial pneumothorax has been induced, the pleura can be inspected with the aid of a thoracoscope and further assistance in diagnosis obtained.

PLEURAL ASPIRATION AND BIOPSY

Pleural effusions may be drained by inserting a wide-bore needle into the fluid-filled pleural space through one of the rib spaces, under local anaesthesia. The needle is inserted perpendicular to the skin and pleura, just above a rib margin. Aspirations may be *therapeutic*, to relieve respiratory embarrassment due to a large effusion, or *diagnostic*, to remove fluid for examination.

Pleural fluid can be examined macroscopically and microscopically. Full details cannot be given here, but the colour, consistency and quantity should be noted. A *trasnudate* from the capillaries, as occurs in cardiac and renal disease, can be distinguished from an *exudate* resulting from pleural inflammation by its lower protein content (<30g/l) and specific gravity (usually <1.015). Frankly blood-stained effusions occur with carcinoma, pulmonary infarction and trauma. In tuberculous effusions the fluid is straw-coloured and copious (often well over 1 litre) and may coagulate on standing; under the microscope many leucocytes are seen, lymphocytes often predominating. Tubercle bacilli are rarely seen, but can more commonly be cultured. In *empyema*, pus is aspirated which may be full of white cells and organisms.

Needle biopsy of the pleura may also be useful in establishing the diagnosis of the cause of a pleural effusion. In a high proportion of patients the presence of carcinoma or tuberculosis may be detected. Biopsy of lung can also be performed and is useful in establishing a histological diagnosis in diffuse lung diseases, such as fibrosing alveolitis. Tissue may be obtained by means of a needle or drill biotome inserted percutaneously or by means of a transbronchial biopsy using the fibreoptic bronchoscope.

LUNG FUNCTION TESTS

In recent years, tests of lung function of increasing complexity have been introduced, which are beyond the scope of this chapter, but some of the simple tests useful in clinical practice will be described. It must be stressed that lung function tests enable the clinician to make a *physiological* rather than a *pathological* diagnosis. That is to say, they will indicate that there is obstruction to air flow, but not that the patient has a bronchial carcinoma. Also, they are more likely to be abnormal if there is a diffuse process affecting the lung than if there is merely a localized lesion. They may be useful under the following circumstances:

1 To give an objective assessment of a patient's disability
2 To follow the progress of a disease and the effect of treatment
3 To try to differentiate possible causes of a patient's dyspnoea
4 To aid the management of cases of respiratory failure
5 To assess patients prior to anaesthesia and surgery, particularly thoracic surgery leading to lung resection.

Vital capacity and spirometry

The simplest and still perhaps the most valuable tests are the measurement of the patient's *vital capacity* and the recording of the *expiratory spirogram*. These can be measured by various types of *spirometer* and recorded graphically (Fig. 8.10). The patient inhales maximally and then breathes out as hard and as fast as he can. Measurements are then made of the amount of air he expels and the speed at which he does so. The amount of air expelled by maximal voluntary effort is the *vital capacity*. In normal subjects three-quarters of this air is expelled within the first second and all within about three seconds. Thus the normal curve is steep. In diseases such as asthma, bronchitis and emphysema there is obstruction to the flow of air out of the lungs, owing to collapse or constriction of the airways, or intraluminal obstruction owing to mucus or oedema, so that the curve is flattened (Fig. 8.10). On scrutiny of the curves, this flattening is apparent, but a numerical value can be given to the degree of flattening by recording the volume expired in one second. This volume (*forced expiratory volume* at one second, or FEV_1) is then expressed as a ratio of the *vital capacity* (VC). This ratio (FEV_1/VC) is called the FEV% and should exceed 70% in healthy individuals under 60 years of age. If the percentage is below this figure, the patient may be described as suffering from *airways obstruction*. The test may be repeated after the use of a bronchodilator aerosol, and, if the FEV_1 improves, the *airways obstruction* is said to be *reversible*. In some patients, treatment for several days with oral bronchodilators or even steroids may be needed to demonstrate reversibility. Broadly speaking, in asthma and bronchitis the obstruction is partly reversible by bronchodilators, whereas in emphysema it is not. However, the distinction between these conditions is not as clear as might be supposed. Alternatively the maximum expiratory flow rate can be measured by means of a peak flow meter. This portable instrument (Fig. 8.11) directly measures the expiratory flow rate, which is reduced in airways obstruction. The other principal abnormality which can be recognized from the expiratory spirogram is pulmonary *restriction*. This may result from limitation of movement of the chest wall (e.g. kyphoscoliosis) or diseases causing loss of lung volume (e.g. pulmonary fibrosis). In these conditions the vital capacity is reduced but the shape of the trace is similar to normal (Fig. 8.10). The ratio FEV_1/VC remains normal (more than 70%) and the peak expiratory flow rate measured by the peak flow meter is also normal.

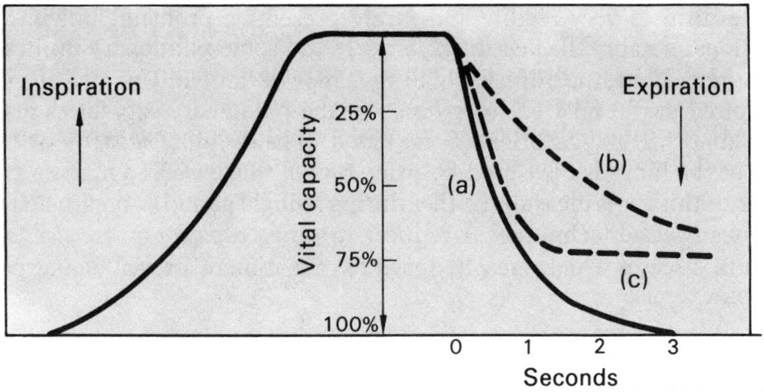

Fig. 8.10 The expiratory spirogram: (a) normal; (b) airway obstruction; (c) restriction.

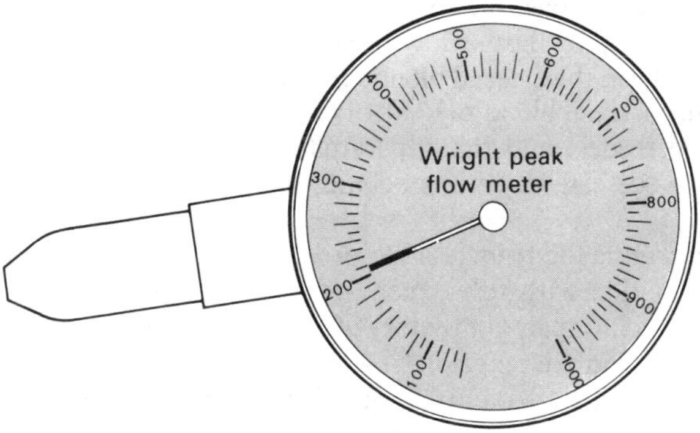

Fig. 8.11 A Wright peak flow meter.

Diffusion and distribution

Having entered the lungs, air is normally fairly evenly distributed throughout them. Similarly the blood entering the lungs from the pulmonary arteries has a quite even distribution, although in health both ventilation and perfusion are greater at the bases compared with the apices of the lungs. Modern radio-isotope techniques can be used for looking at the pattern of perfusion or ventilation; some centres can perform simultaneous ventilation–perfusion scans. In disease both ventilation and perfusion can be quite uneven and may lead to abnormal gas exchange.

Oxygen and carbon dioxide must pass freely between alveoli and pulmonary capillaries. The passage of these gases occurs largely by diffusion. Carbon dioxide diffuses very readily and rarely presents a problem; but in certain conditions, notably the *interstitial fibroses*, and some pulmonary infiltrations, such as *sarcoidosis*, the diffusion of oxygen may be limited. Unequal *distribution* of inspired gas in relation to *perfusion* of the pulmonary capillaries may also cause abnormal oxygenation of the blood. The *diffusing capacity* or *transfer factor* of the lungs is measured by using *carbon monoxide* as a marker gas; the uptake of this gas is measured either during a single period of breath holding or by a steady-state technique. A reduced *diffusing capacity* or *transfer factor* is found in diseases which cause reduced oxygenation of arterial blood, particularly on exercise.

The blood gases

The overall function of the lungs is to allow oxygen to reach the tissues of the body via the blood to facilitate aerobic respiration; also a waste product of metabolism, carbon dioxide, is excreted from the lungs and ventilation plays an important part in acid—base regulation of the body. The effectiveness of gas exchange can be assessed by measuring the *partial pressure* of oxygen (PO_2) and carbon dioxide (PCO_2) in the arterial blood, and acid–base status can be investigated by measuring arterial blood pH. All of these parameters can be measured by appropriate electrodes, and the apparatus is available in most hospitals. Also the arterial PCO_2 can be estimated indirectly by a simple rebreathing method.

Alveolar ventilation is the principal factor which determines arterial PCO_2. Alveolar hypoventilation with subsequent *respiratory failure* may result from drugs or diseases which impair ventilatory effort as well as from lung diseases. Normal arterial PCO_2 is in the range of 4.7–6.0 kPa (34–45 mmHg); a low PCO_2 may result from alveolar hyperventilation. Normal arterial PO_2 is 11.3–14.0 kPa (80–100 mmHg) and will be reduced in many lung diseases as well as in cardiac conditions which cause shunting of venous blood to the arterial circulation. The pH of arterial blood is normally kept within the tight limits of 7.38–7.42 but may be altered by renal failure and other metabolic disorders such as diabetic ketoacidosis. Blood gas and pH measurements are widely used in clinical medicine and, indeed, to try to manage respiratory failure without them is analagous to treating diabetic coma without doing blood sugar measurements.

Other tests

Many other physiological tests of lung function are available including measurements of lung compliance, airway resistance and gas mixing in the lung. Exercise testing may be needed in some cases to assess fully every aspect of lung function.

IMMUNOLOGY

Skin tests can be valuable in the diagnosis of chest disease. Allergic asthma is associated with type 1 hypersensitivity and immediate skin reactions to allergens such as grass pollen and house dust mite. Delayed hypersensitivity (type 4) is shown by Mantoux tests used to detect the presence of tuberculous infection (previous or recent). The Kveim test is relatively specific for sarcoidosis. Here an intradermal injection of antigen is made and the site of the lesion is biopsied for histological examination six weeks later. Antibody levels in serum can now be measured and are of use in diagnosis of many conditions. Precipitating antibodies are present in patients with some fungal diseases, and specific reaginic antibodies (IgE) can now be accurately measured. IgE levels are often raised in asthma, particularly if this is due to allergy.

9
The cardiovascular system

Clinical assessment of the cardiovascular system requires a rational approach in order to analyse the available information in a coherent manner. In every case, the clinician must integrate the facts available from the history, the examination and the investigation in such a way as to reach a conclusion about the structure and function of the heart and the pulmonary and systemic vascular trees. In this respect, the clinical approach to the cardiovascular system has many similarities with that to the nervous system.

GENERAL CONSIDERATIONS

The experienced clinician always precedes auscultation by a careful assessment of the arterial and venous pulses together with any abnormality of the praecordial impulse. Many students give insufficient time and attention to these features of the cardiovascular system. The detection of abnormalities in these areas not only provides invaluable evidence about the nature of any cardiac abnormality, but often provides critical information on the functional severity of any lesion which may be present. Thus, by the time the examiner has reached the stage of auscultation, the salient points of the history and the previously established clinical observations frequently suggest findings which may then be detected by stethoscope. By contrast, the beginner's mind may be so filled with anxiety at the thought of failing to hear some unspecified sound that no logical analysis of the auscultatory abnormalities is made. In auscultation of the heart it is important to have some idea what abnormalities you expect to find.

For these reasons, it is best to examine the cardiovascular system in the following order: arterial pulses, blood pressure, venous pulses, praecordium and finally auscultation. However, before proceeding to this examination certain general points should be noted.

GENERAL EXAMINATION IN RELATION TO THE CARDIOVASCULAR SYSTEM

Anaemia, often recognized by pale mucous membranes, is an important cause of angina. Right ventricular failure causes *enlargement of the liver* and *ascites*. The location of *oedema* depends on the patient's posture. It is always most apparent in dependent parts so that, in a relatively mobile patient, it is most readily detected by pressure over the distal end of the tibia. However, in the patient confined to bed, oedema will tend to collect over the sacrum and the dorsal spine. If the patient is lying in the supine position, oedema can easily be overlooked if it is not specifically sought.

The presence of *finger clubbing* in association with *peripheral and central cyanosis* suggests there is a right-to-left intracardiac or intrapulmonary shunt. In patients with infective endocarditis, *finger clubbing and splenomegaly* may be present. Microvascular embolic phenomena, probably due to antigen–antibody reactions are manifest by *splinter haemorrhages* in the nail beds of the fingers and toes, and small *petechial haemorrhages* in the conjunctivae. Larger emboli, probably fragments of vegetations from an infected valve, may present as painful erythematous lumps in the pulps of the fingers and toes, palms of the hands and soles of the feet (*Osler's nodes*). The equivalent phenomenon in the retinal circulation, seen on examination of the optic fundi, is called *Roth's spot*.

Patients with left ventricular failure may be *breathless* at rest to the extent that they cannot complete a sentence without pausing for breath. In these patients *crepitations* (see p. 184) can often be detected at the lung bases.

ANATOMICAL LANDMARKS

The *praecordium* is the term used to indicate the anterior aspect of the chest which overlies the heart. It is often convenient to refer to a point on the chest wall, and certain landmarks, some natural and some artificial, are commonly used for this purpose.

The ribs and interspaces on either side form convenient horizontal landmarks. In order to count them, feel for the ridge which marks the junction of the manubrium with the body of the sternum, known as the angle of Louis, or sternal angle. When this has been found, run the finger outwards until it reaches the second costal cartilage, which articulates with the sternum at this level. The space immediately above this is the first intercostal space. The spaces should then be counted downwards well away from the sternum, where they are more easily felt.

The distance of any given point from the midline of the body may be referred to as a series of vertical lines. These are the *midclavicular line*, defined as the vertical line dropped from the centre of the clavicle, or, what amounts to the same thing, the line midway between the middle of the suprasternal notch and the tip of the acromion; and the *anterior, mid-*, and *posterior axillary lines*, descending respectively from the anterior border, the centre and the posterior border of the axilla.

ARTERIAL PULSES

The presence or absence of the main peripheral pulses—the radial, brachial, carotid, femoral, popliteal, posterior tibial, and dorsalis pedis pulses—should be noted. The volume of each is compared with the other side.

The following observations should then be made with regard to cardiac function (disease of the peripheral vessels is considered later in this chapter):

1 Rate of pulse
2 Rhythm
3 Character
4 Volume
5 Presence or absence of delay of the femoral pulses compared with the radials

To assess the rate and rhythm, the radial pulse at the wrist is generally used. It is best felt with the tips of the fingers, the patient's forearm being pronated and the wrist slightly flexed. When the character and volume of the arterial pulse are being analysed, one should examine the carotid artery, which is the closest pulse to the ascending aorta; here, modifications to the waveform by the vessels of the peripheral arterial system are kept to a minimum. The patient's right carotid should be palpated with the examiner's left thumb and the left carotid with the examiner's right thumb. Carotid pulses must always be examined sequentially, *never* simultaneously, since bilateral carotid compression may lead to syncope.

The blood pressure cannot be measured accurately without a sphygmomanometer (see p. 204). The terms 'good', 'bad', 'strong' and 'weak' in relation to the pulse lack precision and should be avoided.

Rate

The rate of the pulse is stated as so many beats a minute. It is counted, not when the fingers are first laid upon the pulse, but when any quickening due to nervousness in the patient has subsided and the pulse has resumed its normal rate. It is, therefore, good practice to feel the radial pulse gently while eliciting the routine parts of the history. Count the beats for not less than half a minute. In cases of atrial fibrillation, the pulse rate counted at the wrist will not indicate the true rate of ventricular contractions. In such cases, the rate of the heart beat should be counted by auscultation at the apex, and the difference between this rate and the pulse rate at the wrist recorded. This difference is referred to as the *pulse deficit*. It is explained as follows. Atrial fibrillation is characterized by a varying length of diastole. When diastole is short, filling of the left ventricle may be so poor that on the subsequent systole there is insufficient stroke volume to cause opening of the aortic valve. The arterial pulse is therefore non-existent. As diastole becomes longer, the stroke volume gradually increases; a pulse might be recorded in the central aorta, yet not be sufficiently large to reach the periphery at the radial artery. Following a long diastole (a slower heart rate) the strength of the subsequent systolic stroke volume is increased.

The resting heart rate shows considerable variation, ranging between 50 and 120 beats per minute. The parasympathetic and sympathetic components of the autonomic nervous system have a major effect on heart rate. The pulse rate is increased by exercise, fever and in thyrotoxicosis. It is also increased in abnormal tachyarrhythmias. Regular athletic training and myxoedema are the commonest causes of bradycardia. Abnormalities of function of the sinus or atrio-ventricular nodes may reduce the heart rate to below 50 beats per minute.

Rhythm

Decide next whether the rhythm is regular or irregular. If it is irregular, decide if it is completely irregular, whether the irregularity has a recurring pattern, or whether an otherwise regular rhythm is occasionally interrupted by some slight irregularity. The pulse of atrial fibrillation is completely irregular. The irregularity is usually obvious when the rate is rapid, but becomes less easy to recognize when the rate has been slowed by digitalis. If the rhythm has a recurring pattern, or there are occasional irregularities, these are likely to be due to extrasystoles. An extrasystole is a beat which occurs prematurely, is of reduced volume and is followed by lengthened diastole—clinically appreciated as a 'pause'. Disorders of rhythm are described more fully under 'Electrocardiography' (p. 236).

Character

Study the character or form of the arterial pulse wave (Fig. 9.1) by palpation of the carotid pulse. It is best felt with the thumb, pressing backwards at the medial border of the sternomastoid at the level of the thyroid cartilage. It is not usually possible to detect slight variations from the normal, but in certain diseases the character of the pulse is detectably abnormal. The most important of these are as follows:

Slow rising pulse The arterial pulse in aortic stenosis (Fig. 9.2) is typically 'parvus et tardus'—of small volume with a late systolic peak. There is often a thrill in the carotid pulse and with practice the 'slow rising' characteristic can be appreciated. This slow rising pulse used to be known as an anacrotic pulse.

Collapsing (water-hammer) pulse A collapsing pulse is characterized by a rapid upstroke and descent of the pulse wave. It occurs most often in aortic regurgitation. The abrupt upstroke is due to the greatly increased stroke volume. The collapsing character is caused by two factors: firstly the diastolic leak back into the left ventricle and secondly the rapid run-off to the periphery because of a low systemic vascular resistance. This type of pulse may also be seen with patent ductus arteriosus, ruptured sinus of Valsalva or large arterio-venous communications.

Bisferiens pulse Bisferiens pulse is a combination of the slow rising and collapsing pulses occurring when aortic stenosis and incompetence are present.

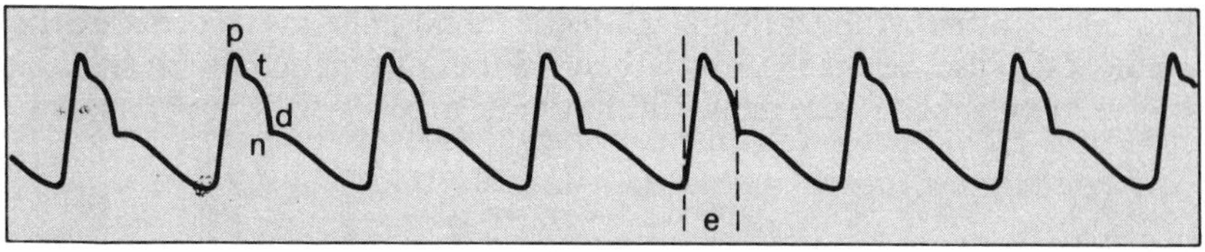

Fig. 9.1 A normal arterial pulse tracing. p: percussion wave; t: tidal wave; n: dicrotic notch; d: dicrotic wave; e: period of ventricular systole (aortic valve open).

Pulsus paradoxus This term describes the marked diminution in arterial pressure which occurs in patients with a large pericardial effusion or severe asthma. The term is confusing because this diminution is merely an accentuation of the normal physiological finding of a fall in peak arterial pressure of 5–10 mmHg during inspiration. The 'paradox' is that heart sounds may still be heard on auscultation over the praecordium at a time when no pulse is palpable at the radial artery. In patients with a large pericardial effusion the pericardial fluid acts as a restraint on the total intracardiac volume. Thus when right ventricular volume increases with inspiration, the left ventricular volume falls

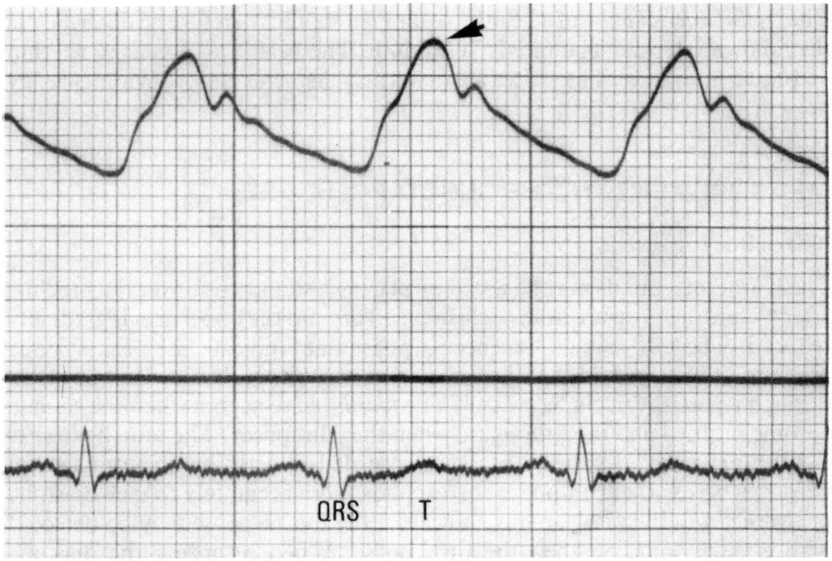

Fig. 9.2 A pressure recording from the aorta in a patient with aortic stenosis. The upstroke of the pressure pulse is slow and the peak (arrow) is delayed compared with the normal arterial pulse (Fig. 9.1). The onset of systole is indicated by the QRS complex on the ECG tracing beneath the pressure pulse.

and the arterial pulse volume decreases. This is an extremely important physical sign indicating the presence of *cardiac tamponade*.

Pulsus alternans When the ventricle beats strongly, then weakly, in successive beats of normal rhythm, alternation is present. When this condition is discovered, provided no abnormal rhythm is present, it may be inferred that the left ventricular muscle is severely damaged.

Volume

Estimate the volume of the pulse. This gives a rough guide to the pulse pressure, which depends on the stroke volume and the compliance of the arteries. With normal vessels the pulse volume gives an indication of the stroke volume. In older subjects the vessels are more rigid (less compliant) causing a widened pulse pressure for the same stroke volume.

Delay

Delay of the femoral compared with the right radial pulse is found in coarctation of the aorta.

The *typical arterial pulse* of a healthy adult man should therefore be described in the following terms. The rate is 70/minute. The beats are regular in rhythm and equal in volume. The pulses are of normal character and are symmetrically present.

MEASUREMENT OF THE BLOOD PRESSURE

Korotkoff sounds

The Korotkoff sounds may be heard by placing a stethoscope over the brachial artery while the pressure in an occlusion cuff around the upper arm is gradually reduced. The *first* sounds that occur (phase one) indicate the peak systolic pressure. The *second* and *third* phases are due to the turbulent flow of blood through a partially occluded vessel. The *fourth* phase occurs when the sounds become muffled and the *fifth* phase when they disappear. The fourth phase is 7–10 mmHg above diastolic pressure recorded directly by an intra-arterial needle, whereas the fifth phase corresponds more accurately to true diastolic pressure. In individual patients, however, the fourth phase may be detected with greater precision than the fifth phase. When recording the diastolic pressure both phases should be noted if they have been clearly heard.

The sphygmomanometer

Certain details are important in the use of the sphygmomanometer. The patient should be sitting or lying at ease. The manometer is placed so as to be at the same level as the observer's eye. All clothing should be removed from the arm. The cuff should be applied closely to the upper arm, with the lower border not less than 2.5 cm from the cubital fossa.

The radial pulse is palpated while the cuff is inflated to a pressure of 30 mmHg above the level at which radial pulsation can no longer be felt. The stethoscope is then placed lightly over the brachial artery. The pressure in the cuff is lowered, 5 mmHg at a time, until the first sounds are heard. This is the systolic pressure. Continue to lower the pressure in the cuff until the sounds suddenly become faint. This is the diastolic pressure (fourth phase). Continue to reduce the pressure and between 1 and 10 mmHg lower the sounds disappear completely (fifth phase).

Occasionally the sounds disappear at a point below 200 mm for a period and then reappear, finally disappearing at the point of diastolic pressure. Thus the sounds may first appear when the mercury falls to 210 (systolic pressure), disappear from 180 to 160 (silent gap), reappear and finally disappear at 120 (diastolic pressure). This phenomenon of a silent gap is found in certain patients with hypertension; its significance is unknown, but its occurrence makes it important that the armlet pressure at the start of the examination should always have been sufficient to obliterate the radial pulse.

The systemic arterial pressure is significantly affected by exertion, anxiety, excitement and changes in posture. It should therefore be observed when the patient has been resting quietly. Check that the width of the cuff is correct. For an adult, the standard cuff width is 12.5 cm. If a narrower cuff is used, the recorded pressures will be falsely high. In obese patients it is essential to use a wider cuff such as a thigh cuff to measure the occlusion pressure in the upper arm. In nervous patients the first reading is often high; a second reading when the patient has become accustomed to the procedure and is more relaxed may be more representative. It is useful to note the pulse rate at the same time, as circulating catecholamines will affect both measurements. An elevated pulse rate in the presence of an elevated blood pressure suggests that some of the 'hypertension' is due to a temporary increase in circulating adrenaline and noradrenaline levels.

It is essential to work as quickly as is compatible with accuracy, for compression of a limb itself induces a rise in blood pressure. To reduce this source of error when successive estimations are to be made, the air pressure in the armlet should always be allowed to fall to zero as soon as each reading has been taken. It is important to measure the blood pressure in patients taking hypotensive drugs or otherwise suspected of postural hypotension (in both the recumbent and the standing positions).

For children, there are a variety of cuffs of different widths. Select the size which covers most of the upper arm but leaves a gap of 1 cm below the axilla and above the antecubital fossa. In suspected coarctation of the aorta it may be useful to compare the systolic blood pressure in the arm with that in the leg; the patient lies face downwards and an 18 cm cuff is applied above the knee and auscultation carried out over the popliteal artery.

Normal blood pressure The average systolic pressure in healthy adults is 100–140 mmHg, the average diastolic pressure, 60–90 mmHg. In children it is closer to the lower end of the scale, and in the elderly it reaches or even exceeds the higher figure. The difference between the systolic and the diastolic pressures—the pulse pressure—is 30–60 mmHg.

Abnormal blood pressure Abnormal blood pressure must be considered in relation to the patient's age. A blood pressure of 140 over 90 would indicate quite severe hypertension in a child while much higher systolic pressures in an elderly patient is inevitable due to loss of elasticity in the peripheral arterial system. The increased rigidity due to degenerative changes (arteriosclerosis) causes the systolic pressure peak to be particularly elevated.

THE VENOUS PULSE

The neck veins

The importance of studying the level of pressure in the internal jugular veins lies in the fact that these vessels are usually in direct communication with the right atrium. In this way the pressure changes within the heart may be predicted by simple clinical observation. It may be easier to recognize the pulsation in the external jugular veins than in the internal jugular system, but using the former is a less reliable means of predicting pressure changes in the right atrium. There are two reasons for this. Firstly, the presence of venous valves within the external jugular system prevents it being a pure conductor of more central pressure changes. Secondly, the external jugular system passes through more fascial planes than the internal system and so is more likely to be affected by extrinsic compression from other structures in the neck and upper thorax.

The venous pulse (Fig. 9.3) has three positive waves, *a*, *c*, and *v*, and two negative waves or descents, *x* and *y*. The *a* wave is due to atrial contraction. This is followed by the *x* descent, which is interrupted by a small *c* wave (which is rarely visible on inspection of the neck veins). The *c* wave coincides with the onset of ventricular systole and results from the movement of the tricuspid valve ring into the right atrium as the right ventricular pressure rises. The *v* wave indicates a passive rise in pressure as venous return to the atrium continues during ventricular systole while the tricuspid valve is closed. When the tricuspid valve opens, blood enters the right ventricle rapidly and there is consequently a lowering of the right atrial pressure—the *y* descent.

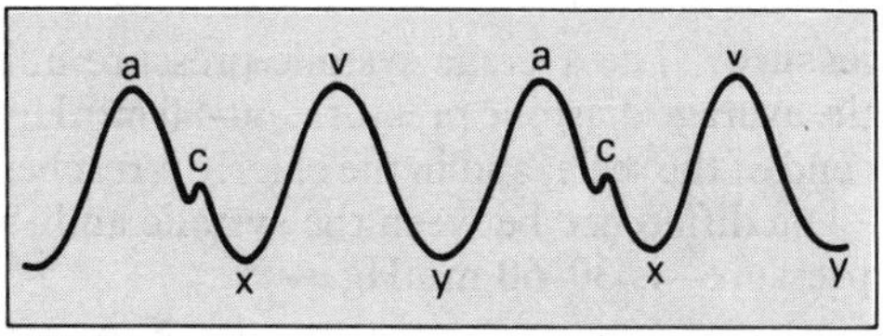

Fig. 9.3 The normal venous pulse (see text).

Examination

Examine the neck veins with the patient in a good light, and reclining at an angle of about 45° (Fig. 9.4). The neck should be supported so that the neck muscles, especially the sternomastoids, are relaxed. The veins normally show slight pulsation, and three small waves (the *a*, *c* and *v* waves) can be distinguished in each cardiac cycle. There is, however, a mean level, and the perpendicular height of this level above the right atrium indicates the mean hydrostatic pressure within the right atrium (6–8 cm water). In health this level is the same as that of the sternal angle, whatever the position of the patient. The

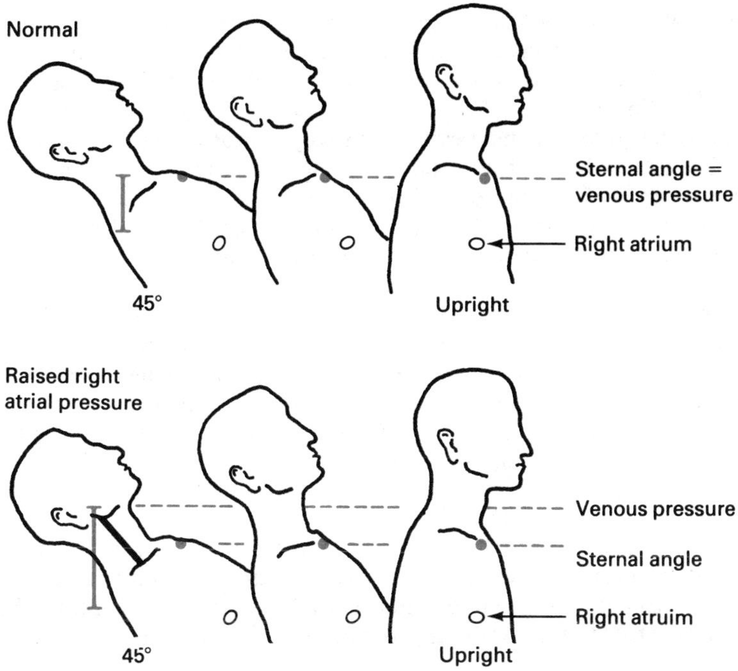

Fig. 9.4 In the normal subject lying with the upper part of the body at an angle of 45° to the horizontal, the peaks of the right atrial pressure waves are just visible in the internal jugular vein. As indicated in the upper diagram, the distance between the right atrium and the sternal angle remains relatively constant regardless of the position of the thorax. However, when the upright position is assumed, the tops of the right atrial pressure waves, whilst reaching the sternal angle, are hidden from the observer's view by the part of the thoracic cage which is now situated above the sternal angle.

When the venous pressure is grossly elevated (lower diagrams) the top of the right atrial pressure waves lies above the angle of the jaw. This may make it difficult to observe their pulsatile nature when the patient is positioned at 45°. When the patient is upright the top of the right atrial pressure wave becomes visible in the mid or lower portion of the neck.

sternal angle is therefore a convenient reference point for measuring or estimating the right atrial pressure. This means that in a healthy person reclining at an angle of 45°, the mean level will be invisible, because it is just below the clavicle, but the *a*, *c* and *v* waves may appear above the clavicle.

Arterial pulsation may also be visible in the neck and has to be distinguished from venous pulsation. The venous pulse has a definite upper level, though it may be necessary to sit the patient up higher or lay him lower to find it. This level falls during inspiration when blood is drawn into the heart. When the patient's neck is viewed from the end of the bed the venous pulse is seen to have a dominant inward motion, towards the midline (the *y* descent), whereas the arterial pulse exhibits a dominant 'outward' wave. In addition it is usually impossible to palpate any impulse from the venous waves, whereas the much higher pressure arterial pulses are readily felt by very slight pressure of the examiner's finger.

A raised jugular venous pressure is usually indicative of right heart failure. Occasionally it is due to obstruction of the superior vena cava, in which case the normal pulsations of the venous pulse are absent. A slight rise in venous pressure also occurs with an increase in the circulating blood volume, as in pregnancy, acute nephritis or over-enthusiastic treatment with intravenous fluids.

The venous pulse is usually seen quite easily by the methods described, but occasionally difficulties occur. The mean venous pressure may be so high, for instance, that the pulsation is obscured within the cranium when the patient is semi-recumbent, and is visible only high in the neck when he sits upright. In patients with a very low right atrial pressure the pulsation may be visible only when the patient lies completely flat.

The *a* wave is prominent when right ventricular hypertrophy leads to increased resistance to filling. This is found in pulmonary stenosis or pulmonary hypertension as a result of increased ventricular work associated with pressure overload. In theory a large *a* wave is present in tricuspid stenosis but most patients with this condition are in atrial fibrillation and therefore there is no *a* wave. Atrial flutter, however, does cause sufficient atrial activity for rapid

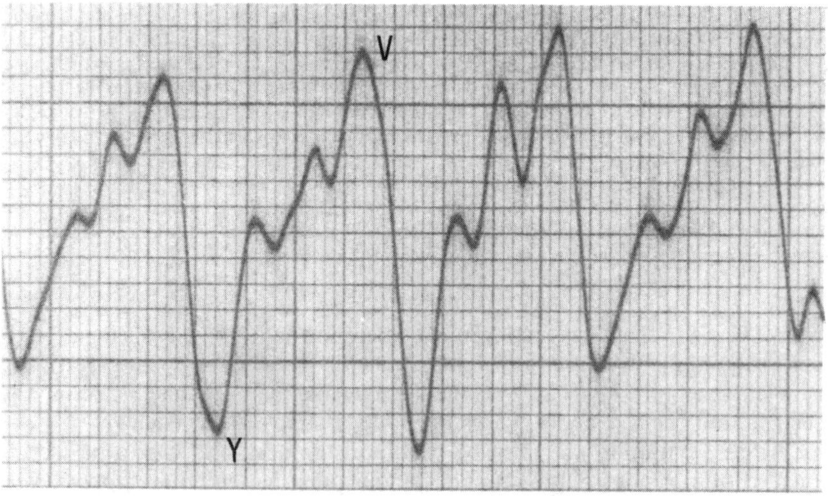

Fig. 9.5 Right atrial pressure trace showing the typical waveform found in patients with an elevated right atrial pressure. Notice that the most dramatic abnormality is the abrupt fall in pressure associated with the *y* descent. On examination of the neck veins this would be observed as a rapid impulse inwards towards the midline.

waves to be noted. In tricuspid regurgitation, the *v* wave is replaced by a large systolic wave due to regurgitation of blood into the right atrium during right ventricular systole. The systolic *v* wave is followed by a particularly prominent *y* descent (Fig. 9.5).

In complete heart block (complete atrioventricular dissociation) regular *a* waves can be seen in the neck while carotid pulsation occurs at a slower independent rate. From time to time atrial contraction occurs when the atrioventricular valves are closed during ventricular systole. All the force of right atrial contraction is transmitted backwards into the veins, to give a 'cannon wave'. If the arterial pulse is slow, the neck veins should be carefully examined for more rapid, regular *a* waves and 'cannon waves'. Cannon waves are also seen in atrioventricular junctional rhythm when the atrium and ventricle are activated simultaneously, and the atrium contracts on a closed atrioventricular valve.

THE PRAECORDIUM

Inspection and palpation

Deformities of the chest wall can affect the physical signs found in the examination of the heart. The commonest finding associated with these deformities is an ejection systolic murmur, which may be wrongly attributed to organic heart disease. The presence of kyphosis, scoliosis or sternal depression should therefore be noted.

Next identify the apex beat and assess the cardiac impulse. It should be emphasized that the term cardiac impulse does not refer only to the character of the apex beat but includes other pulsations and palpable murmurs (thrills) and heart sounds.

The cardiac impulse

It is customary to locate the apex beat, which is the lowest and outermost point of definite cardiac pulsation, and to delineate its position in terms of the particular intercostal space and distance from the midline in which it is felt. The normal position of the apex beat is 9 cm from the midline, or 1 cm internal to the midclavicular line in the fifth intercostal space.

The position of the apex beat is a valuable physical sign, if its limitations are understood.

Firstly, it must be felt with the patient sitting or lying quite straight. The apex beat of a normal person may be felt in the anterior axillary line, if the person is lying on his left side.

Secondly, it must be realized that the commonest cause of displacement of the apex beat is a deformity of the thoracic cage, usually scoliosis.

A real displacement of the apex beat may be due to disease of the surrounding viscera, which 'push' or 'pull' it from its usual site. Instances of 'pushing' are found in pleural effusion and pneumothorax, and of 'pulling' in pulmonary fibrosis and collapse of the lung. It may also be due to disease of the heart, when displacement of the apex beat may indicate enlargement, particularly of the left ventricle. Of equal importance in this respect is palpation over the left ventricle, the right ventricle, and the pulmonary artery to determine the character of the cardiac impulse, from which information can be gained about the function of the ventricles.

The *left ventricle* normally produces the apex beat. When it is hypertrophied, the beat becomes more forceful and may extend outwards towards the axilla.

The *right ventricle*, when hypertrophied, can be felt by placing the hand firmly over the praecordium just to the left of the sternum, when a definite 'lift' will be detected.

The *pulmonary artery* can be palpated in the second left intercostal space when it is dilated as in pulmonary hypertension.

If an hypertrophied left ventricle is present, an attempt should be made to differentiate between that resulting from obstruction to outflow (pressure overload) and that associated with excess filling of the ventricle (volume overload). Pressure overload, due to aortic stenosis or systemic hypertension, causes a forceful sustained heave. On the other hand, the volume overload occurring in aortic or mitral regurgitation is followed by easy and rapid (hyperkinetic) ejection of blood from the ventricles, producing an equally forceful but less sustained impulse.

Failure to detect an apex beat is usually due to obesity, but may be a feature in patients with pleural or pericardial effusions. Dextrocardia is an extremely rare malformation.

Other pulsations

In addition to the arterial and venous pulses already described, pulsations may also be noted at the root of the neck, the front of the chest, and the epigastrium.

In the *suprasternal notch* the pulsation is usually systolic in time, and when well marked may be an indication of unfolding or aneurysm of the arch of the aorta.

In the *neck* various pulsations may be observed. The carotid pulsation may be visible in anxious or agitated patients, in diseases which cause overactivity of the heart, such as thyrotoxicosis, and in cases of aortic regurgitation, hypertension or aneurysm of the aorta. In hypertension or in patients with large-calibre arterial vessels, the right carotid sometimes shows abnormal pulsation due to kinking.

In the *chest wall*, a rare source of pulsation is an aneurysm of the aorta. The position of the impulse varies according to the part of the aorta which is diseased. If the *ascending aorta* is affected, the pulsation is chiefly to the right of the sternum, whilst the *aortic arch* gives rise to less distinct pulsation under the manubrium sterni, and the *descending aorta* still more to the left.

In *coarctation of the aorta* a collateral arterial circulation develops, and pulsation may be detected in the anastomotic channels overlying the scapulae. These are palpable over the posterior chest wall and may even be visible on inspection.

Pulsation in the *epigastrium* is most commonly due to nervousness or excitement in a thin person. Occasionally it is due to pulsation of the liver in heart failure with tricuspid regurgitation. Aneurysms of the abdominal aorta may present as an expansile swelling in the epigastrium.

Thrills

The physical property of a sound or murmur which makes it 'loud' will also allow it to be detected by palpation. A palpable murmur is called a thrill and transmits to the hand a sensation like the purring of a cat. The character, timing and variation with respiration of thrills are the same as those of the corresponding murmurs and are discussed with murmurs. The palpable impulse from a loud high pitched sound will be brief with a 'sharp' quality. A third or fourth sound is often easier to feel than to hear. The loud first sound of mitral stenosis is often palpable and the sounds of aortic and pulmonary valve closure are palpable in systemic and pulmonary hypertension respectively.

PERCUSSION

Percussion of the heart is now seldom carried out, adds little to the clinical assessment and has been superseded by the chest X-ray and echocardiography.

AUSCULTATION

Auscultation of the heart often presents difficulties for the beginner. As with other skills, it requires a great deal of practice and constant repetition. The skilled examiner listens for specific findings, focusing attention on particular parts of the cardiac cycle. An understanding of the events of the cardiac cycle (Fig. 9.6) is a useful basis for auscultation. A common error is to wrongly identify systole and diastole. Palpation of the carotid artery provides a systolic time reference and it is always wise to feel the carotid artery while auscultating; the delay in the radial pulse may cause confusion.

The stethoscope The stethoscope should combine both a bell-type chest piece and a diaphragm. High-pitched sounds such as aortic diastolic murmurs

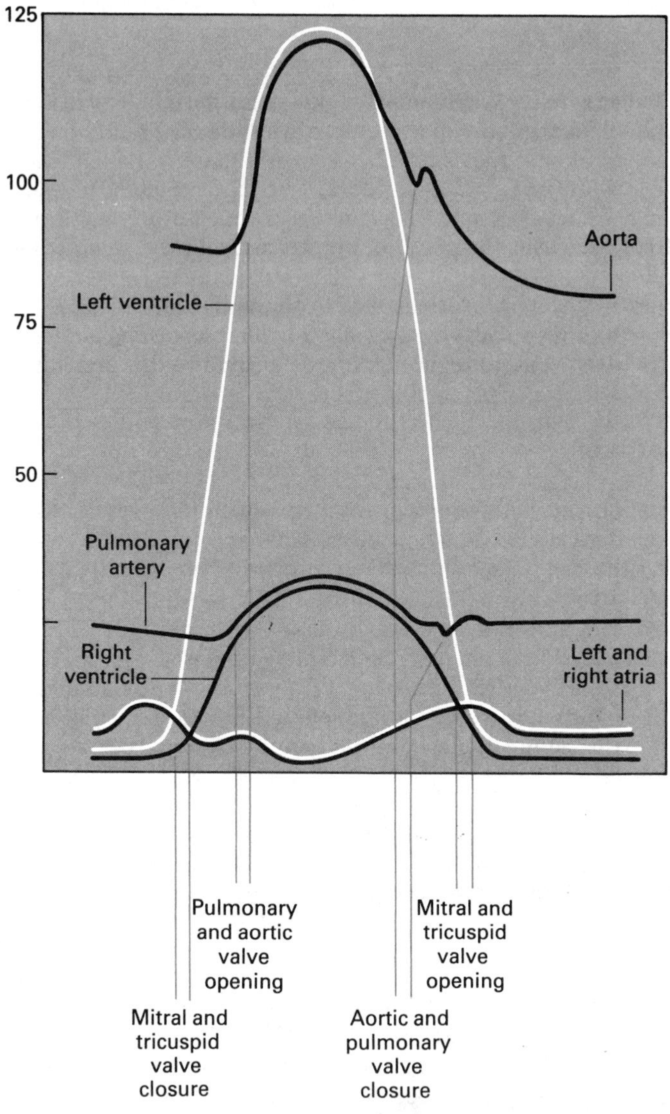

Fig. 9.6 The cardiac cycle. Normally the onset of left ventricular systole precedes the onset of pressure rise in the right ventricle. The mitral valve therefore closes before the tricuspid valve. Because the pulmonary artery diastolic pressure is lower than aortic diastolic pressure, the pulmonary valve opens before the aortic valve. It follows that pulmonary ejection sounds occur closer to the first heart sound than do aortic ejection sounds. During systole the pressure in the ventricles slightly exceeds the pressure in the corresponding great arteries. Towards the end of systole the ventricular pressure falls below the pressure in the great arteries and when diastolic pressure is reached the semilunar valves close. Normally aortic valve closure precedes pulmonary valve closure. The mitral and tricuspid valves begin to open at the point at which the ventricular pressures fall below the corresponding atrial pressures.

are heard better with the diaphragm, and low-pitched sounds such as the third heart sound or mitral diastolic murmurs with the bell.

Auscultatory areas

Certain areas are customarily called by the name of the valve from which murmurs and sounds arise:

1 The *mitral area*, which corresponds to the apex beat.
2 The *tricuspid area*, which lies just to the left of the lower end of the sternum.
3 The *aortic area*, which is to the right of the sternum in the second intercostal space.
4 The *pulmonary area*, which is to the left of the sternum in the second intercostal space.

Auscultation should not necessarily be confined to these areas, and sounds heard in a particular area do not necessarily come from that particular valve; for example, murmurs originating at the aortic valve are frequently best heard at the mitral area.

Heart sounds

The events of the cardiac cycle are illustrated in Fig. 9.6. At the onset of ventricular systole, the mitral and tricuspid valves close consecutively to give the first heart sound. Opening of the pulmonary and aortic valves occurs next and is normally inaudible. The closure of the aortic and pulmonary valves gives rise to the two components of the second sound. It will be seen that because of the lower pressure in the right ventricle compared with the left, closure of the pulmonary valve follows that of the aortic valve. After a brief period the mitral and tricuspid valves open inaudibly in the normal heart.

Abnormal heart sounds

In disease the following deviations from the normal may occur:

1 The sounds may have a different intensity, either increased or decreased.
2 The sounds may be abnormally split.
3 Low-frequency sounds in diastole—third or fourth sounds—may be heard.
4 Additional sounds, often related to abnormal valves, may be heard.

Alterations in intensity

In patients with thick chest walls, and in those with a serious degree of emphysema, the heart sounds may scarcely be audible, though there is no heart disease. Conversely, in the presence of serious heart disease the sounds may be quite normal. Thus alterations in the intensity of the heart sounds are significant only when considered in relation to all the other features of the case. For example, in pericardial effusion, the heart sounds are distant or inaudible.

Accentuation of the first sound is often present in mitral stenosis and in tachycardia from any cause. The intensity of the first sound varies strikingly in complete atrioventricular block.

Accentuation of the sound of aortic or pulmonary valve closure is found when there is systemic or pulmonary hypertension. In calcific aortic stenosis the aortic component of the second sound is soft, and in severe pulmonary stenosis the pulmonary component (P_2) is soft.

Splitting

The mitral valve closes slightly before the tricuspid valve, and this gives rise to splitting of the first sound. This splitting is often difficult to detect by auscultation because the two sounds are separated by a short interval. When it is heard, splitting of the first sound is not a sign of heart disease and is of importance only because its two components may be confused with an atrial sound followed by a first sound, or with a first sound followed by an ejection click.

Splitting of the second sound is much easier to appreciate because the aortic and pulmonary valve closure sounds (A_2 and P_2) are more widely separated. Aortic valve closure (A_2) is audible in all areas. Pulmonary valve closure (P_2) is normally audible only in the pulmonary area and for a short distance down the left sternal edge. When P_2 is loud it is also audible over a wider area of the praecordium. It follows that splitting of the second sound is usually heard only at and close to the pulmonary area. Splitting is most easily heard in children, and may not be audible in older adults, especially men, when muscle noise, a thick chest wall, and emphysema make P_2 inaudible. Normally P_2 follows A_2, and the splitting is widest during inspiration and narrowest in expiration (physiological splitting). Splitting of 0.06 second during inspiration and 0.02 second (a very close split or single sound) in expiration would be average for a child or young adult.

The mechanism of splitting of the second sound is as follows. During inspiration blood is drawn into the thorax and the right ventricular stroke volume increases. The duration of right ventricular systole therefore lengthens, and P_2 is therefore slightly delayed. Conversely the left ventricular stroke volume falls during inspiration, because the greater negative pressure within the thorax enlarges the capacity of the left atrium and pulmonary veins and reduces left atrial pressure and hence left ventricular filling and stroke volume. Thus left ventricular systole is shortened and A_2 is earlier. During inspiration, then, A_2 occurs earlier and P_2 later, so that splitting of the second sound widens. During expiration the changes are exactly opposite and the splitting narrows. Movement of P_2 is considerably greater than that of A_2.

Third and fourth heart sounds

In addition to the first and second heart sounds which are both of a high frequency, lower frequency sounds may be heard in diastole. These additional sounds are known as the third and the fourth (or atrial) sounds. When either of these additional sounds is present they give a cadence containing three beats rather than the normal two beats—'lub' and 'dub'.

Both of these low frequency sounds are caused by abnormal filling patterns in the left ventricle. The third heart sound occurs in early diastole at the time of maximal ventricular filling. This occurs about 0.15 second after the second heart sound. The fourth heart sound occurs when the bolus of blood is delivered into the ventricle from atrial contraction. It follows that this sound is found only in patients in sinus rhythm.

The third heart sound may occur in healthy young adults and is also a particular feature of pregnancy. In any other clinical setting, however, the presence of a third heart sound indicates abnormal left ventricular filling. The most important causes of this are left ventricular failure and mitral regurgitation.

Fourth heart sounds are caused by an increased stiffness or non-compliance of the ventricles. Atrial contraction as a consequence produces a sudden increase in pressure in the ventricle, rather than the ventricle increasing its volume to accommodate the extra blood delivered by atrial systole. When the heart rate is rapid, diastole is shortened and the third and fourth heart sounds may coincide. When this occurs the amplitude of the sound increases and is more easily detected, giving rise to a summation gallop rhythm, so called because it gives the auditory impression of a galloping horse. Third or fourth heart sounds may originate from either right or left ventricles. These diastolic sounds are always best heard with the bell of the stethoscope and auscultation should routinely include a search for these sounds with the patient turned slightly on to the left side.

In constrictive pericarditis a very loud low frequency diastolic sound is characteristically audible. This is known as a pericardial 'knock'. The presence of this sound always coincides with the very abrupt halt to early diastolic filling which is the distinctive abnormality of pericardial constriction.

Additional sounds

Ejection systolic clicks arise from the opening of the semilunar valves, either aortic or pulmonary (Fig. 9.6). These sounds therefore occur in early systole, mimicking splitting of the first heart sound. Aortic ejection sounds are well heard throughout the praecordium but are best appreciated at the apex, where they are preceded by the first heart sound at its loudest intensity. The valve is abnormal although this may be trivial, for example a bicuspid aortic valve without stenosis. Pulmonary ejection sounds become much softer on inspiration but are loud and sharp on expiration.

When one of the great arteries is dilated, for example the pulmonary artery in pulmonary hypertension, a systolic ejection sound can frequently be heard. A similar sound occurs in longstanding untreated hypertension. These hypertensive ejection sounds may be due to secondary changes in the corresponding semilunar valves.

Opening of the mitral and tricuspid valves occurs in early diastole shortly after the second heart sound (Fig. 9.6). Normally these valves open silently but when the valve leaflets are abnormal, as in rheumatic, mitral or tricuspid stenosis, a sound is associated with the opening movement. This sound is analogous to the systolic clicks of the aortic or pulmonary valve opening, but, by tradition, the sounds are known as opening snaps when they are related to the mitral or tricuspid valves. The presence of an opening snap is indicative of a pliable valve leaflet.

Loud extra sounds or clicks occur in mid-systole in association with prolapse of the mitral valve. These mid-systolic clicks may or may not be associated with a late systolic murmur. The presence of a mid-systolic click leads to a cadence which resembles that of a third heart sound. The two can be distinguished by the high frequency of the mid-systolic click and the low frequency of the third heart sound. Mid-systolic clicks arise from the halting of the mitral leaflet as it prolapses into the left atrium during systole.

Murmurs

Murmurs are due to turbulence in the blood flow at or near a valve or an abnormal communication within the heart. It follows that a loud murmur may originate from a rather small orifice such as a ventricular septal defect. Equally a soft murmur may originate from a large abnormal orifice as in very severe aortic regurgitation. Thus while it is important to note the intensity of a murmur, one should not make immediate deductions about its importance solely from its loudness. Not all murmurs are produced by a structural disorder of the heart; they may be due to abnormally rapid flow of blood through a normal valve. Such murmurs are called *flow murmurs*. Murmurs also occur at the site of arterial stenoses, when they are traditionally called *bruits*. In examining a murmur the following points must be noted:

Time of occurrence Murmurs may be systolic, diastolic or continuous throughout systole and diastole. Murmurs can only be timed reliably if the carotid arterial pulse is palpated during auscultation so that systole can be determined. *Systolic murmurs* are either *pansystolic*, as in mitral or tricuspid regurgitation and ventricular septal defect, or *ejection*, when they arise either from the pulmonary or aortic outflow tracts. Pansystolic murmurs start immediately with the first heart sound and continue through to the second heart

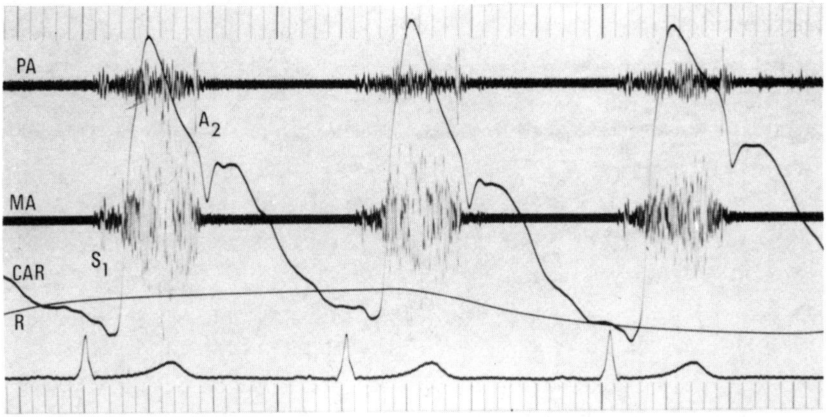

Fig. 9.7 Phonocardiograms recorded from the pulmonary area (PA) and mitral area (MA) together with the carotid pulse (CAR) and respiration (R) in a patient with mitral regurgitation. The ECG is shown at the bottom of the tracing. A systolic murmur can be seen in the phonocardiogram recorded at the mitral area. The murmur starts immediately after the first heart sound (S_1) and continues right up to and including the second heart sound (A_2). In this example the presence of the pansystolic murmur at the mitral area obliterates A_2, which would have been audible only in the pulmonary area.

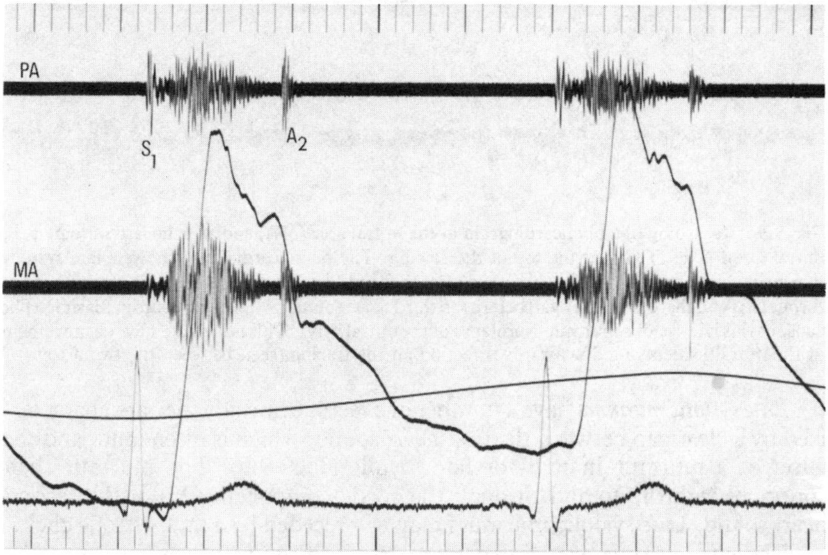

Fig. 9.8 Phonocardiograms recorded from the pulmonary area (PA) and mitral area (MA) in a patient with an ejection systolic murmur. The carotid pulse and respiration are recorded in a manner similar to Fig. 9.7. The diamond shape of an ejection systoliç murmur can be clearly seen. A clear gap is visible between the end of the murmur and the beginning of A_2.

sound (Fig. 9.7). Typically they have a uniform intensity. By contrast, ejection systolic murmurs have a diamond-shaped configuration building to a peak in mid-systole (Fig. 9.8). Ejection murmurs typically diminish before the second heart sound.

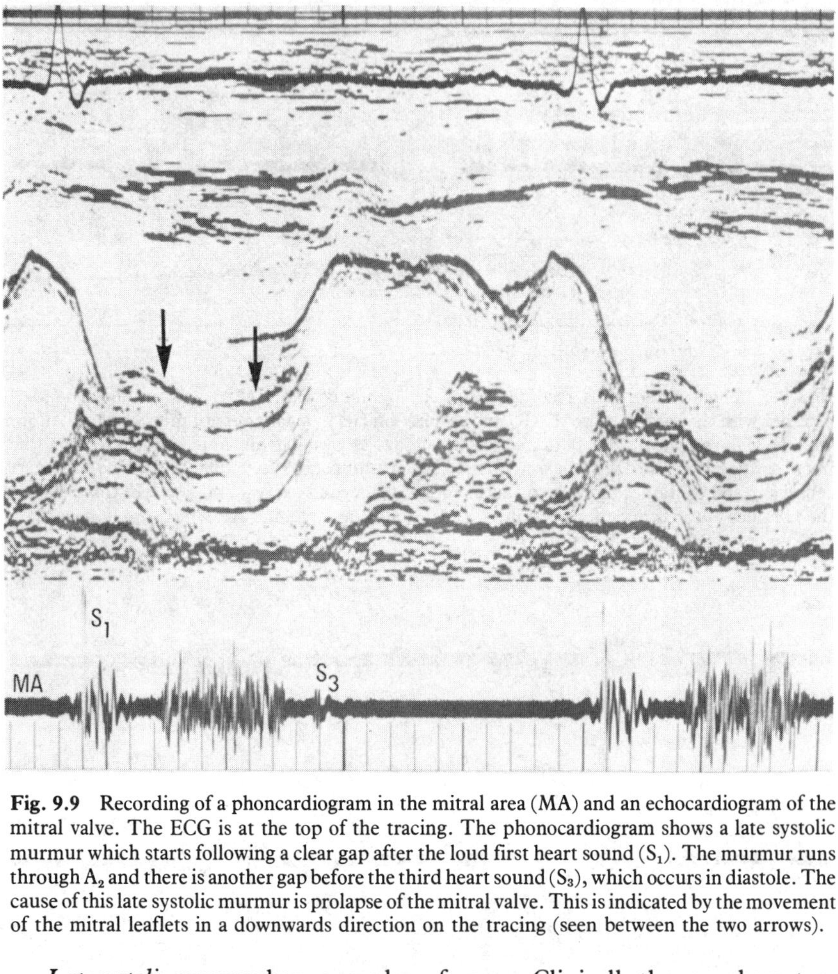

Fig. 9.9 Recording of a phoncardiogram in the mitral area (MA) and an echocardiogram of the mitral valve. The ECG is at the top of the tracing. The phonocardiogram shows a late systolic murmur which starts following a clear gap after the loud first heart sound (S_1). The murmur runs through A_2 and there is another gap before the third heart sound (S_3), which occurs in diastole. The cause of this late systolic murmur is prolapse of the mitral valve. This is indicated by the movement of the mitral leaflets in a downwards direction on the tracing (seen between the two arrows).

Late systolic murmurs have a number of causes. Clinically they are characterized by a clear gap between the first heart sound, which is often loud, and the onset of a murmur in mid- or late systole (Fig. 9.9). The murmur then continues right up to and through the aortic component (A_2) of the second heart sound. Late systolic murmurs may be preceded by a mid-systolic click.

Diastolic murmurs are of two types. *Early diastolic murmurs* start at the second heart sound and occur as a result of aortic or pulmonary regurgitation. *Mid-diastolic murmurs*, in which there is a short gap after the second heart sound before the beginning of the murmur, arise from the mitral or tricuspid valve.

The behaviour of the murmur during respiration The stroke output of the right heart increases during inspiration, while that of the left heart is reduced. It follows that a murmur originating on the right side of the heart will become louder during inspiration.

Point of maximum intensity and direction of selective propagation Murmurs due to pulmonary and tricuspid valve lesions are generally well localized to the areas on the praecordium which have been described earlier as overlying the corresponding valves. Aortic and mitral murmurs, however, may radiate extensively. Aortic systolic murmurs, for instance, may be as loud, if not louder, at the cardiac apex than they are in the aortic area. Systolic murmurs that radiate into the carotid arteries are usually aortic in origin. Pansystolic murmurs due to mitral regurgitation may be heard over a wide area of the chest. The murmur of severe mitral regurgitation is often easily audible in the aortic and pulmonary areas. It follows that the point of maximal intensity should not be regarded as one of the cardinal diagnostic features in aortic stenosis and mitral regurgitation.

The character of a murmur Although formerly stressed, the character of a murmur is now considered an unreliable guide to its origin. Rough murmurs are associated with obstruction to flow through a narrowed valve; blowing murmurs are more typical of an incompetent valve.

In the next paragraphs the haemodynamics in the common forms of valvular disease are presented, and the associated auscultatory signs discussed.

Mitral valve disease

Mitral stenosis

The physical signs found in mitral stenosis are attributable to two separate effects of the rheumatic process on the thin, delicate mitral leaflets. Firstly, the valvulitis causes thickening and fibrosis of the cusps themselves. This process tends to continue throughout adult life and is responsible for the alterations in intensity of the first heart sound and the presence of the opening snap. Secondly, the two leaflets become fused at the edges of the commissures so that the orifice available for blood to pass from the left atrium to the left ventricle becomes reduced. The ensuing turbulence of blood flow causes the mid-diastolic murmur associated with mitral stenosis.

Heart sounds The classical findings in mitral stenosis, before the leaflets become very thickened and calcified, are (a) a first heart sound much louder than normal and (b) an opening snap occurring shortly after (0.06–0.14 s) the

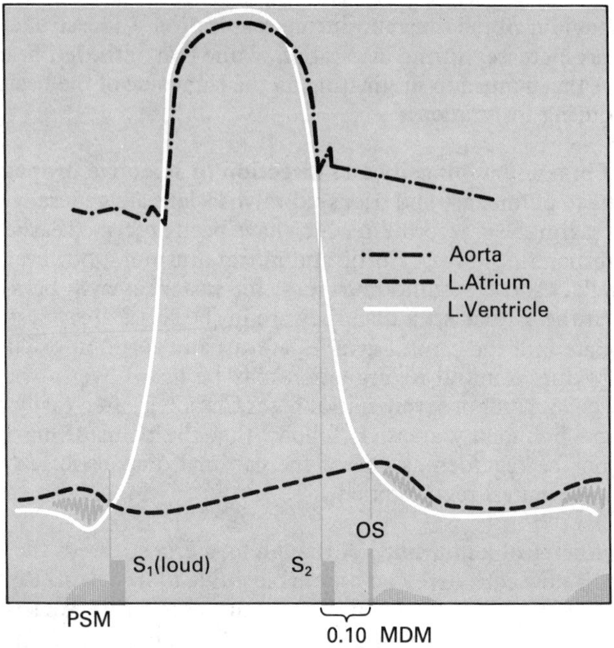

Fig. 9.10 The relationship of diastolic murmurs to the haemodynamics in mild mitral stenosis. The left atrial pressure is only slightly elevated so that mitral valve opening, indicated by the opening snap (OS), is not particularly early in relationship to the second heart sound (S_2).

second heart sound. These cause a striking alteration in the cadence of the heart sounds and once they have been recognized provide the easiest and most sensitive clinical means of detecting mitral stenosis.

The closeness of the opening snap to the second heart sound is a useful indicator of the severity of the mitral stenosis. The reason for this is that the mitral valve opens only after the left ventricular pressure has fallen below the left atrial pressure (Fig. 9.10); consequently the more severe the mitral stenosis the higher is the left atrial pressure and the closer to the second heart sound does the mitral valve open (Fig. 9.11).

In later years, as the mitral valve begins to develop calcification and marked fibrotic thickening, the intensity of both the first heart sound and the opening snap diminishes. A loud first heart sound and opening snap therefore indicates the presence of a relatively pliable and non-calcified valve. Such valves may be suitable for the operation of mitral valvotomy, rather than needing to be replaced, should surgery be indicated.

The mitral diastolic murmur This murmur is typically low pitched and must be sought with the bell of the stethoscope and the patient turned towards the left side. Its *loudness* is accentuated by a brief period of exertion such as the

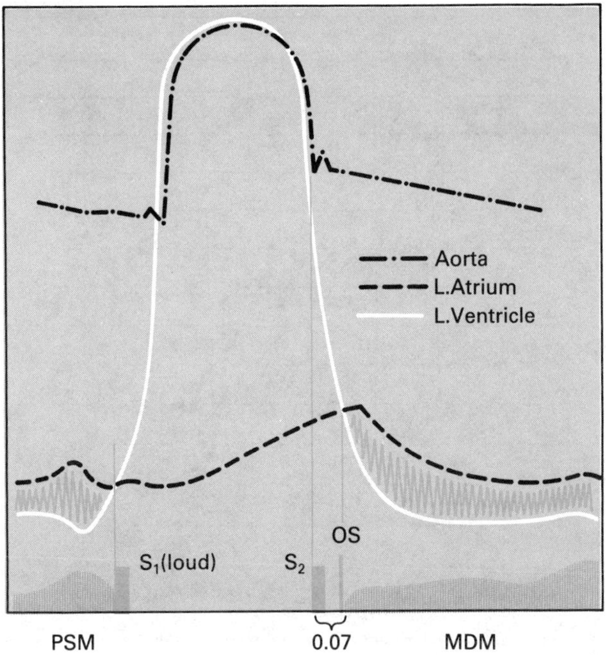

Fig. 9.11 The relationship of murmurs to haemodynamics in severe mitral stenosis. Increasing severity of mitral valve obstruction leads to elevation of the left atrial pressure. Because the left ventricular pressure has less far to fall to reach this elevated atrial pressure, the time from A_2 to the opening snap is shortened.

patient touching her toes five or six times. The *length* of the murmur is an important indicator of the severity of the mitral stenosis. This should be assessed in a cardiac cycle with a long diastole.

If the patient is in atrial fibrillation then the length of diastole may vary greatly. With a short diastole, the diastolic murmur may appear to be full length, but the examiner should wait for a long diastole to assess the length of the murmur. In mild to moderate mitral stenosis a length of diastole equivalent to a heart rate of about 70 beats per minute is often sufficiently long to allow equilibration of left atrial and left ventricular pressures at the end of diastole and hence the murmur does not completely fill this phase of the cardiac cycle.

In patients in sinus rhythm (Fig. 9.12), the mitral stenotic murmur is accentuated at the end of diastole. Two factors contribute to this phenomenon. Firstly, atrial systole increases flow across the stenotic valve from left atrium to left ventricle and this accentuates the loudness of a murmur. Such accentuation is also sometimes noted in patients in atrial fibrillation. In this case identification of the second factor becomes important, namely turbulence caused by the mitral valve starting to close under the influence of the onset of ventricular systole. This occurs before the first heart sound and so gives the

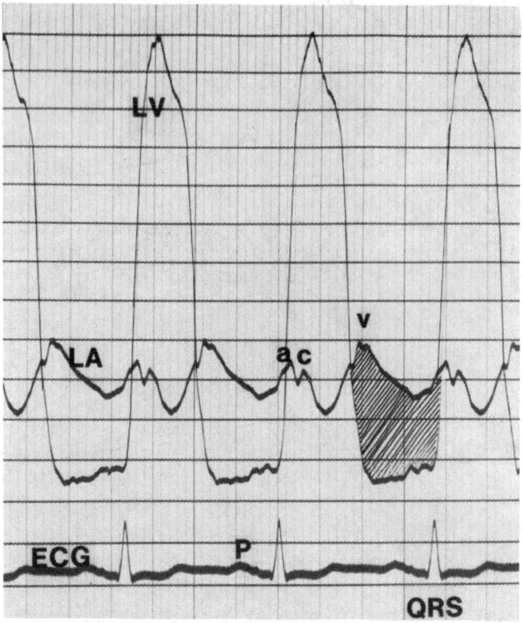

Fig. 9.12 Left atrial (LA) and left ventricular (LV) pressure tracings in a patient with mitral stenosis and sinus rhythm. The *a* and *c* waves together with the *v* wave can be seen in the left atrial tracing. The shaded area between the atrial and ventricular pressures during diastole indicates the size of the gradient across this patient's mitral valve. Each of the horizontal lines represents 10 mmHg; thus the end diastolic gradient is 20 mmHg, although the gradient in early diastole is closer to 35 mmHg.

impression of falling in late diastole. It is, however, due to the start of ventricular systole.

Mitral regurgitation

There are a number of different causes for the mitral leaflets' failure to prevent reflux of blood from the left ventricle to the left atrium during systole. The cusps may be affected by rheumatic disease or mitral valve prolapse; the chordae tendinae may rupture, which leads to part of a cusp being unsupported; or there may be ischaemic damage to a papillary muscle. Irrespective of its cause the characteristic auscultatory finding in mitral regurgitation is a pansystolic murmur.

The mitral pansystolic murmur The regurgitant jet of blood starts as soon as left ventricular pressure exceeds left atrial pressure, that is, immediately after the first heart sound, and continues up to and through the second heart

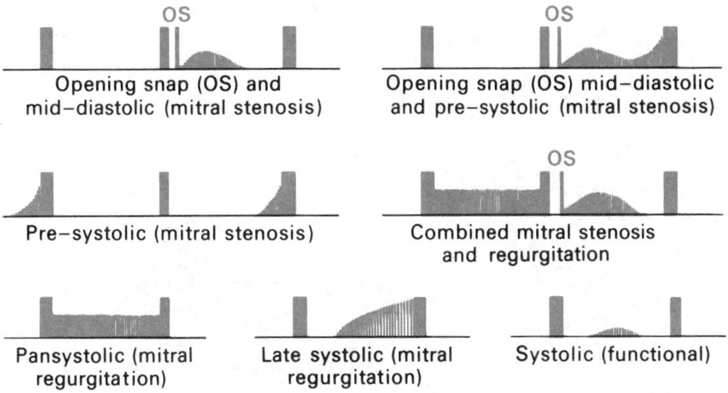

Fig. 9.13 Mitral murmurs.

sound until left ventricular pressure falls below left atrial pressure. These events account for the characteristics of the pansystolic murmur. The murmur is best heard at the mitral area, and it radiates to the axilla and to the back when the anterior leaflet is abnormal. When the posterior leaflet is damaged the regurgitant jet is often directed anteriorly so that the murmur is then loudest over the anterior praecordium and up to the pulmonary area.

The mitral late systolic murmur A late systolic murmur heard at the mitral area is indicative of mild mitral regurgitation and is usually associated with mitral valve prolapse. A late mitral systolic murmur may also be heard in patients with mitral regurgitation due to ischaemic damage to a papillary muscle or to hypertrophic cardiomyopathy.

The various combinations of murmurs associated with mitral valve disease are summarized in Fig. 9.13.

Aortic valve disease

Aortic stenosis

The haemodynamics in aortic stenosis are shown diagrammatically in Fig. 9.14. There is a pressure gradient between the left ventricle and aorta during systole, and the size of this pressure difference is an indication of the severity of the stenosis. The gradient is greatest in the middle of systole, and is relatively small early and late in the systole. The murmur therefore has a 'diamond' shape, starting soft, building to a peak in mid-systole then becoming less loud in late systole immediately before the second sound. All murmurs due to the ejection of blood through abnormal semilunar valves, or to abnormally high blood flow through normal semilunar valves, have this same pattern and are

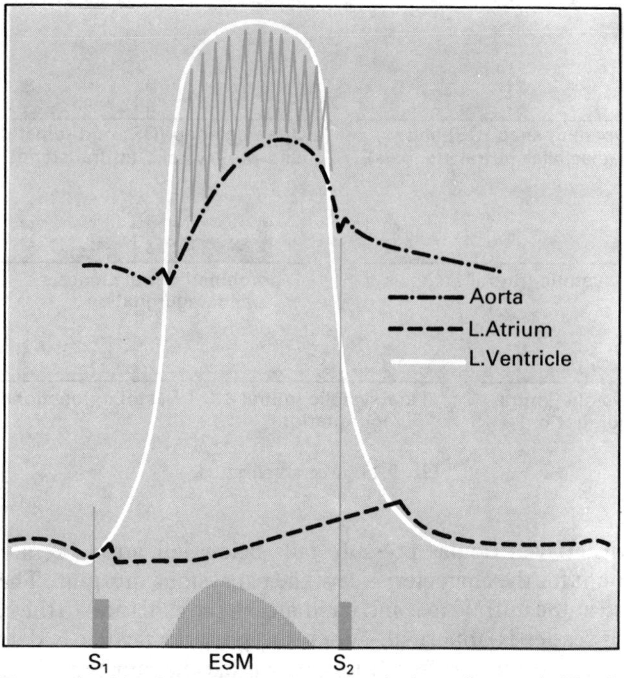

Fig. 9.14 The relationship of murmurs to haemodynamics in aortic stenosis. The slow ejection of blood into the aorta causes a slow rise in aortic pressure. The murmur follows the flow pattern rising to a peak in mid-systole then declining.

called 'ejection' systolic murmurs.

The *aortic ejection murmur* is heard in the aortic area and radiates into the carotids although it is frequently also well heard at the mitral area.

The *aortic ejection click* is produced on opening of the aortic valve in aortic valve stenosis. It is therefore heard just after the first heart sound at the beginning of the ejection murmur. Its presence indicates that stenosis is at the valvular rather than the supra- or subvalvular level. In aortic stenosis A_2 is delayed because of prolonged left ventricular systole. This causes a single S_2 and reversed splitting. Frequently this sign is difficult to detect because A_2, like the ejection click, becomes soft or inaudible when the cusps are heavily calcified. When the valve is rigid from fibrosis or calcification, no click is heard.

Aortic regurgitation

Regurgitant flow at the aortic valve (Fig. 9.15) may be large, and in severe cases can equal the forward flow of blood into the circulation. The stroke output from the left ventricle through the aortic valve into the aorta may therefore be doubled. This increased flow across the valve invariably gives rise to an aortic ejection murmur. Thus an aortic ejection murmur in a patient

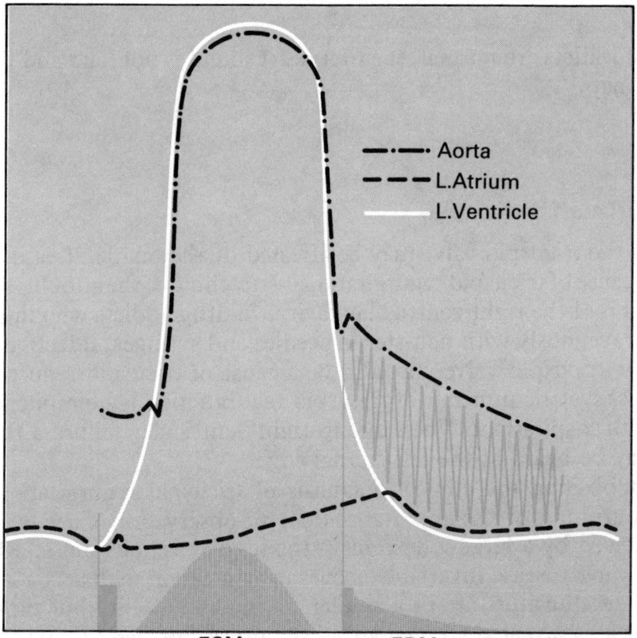

Fig. 9.15 The relationship of murmurs to haemodynamics in aortic regurgitation. The increased systolic stroke volume causes an ejection systolic murmur even though there is no co-existing aortic stenosis. Regurgitation commences as soon as the left ventricular pressure falls below the aortic diastolic pressure, i.e. immediately after aortic valve closure. The early diastolic murmur tails off as the diastolic pressure (and hence the gradient across the valve) diminishes and the left ventricle fills. ESM = ejection systolic murmur. EDM = early diastolic murmur.

with aortic regurgitation does not necessarily indicate the presence of aortic stenosis. The latter is best recognized by the contour of the carotid pulse.

The *early* or *immediate diastolic murmur* of aortic regurgitation starts with the second heart sound and continues for a variable time in diastole. It is a high-pitched murmur, usually soft, and usually requires intent auscultation for its recognition. It is best heard down the left sternal edge when the patient sits forward and breathes out; the examiner must listen with the diaphragm of the stethoscope.

The Austin Flint murmur In severe aortic regurgitation a low-pitched diastolic murmur may be audible at the mitral area. This murmur originates from the anterior leaflet of the mitral valve and is due to the confluence of two streams of blood. On one side there is antegrade flow from the left atrium to the left ventricle, and on the other side there is the regurgitant jet of blood through the incompetent aortic valve impinging on the anterior mitral leaflet. The resulting murmur closely resembles the murmur of mitral stenosis, but since the mitral leaflets are normal, the first heart sound is not loud and there is no opening snap.

Tricuspid valve disease

Although the tricuspid valve may be affected by rheumatic disease, the most common cause of tricuspid regurgitation is stretching of the annulus secondary to dilatation of the right ventricular cavity. In drug addicts who inject themselves intravenously with non-sterile needles and syringes, infective endocarditis of the tricuspid valve may also be a cause of tricuspid regurgitation.

The pansystolic murmur of tricuspid regurgitation is high pitched and is louder with inspiration. When due to right ventricular failure a third heart sound may be heard at the left sternal edge.

In establishing the clinical diagnosis of tricuspid regurgitation, a pansystolic murmur is of less importance than the observation of a giant systolic *v* wave followed by a large *y* descent in the jugular venous pulse. Rheumatic tricuspid valve disease invariably occurs in association with aortic and mitral disease. The murmurs are of a similar timing and quality but typically the opening snap associated with tricuspid stenosis occurs later than the opening snap of mitral stenosis.

A rare congenital disorder of the tricuspid valve is Ebstein's anomaly. The main abnormality in this condition is a great increase in the size of the anterior leaflet of the tricuspid valve. This is associated with a very loud first heart sound followed by a short systolic murmur. There is usually a tricuspid opening snap.

Myxoma

Myxomas are benign tumours of the atria. They most commonly occur in the left atrium but are also encountered in the right. The condition is of importance since it may cause emboli to the systemic circulation in the case of the left-sided tumour and to the pulmonary circulation in the right-sided tumour. Both clinically and haemodynamically a left atrial myxoma mimics mitral stenosis. This is because the tumour mass, which is attached to the inter-atrial septum by a stalk, drops down between the mitral leaflets during diastole causing obstruction of flow from the left atrium to the left ventricle.

The physical signs are variable but a loud first sound is usual and a low-pitched diastolic murmur may be audible. In addition there is often a low-frequency diastolic sound known as a 'tumour plop'. Systolic murmurs may also occur due to the mild mitral incompetence caused by damage to the mitral cusps by the presence and movement of the tumour.

Hypertrophic cardiomyopathy

Hypertrophic cardiomyopathy is a condition of unknown aetiology in which the muscle fibres of the ventricles become inappropriately hypertrophied and distorted. The commonest site for the process to occur is the inter-ventricular septum and only in the later stages of the condition or in particularly severe cases are the free walls of the left and right ventricles involved. Two main functional abnormalities occur as a consequence of the abnormal anatomy.

Firstly, the hypertrophied ventricle becomes much stiffer than normal and this is manifest by the presence of a loud fourth heart sound. Secondly, the inter-ventricular septum, when it contracts, bulges into the outflow tract of the left ventricle thus causing an intra-ventricular gradient. Such gradients do not always occur in hypertrophic cardiomyopathy but when they do they are generally associated with the presence of a systolic murmur. This murmur is essentially ejection systolic in nature but in some patients it may be prolonged until the second heart sound. A degree of mitral regurgitation may be associated with hypertrophic cardiomyopathy due to involvement of the papillary muscles. When present this tends to cause the systolic murmur to extend to the second heart sound.

The pattern of blood flow from the left ventricle is invariably abnormal whether obstruction is present or not. This leads to a typical jerky or sharp carotid arterial pulse. Even when there is severe obstruction the carotid upstroke does not become slow and delayed and this is an important distinguishing feature between hypertrophic cardiomyopathy and aortic valve stenosis.

Pulmonary stenosis

In mild pulmonary valve stenosis the only abnormal signs are found on auscultation (Fig. 9.16). The ejection systolic murmur is loudest in inspiration and best heard in the pulmonary area. It is preceded by an ejection click which is loudest in expiration and may be inaudible during inspiration. This distinguishes it from an aortic ejection click, which is of constant intensity. The second sound behaves normally on inspiration, but the width of splitting is wider than normal because of a delay in pulmonary valve closure.

The pulmonary component of the second sound is delayed in proportion to the severity of the stenosis. If the stenosis is severe, the closure of the pulmonary valve becomes soft or inaudible. The pressure overload on the right ventricle leads to a palpable right ventricular impulse at the left sternal edge.

Right ventricular outflow may be obstructed by inappropriate hypertrophy of the muscle which comprises the outflow tract—infundibular stenosis. In this case an ejection systolic murmur and delay in P_2 will also be heard but there is no pulmonary ejection sound.

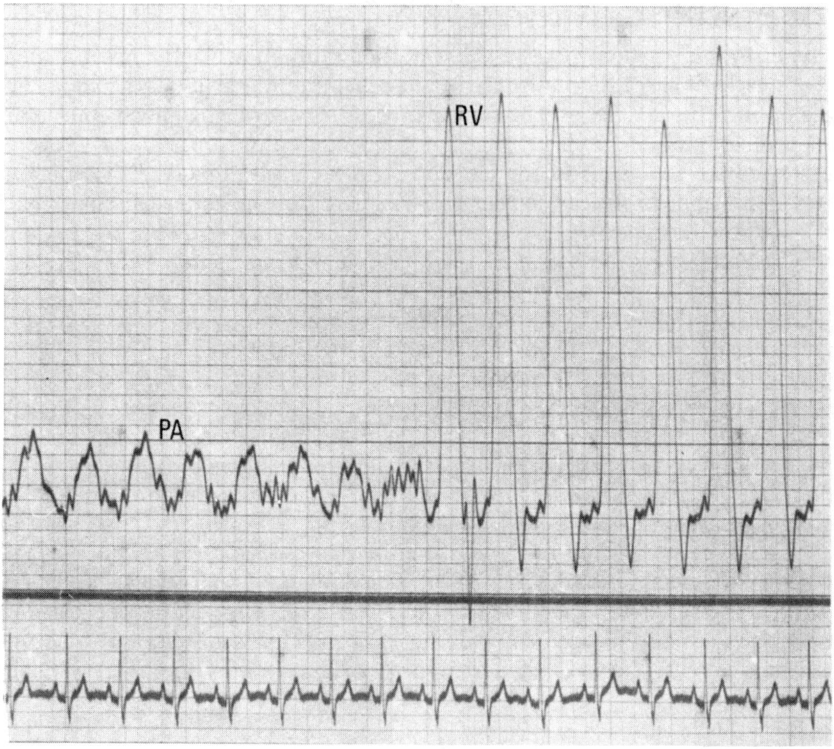

Fig. 9.16 Pressure tracings from a patient with pulmonary stenosis. A catheter has been withdrawn from the pulmonary artery into the right ventricle. The severity of the stenosis is measured by the difference between the peak systolic pressure in the right ventricle and the peak systolic pressure in the pulmonary artery. Each dense horizontal line represents 25 mmHg. The pressure difference in this patient is therefore between 55 and 60 mmHg. Similar principles apply in aortic stenosis; the severity of the stenosis is assessed by the pressure difference between the left ventricle and the aorta.

Left to right shunts

When there is an abnormal communication between the left and right sides of the circulation, blood will flow from left to right provided the pulmonary vascular resistance is not grossly increased. Such communications occur anatomically at the *atrial level* (i.e. atrial septal defect), the *ventricular level* (i.e. ventricular septal defect), and between the *aorta and the pulmonary artery* (i.e. patent ductus arteriosus).

Atrial septal defect

Blood flows through an atrial septal defect from left atrium to right, since normal pressure relationships are maintained within the atria. The blood flow through the defect is often more than twice the flow entering the left ventricle (i.e. the systemic blood flow). The blood entering the right atrium will then be the systemic flow plus the flow from the left atrium through the atrial septal defect, i.e. three times the systemic flow. This increased flow passes from the right atrium to the right ventricle, pulmonary artery, lung vessels and so back to the left atrium.

Because the defect is very large and the pressure gradient very small (about 1 mmHg), there is little turbulence and no audible murmur from blood flowing through the defect itself. The characteristic auscultatory sign is *fixed* splitting of the second heart sound, since the increased right ventricular stroke volume does not vary with respiration. The increased blood flow through the pulmonary valve produces a functional ejection pulmonary systolic murmur which is moderately loud. A functional tricuspid flow murmur is often present. It is mid-diastolic, of low frequency and best heard at the lower end of the sternum.

Ventricular septal defect

Ventricular septal defects are rarely as large as atrial septal defects and usually less than 1 cm in diameter. The right ventricular systolic pressure is normally about one-fifth of that in the left ventricle, so there is a pressure gradient from left ventricle to right throughout systole.

In mild cases, in which the defect has the cross-sectional area of a pencil lead, the only abnormal sign is a loud pansystolic murmur, best heard at the lower end of the sternum. The murmur is usually accompanied by a thrill.

In more severe cases there is evidence of increased blood flow through the pulmonary vasculature and the left heart. In addition to the pansystolic murmur and thrill there may be a short soft mid-diastolic murmur due to the increased flow of blood through the mitral valve. Splitting of the second sound is normal, though A_2 may be difficult to hear as it tends to be obscured by the pansystolic murmur which extends to P_2. When there is pulmonary hypertension the second sound becomes single and loud.

Patent ductus arteriosus

The communication has the same size range as in ventricular septal defects. A pressure gradient through the communication from aorta to pulmonary artery is present throughout the cardiac cycle and is greatest towards the end of systole. The increased flow affects the left heart and pulmonary circulation exclusively. If the communication is small, a murmur is the only abnormal sign. It is best heard at the pulmonary area in expiration, and is continuous through both systole and diastole. The accentuation of the murmur about the time of the second sound gives it a particular character, and it is sometimes described as a machinery murmur. In addition to the continuous murmur, a short soft functional mitral diastolic murmur may be present.

Patent ductus arteriosus is the most common but not the only cause of a continuous murmur. Pulmonary arteriovenous fistulae, coronary arterio-venous fistulae or communications between the ascending aorta and pulmonary artery will produce similar physical signs. Particular care should always be taken not to confuse the murmurs of a patent ductus arteriosus with a venous hum.

Fallot's tetralogy

Fallot's tetralogy consists of pulmonary stenosis, ventricular septal defect, right ventricular hypertrophy and overriding of the aorta, i.e. the aorta arises astride the ventricular septal defect. The essential features are pulmonary stenosis of at least moderate severity and a large ventricular septal defect, so that the pressure in the two ventricles is equal in systole. The right ventricular output is ejected partly into the pulmonary artery through the pulmonary stenosis, and partly into the aorta through the ventricular septal defect. The admixture of deoxygenated blood with the left ventricular output makes the patient cyanosed.

The auscultatory signs are a pulmonary ejection murmur and a single second sound. P_2 is inaudible both because of the low blood flow in the pulmonary artery and because of the associated pulmonary stenosis.

Coarctation of the aorta

In coarctation of the aorta there is a stricture of the aorta at or near the insertion of the ligamentum arteriosum. The arterial pressure proximal to the coarctation is increased, so that the blood pressure in the arms is greater than that in the legs. The radial and femoral pulses should be felt simultaneously. Normally the timing of the pulse wave is identical in these vessels. In coarctation the femoral pulse is delayed and diminished, or absent. The raised arterial pressure leads to left ventricular hypertrophy, which can be detected clinically. There is often an ejection click and an aortic ejection systolic murmur because of an associated congenital bicuspid aortic valve. Collateral vessels linking the subclavian arteries, which arise above the aortic stricture, with intercostal arteries arising below the stricture can usually be felt above the scapulae, and are best seen with the patient bending forwards in a good light.

Pulmonary hypertension

There are a number of important physical signs in addition to the auscultatory abnormalities which indicate the presence of pulmonary hypertension. A prominent *a* wave is visible in the venous pulse even though the mean level of the venous pressure is not elevated. This *a* wave is due to the stiff (non-compliant), thickened right ventricular wall which invariably develops in response to the presence of severe pulmonary hypertension. The carotid arterial pulse volume is small. On palpation of the praecordium a prominent parasternal impulse due to right ventricular hypertrophy is palpable.

Pulmonary hypertension by itself does not lead to any systolic or diastolic murmurs. The most important finding is that pulmonary valve closure (P_2) is accentuated and may be palpable. In a number of cases, a pulmonary ejection click can also be heard. In severe long-standing pulmonary hypertension the dilatation of the pulmonary artery may lead to secondary pulmonary valve regurgitation. This presents as a high-pitched early diastolic murmur loudest in the pulmonary area and radiating down the left sternal border. Pulmonary incompetence is very rarely found other than in association with pulmonary hypertension or following pulmonary valvotomy.

Flow murmurs

Systolic flow murmurs are due to turbulent, increased flow of blood across a normal valve, and thus *do not indicate valvular disease*. Such murmurs are always of an ejection pattern. Flow murmurs may have either a grunting or a musical component and their timing is generally earlier in systole than murmurs due to an organic obstruction to outflow. Flow murmurs may arise from either the left or right ventricular outflow tracts. Flow murmurs are never associated with any abnormality in the electrocardiogram, but may sometimes be due to an abnormality of the thoracic wall, such as a depressed sternum.

Flow murmurs are most commonly encountered in children and young adults or in the elderly. They also occur whenever there is an increased stroke volume, such as in anaemia, thyrotoxicosis, systemic hypertension, or in chronic anxiety.

Exocardial sounds and murmurs

Venous hum

Sometimes in children a continuous murmur can be heard in the neck and upper chest which is due to kinking and partial obstruction of one of the larger veins in the neck, thus preventing the continuous flow of blood through the vein. The origin of the murmur should be suspected because of the youth of the patient and the loudness of the murmur in the neck. The hum can be obliterated by pressure on the neck, which produces complete obstruction of the vein, or by altering the position of the neck so as to relieve the venous obstruction. It is particularly important to exclude a venous hum if a diagnosis of patent ductus is being considered.

Pericardial rubs

Pericardial rubs have a characteristic high-pitched sound which has been likened to the noise emitted by compression of new leather. They are generally loudest in systole but often have an additional diastolic component. Because part of the pericardium is in contact with the lung there may also be a marked respiratory element. Pericardial rubs are one of the most evanescent of physical signs and vary greatly from hour to hour. The presence of a pericardial rub indicates that two inflamed layers of pericardium are in contact. The development of an effusion will separate the two layers of pericardium and hence lead to the disappearance of the rub.

ISCHAEMIC HEART DISEASE

The arteries of the coronary circulation are at risk of developing atherosclerosis, which may partially or completely occlude their lumen; this disease process is a major cause of mortality and morbidity in many countries. Characteristically coronary artery disease is symptomless for many years. It may present as a chronic intermittent impairment of blood supply to the myocardium, resulting in the symptom of angina, or as an acute disorder when a coronary vessel is completely occluded. The latter generally occurs because of intraluminal thrombosis at the site of an atheromatous plaque, leading to death of the myocardium supplied by that vessel—myocardial infarction (see Fig. 9.32).

The diagnosis of coronary artery disease depends greatly on an accurate history. The symptom of angina pectoris may be described by the patient as a 'pain', 'tightness', 'unpleasant sensation' or even a feeling of breathlessness. It characteristically occurs in the upper chest, radiating to both the left and the right side of the sternum often in a band-like or constricting fashion. The pain may also radiate down the inner aspect of the left arm, into the left elbow and the little finger of the left hand. Less commonly it radiates to a region between the scapulae or up into the lower jaw, especially around the teeth.

The pain is characteristically provoked by exertion or, in some cases, by emotional stress. It occurs *during* rather than at the end of exercise. Rest alleviates the pain and it may be possible for the patient to walk much further during a subsequent period of exercise after resting—the warm up effect. The pain is typically more severe or more easily provoked in cold weather, especially if windy. Nitroglycerine relieves the pain within 5 to 10 minutes of starting to suck a tablet.

When typical cardiac pain lasts for more than 30 minutes the possibility of a diagnosis of myocardial infarction arises. In this instance the characteristics of the pain are similar to that of angina but it is generally more severe, is not relieved by nitroglycerine, and is often associated with nausea or vomiting and with profuse sweating.

Unstable angina describes a clinical pattern in which angina occurs either at rest or with very minimal exertion but without progressing to myocardial infarction. Because the major characteristic of angina, namely, its relationship to physical exertion, is absent, it is sometimes difficult to distinguish unstable angina from pain which is not in fact of cardiac origin. Severe or unstable angina is often worse first thing on waking in the morning or after a heavy meal; it may also occur during sleep with or without accompanying nightmares.

Physical examination in patients with angina due to coronary artery disease is generally unrewarding, but it is always important to exclude the diagnoses of aortic stenosis, hypertrophic cardiomyopathy or severe pulmonary hypertension in patients who give this history. There may be signs of generalized arterial disease.

Important general conditions which may precipitate angina are anaemia and myxoedema. The physical signs associated with these conditions should be sought in every patient with angina. There may be clinical evidence to indicate hyperlipidaemia. Lipid deposits may occur as xanthelasmata in the upper or lower eyelids or they may be found on palpation of tendons, particularly the Achilles, triceps and extensor tendons of the hand. Lipid may be deposited in the cornea at its margin with the conjunctiva—the *arcus*. There is a slight gap between the lipid deposit and the conjunctiva itself.

On auscultation the only abnormality in coronary disease is the presence of a fourth heart sound, which is due to an increase in stiffness of the left ventricular muscle when it has an inadequate blood supply. This may be a chronic finding but it also occurs typically during the acute phase of myocardial infarction.

Mitral regurgitation may occur as a complication of ischaemia, or infarction, of the papillary muscles. Usually the degree of regurgitation is not severe and the typical finding is of a soft late systolic murmur. Occasionally ischaemic rupture of a papillary muscle leads to very severe mitral regurgitation with a loud pansystolic murmur. A similar physical finding presents in association with a ventricular septal defect due to rupture of the interventricular septum, and on clinical grounds alone it may be difficult to distinguish these two diagnoses. In general, mitral regurgitation is more commonly associated with disease of the right or left circumflex coronary arteries, whereas an acquired ventricular septal defect is usually associated with disease of the left anterior descending coronary artery.

The right ventricle is largely supplied by the right coronary artery and there is often a mild degree of right ventricular dysfunction associated with inferior myocardial infarction. This is manifest clinically as a 2–3 cm elevation of the jugular venous pressure, but this is usually a transitory phenomenon.

THE PERIPHERAL VASCULAR SYSTEM

Examination of the peripheral vascular system, including both the arterial and venous system, is often carried out as part of the general examination. It is of particular importance in patients with symptoms of arterial or venous disease of the limbs, and in those with cerebral or coronary arterial disease. Further, many patients with hypertension or diabetes mellitus have associated arterial disease, and degenerative vascular disease is common in the elderly. Special attention must therefore be paid to the arterial system in these patients.

Peripheral arterial system

Intermittent claudication is the term used to describe the cramp-like aching pain felt in the calf muscles during exercise. The pain occurs only during exercise, often after walking a certain distance, and it gradually ceases when the patient stops walking. It is ischaemic pain due to failure of the peripheral arterial system to allow a sufficiently increased blood flow to the legs to match the metabolic demands of muscular work. In certain forms of inflammatory arterial disease, e.g. polyarteritis nodosa or temporal arteritis, similar ischaemic pain may occur in other muscles. Intermittent claudication of the legs is not associated with numbness or tingling in the feet or legs unless the blood supply of the cauda equina or of the spinal cord is affected.

Impaired blood supply to a limb can be assessed by its lowered skin temperature and by its impaired nutritional status. Temperature differences can be reliably assessed only when the limbs have been exposed to a constant room temperature for 10–20 minutes. In an ischaemic leg the skin of the foot is cold and pale or cyanosed, and capillary filling after blanching with light finger pressure is delayed. *Reactive hyperaemia* is also delayed. This can be demonstrated with the patient lying down. The leg is elevated for several minutes to allow the venous pool of blood in the leg to drain into the circulation, and then the patient sits up and allows the leg to hang over the edge of the bed. Normally the foot will flush pink in about 10 seconds; the flush takes a longer time to appear if blood flow is inadequate.

When there has been chronic arterial insufficiency the skin becomes thin and shiny, often losing its hair, and the nails become brittle. Late manifestations of severe arterial insufficiency are chronic ulceration and even gangrene, especially of the distal parts of the toes or feet, the dead area becoming shrivelled, blackened and often demarcated from neighbouring healthy tissue by a thin red zone of inflamed tissue. In *acute interruption of arterial flow* to a limb, as in embolic or thrombotic occlusion of a femoral artery, the affected leg becomes colder than the normal limb, the peripheral pulses below the level of obstruction disappear, and the skin, which is at first white, becomes blue and, later, gangrenous.

Diminished or absent pulsation of vessels is of great value in localizing arterial lesions, both acute and chronic. In the legs the femoral, popliteal, posterior tibial and dorsalis pedis pulses should be carefully palpated with slightly flexed fingers, and their pulsation compared with that in the contralateral vessels. Using the bell of the stethoscope a careful search for the hissing systolic sound (arterial bruit) associated with partial obstruction should be made in both femoral arteries, in the abdomen (aortic bruits) and in the loins (renal artery bruits).

In patients with claudication, the distal pulses should also be examined after exercise since the diversion of blood flow to exercised muscle may cause previously detectable pulses to disappear, indicating restriction of flow in the affected limb.

In the arms the brachial and radial pulses should be similarly assessed and bruits listened for over the subclavian vessels. The carotid arteries should be carefully examined; it is particularly common to find systolic bruits in these vessels. Arterial pulsation in the limbs can be assessed quantitatively with a Döppler ultrasonic flow meter.

Spasm of arterioles may occur in the presence of normal peripheral pulses. This is usually seen in the hands; the digital arteries go into spasm in response to cold or to emotional stimuli so that the fingers become white and then cyanosed. When the spasm passes off, the fingers become hyperaemic and pink. This sequence of changes is termed *Raynaud's phenomenon*. Very rarely it may lead to superficial necrosis of the skin of the fingers.

In patients with arterial disease it is important to remember that the arterioles, capillary bed and small veins can be inspected directly in the retina by ophthalmoscopy (see p. 395). Some patients with hyperlipidaemia show an 'arcus' and xanthelasmata (see Plate IV). Lipid deposits within tendons may be detected in the Achilles, triceps and extensor tendons to the fingers.

Peripheral venous system

Varicose veins should be looked for with the patient standing. Superficial varicosities are then obvious. The efficiency of the valves of the long saphenous vein should be assessed by Trendelenburg's test. With the patient lying, the saphenous vein is emptied by elevating the leg. The upper end of the vein is then occluded by finger pressure on the saphenous opening. While the examiner maintains this pressure, the patient stands. If the valves are incompetent the vein will fill from above when the pressure is released.

Venous thrombosis is rare in healthy mobile subjects but may sometimes occur in women taking oral contraceptives. However, it is a frequent complication of enforced bed rest, particularly after surgery. Congestive cardiac failure also leads to venous stasis and thrombosis. The affected limb is swollen, tender and warmer than normal. Dilated superficial veins may be seen which do not collapse when the leg is elevated. Forceful dorsiflexion of the foot will cause pain in the calf (Homans' sign). Sometimes extension of deep venous thrombosis upwards to the thigh may lead to a tender, hard, palpable femoral vein.

Studies with radioactive fibrinogen, which is taken up by the forming thrombus, and venography have shown that quite extensive venous thrombosis can occur without significant physical findings. Pulmonary embolism may be the first clinical manifestation of a deep vein thrombosis in the leg.

ROUTINE CARDIOVASCULAR EXAMINATION

A record of a normal examination of the cardiovascular system should be constructed along the following lines.

The arterial pulse is of regular rate and rhythm and the carotid upstroke is normal. The blood pressure in the right arm with the patient lying is 120/80.

The venous pressure is not elevated and there are no abnormal pulsations on palpation of the praecordium. On auscultation the first heart sound is normal and splitting of the second sound can be identified. There are no murmurs and no additional heart sounds.

The peripheral pulses in the upper and lower limbs are all present and equal as are the carotid pulses. There are no bruits.

ELECTROCARDIOGRAPHY

The electrocardiogram (ECG) is a recording from the body surface of the electrical changes that occur within the heart during the cardiac cycle. An outline of this technique is presented here.

The main areas in which the electrocardiogram (ECG) can prove useful are:

1 Analysis of abnormal rhythms.
2 Detection and localization of changes in the myocardium due to coronary artery disease.
3 Detection of hypertrophy of the walls of the atria and ventricles.
4 Detection of changes in electrical activity due to pericardial disease.
5 Detection of changes in electrical activity of the heart consequent on general metabolic changes.

Additional valuable information may be obtained by recording the electrocardiogram during physical exercise (see Exercise Tests, p. 251).

Definitions

The points of electrical contact—electrode positions—are the four limbs together with specific positions on the thorax. The limb leads are arranged so as to provide an analysis of the vector of the electrical forces arising in the heart. The standard limb leads are as follows:

Bipolar	Lead I	right arm – left arm
	Lead II	right arm – left leg
	Lead III	left arm – left leg
Unipolar	aVR	right arm
	aVL	left arm
	aVF	left foot

The standard placements of the chest leads are shown in Fig. 9.17. Leads II, III and aVF record changes on the inferior or diaphragmatic surface of the heart, leads I and aVL changes from the lateral border of the heart, and the chest leads overlie the inter-ventricular septum and the anterior wall of the left ventricle.

Atrial depolarization is the source of the changes in electrical potentials which cause the P wave. The QRS complex is due to ventricular depolarization and the T wave to ventricular repolarization (Fig. 9.18). Atrial repolarization is associated with very small electrical changes which are not recorded on the conventional surface electrocardiogram. The Q wave is an initial negative deflection in the QRS complex.

The P–R interval (measured from the beginning of the P wave to the beginning of QRS complex) is normally less than 0.2 second. The duration of the normal QRS complex is less than 0.12 second (Fig. 9.19).

Reading and interpretation of the electrocardiogram

The electrocardiogram must be examined systematically. A convenient method is as follows:

1 Determine the cardiac rate and rhythm.
2 Assess the P–R interval and the width of the QRS complex.
3 Examine the P wave and the QRS complex.
4 Examine the S–T segment and T wave.

The electrocardiogram in disorders of cardiac rhythm

Because it provides a record of both atrial excitation (P waves) and ventricular excitation (QRS complex) the electrocardiogram is useful in analysing cardiac dysrhythmias. P waves are usually best seen in lead II or in the right-sided chest leads (V_1) and these leads should therefore be studied particularly carefully when there is a disorder of cardiac rhythm.

In health the heart beat is initiated in the sinoatrial node (pacemaker), which lies near the junction of the superior vena cava and the right atrium. The impulse spreads through both atria and thence to the atrioventricular (AV) node. From the AV node the impulse is conducted down the bundle of His and from there to the Purkinje fibres in the left and right bundle branches.

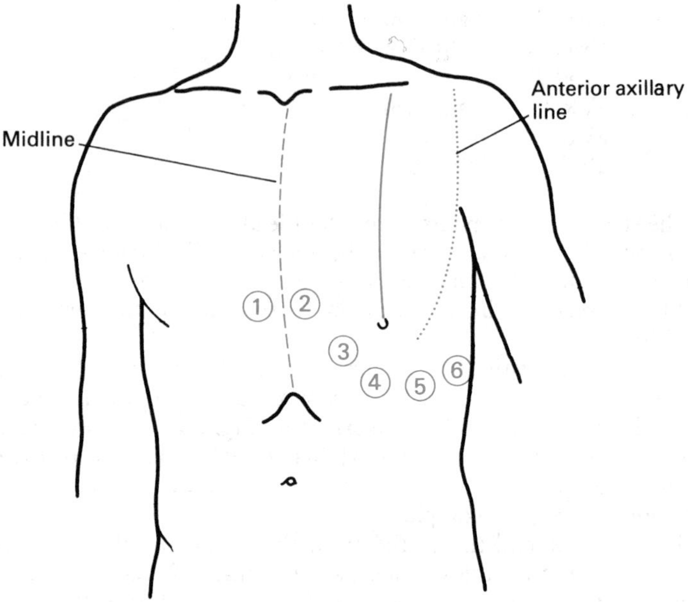

Fig. 9.17 The positions of the electrode in chest lead recordings.
V_1 Fourth intercostal space at the right sternal edge.
V_2 Fourth intercostal space at the left sternal edge.
V_3 Halfway between V_2 and V_4.
V_4 Mid-clavicular line in the fifth intercostal space.
V_5 Anterior axillary line horizontal to V_4.
V_6 Mid-axillary line horizontal to V_4 and V_5.

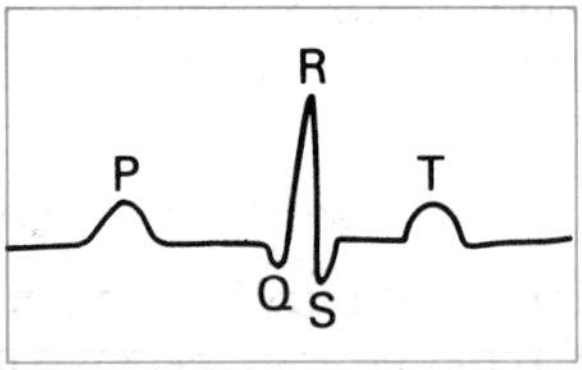

Fig. 9.18 The terminology of the electrocardiogram.

Sinus tachycardia

The cardiac impulse arises normally from the sinus node in sinus tachycardia, and the electrocardiogram is normal in form. The pulse rate is increased above 100 (adults). Sinus tachycardia may result from emotion, exercise, fever, hyperthyroidism and anaemia.

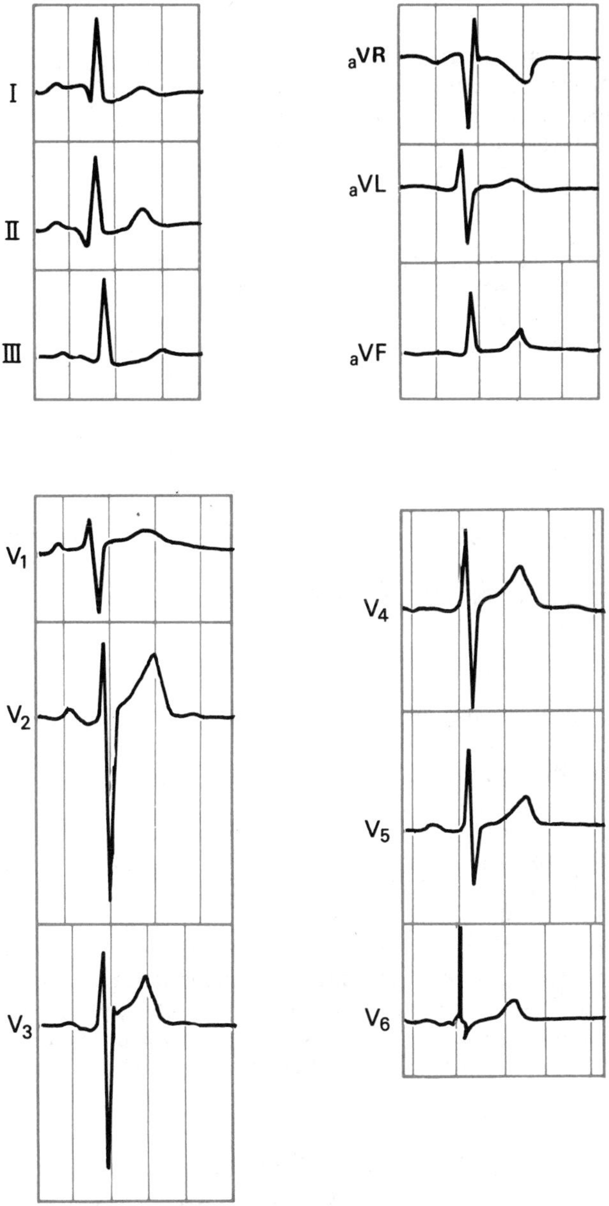

Fig. 9.19 The normal electrocardiogram. Standard leads (I, II, III), V (unipolar) limb leads, V (unipolar) chest leads V_1–V_6.

Sinus bradycardia

Again the electrocardiogram is normal in form, but the heart rate is less than 60/minute. Sinus bradycardia occurs in trained athletes and in patients with increased intracranial pressure, myxoedema and jaundice. It may also be an indication of fibrosis or ischaemia of the sinus node—sinoatrial disease.

Sinus arrhythmia

The cardiac impulse arises normally in the sinoatrial node, the rhythmicity of which varies; the heart rate increases with inspiration and diminishes with expiration (Fig. 9.20). The electrocardiogram is normal apart from variation in the R–R intervals. This arrhythmia is a normal finding in young people; it is increased by deep breathing and abolished by exercise.

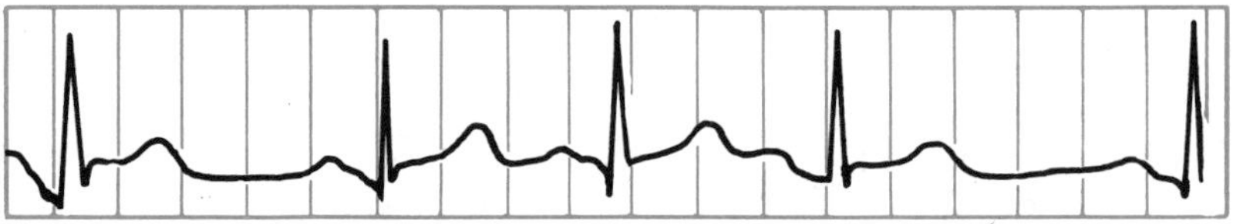

Fig. 9.20 Sinus arrhythmia.

Extrasystoles or ectopic beats

Ectopic beats arise from foci in the atria or ventricles which stimulate the heart before the next sinus beat is due. In ventricular extrasystoles P waves are absent and the QRS complexes are broad, the T wave pointing in the opposite direction to the major deflection of the QRS. The extrasystole comes prematurely and is followed by a pause (the compensatory pause).

The electrocardiogram of an atrial extrasystole shows the P wave to be abnormal in form, but the QRS which follows it is normal. The pause which follows the extrasystole is longer than normal (Fig. 9.21).

Extrasystoles are thus premature beats followed by an abnormally long pause and can be recognized by auscultation or palpation. Extrasystoles occur both in health and in patients with heart disease. If an extrasystole follows each normal beat as in Fig. 9.22 the pulse is said to be coupled (bigeminy). If the patient is being treated with digoxin the possibility of toxicity should be considered.

Atrial tachycardia and atrial flutter

Atrial tachycardia (Fig. 9.23) and atrial flutter (Fig. 9.24) are due to the presence of an ectopic focus in the atrium which beats regularly at a rapid rate. The P waves are abnormal in shape, but the QRS complexes are usually

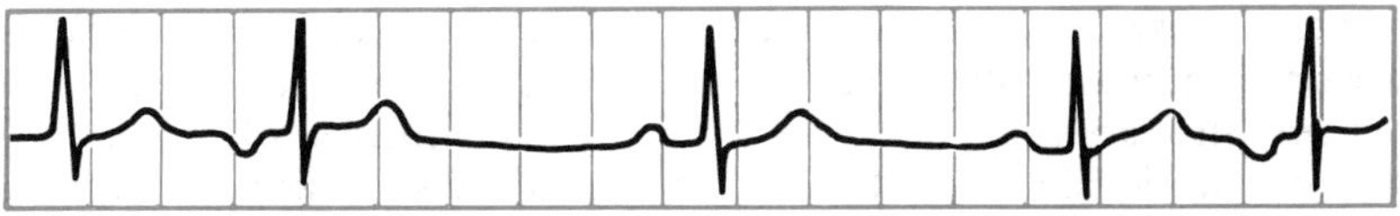

Fig. 9.21 Atrial extrasystoles. Note the abnormal (inverted) P wave. The R–R interval is longer after the extrasystole than in the normal cycle.

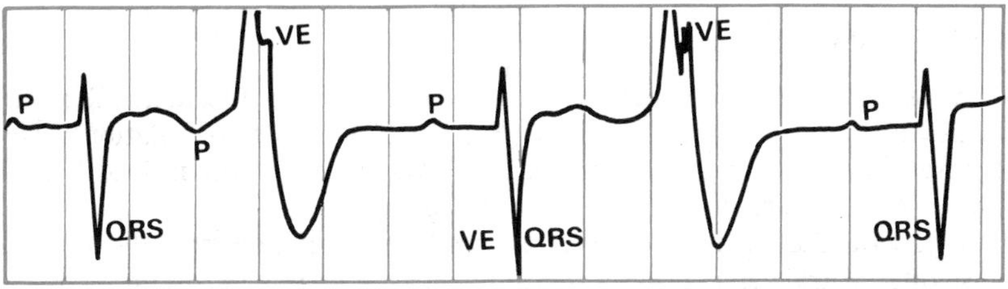

Fig. 9.22 Ventricular extrasystoles. Note there is no P wave before the second extrasystole, and there is an abortive P wave just before the first extrasystole. VE: ventricular ectopic beat.

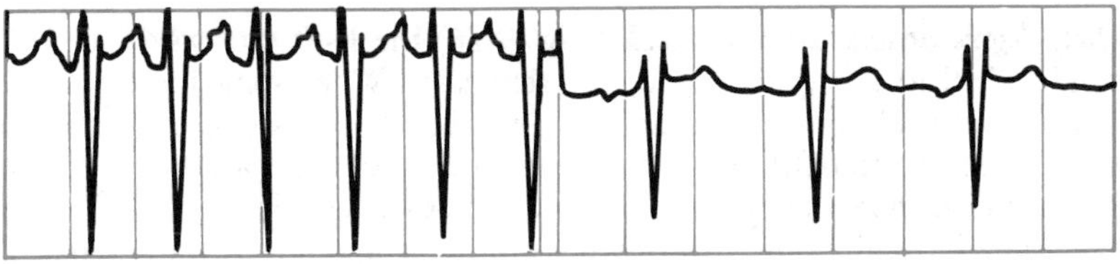

Fig. 9.23 Atrial tachycardia. During attack, pulse rate 225; after attack, sinus tachycardia, pulse rate 130.

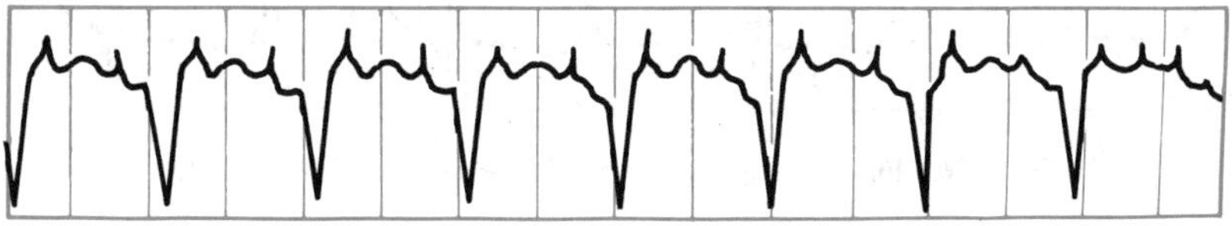

Fig. 9.24 Atrial flutter, 2:1 block. Atrial rate about 300. Note the two spiked flutter waves to each ventricular complex.

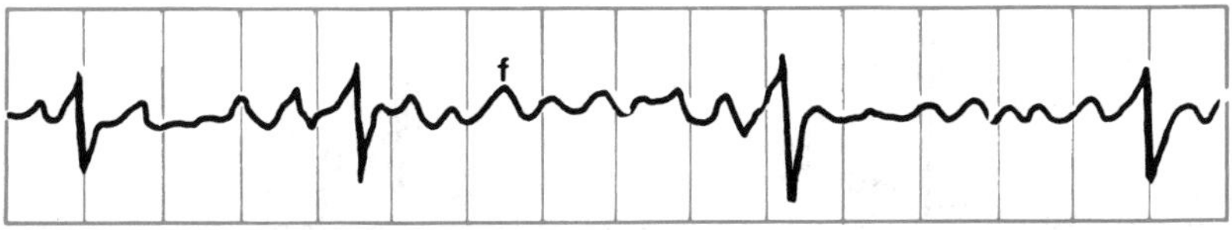

Fig. 9.25 Atrial fibrillation. Note the *f* waves and irregular ventricular rhythm.

normal; however, at faster rates a bundle branch block pattern (p. 245) may develop. As a rule not all atrial impulses are conducted to the ventricles. Often alternate beats are conducted, when 2:1 atrioventricular block is said to be present. Occasionally 3:1 or 4:1 block is present and sometimes the degree of block varies.

Atrial flutter and tachycardia may occur in the absence of other cardiac abnormalities, or in thyrotoxicosis and rheumatic or ischaemic heart disease.

Atrial fibrillation

There is no coordinated atrial activity (either electrical or mechanical) in atrial fibrillation. The electrocardiogram (Fig. 9.25) shows *f* (fibrillation) waves representing the atrial activity instead of P waves, especially in lead V_1. The QRS complexes are normal but occur irregularly.

Atrial fibrillation is recognized clinically by complete irregularity of the pulse rate. Mitral valve disease, ischaemic heart disease and thyrotoxicosis are the commonest causes of atrial fibrillation.

Atrioventricular block (heart block)

In *first degree atrioventricular block* (Fig. 9.26) the P–R interval exceeds 0.2 second and all atrial impulses reach the ventricles. When some impulses fail to reach the ventricle but others do reach it, then there is *second degree atrioventricular block*. In *third degree atrioventricular block (complete)* the atria and ventricles beat independently i.e. they are dissociated (Fig. 9.27). The ventricular rate is usually slow, 20–40 beats/minute, and often erratic and may fail completely—ventricular standstill.

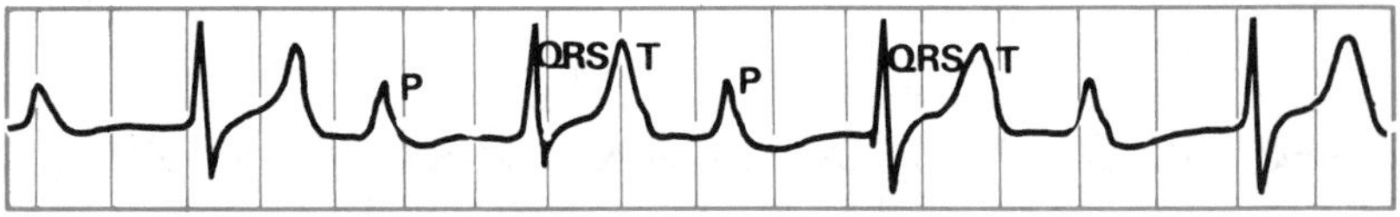

Fig. 9.26 First degree heart block. P–R interval = 0.42 second.

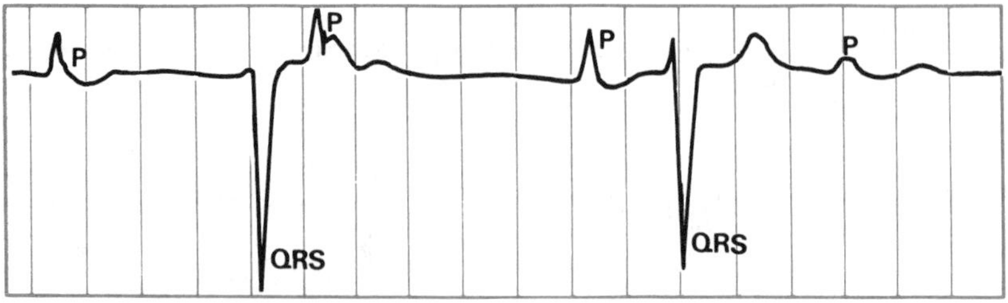

Fig. 9.27 Complete heart block. Atrial rate 55; ventricular rate 39.

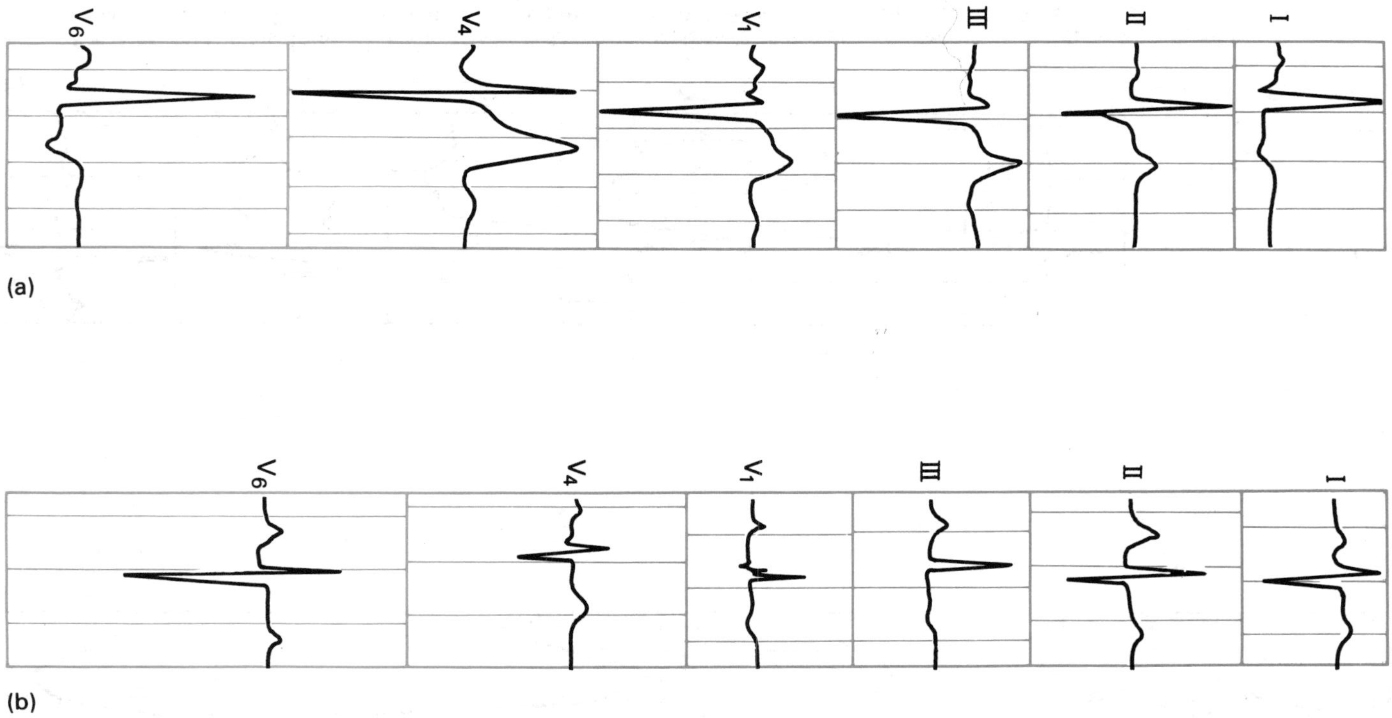

Fig. 9.28 (a) Left ventricular hypertrophy. Note the deep S wave in V_1; the tall R wave in V_6; and S–T depression and T wave inversion in lead I and V_6. (b) Right ventricular hypertrophy. Note the tall R wave in V_1; deep S wave in V_6; and T wave inversion in lead III and V_1. In this tracing the T wave is normal in lead II, though it is usually flat or inverted in right ventricular hypertrophy. The P wave in V_1 is sharp and peaked, suggesting right atrial hypertrophy.

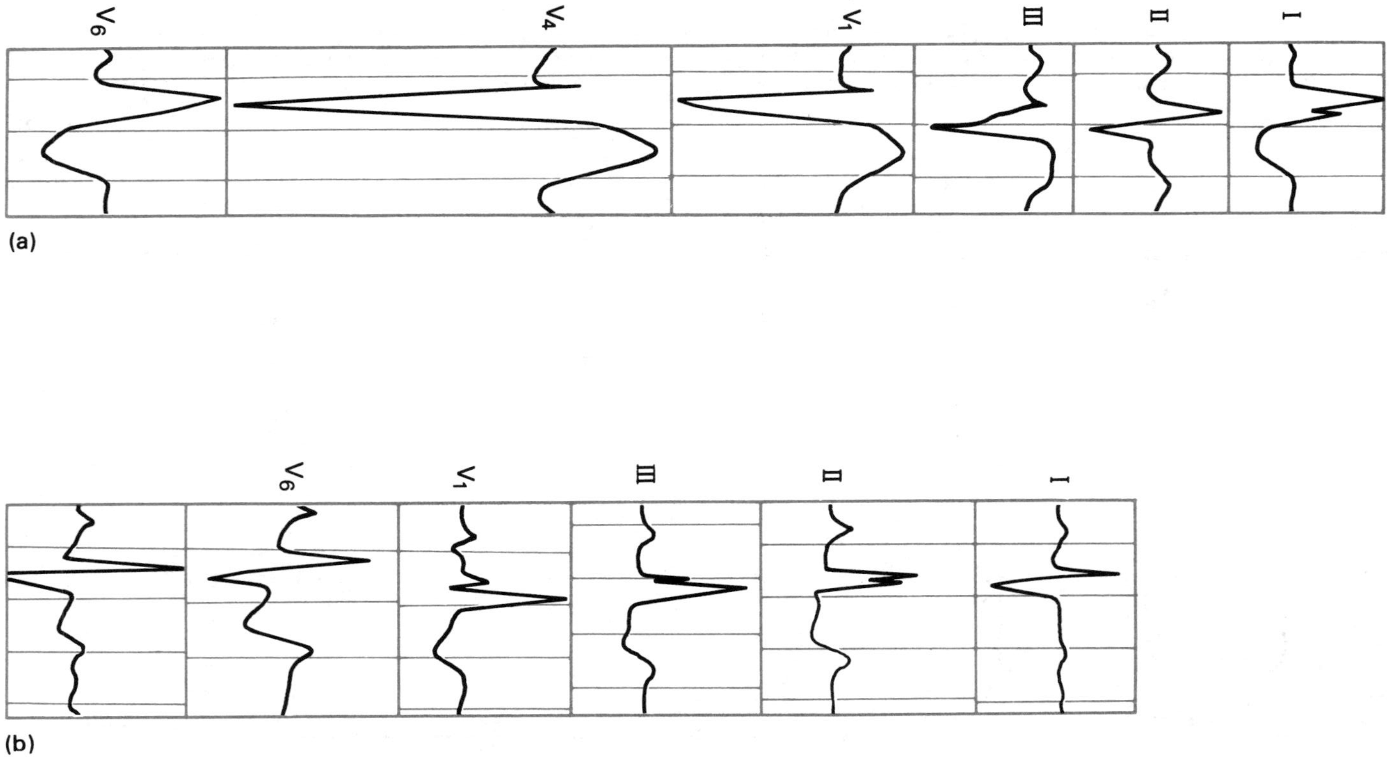

Fig. 2.29 (a) Left bundle branch block. Note the wide QRS complexes (0.15 second) and deep wide slurred R wave in V_6. (b) Right bundle branch block. Note the wide QRS complexes (0.15 seconds), RSR pattern in V_1 and deep wide S wave in V_6.

Ventricular fibrillation

A similar mechanism operates in the ventricles as in the atria with atrial fibrillation. There are no distinct QRS complexes, but bizarre undulations of irregular height and rate. There is no effective cardiac output; loss of consciousness rapidly develops and this rhythm is fatal unless treated promptly.

The electrocardiogram in some other conditions

Ventricular hypertrophy

Ventricular hypertrophy is diagnosed principally from the chest leads and in particular V_1 and V_6. Fig. 9.28 shows the appearance of the QRS complexes in V_1 (over the right ventricle) and V_6 (over the left ventricle). It must be appreciated that the QRS complex from any lead represents the algebraic sum of the electrical activity of both ventricles (compare with the normal ECG in Fig. 9.19). At any point in time the ECG will show an R wave (positive deflection) if the resultant current vector is directed towards the electrode and an S wave (negative deflection) if the resultant vector is going away from the electrode. Ventricular hypertrophy is associated with an increase in the electrical activity of depolarization. As a result there is an increase in the magnitude of the QRS deflections best seen in the chest leads.

Left ventricular hypertrophy As the left ventricle lies to the left and posteriorly there is an increase in the size of the R wave in the left chest leads (V_5–V_6) and an increase in the S wave in the right chest leads (V_1–V_2) (see Fig. 9.28a).

Right ventricular hypertrophy The R wave in the right chest leads is increased and there is a deeper S wave in the left chest leads, as the increased electrical activity is associated with the anteriorly placed right ventricle (Fig. 9.28b).

In addition, both types of ventricular hypertrophy may show a ventricular strain pattern. There is an abnormality of ventricular repolarization associated with hypertrophy. It causes the T wave to point away from the affected ventricle giving S–T depression and T wave inversion in leads I, aVL and the left chest leads in left ventricular hypertrophy, and in leads V_1, V_2, II and III in right ventricular hypertrophy. Other causes of T wave changes are mentioned on p. 246.

Bundle branch block

In bundle branch block (Fig. 9.29), owing to an interruption of one of the bundle branches, conduction to one ventricle is delayed. The QRS duration is greater than 0.12 second. For example, if the left bundle is interrupted, conduction to the left ventricle is delayed and it becomes activated at a time when it is no longer opposed by the right ventricle, and therefore produces large deflections, as in hypertrophy of the left ventricle.

Myocardial infarction

Myocardial infarction alters the electrocardiogram by the successive production of abnormalities in the S–T segments, the development of Q waves and T wave inversion (Fig. 9.30).

It should be noted that within the first two hours of infarction the electrocardiogram may be virtually normal. Subsequently the S–T segments become raised (Fig. 9.30b). In a few days the T waves become inverted (Fig. 9.30c). The S–T segment gradually returns to the base line, taking several weeks to do so. T wave inversion may eventually return to normal (Fig. 9.30d), but some inversion usually persists. Abnormal Q waves are usually permanent.

The presence of Q waves indicates a full-thickness infarct and is usually associated with complete occlusion of a coronary vessel. If only T wave changes occur then this is described as a subendocardial or partial thickness infarction. The leads showing Q waves or S–T and T wave change are determined by the site of the infarct. The electrocardiograms illustrating classical anterior and inferior infarction (Fig. 9.31) are tracings taken several weeks after the infarction.

In *anterior infarction* the changes are seen in leads I and V_1 to V_5. In *inferior infarction* the changes are seen in leads II and III and aVF. In *lateral infarction* the changes occur in leads I, aVL, V_5 and V_6 (Table 9.1).

Table 9.1 The relationship between myocardial regions, coronary vessels and the electrocardiogram

Myocardial region	Coronary vessel	ECG leads	
Anteroseptal	Left anterior descending	V_1–V_5	} V_6[2]
Lateral	Left circumflex	I, aVL	
Inferior	Right coronary 90% (circumflex 10%)[1]	II, III, aVF	

[1] In a heavily left dominant system with a small or insignificant right coronary circulation, the inferior wall of the left ventricle may be supplied by the left circumflex vessel.

[2] V_6 (apex) may be supplied by any of the three vessels, depending on the anatomy of the coronary tree.

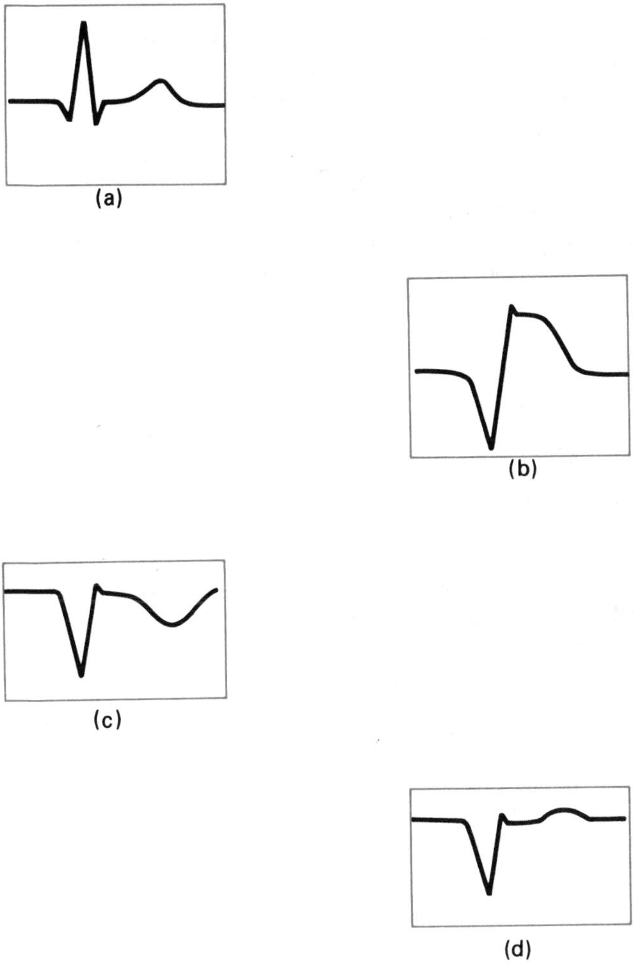

Fig. 9.30 The evolution of the changes in the QRS complex, S–T segment and T wave after cardiac infarction. (a) Normal pattern. (b) A few hours after infarction: a Q wave is present and the S–T segment is elevated (Pardee's sign). (c) After a time the S–T segment returns to the base line and the T wave becomes steeply inverted. (d) After a further period the T wave becomes inverted, flat and finally upright. Note that the Q wave persists.

Plate I Intestinal Parasites

1 *Entamoeba histolytica*. Fully developed four-nucleated cyst, containing chromatid bodies, as seen in saline preparations. × 1500
2 *Entamoeba histolytica*. Four-nucleated cyst as seen in iodine preparation. × 1500
3 *Entamoeba histolytica*. Active form, containing included red blood cells, as seen in saline preparations. × 1500
4 *Iodamoeba bütschlii*. Cyst, as seen in saline preparations. Note the unstained glycogen vacuole. × 1500
5 *Entamoeba coli*. Fully developed eight-nucleated cyst, as seen in saline preparations. × 1500
6 *Entamoeba coli*. Eight-nucleated cyst stained by Lugol's iodine solution. × 1500
7 *Entamoeba coli*. Active form, as seen in saline preparations. × 1500
8 *Iodamoeba bütschlii*. Cyst stained by Lugol's iodine solution. × 1500
9 *Giardia lamblia*. Cyst form, stained by Heidenhain's haematoxylin. × 1500
10 *Giardia lamblia*. Active form, stained by Heidenhain's haematoxylin. × 1500
11 *Trichomonas hominis*. Stained by Giemsa's method. × 1500
12 *Isospora belli (I. hominis)*. Undeveloped oocyst as passed in human faeces. × 500
13 *Balantidium coli*. Active form stained by Heidenhain's haematoxylin. × 350
14 Ova of *Ankylostoma duodenale* (hookworm). × 500
15 Ova of *Enterobius vermicularis* (threadworm). × 500
16 Ova of *Taenia solium* and *T. saginata* (tapeworms). × 500
17 Ova of *Trichuris trichiura* (whipworm). × 500
18 Ova of *Ascaris lumbricoides* (roundworm). × 500
19 Ova of *Schistosoma haematobium*. × 300
20 Ova of *Schistosoma japonicum*. × 300
21 Ova of *Schistosoma mansoni*. × 300

All magnifications approximate

Drawings by W. Cooper

Plate I Intestinal Parasites

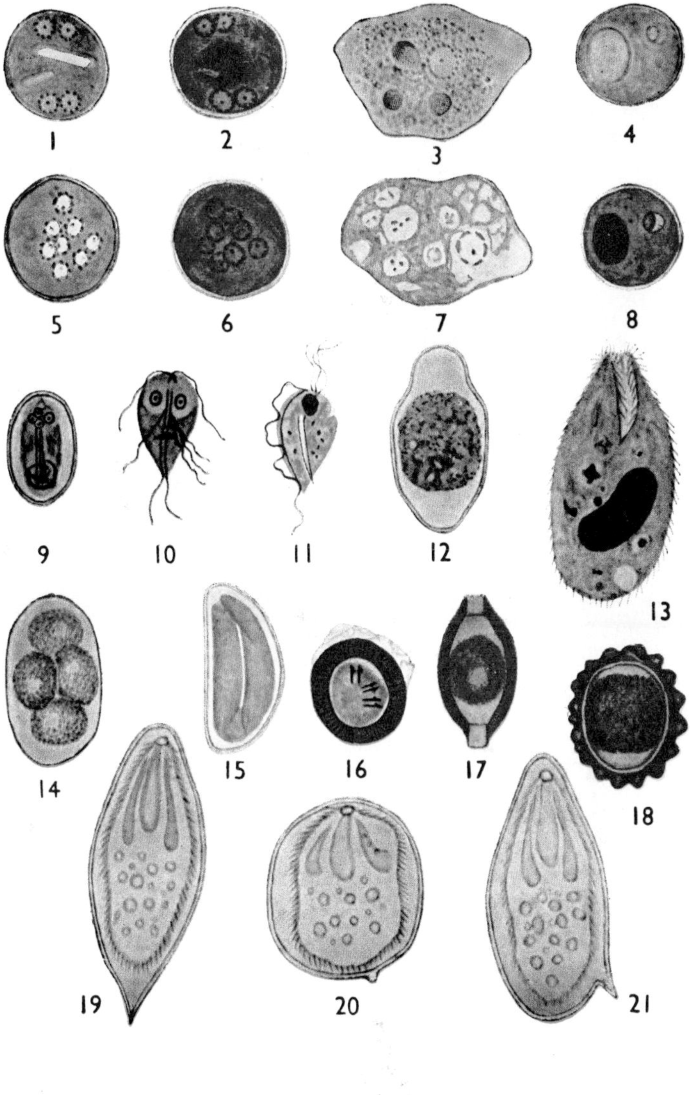

Plate II The Eye

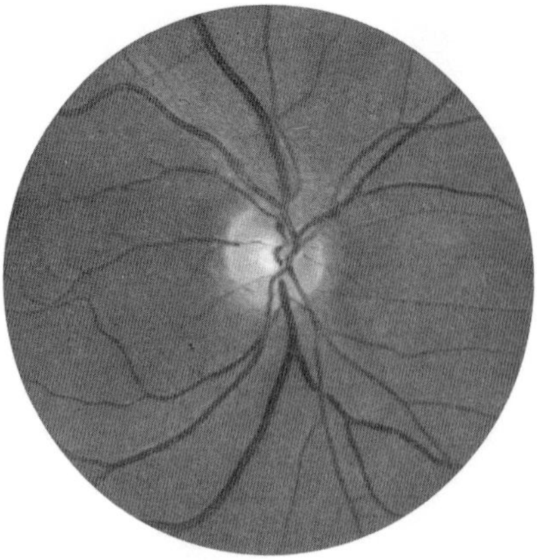

Normal fundus Note the yellowish colour of the optic disc and the retinal veins (the larger, darker vessels) and arteries leaving the centre of the disc superiorly and inferiorly. A single arterial branch passes laterally to supply the macular part of the retina

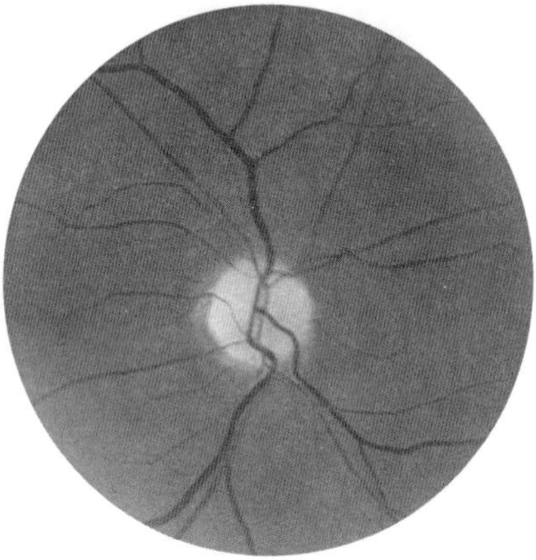

Primary optic atrophy The disc is pale and whiter than normal, and its edges are unusually sharply demarcated from the retina. The retinal vessels are slightly attenuated

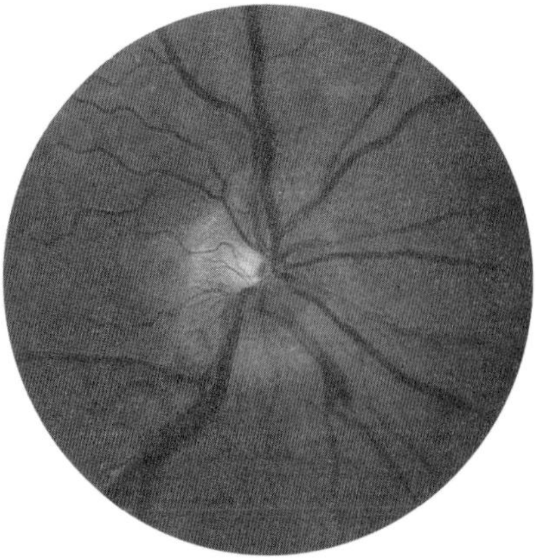

Papilloedema See Fig. 13.1 (p. 398) for description

Plate III The Eye

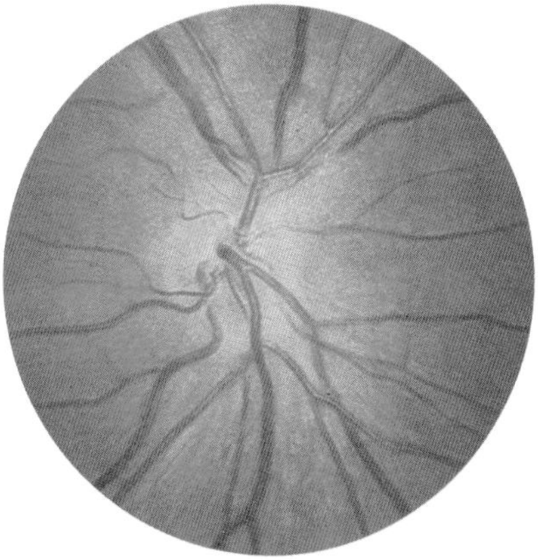

Pseudopapilloedema See Fig. 13.2 (p. 398) for description

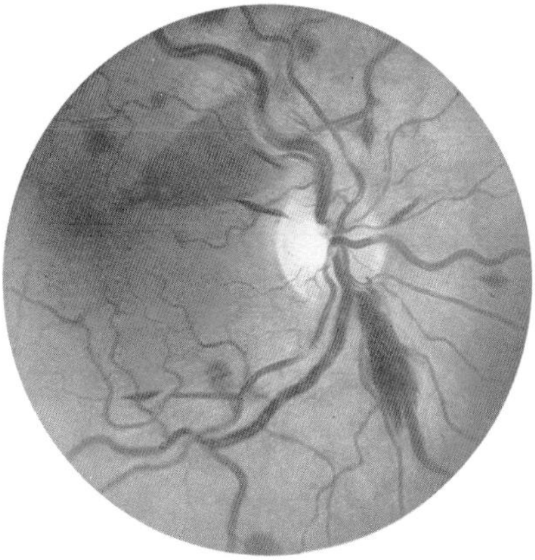

Central retinal vein occlusion The retina shows choroidal and retinal haemorrhages. The venous occlusion was due to chronic myelocytic leukaemia

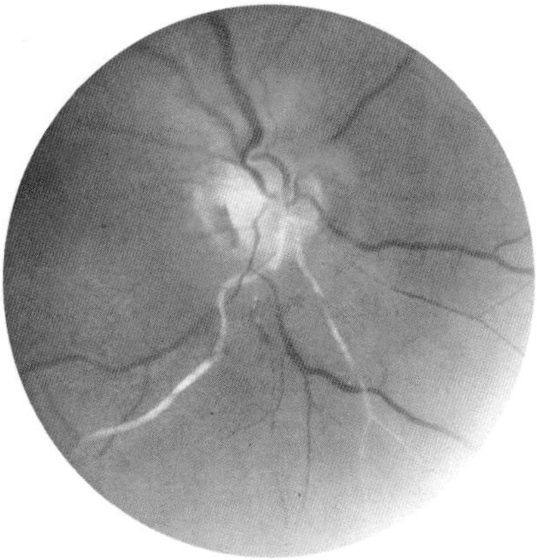

Retinal emboli Cholesterol emboli in the retinal arteries of a patient with atheromatous disease of the internal carotid artery in the neck

Plate IV The Eye

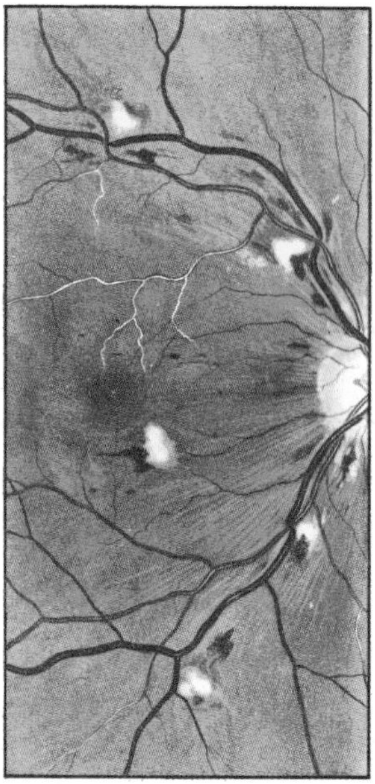

Hypertensive retinopathy The arteries are irregular in calibre and show 'silver wiring'. Arteriovenous nipping is present. Characteristic 'flame-shaped' haemorrhages and 'cotton wool' exudates can be seen

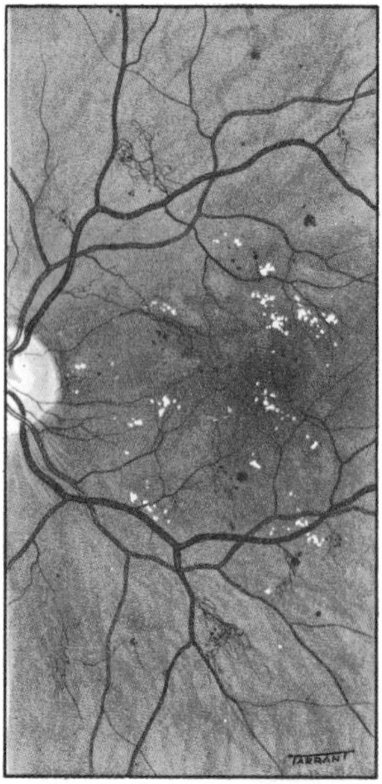

Diabetic retinopathy Micro-aneurysms (tiny red dots), round haemorrhages, waxy exudates and areas of new vessel formation are characteristic of this condition. In many patients hypertensive retinopathy is also present

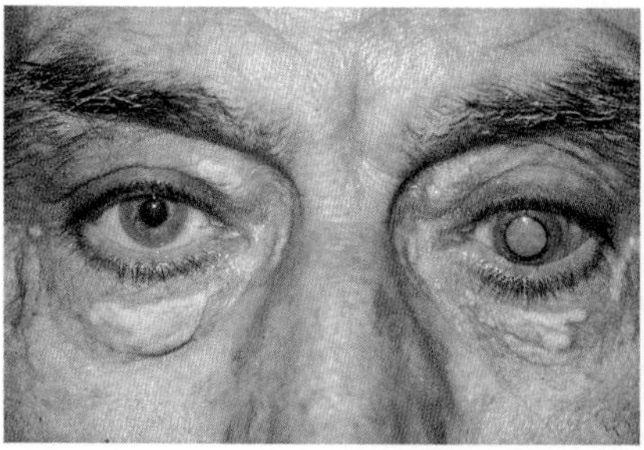

Xanthelasmata palpebrarum and cataract Yellow xanthelasmata are prominent below both eyes and in the upper lids. There is a mature left cataract (not directly related to the xanthelasmata)

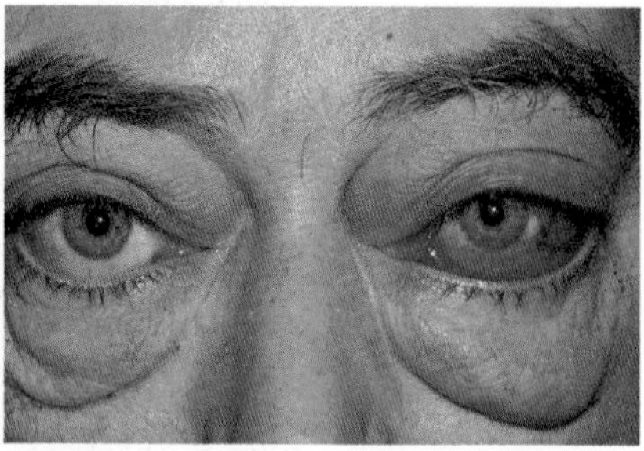

Thyroid eye disease There is slight proptosis and eye movements are limited. The peri-orbital tissues are swollen and there is chronic inflammation of the right eye. Note that lid retraction is not a necessary feature of thyroid eye disease, which may occur in the euthyroid state

Plate V Some Skin Disorders

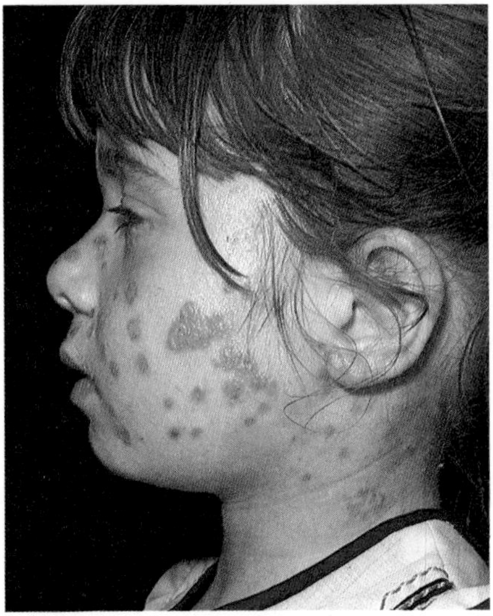

Impetigo

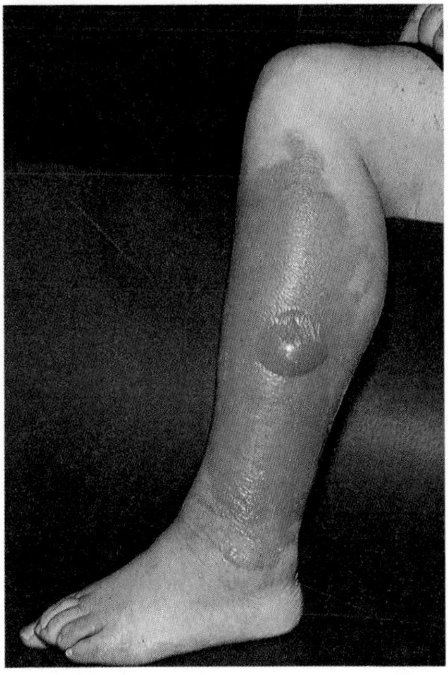

Erysipelas

Plate VI Some Skin Disorders

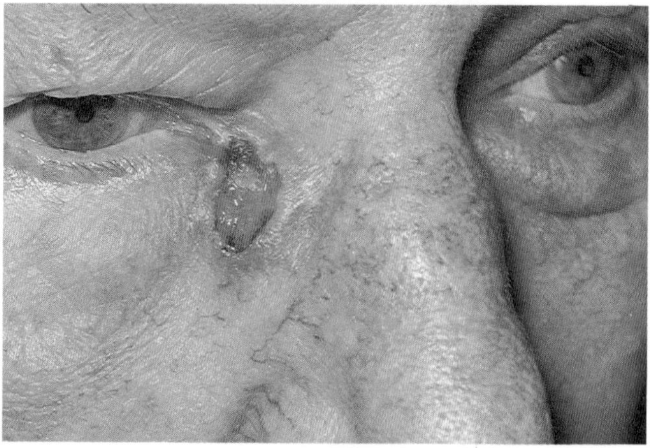

Basal cell carcinoma

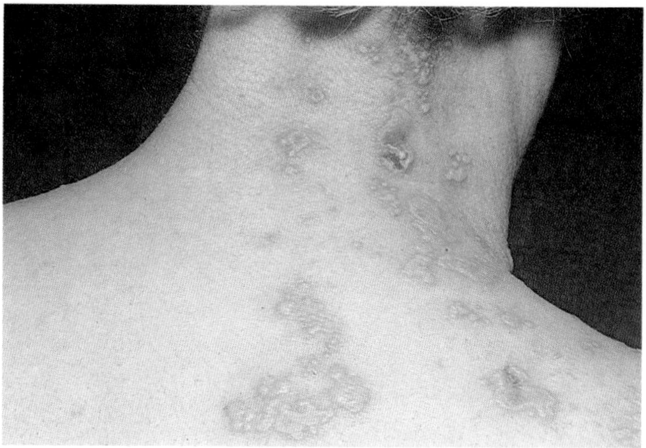

Herpes zoster

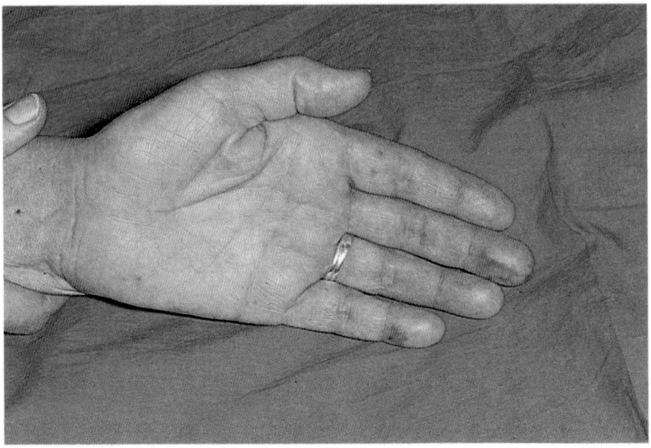

Bacterial endocarditis The lesions in the finger tips are due to embolic occlusion of branches of the digital arteries

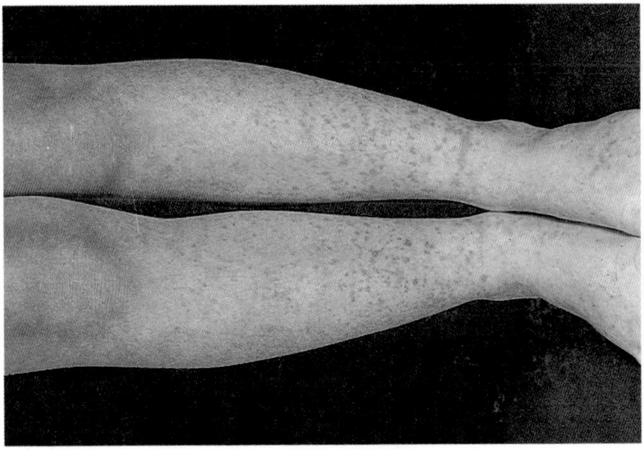

Purpura in Henoch–Schönlein disease

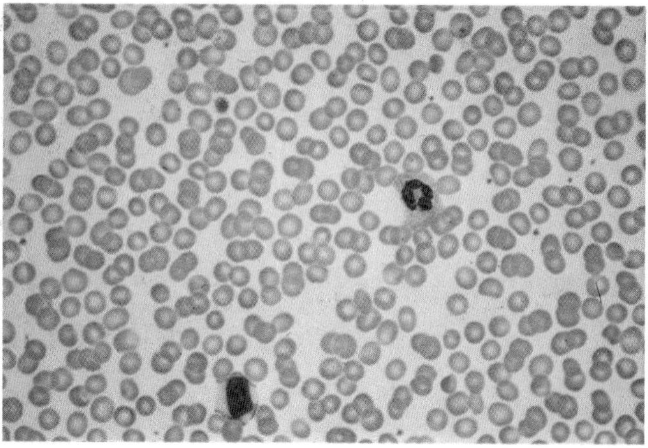

Normal peripheral blood The red cells show little variation in size or shape. A neutrophil granulocyte and a lymphocyte are visible and platelets are scattered through the film

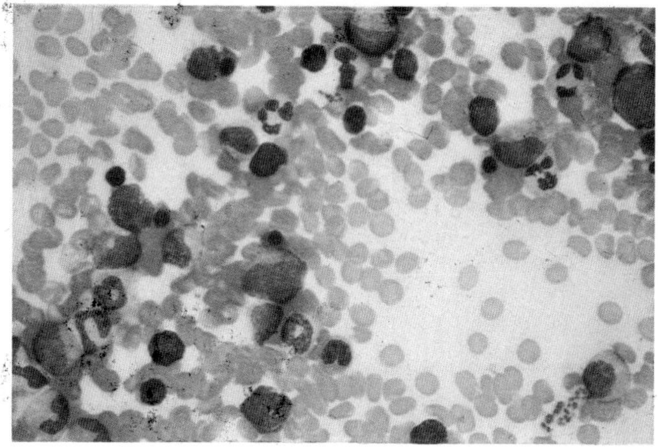

Normal bone marrow aspirate Nucleated red cells, granulocyte precursors and mature cells are present

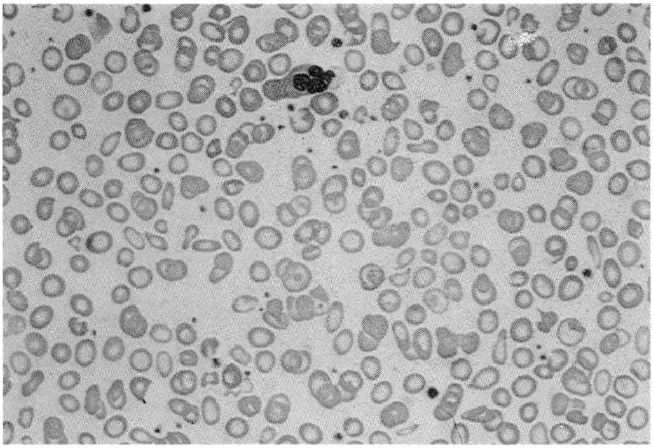

Iron deficiency anaemia (peripheral blood) Hypochromia, microcytosis, anisocytosis and target cells are shown

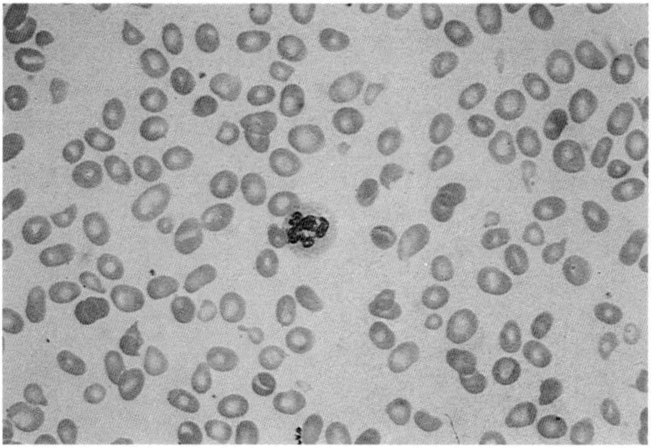

Macrocytic anaemia (peripheral blood) Macrocytosis, anisocytosis, poikilocytosis and target cells are shown

Plate X The Blood

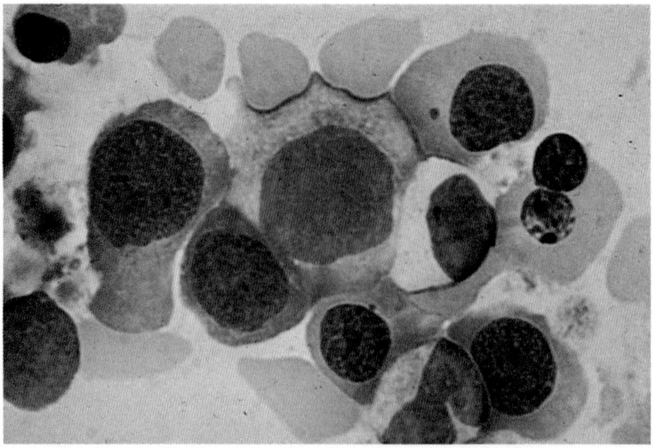

Megaloblastic bone marrow The majority of cells are megaloblastic erythroblasts showing failure of nuclear development and abnormal nuclear morphology

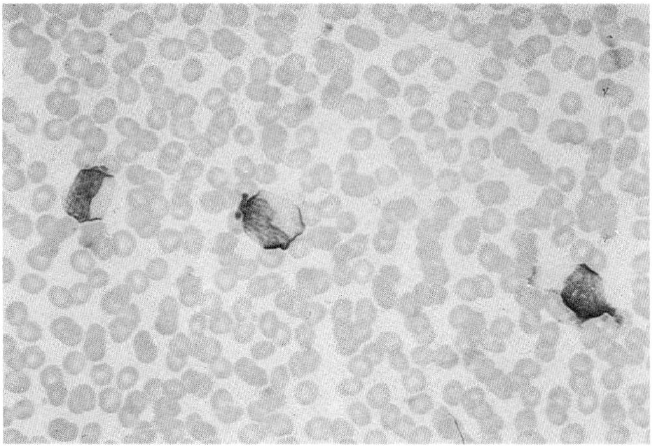

Glandular fever (peripheral blood) Atypical mononuclear cells are visible

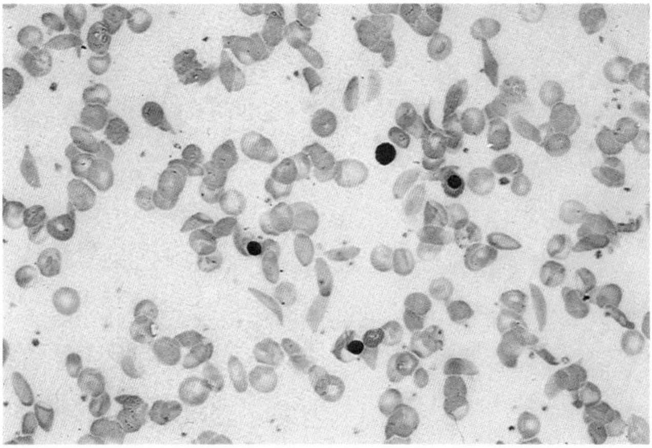

Sickle haemoglobin disease (peripheral blood) In homozygous disease (HbSS), sickle cells and target cells are present together with occasional nucleated red cells. Heterozygotes (HbSA) have a normal peripheral blood

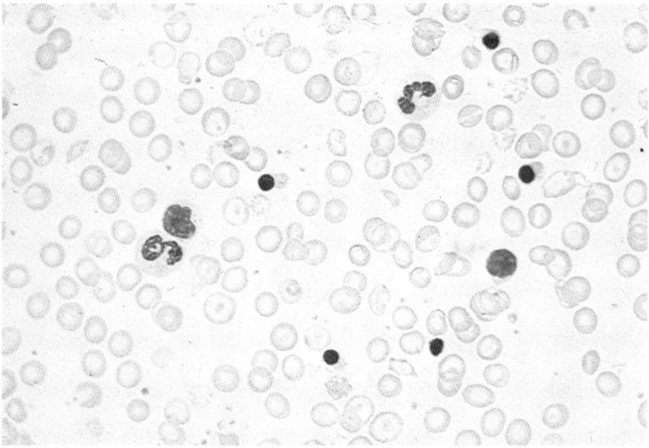

β-Thalassaemia major (peripheral blood) There is hypochromia, microcytosis and anisocytosis. Target cells and nucleated red cells are numerous. In β-thalassaemia minor the peripheral blood looks like that of iron deficiency

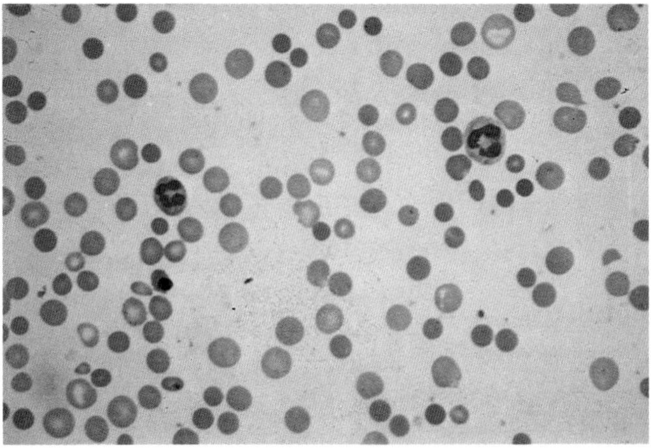

Spherocytosis (peripheral blood) Microspherocytes are small, dense red cells characteristic of hereditary spherocytosis and autoimmune haemolytic anaemia. In addition this film contains polychromatic macrocytes, which are present in many forms of haemolytic anaemia

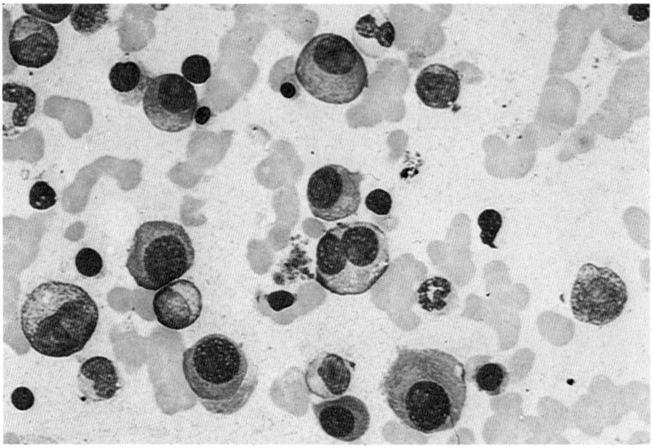

Myelomatosis (bone marrow) The marrow is infiltrated with plasma cells and one binucleate form is present. The red cells show rouleaux formation

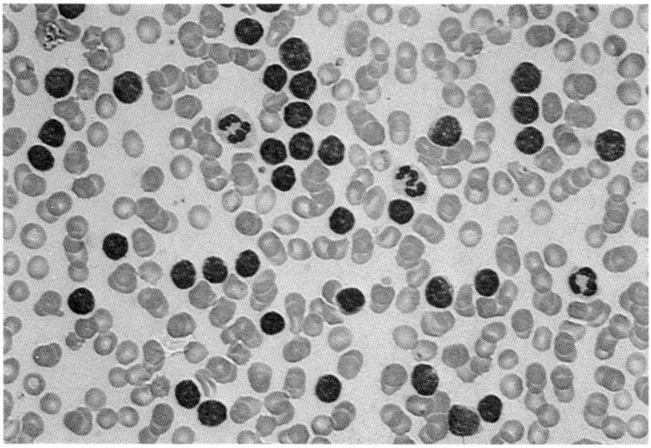

Chronic lymphocytic leukaemia (peripheral blood) The white cell count is increased and most of the white cells are small lymphocytes

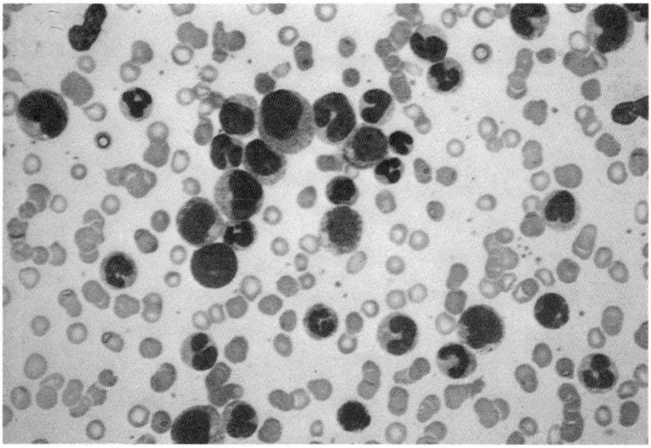

Chronic granulocytic (myeloid) leukaemia (peripheral blood) There is an increased number of granulocytes, most of which are mature neutrophils. A few more primitive cells are also present

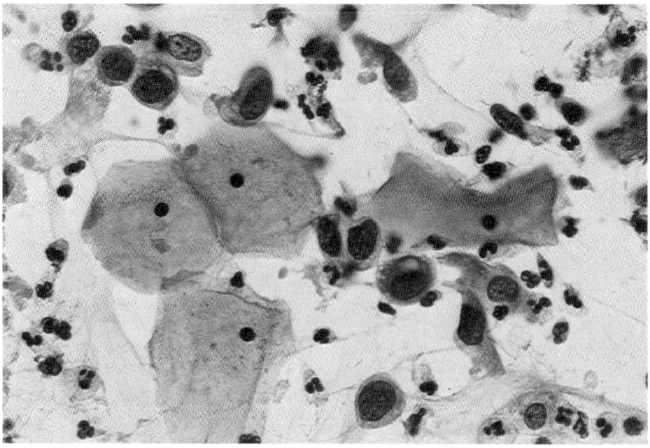

Smear from uterine cervix Cells scraped from the uterine cervix. There are several abnormal small squamous cells indicating in situ carcinoma of the cervix. Large pink-stained normal superficial squamous cells and many inflammatory cells are also included. Papanicolaou stain. × 160

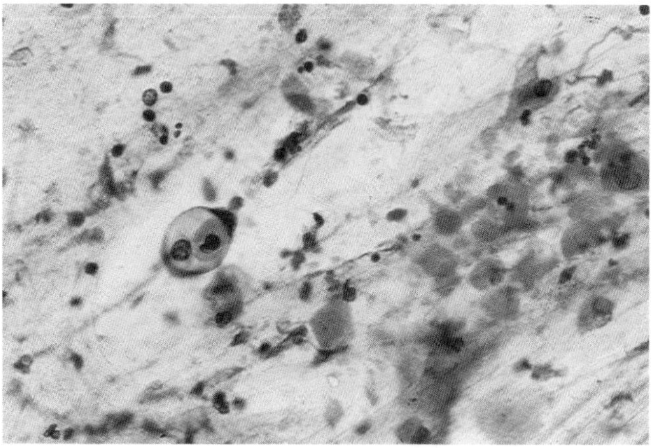

Sputum cytology A squamous pearl and numerous anucleate abnormal keratinized squamous cells in sputum from a patient with squamous cell carcinoma of the lung. Haematoxylin and eosin. × 160

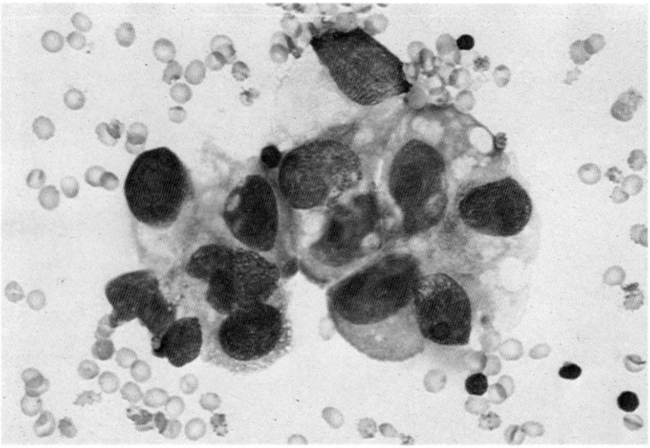

Ascites cytology A group of tumour cells showing random orientation and large abnormal nucleoli indicating malignancy. Ascitic fluid from a patient with ovarian carcinoma. May–Grünwald–Giemsa stain. × 160

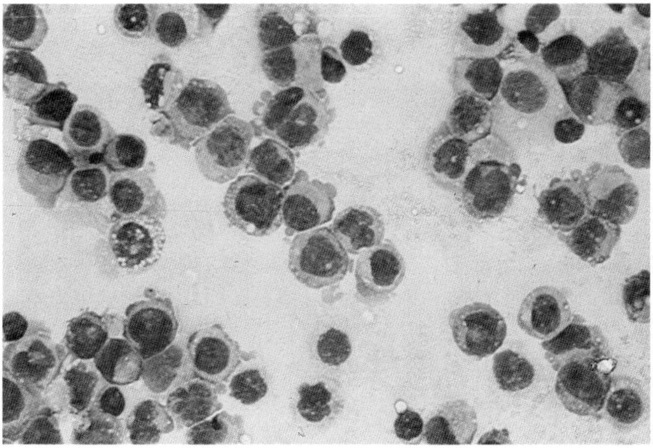

Cerebrospinal fluid cytology Cell deposit from cerebrospinal fluid almost exclusively comprising carcinoma cells shed from the leptomeninges. Metastasis to meninges from primary carcinoma of the breast. May–Grünwald–Giemsa stain. × 160

Plate XVI Parasites of the Blood

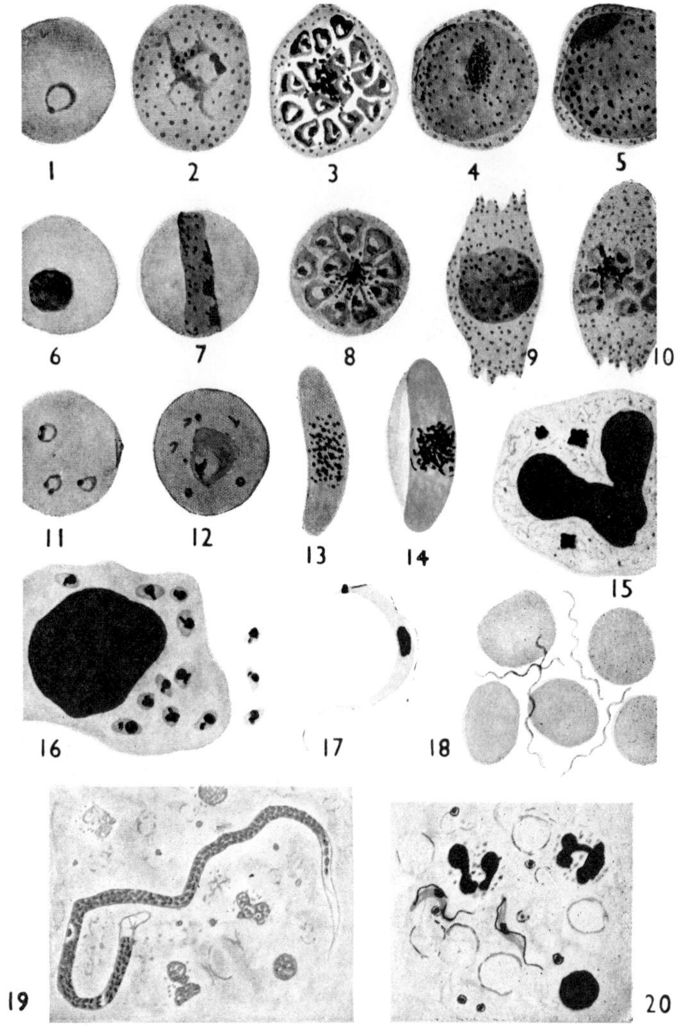

Plate XVI Parasites of the Blood

1. *Plasmodium vivax*. Ring stage. × 2000
2. *Plasmodium vivax*. Amoeboid form. × 2000
3. *Plasmodium vivax*. Fully developed schizont. × 2000
4. *Plasmodium vivax*. Male gametocyte. × 2000
5. *Plasmodium vivax*. Female gametocyte. × 2000
6. *Plasmodium malariae*. 'Compact' form. × 2000
7. *Plasmodium malariae*. 'Band' form. × 2000
8. *Plasmodium malariae*. Fully developed schizont. × 2000
9. *Plasmodium ovale*. Female gametocyte. × 2000
10. *Plasmodium ovale*. Fully developed schizont. × 2000
11. *Plasmodium falciparum*. Red blood corpuscles containing various types of young ring. × 2000
12. *Plasmodium falciparum*. 'Old' ring, showing altered staining reaction and Maurer's dots. × 2000
13. *Plasmodium falciparum*. Male gametocyte or crescent. × 2000
14. *Plasmodium falciparum*. Female gametocyte or crescent. × 2000
15. *Plasmodium falciparum*. Pigment in polymorphonuclear leucocyte. × 2000
16. *Leishmania donovani* from a spleen smear. Some lying free and others within the cytoplasm of an endothelial cell. × 2000
17. *Trypanosoma cruzi*. Adult form as seen occasionally in the blood of patients suffering from Chagas' disease. × 2000
18. *Borrelia recurrentis*. × 2000
19. *Filaria loa*. × 600
20. *Trypanosoma rhodesiense* as seen in a thick blood film of patients suffering from trypanosomiasis. × 1000

Drawings by W. Cooper

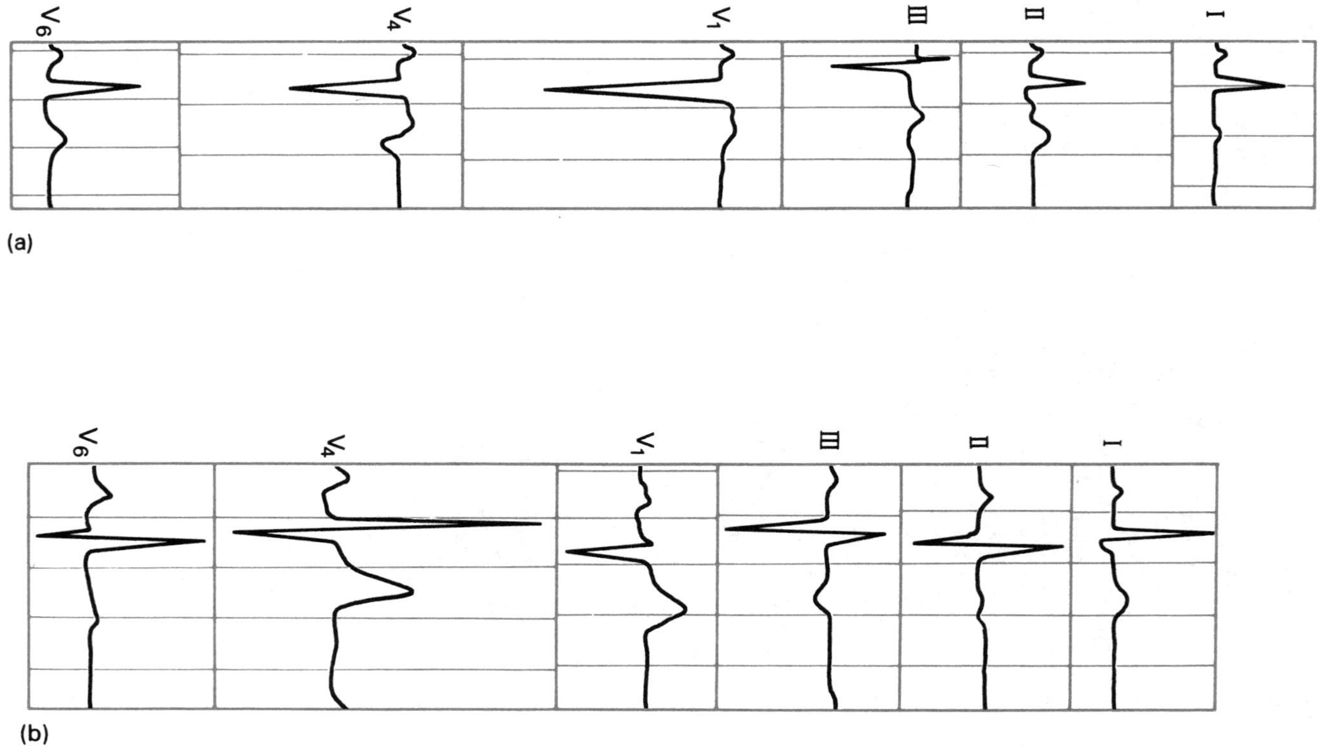

Fig. 9.31 (a) Anterior cardiac infarction. Note the Q wave in V_1 and V_4. (b) Inferior cardiac infarction. Note the Q waves in leads II and III. The T wave is slightly inverted in lead II and inverted in lead III. V_6 also shows a Q wave and a low T wave, so this is really inferolateral infarction.

P wave changes

Because the sinoatrial node is located in the right atrium, right atrial depolarization precedes left atrial depolarization. Left atrial hypertrophy therefore causes a broadening of the P wave. This is best seen in standard lead II, where the delayed left atrial depolarization appears as a second positive deflection. This gives an M-shaped configuration to the P wave and this is often called a P mitrale; severe mitral valve stenosis, provided the patient maintains sinus rhythm, produces this typical appearance of the P wave. Left atrial hypertrophy can also be noted in leads V_1 and V_2; in these leads the left atrial hypertrophy appears as a terminal negative deflection of the P wave.

In contrast, right atrial hypertrophy leads to a peaked appearance of the P wave in both leads II and V_1. This appearance is sometimes known as P pulmonale since pulmonary hypertension is one of the important causes of right atrial hypertrophy.

EXERCISE TESTS

Because the major physiological disorder associated with coronary artery disease is a failure of adequate blood supply in response to increased demand, it follows that an electrocardiogram recorded at rest has limited value in predicting a disorder which has its maximum effect during exertion. The objective of an exercise test is, therefore, to stress the patient on either a treadmill or a bicycle ergometer, and to record the electrocardiogram during and immediately after the period of exercise. The protocol calls for an increasing level of work to be done until either angina develops or a heart rate of between 140 and 175 is reached, depending on the patient's age and sex. In the presence of coronary artery disease the S–T segment is often depressed when the myocardium is ischaemic (Fig. 9.32). The presence of S–T segment depression with either a horizontal or downward sloping configuration is then very suggestive of myocardial ischaemia.

Exercise testing cannot at present definitively deny the presence of coronary artery disease (Fig. 9.32) nor is it absolutely specific in predicting its presence. In attempts to increase the clinical usefulness of exercise testing in detecting coronary artery disease the technique has been combined with methods for imaging the heart with radioactive tracer elements. In this way the myocardial perfusion during exercise and subsequently at rest is compared and it is possible to detect areas which were underperfused during exercise. Further refinements of the non-invasive investigation of ischaemic heart disease are currently under investigation. At present coronary arteriography (Fig. 9.32c) may be regarded as demonstrating abnormal anatomy and the investigations described above in this section as demonstrating altered physiology.

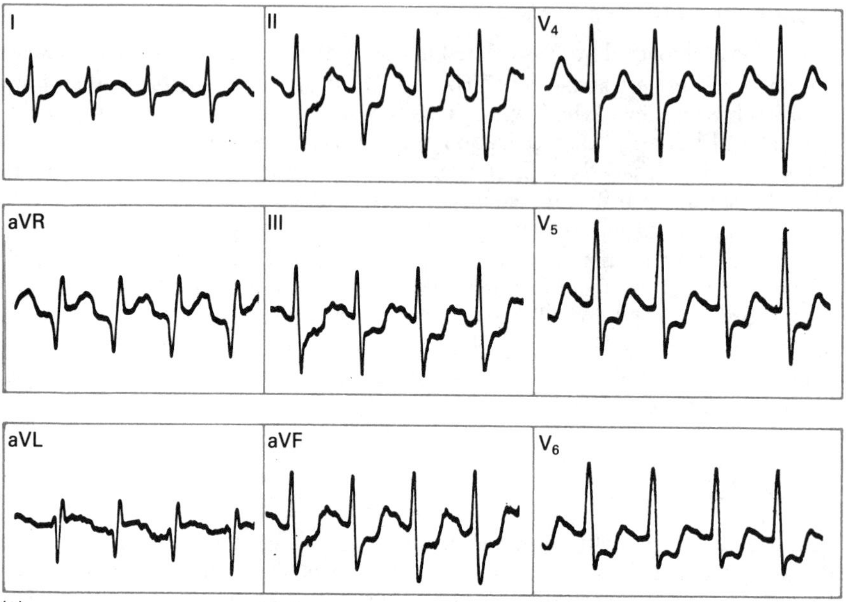

(a)

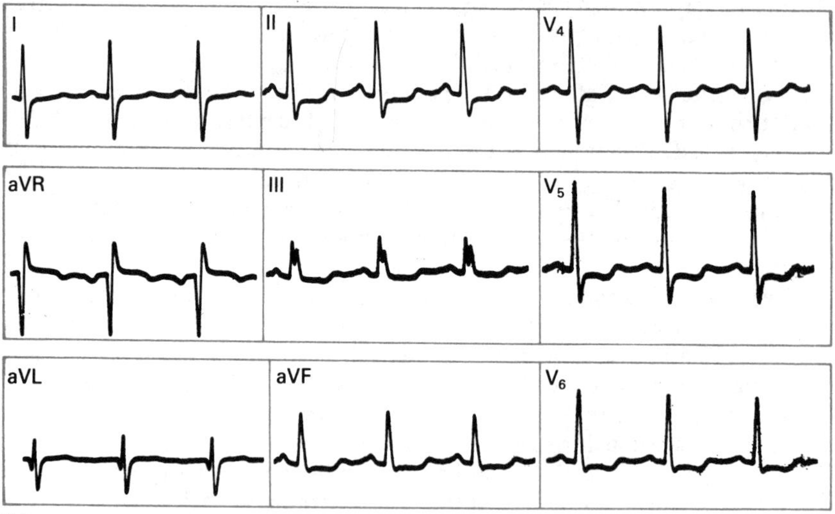

(b)

Fig. 9.32 A positive exercise test in a patient who was subsequently shown to have a severe stenosis in the left main coronary vessel. The tracing recorded immediately after exercise (a) shows a heart rate of 160 beats per minute with marked depression of the S–T segments in the inferior (II, III and aVF) and anterior (V_5 and V_6) leads. After ten minutes (b) the S–T segment had returned towards normal although there is still some slight depression remaining.

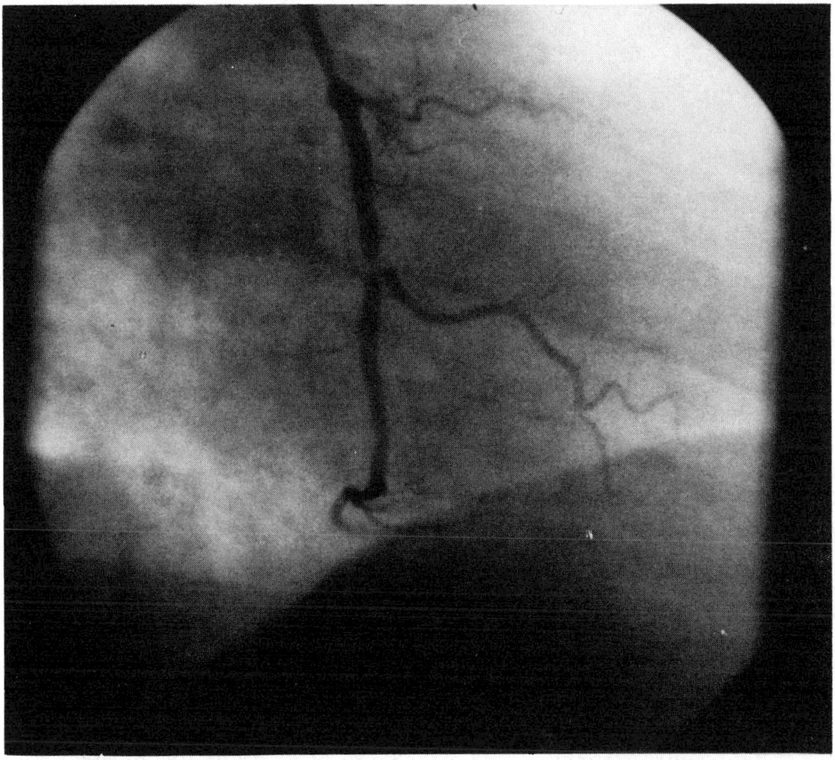

(c)

Fig. 9.32(c) Coronary angiography. There is a stenosis in the right coronary artery at a major branch. The illustration is taken from a cine radiograph made as part of the investigation. The patient presented with angina but cardiac infarction had not occurred.

RADIOGRAPHIC EXAMINATION

In addition to the standard posteroanterior X-ray of the chest much information may be gained by taking more penetrated films of the posteroanterior and right lateral views.

Screening of the heart is primarily of value in visualizing calcification in valves; it is occasionally useful in detecting the presence of a left ventricular aneurysm.

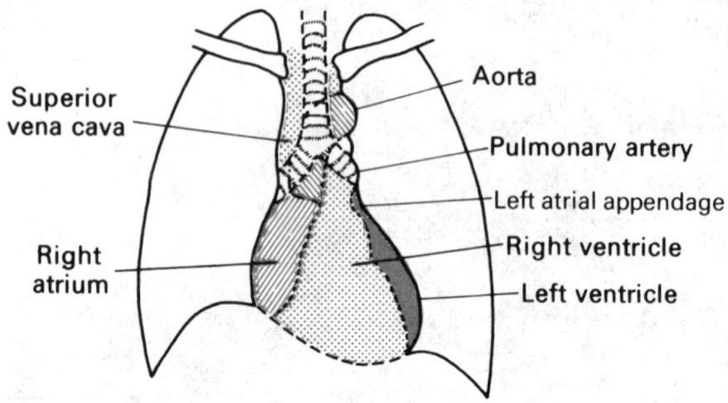

Fig. 9.33 The cardiac silhouette in the anteroposterior position. This is particularly useful in studying the outflow from the left atrium, the pulmonary artery and the aortic knuckle.

The normal cardiac outline

The heart (Fig. 9.33) is seen as a flask-shaped shadow, lying between the translucent lungs, about one-third of its area to the right of the midline and two-thirds to the left. The apex of the heart is internal to the mid-clavicular line.

The right border of the normal cardiac shadow is formed, from above downwards, by two curves:

1 A slightly curved portion—the outer edge of the superior vena cava with the ascending aorta.

2 A more convex portion—the outer border of the right atrium, the lower margin of which lies at the diaphragm.

The left border comprises from above downwards:

1 The prominent knuckle produced by the arch of the aorta as it passes backwards, slightly to the left, then downwards.

2 The straighter line of the pulmonary artery.

3 The left atrial appendage.

4 The wide sweep of the left ventricle, ending at the apex, where it rests on the diaphragm.

In the overpenetrated posteroanterior film the left atrium can be seen, especially if enlarged, and the aorta is particularly well shown. Calcification in the pericardium or valves may be apparent. The right lateral film is of value in localizing valve calcification and in addition is helpful in right ventricular hypertrophy when the anteriorly placed right ventricle lies closer to the sternum than normal.

Common alterations in disease

Position of the heart in the chest

Displacement of the heart as a whole is seen in pleural effusion, pneumothorax and fibrosis of the lung. In distension of the stomach and obesity, the heart is raised with the diaphragm and the apex tilted upwards. The common type of scoliosis (convexity of the curve to the right) is a frequent cause of displacement of the heart to the left. In narrow chests the heart often lies centrally and seems small and slender.

Shape and size of heart

Examination of the heart shadow indicates the overall heart size but it can be difficult to identify precisely which cardiac chamber is enlarged. In left ventricular enlargement, as found with aortic valve disease or hypertension, there is a prominent convexity curving below the diaphragm and forming an obtuse angle (Fig. 9.34). In right ventricular enlargement the outline of the apex is turned up and the heart shadow makes an acute angle with the diaphragm. More commonly it is only possible to indicate that there is an increase in ventricular mass without being able to predict accurately which chamber is responsible.

There are four ways by which left atrial enlargement may be detected:

1 Prominence of the left atrial appendage at the left border of the heart (Fig. 9.35).

2 A double shadow seen through the right atrium. This is the caudal edge of the enlarged left atrium, which does not extend down to the diaphragm as does the right atrium.

3 Upward displacement of the left main bronchus so that it runs horizontally.

4 A barium swallow to outline the oesophagus will reveal the extrinsic compression caused by left atrial enlargement.

Shape and size of the aorta

Dilatation of the ascending aorta is an important abnormality. It is most usually due to weakening of the media in the aortic wall. In patients with Marfan's syndrome, cystic medial necrosis frequently causes severe aortic dilatation. A less common cause is syphilitic aortitis. Irrespective of the cause of aortic dilatation, if the aortic root is involved the function of the aortic cusps may be disturbed so that aortic incompetence results.

At any site of obstruction in the circulation the phenomenon of *post-stenotic dilatation* is likely to occur. In patients with aortic valve stenosis post-stenotic dilatation of the ascending aorta is particularly prominent in the first two to

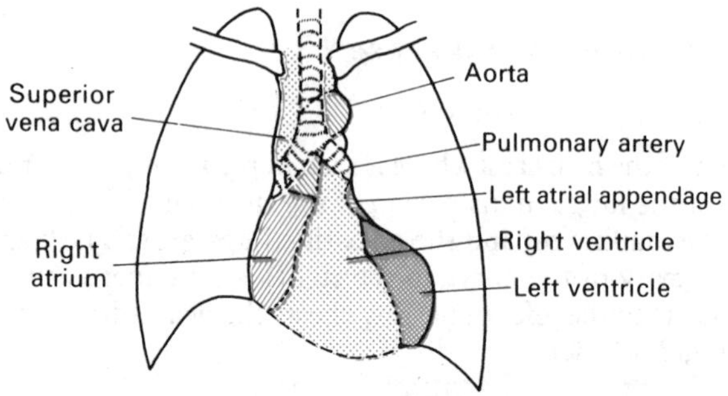

(a)

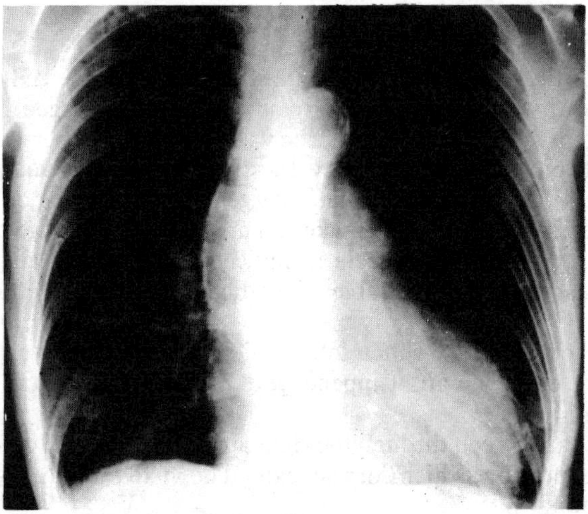

(b)

Fig. 9.34 (a) Diagram of cardiac outline in left ventricular enlargement. (b) Radiograph showing the characteristic shape of left ventricle enlargement in this patient with syphilitic aortic regurgitation. Thin egg-shell calcification is seen in the aortic wall.

three inches above the aortic valve and can easily be recognized on the right side of the aortic shadow on the chest X-ray.

Unfolding of the aorta affects both the ascending and descending portions. It is most often seen in patients with hypertension.

The superior vena cava

In patients with right ventricular failure the shadow of the superior vena cava may be more prominent than normal.

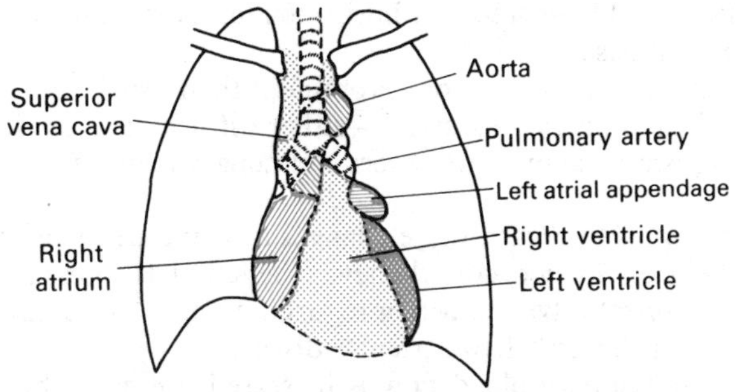

(a)

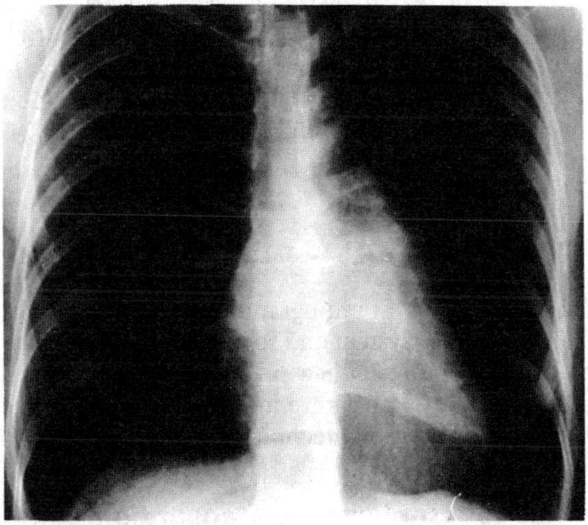

(b)

Fig. 9. 35 (a) Diagram of cardiac outline in mitral stenosis showing prominence of left atrial appendage at left heart border. (b) Radiograph of mitral stenosis. Note the characteristic bulging of the left heart border associated with left atrial enlargement.

The pulmonary artery

The main pulmonary artery is enlarged in pulmonary hypertension. Pulmonary stenosis leads to post-stenotic dilatation and this is detected radiologically as enlargement of the main pulmonary artery.

The pulmonary vasculature

There are four important indicators of raised left atrial pressure:

1 Prominent pulmonary vascular shadows at the hila.

2 Kerley B lines. These are short horizontal lines extending out to the lung edges at the lung bases.
3 The upper lobe veins are more prominent than usual.
4 Interstitial pulmonary shadowing—either diffuse hazy shadowing or the 'bat's wing' appearance of acute severe pulmonary oedema.

It is quite incorrect to regard these changes as being necessarily due to 'left ventricular failure'. They occur whenever the left atrial pressure is elevated, whether due to mitral valve stenosis or regurgitation, left atrial myxoma, aortic valve disease or primary left ventricular disease.

When the pulmonary blood flow is increased, the main branches of the pulmonary artery are increased in size—*pulmonary plethora*. This occurs when there is a left to right shunt in the circulation, e.g. atrial septal defect, ventricular septal defect or patent ductus arteriosus. It is especially obvious when some of the branches are seen end-on near the hilum. Conversely, in Fallot's tetralogy the vascular markings in the lung fields are inconspicuous—*pulmonary oligaemia*.

SPECIAL INVESTIGATIONS

Electrocardiography and chest radiography are essential in the proper assessment of the cardiovascular system and so are considered as part of the routine examination. The need to establish precisely the diagnosis and functional status of patients, frequently as a preliminary to cardiac surgery, has stimulated the development of special techniques.

External pulse recording and phonocardiography

Using suitable transducers, carotid and venous pulsation can be displayed along with the cardiac impulse (apex cardiography) and the recordings of heart sounds and murmurs. This is useful in confirming the time relationships of the physical signs and should be considered an adjunct to the physical examination. However useful in assisting interpretation, these techniques do not elicit new information; phonocardiography will not reveal significant heart murmurs that cannot be heard by auscultation.

Echocardiography

Ultrasound is increasingly used as a diagnostic technique and has become of particular importance in the field of cardiology. The fact that the heart is continually moving and that abnormalities of motion are of diagnostic importance gives echocardiography a particular advantage over other imaging techniques (Fig. 9.36).

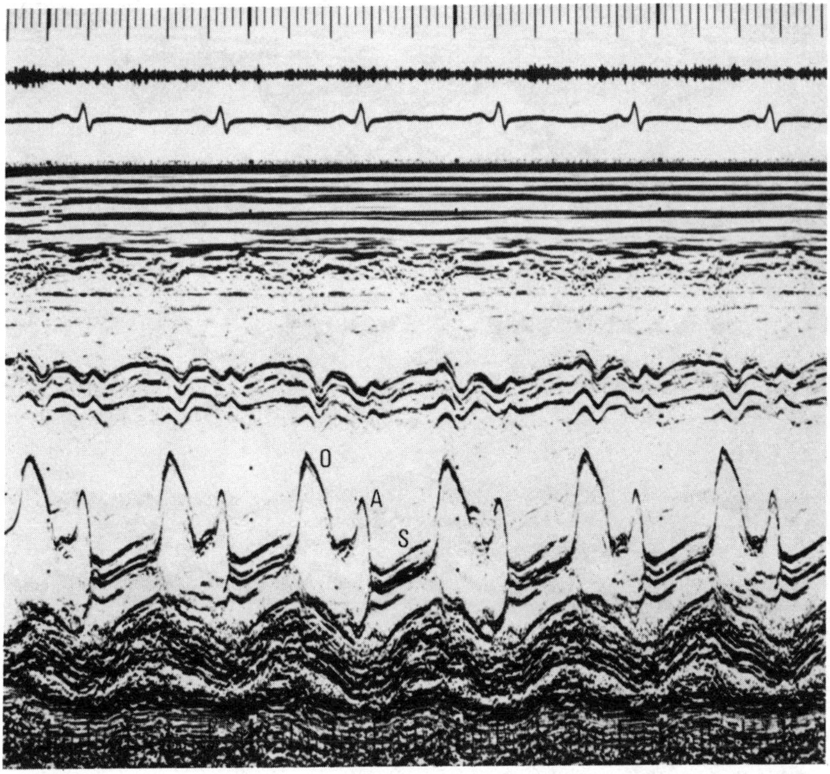

Fig. 9.36 Echocardiogram of a normal mitral valve. The anterior and posterior leaflets are shown moving in opposite directions during diastole. Following the rapid opening of the leaflets in early diastole (O) the leaflets move towards a closed position and then re-open again under the influence of atrial systole (A). During ventricular systole the leaflets are seen as a series of parallel lines moving gradually up the tracing (S).

There are a number of abnormalities that echocardiography is particularly useful in detecting:

1 On the chest X-ray a pericardial effusion causes non-specific enlargement of the cardiac shadow. On ultrasound the fluid shows up as an echolucent area between the epicardium and endocardium (Fig. 9.37).

2 Rheumatic mitral valve disease leads to a characteristically abnormal echocardiographic appearance of the valve (Fig. 9.38): the anterior mitral leaflet, having opened rapidly at the beginning of diastole, moves slowly if at all towards the closed position. If there is any significant fusion of the anterior and posterior leaflets at the commissures, then the ability of the posterior leaflet to move independently from the anterior leaflet is lost. Thus in diastole, instead

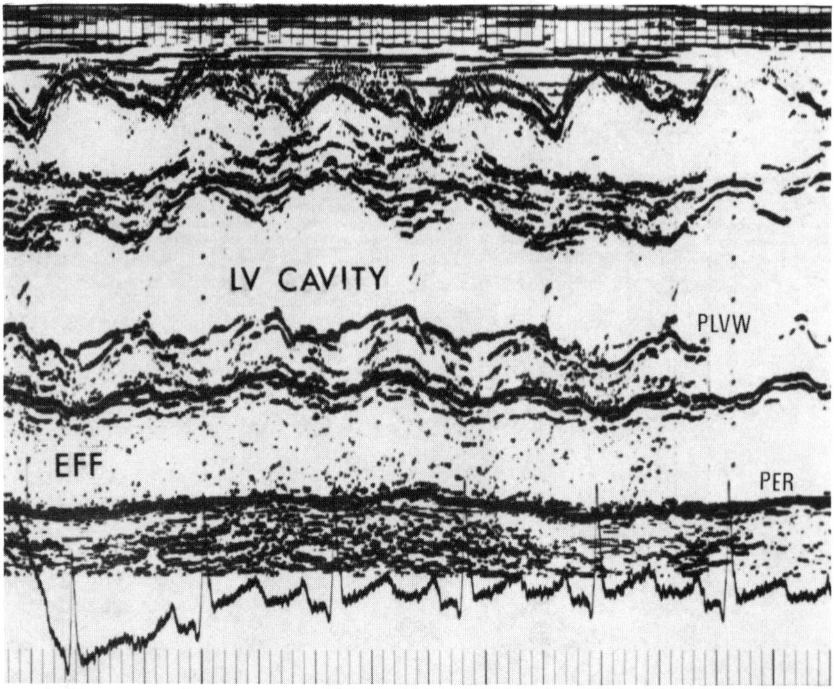

Fig. 9.37 Echocardiogram from a patient with a pericardial effusion (EFF). This is seen as a relatively echo-free space lying above the pericardium (PER). The effusion and pericardium both lie below the left ventricular cavity and the posterior left ventricular wall (PLVW).

of the leaflets moving in opposite directions, the posterior leaflet moves anteriorly in parallel with the anterior leaflet. The rheumatic process leads to considerable thickening of the valve structure and this too can be detected echocardiographically.

3 Echocardiography makes it possible to study a direct image of the left ventricle. The size of the cavity in end systole and end diastole can be measured and this permits the quantification of both volume overload of the left ventricle, in which the end diastolic dimension is increased, and also left ventricular disease, which leads to dilatation of the cavity in both systole and diastole.

4 Hypertrophic cardiomyopathy is characterized by thickening of the interventricular septum. Using echocardiography it is possible to measure the thickness of this structure with accuracy. In addition, abnormalities of motion of the mitral and aortic valves found in this condition are well displayed.

5 Calcium in the aortic valve leading to aortic stenosis is recognized on the echocardiogram as an increase of reflected echoes from the abnormal valve structure. Aortic regurgitation leads to a jet of blood impinging on the anterior

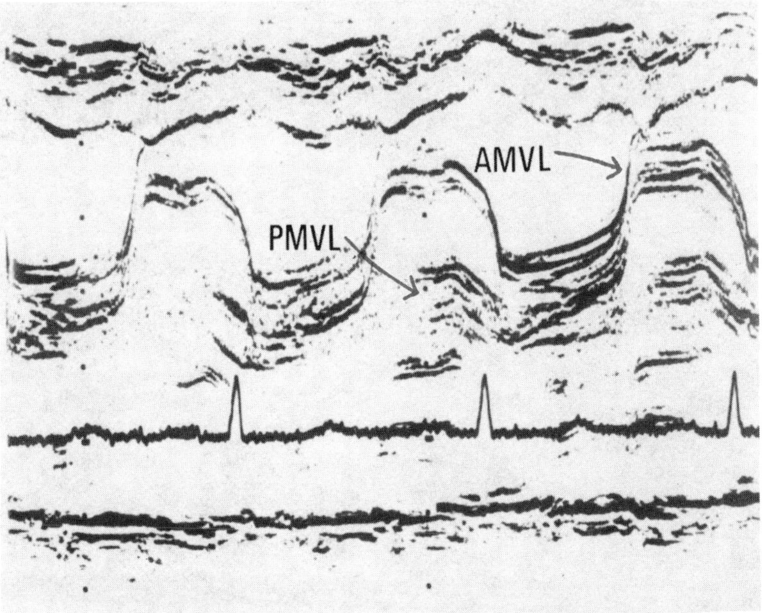

Fig. 9.38 Echocardiogram from a patient with mitral stenosis. In contrast to the normal mitral valve (Fig. 9.36) the anterior and posterior leaflets both move in the same direction during diastole. Both leaflets are thickened and this is shown by an increased number of lines running parallel to each other. The rate of closure of the leaflets in diastole is much slower than normal. (AMVL, anterior mitral valve leaflet; PMVL, posterior mitral valve leaflet.)

mitral leaflet and its presence can be predicted from the finding of a fine fluttering motion of the echocardiographic image of this part of the mitral valve.

6 The presence of various abnormal masses within the heart can be detected by echocardiography. The commonest of these is a vegetation associated with infective endocarditis and usually attached to one of the valves (Fig. 9.39). Cardiac tumours can also be diagnosed and the most important of these, although rare, is an atrial myxoma.

Cardiac catheterization

Cardiac catheterization is carried out when it is necessary to obtain detailed information about the heart, aorta and coronary vessels which cannot be obtained from clinical and other non-invasive methods. The technique carries a small risk of both morbidity and mortality and therefore should be under-

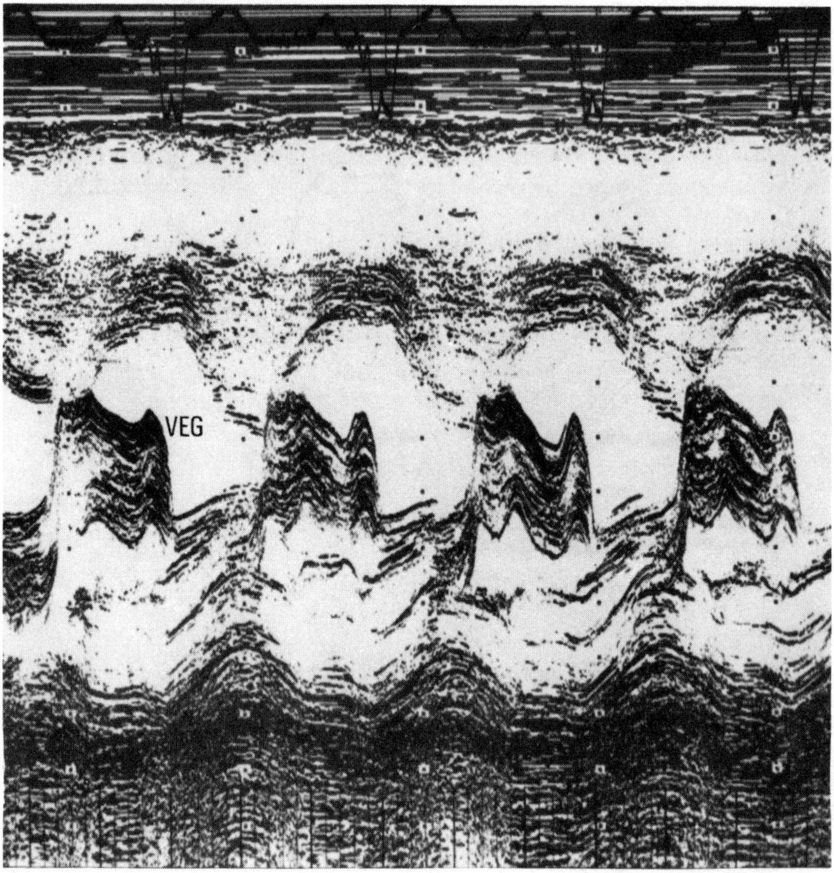

Fig. 9.39 Echocardiogram of the mitral valve in a patient with a vegetation (VEG) attached to the anterior mitral leaflet.

taken only following a full assessment which defines the objectives of the procedure.

Cardiac catheterization provides information about the pressures in the different cardiac chambers and also allows angiography to be carried out. There are two peripheral sites at which the circulation may be conveniently entered—the femoral artery and femoral vein, and the brachial artery and brachial vein.

Measurement of the pressure difference in the two chambers on either side of a stenotic valve indicates the severity of the obstruction to forward flow in the circulation. The pulmonary artery pressure can be reliably determined only by right heart catheterization; measurement of the right atrial pressure should correlate well with the clinical assessment of the venous pressure. A left ventricular angiogram and an aortogram are the means by which mitral and aortic regurgitation respectively are demonstrated.

Coronary angiography (see Fig. 9.32c), in which the ostia of the left and right coronary arteries are selectively cannulated, is at present the only means by which the details of the effect of atheroma on the coronary circulation may be documented. This is an essential investigation prior to coronary artery vein graft surgery.

In addition to the above applications, cardiac catheterization plays an important role in congenital heart disease. By sampling the oxygen saturation at different points in the circulation the anatomical site of intracardiac shunts can be defined and the size of the shunt may be quantified.

10
The nervous system

The aim of a neurological examination is to determine the site and nature of disease of the nervous system. In simplified form it is also an essential part of any routine clinical examination. Clinical examination of the nervous system should be thought of as a technique for precisely delineating the patient's disability in physiological and anatomical terms. It gives information about the condition at the time of the examination but gives no clue as to the natural history nor, therefore, to the pathogenesis of the disorder. For the latter, precise history taking is of particular importance since it alone enables the evolution of the disease to be studied.

A detailed neurological examination is an ordeal for ill patients and a test of concentration and cooperation for those in good general health; such detail is usually unnecessary and care should always be taken not to fatigue the patient unduly. Overlong examination may defeat its own ends, especially when sensation is being investigated, by leading to variable and incongruous findings. It may sometimes be preferable to conduct the examination in more than one session.

The order of examination outlined in this chapter need not be rigidly adhered to. For example, if a patient is complaining of sciatic pain, it is appropriate to begin with the examination of the lower limbs and lumbar spine. An abbreviated scheme for routine use is set out at the end of the chapter. Observation of the patient's ordinary activity, for example the way he walks into the room and undresses for examination, is often helpful in deciding how to begin the examination. Always ask a patient examined in bed to undertake as much activity as possible; it is particularly important to see the patient trying to stand and walk, even if this seems difficult.

ANATOMY AND PHYSIOLOGY

The dominant hemisphere is that which plays the major part in control of a person's abstract activities, especially of language. The left hemisphere is dominant in almost all right-handed people and in most left-handed people.

The motor system

The lower motor neurones

Muscular movement depends ultimately on the integrity of the lower motor neurones. The lower motor neurones consist of the anterior horn cells or homologous cells in the brain stem, their efferent nerve fibres, which pass via the anterior spinal nerve roots and peripheral nerves to the muscles, and the muscle fibres innervated by these nerve fibres and their terminal axonal branches. If this final common pathway is interrupted at any point, *weakness*, *fasciculation*, *muscle wasting*, *loss of tendon reflexes* and *hypotonia* occur. These are the cardinal signs of a lower motor neurone lesion.

Although various reflex movements operate at a spinal level, the initiation of voluntary movements and the maintenance of posture and muscle tone depend on neural activity in higher centres, especially the corticospinal and extrapyramidal systems and the cerebellum. These patterns of activity can only reach the muscles if the final common path is intact.

The corticospinal system

The corticospinal (pyramidal) system consists of the pathways which directly link the pyramidal cells in the fifth layer of the motor cortex with the motor neurones in the brain stem and spinal cord. The corticospinal tracts contain these fibres and also fibres which arise from the postcentral cortex and from subcortical structures. The motor area of the cortex occupies the anterior aspect of the central sulcus (rolandic fissure) and the adjacent parts of the precentral gyrus. There is localization of function in the motor cortex, different parts of the opposite side of the body being separately represented. Those parts of the body which carry out the most skilled movements, for example the fingers and thumb, have the largest areas of cortical representation. The areas for tongue, jaw and facial movements lie in the inferior part of the motor cortex, those for the arm, trunk and leg following successively as the motor area ascends on to the vertex and medial aspect of the hemisphere (Fig. 10.1).

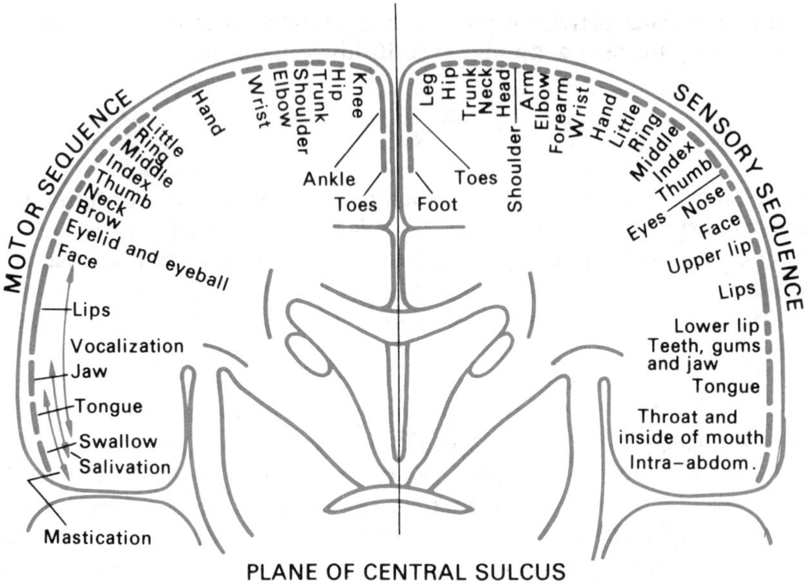

Fig. 10.1 Rasmussen and Penfield's diagram of localization in the motor (left) and sensory (right) cortex.

The fibres of the corticospinal tracts descend from their cells of origin into the internal capsule, occupying the anterior two-thirds of the posterior limb. Here the order of representation of the body is face, shoulder, elbow, hand, trunk and lower limb from before backwards. The corticospinal fibres then descend to occupy the middle three-fifths of the cerebral peduncles in the mid-brain. In the pons, the tract becomes broken into scattered bundles by the transverse pontine fibres and nuclei pontis. In the upper part of the medulla the corticospinal fibres occupy the pyramids, protuberances on the anterior aspect of the brain stem. In the lower part of the medulla the majority of the corticospinal fibres decussate with those of the opposite side and pass posteriorly into the spinal cord to form the crossed lateral corticospinal tracts. A smaller number of fibres do not decussate, but continue downwards in the anterior columns as the direct corticospinal tracts, which decussate at segmental levels in the anterior commissure. The corticospinal fibres terminate in the grey matter of the brain stem motor nuclei or in the anterior horns of the spinal cord.

The corticospinal system is concerned with the initiation of voluntary and skilled motor acts, particularly of fine distal movements. The paralysis resulting from lesions affecting corticospinal fibres *alone* consists initially of weakness of the contralateral side of the body. Rapid improvement usually occurs, resulting in residual impairment of fine and rapid distal movements of the digits, as in picking up a small object, and mild weakness of hip flexion and shoulder abduction. The more familiar occurrence of widespread paralysis of one side of the body (*hemiplegia*) or of a single limb (*monoplegia*) is usually the result of a more extensive lesion affecting extrapyramidal or other subcortical structures in addition to the corticospinal fibres themselves. Even in cases of dense hemiplegia, movements of the head and trunk (axial movements) usually escape altogether. The nervous pathways for such postural movements are predominantly under subcortical control and are represented bilaterally.

Since, in clinical practice, most lesions of the corticospinal system also damage neighbouring extrapyramidal nuclei and pathways, the distinctions drawn above are rarely of clinical importance. All such cases are loosely grouped as 'corticospinal lesions'. the classical signs of such a lesion (an *upper motor neurone lesion*) are *weakness*, which predominantly affects fine, distal movements, hip flexion and shoulder abduction, *spasticity, increased tendon reflexes*, and an *extensor plantar response* (p. 328).

When the corticospinal system is suddenly damaged or destroyed, as by haemorrhage or injury, there is a temporary depressant effect on the anterior horn cells (neuronal shock). Paralysis is accompanied at first by loss of muscle tone and absent or reduced tendon reflexes. The characteristic hypertonia and increased reflexes of a corticospinal lesion appear after a few hours or days.

The extrapyramidal system

The term *extrapyramidal system* refers to those parts of the nervous system, excluding the motor cortex and corticospinal pathways, which are concerned with movement and posture. The system includes the basal ganglia, the subthalamic nuclei; the substantia nigra, the red nuclei and other structures in the brain stem. The connections of these extrapyramidal centres are complex and include fibres from the cerebral cortex and the thalamus. There are no direct pathways from the basal ganglia to the spinal cord; the connections with the lower motor neurones are indirect, via several paths arising in the brain stem. These include the dentatorubrospinal, reticulospinal, vestibulospinal and olivospinal tracts.

The extrapyramidal system is important in the control of posture and in the initiation of movement, especially those movements which affect postural mechanisms such as sitting, standing, turning over in the lying position, walking and running. Complex volitional movements, such as reaching for an object, require both postural adjustments and fine distal movements, which are themselves broadly speaking under corticospinal control.

Diseases affecting the extrapyramidal system are characterized by difficulty in initiating voluntary movement, by impairment of orienting and balancing reflexes, by alterations in muscle tone and by the appearance of involuntary movements. Muscle power is rarely weakened.

The cerebellum

The cerebellum receives afferent fibres from the spinal cord, vestibular system, basal ganglia and cerebral cortex. It influences the lower motor neurones mainly through its connections, via the thalamus, with the basal ganglia and cerebral cortex.

Lesions of the cerebellum cause muscular hypotonia and incoordination (*ataxia*). Paralysis is not a feature of cerebellar disease. Lesions of the cerebellar vermis cause a characteristic ataxia of the trunk, so that the patient has difficulty sitting up or standing. In such patients there may be little or no incoordination of the limbs.

The sensory system

Sensory input reaches the nervous system from specialized receptors and free nerve endings in the skin and superficial tissues; from other receptors, such as muscle spindles, Golgi tendon organs, pacinian corpuscles and free nerve endings in muscles; and from other specialized receptors in the joints. All afferent fibres enter the central nervous system through the posterior root ganglia and the posterior roots. Disease of these 'first sensory neurones' may thus affect all modalities of sensation. It must be remembered, however, that much sensory input is concerned with the reflex control of posture and movement and as such does not reach consciousness or is not consciously perceived. Thus the conscious recognition of posture and position of a limb (kinaesthesis) is dependent on input from cutaneous and joint receptors and especially from muscle spindles. However, the major role of muscle spindles and tendon organs is in the control of voluntary and reflex movements.

After they have entered the spinal cord, the various sensory fibres are rearranged and grouped into other systems. The majority of these afferent fibres terminate in the grey matter of the posterior horn at or near the level at which they enter. The secondary sensory fibres arise from these cells in the posterior horn. Some of these cross immediately, or within a few segments, to the opposite lateral and anterior columns of the cord and so ascend to the brain stem as the anterior and lateral spinothalamic tracts. Impulses from which the sensations of pain and temperature are derived ascend in the *lateral spinothalamic tract*, the fibres from the lower part of the body being placed laterally and those from the upper part medially. Other afferent fibres do not synapse in the grey matter of the posterior horns of the spinal cord, but ascend in the ipsilateral posterior columns: these posterior column fibres carry impulses upon which depend the appreciation of position, movement, size, shape, discrimination and texture, and vibration (which should be regarded only as touch rapidly applied). The medial of the two posterior columns, the *fasciculus gracilis*, contains fibres originating in the lower part of the body, whereas the lateral, the *fasciculus cuneatus*, carries fibres predominantly from the upper limbs. It should be noted, therefore, that somatotopic lamination of fibres in the posterior columns is the converse of that in the lateral spinothalamic tracts.

At any level of the spinal cord, therefore, there are two major groups of sensory fibres conveying sensory information towards the brain: one in the anterior and lateral columns carrying pain and temperature from the opposite half of the body, and a second in the posterior column, conveying the appreciation of posture, weight, size, shape and other qualities of sensation from the same side of the body. A unilateral lesion of the spinal cord, therefore, results in loss of pain and thermal sensibility below the level of the lesion on the opposite side of the body, while on the side of the lesion there is, in addition to spastic paralysis, disturbance of the sense of position and of movement and loss of recognition of weight, size, shape, touch and vibration. This group of clinical signs is called the *Brown–Séquard syndrome*.

At the upper end of the spinal cord the posterior column fibres terminate in the gracile and cuneate nuclei. The fibres of the secondary sensory neurone originate in these nuclei and immediately cross to the opposite side of the medulla in the sensory decussation. In the medulla, therefore, *all* sensory impulses are carried in sensory tracts situated on the opposite side to that from which they arise. But even here all do not run in a single pathway: spinothalamic fibres pass through the lateral part of the medulla, while the posterior columns enter the medial lemniscus. Higher in the brain stem the two sensory pathways are joined by the secondary sensory fibres from sensory cranial nerve nuclei. Finally the fibres of the medial lemniscus and spinothalamic tract terminate in the thalamus. All secondary sensory fibres synapse in the thalamus. From this level a third system of sensory fibres conveys sensory input through the internal capsule to the cerebral cortex.

The description of the major sensory pathways given above is sufficient for practical use in diagnosis but it is an oversimplification of a complex subject. There are, for example, many afferent pathways other than the two described. Furthermore, these two pathways themselves are not modality specific, in the sense that certain fibres 'carry' vibration sense or other forms of sensation: but rather the interaction of different patterns of impulse in different sized fibres of differing conduction velocity determines the sensation perceived at the highest levels of the nervous system. The importance of spinal mechanisms in the control of the flow of afferent information has recently been emphasized in the 'gate control' theory of sensation. This work has demonstrated, furthermore, the pre-eminent role of the dorsal columns in exploratory, movement-directed behaviour, rather than in the passive reception of sensory input.

The spinal cord

The spinal cord extends caudally to the interspace between the 12th thoracic and 1st lumbar spines; the thecal membranes are continued down as far as the body of the 2nd sacral vertebra. The cervical enlargement reaches to the 7th

Table 10.1 Segmental innervation of the muscles of the upper limb

		CERVICAL SEGMENTS				DORSAL
		5	**6**	**7**	**8**	**1**
SHOULDER	SUPRASPINATUS	■				
	TERES MIN.	■				
	DELTOID	■	■			
	INFRASPINATUS	■	■			
	SUBSCAPULARIS	■	■			
	TERES MAJOR		■	■		
ARM	BICEPS	■	■			
	TRICEPS		■	■	■	
FOREARM	BRACHIO-RADIALIS		■			
	SUPINATOR		■			
	EXTENSOR CARPI RADIAL.		■	■		
	PRONATOR TERES		■	■		
	FLEXOR CARPI RADIAL.		■	■		
	FLEXOR POLLIC. LONG.		■	■		
	ABDUCT. POLL. LONG.			■		
	EXTENS. POLL. BREV.			■		
	EXTENS. POLL. LONG.			■	■	
	EXTENS. DIGITOR.			■	■	
	EXTENS. INDICIS.			■	■	
	EXTENS. CARPI. ULN.			■	■	
	EXTENS. DIGITOR. MIN.			■	■	
	FLEXOR DIGITOR. SUBLIMIS			■	■	■
	FLEXOR DIGITOR. PROFUND.			■	■	■
	PRONATOR QUADRAT.			■	■	■
	FLEX. CARPI. ULN.				■	■
	PALMARIS LONG.				■	■
HAND	ABDUCTOR POLL. BREV.		■	■		
	FLEXOR POLL. BREV.		■	■		
	OPPONENS POLL.		■	■		
	FLEXOR DIGIT. MIN.			■	■	
	OPPONENS DIGIT. MIN.			■	■	
	ADDUCT. POLL.				■	■
	PALMARIS BREV.				■	■
	ABDUCTOR DIGIT. MIN.				■	■
	LUMBRICALES				■	■
	INTEROSSEI				■	■

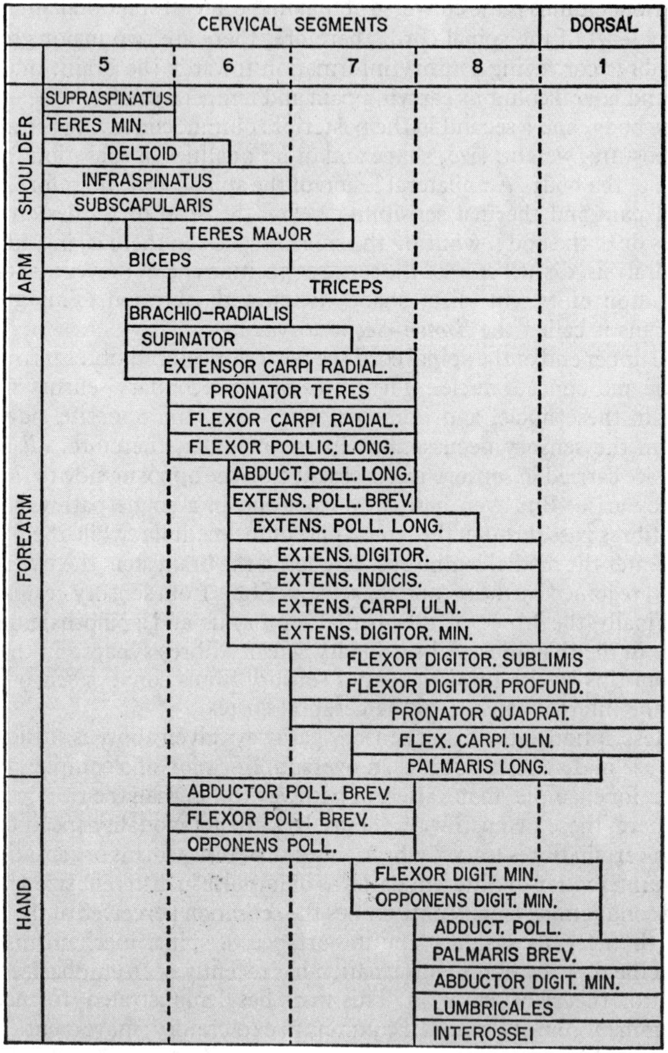

Table 10.2 Segmental innervation of the muscles of the lower limb

		D12	L1	L2	L3	L4	L5	S1	S2
HIP	ILIO-PSOAS	X	X	X	X	X			
	TENSOR FASCIÆ					X	X		
	GLUTEUS MEDIUS					X	X	X	
	GLUTEUS MINIMUS					X	X	X	
	QUADRATUS FEMORIS					X	X	X	
	GLUTEUS MAXIMUS					X	X	X	X
	OBTURATOR INTERN.						X	X	X
THIGH	SARTORIUS			X	X				
	ADDUCT. LONG.			X	X				
	QUADRICEPS			X	X	X			
	GRACILIS			X	X	X			
	ADDUCTOR BREVIS			X	X	X			
	OBTURATOR EXT.				X	X			
	ADDUCT. MAGN.				X	X			
	ADDUCT. MINIM.				X	X			
	SEMITENDINOSUS					X	X	X	
	SEMIMEMBRANOSUS					X	X	X	
	BICEPS FEMORIS					X	X	X	X
LEG	TIBIALIS ANT.					X	X		
	EXTENS. HALL. LONG.					X	X	X	
	EXTENS. DIGIT. LONG.					X	X	X	
	SOLEUS					X	X	X	X
	GASTROCNEMIUS					X	X	X	X
	PERONEUS LONG.						X	X	
	PERONEUS BREV.						X	X	
	TIBIALIS POST.						X	X	X
	FLEXOR DIGITOR. LONG.						X	X	X
	FLEXOR HALLUC. LONG.						X	X	X
FOOT	EXTENS. HALL. BREV.					X	X	X	
	EXTENS. DIGIT. BREVIS					X	X	X	
	INTRINSIC MUSCLES OF THE FOOT						X	X	X
	INTEROSSEI							X	X

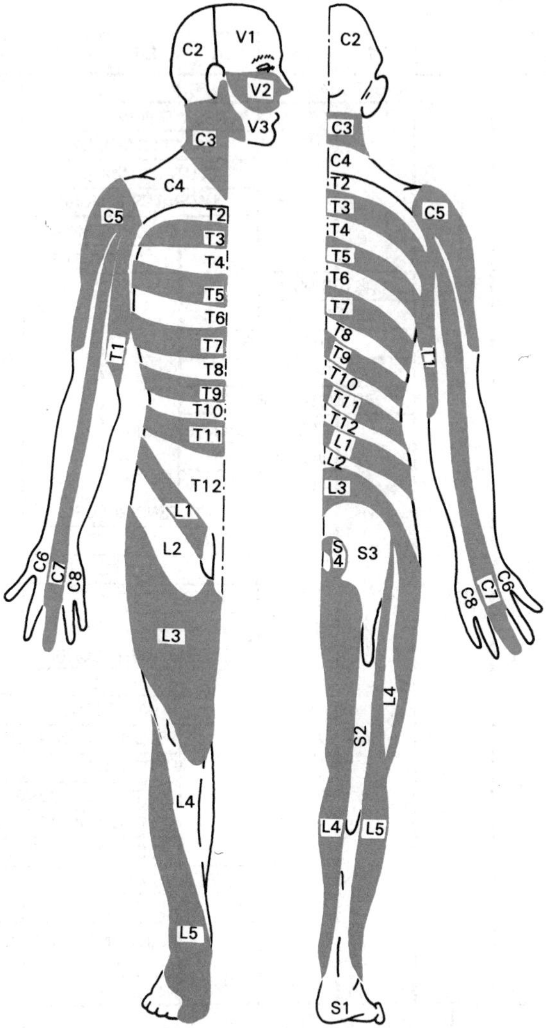

Fig. 10.2 The cutaneous areas supplied by sensory roots. Minor variations are common.

cervical spine. Its largest part is at the level of the 5th and 6th cervical vertebrae. The lumbar segments lie opposite the 10th and 11th thoracic spines and the next interspinous space.

Since the cord ends at the level of the lower border of the 1st lumbar vertebra, spinal segments do not correspond with the vertebrae overlying

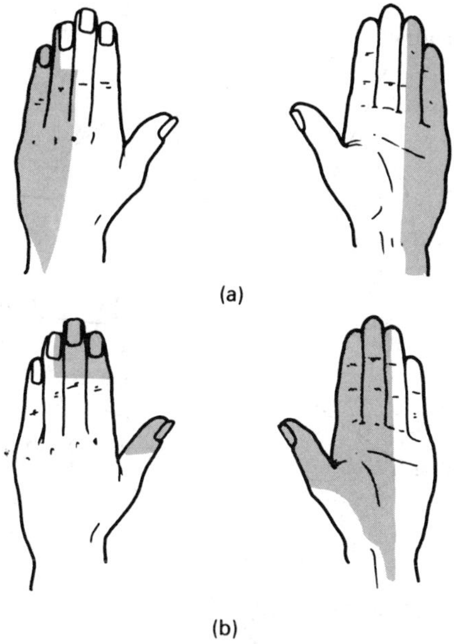

Fig. 10.3 Cutaneous sensory loss. (a) After division of the ulnar nerve above the elbow. (b) After division of the median nerve in the arm. These areas are subject to considerable variation.

them. To determine which spinal segment is related to a given vertebral body, an important concept in assessing patients with spinal cord compression due to vertebral disease:

For the cervical vertebrae, add 1.
For thoracic 1–6, add 2.
For thoracic 7–9, add 3.
The 10th thoracic arch overlies lumbar 1 and 2 segments.
The 11th thoracic arch overlies lumbar 3 and 4 segments.
The 12th thoracic arch overlies lumbar 5.
The 1st lumbar arch overlies the sacral and coccygeal segments.
In the lower dorsal region the tip of a spinous process is on a level with the body of the vertebra below.

The spinal cord is made up of segments, from each of which a pair of anterior (motor) and posterior (sensory) nerve roots arises. The *myotomes* and *dermatomes* supplied by the pairs of nerve roots are shown in Tables 10.1 and 10.2 and in Fig. 10.2. It is important to remember these, since accurate knowledge

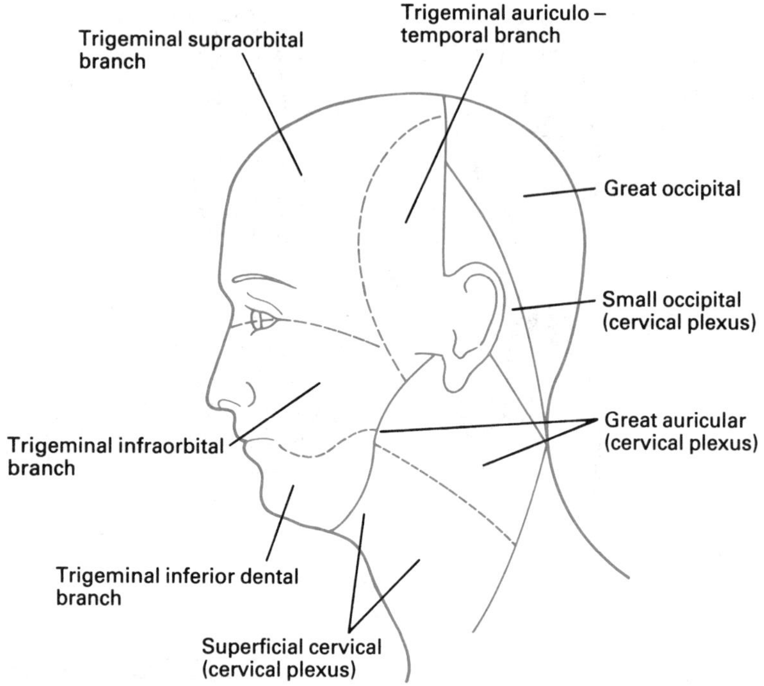

Fig. 10.4 The distribution of the sensory nerves of the head. Compare with the sensory distribution shown in Fig. 10.2.

of them enables quick and easy separation of nerve root and peripheral nerve lesions to be made by simple clinical examination. The sensory loss found after some common peripheral nerve lesions is shown in Figs. 10.3 and 10.4. They should be carefully compared with the patterns of sensory loss shown in Fig. 10.2. Note that C8 and C6 sensory loss extends to the elbow on both ventral and dorsal surfaces of the forearm, but that median nerve sensory loss predominantly affects the palmar surface of the hand. In both ulnar and median nerve lesions sensory loss extends no further proximally than the wrist.

Vascular supply of the brain and spinal cord

The *brain* is supplied by the internal carotid and vertebral arteries (Fig. 10.5). Owing to the position of origin of the left common carotid, an embolus can enter it more easily than it can the artery of the opposite side. Embolic lesions are therefore more frequent in the left than in the right cerebral hemisphere.

The two *vertebral arteries* unite at the lower border of the pons to form the

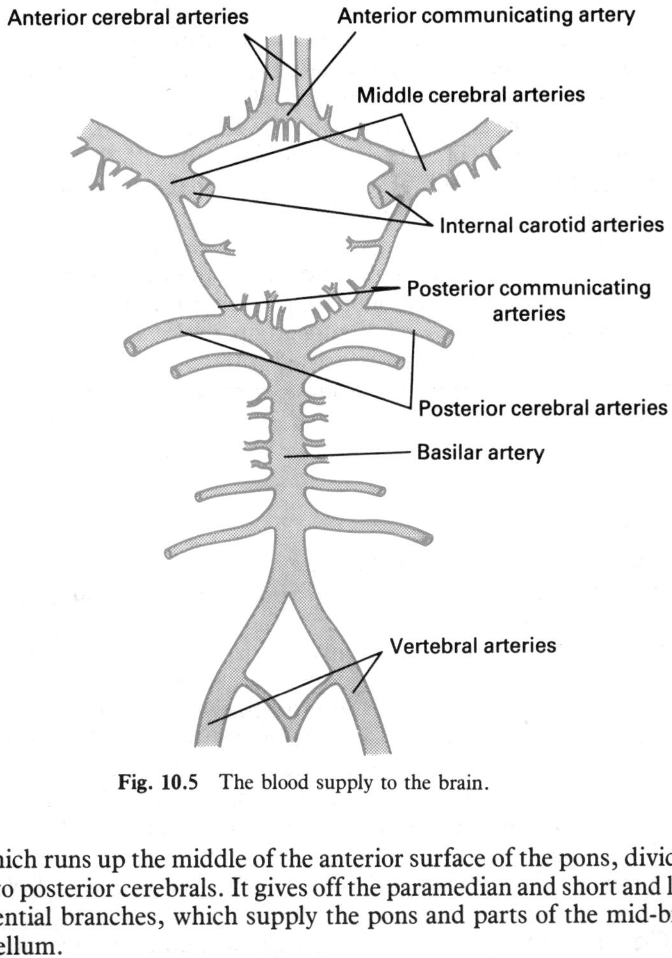

Fig. 10.5 The blood supply to the brain.

basilar, which runs up the middle of the anterior surface of the pons, dividing into the two posterior cerebrals. It gives off the paramedian and short and long circumferential branches, which supply the pons and parts of the mid-brain and cerebellum.

The *posterior cerebral* artery supplies the occipital lobe, the lower part of the temporal lobe and the uncus, the inner part of the crus and the corpora quadrigemina, and the posterior part of the posterior limb of the internal capsule. Occlusion of this artery at its origin will therefore involve the visual cortex and the sensory fibres, but thrombosis often involves the calcarine branch and hence the visual cortex alone.

The *internal carotid artery* gives off the *anterior cerebral* artery, which curves round the anterior end of the corpus callosum, and is chiefly distributed to the inner surface of the cerebral hemisphere as far back as the parieto-occipital fissure. It also supplies the superior frontal gyrus, and gives a branch to the anterior part of the internal capsule and to the basal ganglia.

The *middle cerebral artery*, which lies in the sylvian fissure, is the main branch of the internal carotid artery. Embolism from the internal carotid artery or from the heart, therefore, often involves the middle cerebral artery. The middle cerebral artery gives off *cortical branches*, which supply the frontal lobes, including the motor cortex, and the superior parts of the parietal and temporal lobes. These branches anastomose freely with those of the adjoining anterior cerebral and posterior cerebral arteries so that occlusion of one of them may sometimes be largely compensated by the establishment of a collateral circulation. The middle cerebral artery also gives off *central branches*, which penetrate into the brain substance and supply the white matter and the basal ganglia. There are two chief groups of these central arteries—an anterior group called the *lenticulostriate*, and a posterior group, the *lenticulo-optic*. The lenticulostriate arteries are particularly associated with hypertensive cerebral haemorrhage. These central arteries also anastomose with one another.

Venous blood leaves the brain in the *venous sinuses*. Blood from the interior of the brain enters the cerebral veins, which end in the straight sinus.

Spinal arteries

The *anterior* and *posterior spinal arteries* arise from the vertebral arteries and travel caudally in the pia mater, the former in the anteromedian fissure and the two latter alongside the posterior nerve roots. Although they have a long and tortuous course, they do not diminish in size, being reinforced by radicular tributaries from the intercostal and lumbar arteries, particularly from a large lumbar radicular vessel, the artery of Adamkiewicz. The anterior spinal artery supplies most of the spinal cord, only the posterior parts of the posterior horns and columns being supplied by the posterior spinal arteries. Both anterior and posterior spinal arteries function as anastomotic vessels linking the radicular feeding vessels. Flow does not, therefore, occur in any one direction in these vessels but varies, or may even reverse, in response to local factors such as changes in posture and variations in intra-abdominal and intrathoracic pressure.

The main *veins of the spinal cord* are situated dorsally and ventrally in the midline. Like the arteries, they communicate by radicular branches with the lumbar and intercostal veins, and empty into the vertebral veins. The blood in them flows upwards; hence in compression of the spinal cord, e.g. by tumour, there is venous engorgement below the level of compression. This may very rarely result in a secondary, haemorrhagic, venous infarction of the spinal cord with paralysis and loss of sensation below the level of the lesion. *However, if spinal compression is treated promptly, before cord infarction has occurred, recovery can occur.*

MENTAL FUNCTIONS

It is important to analyse the patient's intellectual state early in the examination, even if the analysis is limited to a subjective assessment of personality, memory, education and abstractional ability formed during the process of history taking, since this assessment is helpful in the subsequent investigation of symptoms. For example, if the patient's memory is impaired, only a limited value can be attached to his account of his illness or the state of his previous health. If he is comatose or unable to understand speech, any attempt to investigate the state of his sensory functions is likely to be frustrated. If for any reason the patient's own history is incomplete, it is essential to obtain a history from the relatives or friends.

Appearance and behaviour

The patient's bearing or actions when lying in bed are important. Note whether there is any disturbance of consciousness such as confusion, stupor or coma. Is he unduly disturbed or apathetic, or in a state of agitation or confusion? Is his attention easily held or fleeting? Does he show a reasonable degree of interest in his surroundings? How does he react to your approach and greeting? Is he well-groomed or unkempt? What is the condition of his hair and hands? Any other unusual features in his behaviour (e.g. facial tics or any inappropriate behaviour) should be noted.

Note whether his conversation flows easily or not: whether he is mute, answers only by monosyllables or is over-talkative. Do his remarks hold together as replies to questions? Do they show looseness of association? Do they show *flight of ideas* (a rushing stream of ideas with some connection) or *thought disorder*, when one remark follows another without logical connection? (See Chapter 3.) Does he keep on repeating your questions or his own remarks (*perseveration*)? He may use strange words (*neologisms*) or real words strung together oddly (*word salad*).

Emotional state

It is important to note his mood. Is he happy or distressed? Is he happier than his condition would warrant (*elation* or *euphoria*) or filled with despair or dismay (*depression*)? Does his conversation lead you to feel that there is flattening of emotion, e.g. he speaks of family or financial success without pleasure or in an incongruous manner (he laughs after relating a misfortune or breaks into tears when given some pleasant news)? Is he able to enjoy anything? Does he feel that nothing is worthwhile? Does he feel fed up with life, or so fed up that he might as well end it (so that there is a risk of suicide)? Does the play of his features suggest that he enjoys a private world of his own, such as smiling or grimacing at odd times? Does he appear perplexed? Find out whether persons or things seem as real as they should, or whether they seem changed in some mysterious way (*depersonalization*). It is, however, unwise to ask leading questions about depersonalization, as neurotic patients will often respond affirmatively. Note whether the patient seems irritable or resentful, or whether he receives your words with suspicion.

Inquiries should be made about the patient's *sleep*. Does he sleep too much or too little? If too much, is any particular action likely to precipitate the hypersomnia? If too little, is the difficulty that of going to sleep, of waking frequently, or waking early in the morning and being unable to go to sleep again? Where there is no physical cause for the insomnia, such as pain, cough, asthma or the wearing of some uncomfortable plaster, the insomnia is likely to be due to some psychological disorder, e.g. the restlessness of mania, the early waking of depression, or the turmoil of the mind with difficulty in getting off to sleep found in anxiety states.

Inquire about *dreams*. These are frequent and sleep-disturbing in the anxiety states, whether the source of the anxiety is apparent or not. In these conditions sleep is not refreshing and the patient may complain of being as tired in the morning as at night.

Delusions and hallucinations

Delusions are false beliefs which continue to be held despite evidence to the contrary. *Hallucinations* are false impressions referred to the organs of special sense (hearing, seeing, smelling, etc.) for which no cause can be found and which the patient knows to be imagined or unreal events. The patient's conversation may have already indicated that these are present. Note their content and the patient's attitude when you express doubt about what seems so real to him.

Neither delusions nor hallucinations may be voiced spontaneously. They have then to be inquired for; the introduction of this subject may call for considerable tact. Is his mind or his body interfered with by others or by some physical agency, e.g. electricity, radio or TV, or poison? Has he felt that others talk about him or shun him? Are his relatives, neighbours and colleagues at work kind to him or difficult to get on with? Has he ideas of supernatural power or inordinate wealth or, conversely, does he feel that he is weakened physically, morally or financially? Has he feelings of guilt? Does he think that he caused his own illness?

Hallucinatory experiences may be carefully hidden. Auditory and visual hallucinations are commonest. Of these visual hallucinations are usually organic and, except in temporal lobe epilepsy, auditory hallucinations are usually due to non-organic psychoses such as schizophrenia. Does he hear or see anything unusual? Does he taste or smell something unexpectedly? Hallucinations may occur only at certain times of the day or in certain places. Delusions which are secondary to hallucinatory experiences must be noted, e.g. that 'the neighbours are against me, because my bedroom smells of gas; my neighbours have caused this'. Notes should be made of any unusual actions on the patient's part prompted by delusions or hallucinatory ideas, e.g. ideas that his wife is in the pay of his enemies, or his clutching at small animals which he 'sees' crawling over his bedclothes.

Orientation in place and time

Does the patient appreciate his surroundings and know where he is, or is he muddled? If he offers an inaccurate answer, is this part of *confabulation*, a filling in of forgotten memories by inappropriately recalled material from previous experiences? Does he know the date approximately, if not correctly? Can he estimate the approximate time without looking at a watch or clock? Does he know why he is in hospital?

Clouding of consciousness

It is important to recognize states of clouded consciousness (see Chapter 3) and to be able to describe and define them to others, particularly in the context of patients with head injury or raised intracranial pressure, who may gradually deteriorate during a period of clinical observation. *Coma* is a state in which the patient makes no psychologically meaningful response to external stimulus or to inner need. In *stupor* the patient, although inaccessible, does show some response, for instance to painful stimuli. Above these deep levels lie various degrees of altered consciousness and lethargy, which may be accompanied by confusion. The questioner must be alert to observe any minor defects in the patient's capacity to grasp what is required of him and what has happened to him. Such defects will usually be manifest in the responses to tests for orientation, recent memory and appreciation of environment.

In *dementia* the patient is confused in time, place and person, and shows impaired abstractional abilities, but is awake and alert; in *delirium* the patient is similarly confused, but shows impaired alertness. Both these abnormal mental states are sometimes termed *organic confusional states* (see Chapter 3).

Memory

Inability to grasp and retain new images and ideas is a feature of acute toxic–delirious reactions and of the subacute and chronic organic psychoses. In these cases recent events may have been registered but cannot be recalled, although later, when recovered, the patient may be able to remember them. However, it is more often the case that, in such patients, events have not been registered.

The degree to which *recent memory* is lost is an index of the severity of organic brain disorder (not necessarily permanent). Inquire about the day of the week and of the month and the names of prominent public figures. Ask the patient to recall what he has read in the paper or seen on television. In formulating questions on these lines, attention should be paid to the patient's educational background and his likely personal interests. Bring up a subject discussed three minutes previously, or give the patient a simple story or address to remember, and note how much is remembered after a short interval or after distraction. These are all tests of recent memory. *Short term memory*, consisting of memory lasting up to a minute or so, required for tasks involving mental manipulations, such as remembering a telephone number while dialling it, is usually spared in patients with recent memory disturbance, for example in Wernicke–Korsakoff syndrome. Short term memory is usually tested by seeing whether the patient can repeat seven digits forwards or five digits backwards or by asking him to spell 'world' backwards.

Long term memory is relatively resistant to the effects of neurological or psychiatric disease but is impaired, as is short term recall, in patients with progressive dementias.

General intelligence

It is always necessary to ascertain the patient's general intelligence since it may be affected by brain injury or disease. The standard which he reached before leaving school, the character of his work, and his work record give a rough-and-ready approximation. Frequent changes of job may indicate mental defect or personality disorder. Frequent changes after an accident or a serious illness in patients with a previously good work record are suggestive of brain damage.

Tests of memory as given above will indicate more serious, specific defects and these can be further exposed by tests of *reasoning*, particularly where the tests show inability to monitor or correct his performance. Ask the patient to take sevens from a hundred (i.e. 100, 93, 86, 79 . . .), or to reverse in his mind's eye the hands of a clock. The absurdities test (e.g. 'What would be wrong if I told you I had three brothers, John, Fred and myself?') indicates grosser disability. People of relatively low intelligence can often give the months of the year parrot-fashion but not which month precedes May and which October, etc.

Tests in which the patient is asked the meaning of rare words or to interpret common proverbs or sayings are commonly used as an index of *abstractional abilities*. *Judgement* may similarly be assessed: 'What would you do if you saw a house on fire or a stamped addressed envelope lying in the road?' In dementia these questions often provoke concrete answers or a confused reply. *Constructional* and *drawing* tests may also be useful. These are briefly described on p. 342.

Released reflexes in dementia

In the demented patient and in other organic confusional states, a number of reflexes, released from the control of higher centres, may be elicited. Some may also be found in patients with large focal lesions; for example, the grasp reflex is characteristically released in patients with contralateral frontal lobe disease. In infancy the presence or absence of these reflexes is used as part of the developmental assessment (p. 468). The most important of these higher level reflexes are the *grasping* and *avoiding responses*, the *palmo-mental reflex*, the *glabellar tap reflex*, and released oral responses such as the *snout response* and tactilely and visually evoked *sucking reflexes*.

Grasping and avoiding responses *Grasping* is elicited by stroking the palmar surface of the patient's hand on its radial aspect, preferably using a firm, distally moving stimulus between the patient's thumb and forefinger. The patient's hand grasps the examiner's and this grasp is not easily inhibited even if the patient is distracted, for example by being asked his address. If traction is applied by simply pulling against the patient's flexed fingers, the patient tends to oppose with an equivalent force. Grasping is typically associated with contralateral frontal lobe disease.

The avoiding response consists of a tendency for the patient's hand to move away from palmar or dorsal stroking or touch. It is usually evoked by stimuli on the ulnar surface of the hand. It is found in patients with contralateral parietal lobe disease, or lesions in its connections.

The palmo-mental reflex consists of a brief contraction of the ipsilateral mentalis muscle, causing puckering of the chin, in response to scratching the skin near the thenar eminence with a key or pin.

Glabellar tap reflex A series of sharp finger taps to the glabella normally elicits only two or three blinks before this response is inhibited, but in patients with diffuse degenerative disorders, especially senile dementia, and also in Parkinson's disease, the response is disinhibited and a blink follows each of a train of stimuli.

Snout reflex Gentle pressure of the examiner's knuckle against the patient's lips causes reflex puckering of the orbicular oris. This is usually associated with similar contraction of the facial musculature evoked by very light taps to the lips with a tendon hammer or with the fingers.

Sucking reflexes Anticipatory opening of the mouth as part of released sucking may be elicited by approaching visual stimuli, e.g. the shining metal end of a tuning fork, or by light contact with the cheeks near the corners of the mouth.

SPEECH

In considering speech disorders, it is essential to distinguish between defects of articulation and enunciation of speech, called *dysarthria*, and disturbances of the structure and organization of language itself, ***aphasia***.

Dysarthria

Defective *articulation* of speech may seem difficult to distinguish from regional or other speech accents but, with practice, this distinction can usually be made quite reliably. Certain constant features of different types of dysarthria can be identified. *Stammering* is a developmental disorder, more common in boys than girls. It is only very rarely due to organic brain disease. In lalling, or 'baby speech', all the difficult consonants are dropped; the patient speaks like a baby. Lalling in adults is usually the result of congenital or infantile deafness. Speech is usually louder than normal in this disorder.

There are four main types of dysarthria:

Cerebellar dysarthria The patient speaks slowly and deliberately, syllable be syllable, as if scanning a line of poetry. The normal prosodic rhythm of syllable, word and sentence production is lost and in extreme forms each syllable is given equal emphasis. Ask the patient to say 'artillery': he will pronounce it 'ar-til-ler-y'. This scanning or staccato disturbance of speech rhythm is the classical form of severe cerebellar dysarthria. It is important to recognize minor, less obvious forms since its presence indicates bilateral disease of the cerebellum or of its brain stem connections.

Pseudobulbar (spastic) dysarthria Individual syllables are slurred, and the precision of consonant pronunciation is lost as in a state of intoxication. Thus 'British Constitution' becomes 'Brizh Conshishushon'. This form of dysarthria is due to bilateral lesions in the corticospinal fibres supplying the muscles of the face, larynx, tongue and respiration, i.e. the lesion is *supranuclear* to, or above the level of, these brain stem nuclei. It is therefore a feature of *pseudobulbar palsy*: the jaw jerk is invariably brisk, and in most patients examination of the limbs reveals evidence of bilateral corticospinal tract lesions, e.g. bilateral extensor plantar responses. *Dysphagia* may be a prominent associated feature, with particular difficulty swallowing liquids, including saliva.

Aphonia Sometimes a patient with a profound pseudobulbar palsy may be unable to make a sound, although conveying by signs that he comprehends perfectly. In hysterical aphonia phonation occurs during spontaneous or voluntary coughing, but in pseudobulbar aphonia coughing is silent.

Bulbar dysarthria Bulbar palsy, due to lower motor neurone lesions affecting the speech musculature, results in non-specific slurring of speech which can usually be readily separated from other forms of dysarthria. There are usually other features of bulbar palsy, particularly *dysphagia*; fluids tend to be regurgitated through the nose and solid foods are difficult to swallow. Palatal air escape may be audible during phonation.

Cortical dysarthria This irregular hesitancy in word production, associated with difficulties in abstract, volitional movements of the lips and tongue, *oro-facial apraxia*, is commonly associated with aphasia due to left frontal and temporal lesions. It never occurs as an isolated abnormality and the term cortical dysarthria should therefore be used with caution.

Aphasia

The word aphasia means a disturbance of the ability to use language, whether in speaking, writing or comprehending. There are several different classifications of aphasia, but these are largely of theoretical interest. In assessing an aphasic patient it is important to relate the functional defect in language to the patient's disability as a whole: how does it affect him? Formal analysis of the aphasia can then be attempted, and this will enable accurate localization of the lesion to be achieved (Fig. 10.6).

Everyday use of language includes:

1 The ability to *use words* in spoken speech. This includes *articulation*, *fluency* (the ability to put words together into phrases and sentences of varying complexity, in various grammatical constructions, without hesitations and errors), *naming* and the accurate *repetition* of complex statements and concepts.
2 The ability to *comprehend* spoken speech.
3 The ability to *read* to oneself (not aloud).
4 The ability to *write*.
5 The ability to comprehend *other symbols*, e.g. mathematical or musical symbols.

Speech defects may readily be analysed in these terms as disturbances of *articulation*, *fluency*, *verbal comprehension*, *naming*, *repetition*, *reading* and *writing*. If a simple rough score is given to each of these categories (Fig. 10.6), a broad analysis of speech function which has some localizing value can be built up. It can be seen, for example, that disturbances of fluency, verbal comprehension, repetition and writing are all prominent in left anterior temporal lobe lesions (amnestic or Wernicke's aphasia). Left frontal lesions affect articulation and fluency more than the other categories of language. Left parieto-occipital lesions impair reading (visual language functions); left parietal lesions impair several other associative functions, but particularly writing. Generally, the lateralization of speech is thought to correspond to handedness, but most left handed people have left hemisphere dominance rather than right.

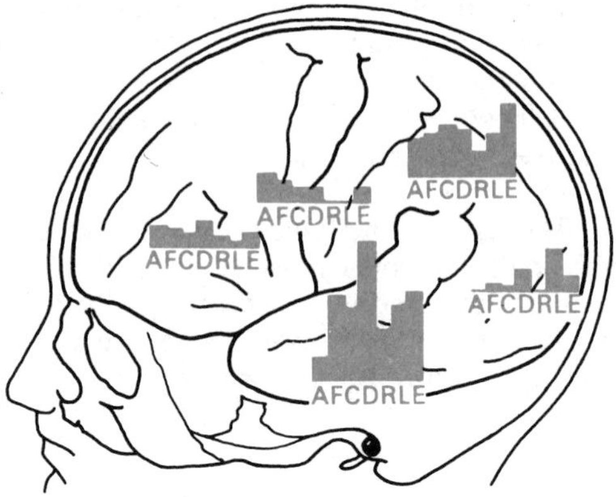

Fig. 10.6 The average degree of disturbance of various language modalities which occurs when there is an isolated lesion of various lobes (frontal, rolandic, parietal, temporal and occipital). A, articulatory disturbances; F, disturbances in the fluency of speech; C, disturbances of verbal comprehension; D, disturbances of naming; R, disturbances of repetition; L, disturbances of reading; E, disturbances of writing.
(After H. Hecaen and R. Angelergues (1964) in Ciba Foundation Symposium on Disorders of Language. London: Churchill.)

Assessment of articulation and fluency, on the one hand, and reading and writing, on the other, enables recognition of lesions in front of and behind the central sulcus (rolandic fissure). This is a useful clinical concept which may be referred to as the *'anterior'* and *'posterior' aphasic syndromes*. The terms *'expressive'* and *'receptive' aphasia* are more or less synonymous but they ignore the equally important functions of reading, writing, repetition, articulation and fluency. In the examination of an aphasic patient, spoken and written speech should be assessed separately.

Assessment of spoken speech

First be sure whether the patient's hearing is adequate. Begin by assessing speech in the context of an ordinary conversation about everyday things or about the patient's illness itself. Note the presence of hesitations, the searching for a forgotten word, and its compensation by the use of a descriptive phrase (paraphasia), *neologisms* (invented or nonsense words), or inappropriately used words or phrases. Note also any articulatory disturbances, particularly clumsiness and difficulty in coordinating movements of lips and tongue (*orofacial* apraxia). Orofacial apraxia is a *bilateral* disturbance of these movements occurring with a *unilateral*, left frontal lesion. It is usually very pronounced when the patient is commanded to put out his tongue or close his eyes and these movements should not, therefore, be used to establish comprehension of speech or the patient's co-operation. Disturbances of fluency are best assessed in spontaneous conversational speech.

The aphasic patient can often use only a few words. These should be noted, as should words or phrases repeated again and again (*perseveration* or *repetitive utterances*).

If he has a considerable vocabulary, first make a note of any examples of slurring, etc., as an indication of disturbed *articulation*. Test him with such words and phrases as 'British Constitution', 'West Register Street', 'biblical criticism', 'artillery'. Then show him common objects—a knife, a pen, a matchbox, etc.—and ask him to *name* them. Sometimes the patient has a general idea of the word he wants to use, but forgets exactly how to pronounce it; he omits some syllables or substitutes others for them, so that the listener may hardly be able to make out what word he wishes to use. These are signs of *amnestic* or *nominal* aphasia.

In anterior aphasias the patient will often be aware of his errors, although unable to correct them. Mistakes in the use of words, e.g. calling a knife a pen, are examples of *word substitution*, a more marked abnormality than *syllabic substitution*. Patients with left posterior lesions, whether in addition to a frontal lesion or occurring alone, show defective ability to monitor their own speech. Their speech not only shows syllabic and word substitutions but it may contain *neologisms*. In extreme examples of this disorder, characteristic of left posterior temporal lesions, speech consists of syllabic neologisms, making no sense at all, *jargon aphasia*. Patients with jargon aphasia tend to talk incessantly, often in relation to inappropriate sounds in their environment, for example in response to a voice on the radio or in another part of the room. Thus patients with left frontal lesions speak hesitantly, with poor fluency, and those with left temporo-parietal lesions speak fluently, but their speech is often devoid of meaning. A further point of difference between these two types of speech defect is that patients with more posteriorly placed lesions show marked difficulties in comprehension of spoken speech. Indeed, this is a marked feature of patients with fluent aphasia, since it is an underlying defect in the adequate monitoring of these patients' own spoken speech.

Speech repetition is a useful test. Patients with left frontal lesions can repeat words and simple phrases, although they may introduce syllabic or other errors, but those with more posterior lesions may be unable even to approach the task. The patient should be asked to repeat a single phrase, clearly stated by the examiner, such as 'Today is Wednesday June 4th; and this is The London Hospital.' Remember never to shout at an aphasic patient: his hearing is normal. If the patient is able to repeat what you say, endeavour to find out whether or not he understands what he is saying. Finally, ask the patient to read aloud and note whether he can find his way about the page, and if speech errors appear.

Assessment of written language

Reading and writing tests are important in the assessment of aphasia.

Reading Reading aloud tests the visual comprehension of language and spoken speech. Reading silently tests comprehension of language through the visual system; this is best tested by asking the patient to obey simple written commands without reading aloud, e.g. 'Touch your nose with your left hand.' When the patient reads aloud, errors in spoken speech can be readily detected since the intended speech pattern is known from the written material. Disturbances of reading are called *dyslexia*.

Writing Ask the patient to write his name; this can often be done when the ability to write is otherwise lost (*dysgraphia*). Ask him some simple question, e.g., 'What is your address?' and get him to write a reply. If he has poor verbal comprehension put your question in writing. If his right hand is paralysed, ask him to write or print with his left. If he writes well, get him to write an account of his illness and note whether he makes use of the wrong word at times or whether there is repeated use (*perseveration*) of any particular word.

Can he write to dictation or copy words and sentences? Try, using a newspaper. If he succeeds, does he understand the meaning of what he writes?

Comprehension of other symbols Write down certain numerals:

2	2	2
+2	+2	+2
—	—	—
4	5	6

and ask him to point out which is correct. Inability to understand and manipulate mathematical symbols, termed *acalculia*, may occur in posterior parietal lesions affecting the dominant hemisphere. If he can read music, test him with musical notes.

Gesture

Many aphasic patients make attempts to use gesture to communicate, but this may be impaired in patients with anterior lesions. Furthermore, many aphasic patients, especially those with Wernicke's (temporal) aphasia, or with posterior, fluent aphasias, do not fully understand complex gestural instructions.

APRAXIA

Occasionally a patient who has neither motor nor sensory paralysis, nor ataxia, cannot perform certain acts, though he can easily execute their component movements. He is consequently unable to make use of objects, though he can recognize their use. This is known as apraxia. It results from damage to the left parietal cortex or parietal white matter of the left or of both hemispheres, or from disease of the connections between the two hemispheres through the corpus callosum. When only the callosal fibres are injured, it affects only the left limbs, i.e. the right hemisphere, but it is more commonly a bilateral disorder.

It may be tested for by asking the patient to use objects or to make or imitate certain movements. For instance he may be given a box of matches and asked to strike a match. If there is apraxia, he may fail to open the box, or to take a match from it, or to strike the match, or may show an inability to recognize which end to strike against the box. It is, of course, important to be sure that the patient understands the request.

THE CRANIAL NERVES

In this section a brief *résumé* of the essential points in the anatomy of each cranial nerve will be given, indicating its function and, in some cases, the symptoms resulting from lesions affecting it. The method for clinical examination of each cranial nerve will be described.

The olfactory (1st) nerve

Anatomy

The central processes of the bipolar sensory cells in the olfactory epithelium pass through the cribriform plate to the olfactory bulb, where the cells of the second olfactory neurones lie. Nerve fibres pass thence to the olfactory area of the cerebral cortex, the uncus of the parahippocampal gyrus.

Testing smell

Have three small bottles containing some oil of cloves, some oil of peppermint and some tincture of asafoetida. Present these to each nostril separately and ask the patient if he recognizes them. Common bedside substances such as soap, fruit or scent may also be used. In testing, avoid the use of such irritating substances as ammonia, for these partially stimulate the trigeminal nerve. In *anosmia* the sense of smell is abolished. Before concluding that this is due to neurological disease exclude local changes in the nose itself, e.g. catarrh. *Parosmia* is the name applied to that condition in which the sense of smell is perverted, so that, for instance, offensive substances seem to have a pleasant odour and vice versa.

Enquire also regarding *hallucinations of smell*. These sometimes constitute the aura of an epileptic fit, originating in the temporal lobe.

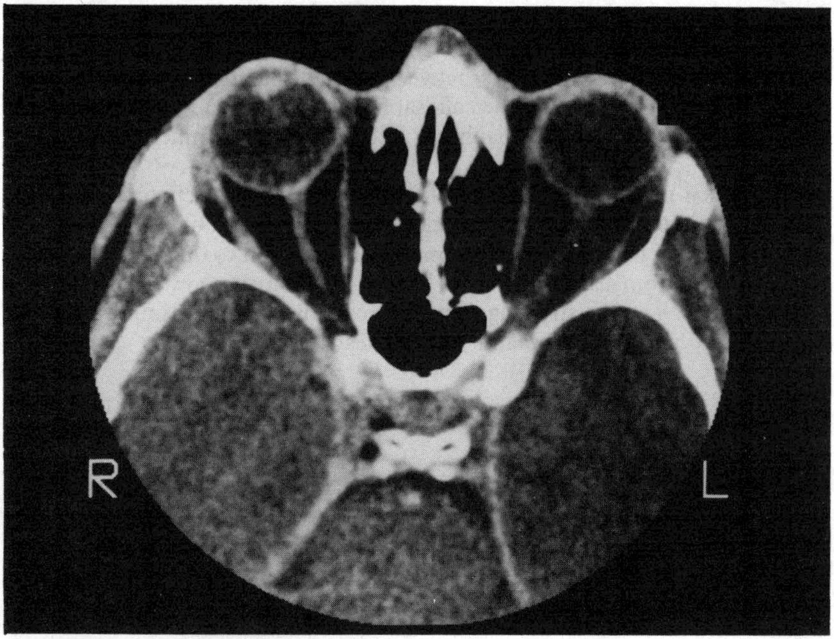

Fig. 10.7 Computerized tomographic (CT) scan of the head in a normal subject. This CT image is orientated in the plane of the orbits. Both eyes are visible. In the right eye the lens appears as a relatively X-ray dense structure. In the orbits the medial and lateral rectus muscle and the optic nerves can be seen forming a cone with its apex at the posterior margin of the orbits. The temporal lobes are situated on either side of the pituitary fossa and optic chiasm. The two orbits are separated by the nose and ethmoid sinuses.

The optic (2nd) nerve

Anatomy

From the retina, the fibres of the optic nerve (Figs. 10.7 and 10.8) pass back to the optic chiasm. Here the fibres from the inner nasal half of each retina, representing the temporal field, decussate, whilst those from the outer temporal half, representing the nasal field, remain on the same side. Each optic tract, *formed after this chiasmal decussation*, therefore consists of fibres from the outer half of the retina on the same side and from the inner half of the retina on the opposite side. Each optic tract passes posteriorly to the lateral geniculate body of the same side and some pregeniculate fibres project to the superior colliculi. The optic radiation originates in the lateral geniculate body on each side, passes through the posterior limb of the internal capsule and then projects posteriorly to the calcarine cortex of the occipital lobe. Those fibres subserving the upper visual fields pass through the white matter of the temporal lobe, whilst those

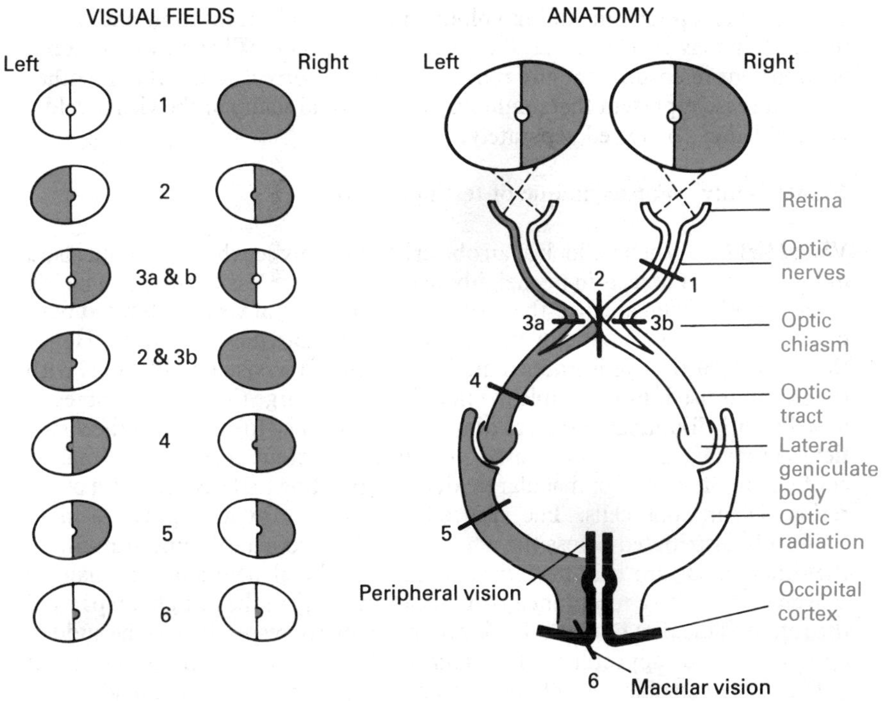

Fig. 10.8 The visual pathways. Lesion at 1 produces blindness in the right eye with loss of direct light reflex. Lesion at 2 produces bitemporal hemianopia often beginning in the central fields as a bitemporal scotomatous defect. Lesions at 3a and 3b produce binasal hemianopia (a rare disorder). Lesions at 2 and 3b produce blindness of the right eye with temporal hemianopia of the left visual field. Lesion at 4 produces right homonymous hemianopia with macular (splitting) involvement. Lesion at 5 produces right homonymous hemianopia with sparing of the macular field. Lesion at 6 produces right homonymous central (macula) hemiscotoma.

mediating impulses from the lower field pass through the parietal lobe. Thus, in the occipital cortex around the calcarine fissure, the left half of the field of vision is represented in the cortex of the right hemisphere and vice versa (Fig. 10.8).

The input from the two homologous fields of the two eyes is represented in adjacent columns of neurones. The most peripheral part of the visual fields is represented anteriorly in the calcarine fissure and the most medial part, the macular field, is represented at the occipital pole (Fig. 10.8).

Test

The *visual acuity* and the *visual fields* must always be examined. Other aspects of visual perception, including colour vision, visual localization and visual recognition may also be tested, if clinically appropriate. When testing vision it is important to ensure that any refractive error is corrected and that no other ocular disease is present that might impair the visual acuity or the visual fields. Each eye must be tested separately.

Visual acuity For technique of testing, see p. 391.

Visual fields When we look at an object, we not only see that object but also a number of other objects in the neighbourhood, more or less distinctly. The full extent of this vision is called the visual field. The field of vision is limited both by the area of the retina and by the margins of the orbit, nose and cheek. Hence the position of the eye is important. The extent of the visual field varies with the stimulus used. For example the field is larger to large than to small objects, or to brightly illuminated than to dimly lit objects. The full extent of the visual field cannot be tested to coloured objects since colour sensitivity is mainly confined to the central or macular field, corresponding to the central part of the retina rich in cone cells. The rod cells, sensitive to white light, are more uniformly distributed across the whole area of the retina. Moving stimuli, on the other hand, are best perceived in the peripheral field since specialized movement-sensitive receptor cells are located mainly in the peripheral parts of the retina. This part of the retina is also particularly responsive to the sudden appearance or disappearance of stationary visual stimuli, but the appreciation of the form of an object is only poorly developed in this part of the field. Form and detail are best perceived in the central field and this aspect of visual function is tested by assessment of the *visual acuity*.

Physiological investigations have disclosed the existence of columns of cells in the visual cortex responsive to precise visual stimuli, for example dark surrounds, linear dark–light junctions oriented in particular planes, and specialized colour-receptive cells. This cortical organization enables the matrix of cells in the retina to function as a very precise transducer of visual information in terms of position, shape, size, colour and movement.

The *visual fields* can be assessed by several methods of varying sophistication, of which the simplest consists of comparing the extent of the patient's visual field with your own; testing the field by *confrontation*. Both eyes should be tested together first (binocular vision), and then each must be tested separately (monocular testing) to exclude a field defect limited to part of the visual field of one eye only.

Confrontation tests Seat yourself opposite the patient, at a distance of about a metre from him. If his *right* eye is to be tested, ask him to cover his left eye with his hand and look steadily at your left eye. Cover your right eye with your right hand and gaze steadily at the patient's right eye. In this way slight movements of the patient's eye, which would introduce error into the test, can be easily detected. Hold up your left hand in a plane midway between the patient's face and your own, at first at almost a full arm's length to the side. Keep moving the fingers of the hand and bring it nearer until you yourself can just perceive the movements of the fingers 'with the tail of your eye'. Ask the patient whether he sees the movements, telling him meanwhile to be sure not to take his own eye off yours. If he fails to see the fingers, keep bringing the hand nearer until he does see them. Test the field in this fashion in every direction—upwards, downwards, to right and to left—using the extent of your own field for the purpose of comparison.

Red pin test This outlines the central field. Since this field may be relatively intact when the fields for other forms of stimulation are seriously constricted, the field for small white objects must also be tested when disease of the visual pathways is suspected. This test can conveniently be done using a pin-head held up in the patient's field in the manner described above. Central areas of impaired vision (*central scotoma*) can be also recognized by this method either because the red or white pin-head cannot be perceived in the scotoma or, in less severe examples, because the intensity of the red colour is reduced in this part of the field.

This method allows the patient's field, including the size of his physiological blind spot (see below), to be compared precisely with the examiner's field. A good rough test in preliminary assessment is to ask the patient to compare the contour and colour of the palm of the examiner's hand held up in the right, left and central fields of each eye separately.

The physiological blind spot is situated to the temporal side of the central point of fixation of the visual field. It corresponds to the point of entry of the optic nerve into the retina; this is the *optic disc*, found slightly to the nasal side of the macula when visualized with the ophthalmoscope. At the optic disc there are no retinal receptor cells and there is thus a small blind spot in the field corresponding to this region. It should always be possible to identify this blind spot when testing the visual field to confrontation with a red pin, and its size should correspond with the examiner's own blind spot when the red pin is held equidistant between the examiner's eye and the patient's eye. The blind spot sometimes appears to be absent in an unco-operative patient, or if the patient is attempting to mislead the examiner. Little reliance can be placed on the visual fields in such patients.

Perimetry The visual field may be mapped using a perimeter. Several types of perimeter are available but all utilize the same principles. The patient is seated comfortably with his chin resting on a chin rest adjusted so that the eye to be tested is oriented at the centre of a hemispherical, illuminated field, upon which spots of light of various intensities, colours or sizes may be projected, or moved, in order to detect the limits of the field and its sensitivity in various parts. In some perimeters, e.g. the Goldmann perimeter, the examiner can observe the patient's eye through a small telescopic eyepiece in the centre of the hemisphere, in order to detect any movement of the patient's eye away from fixation on the central point of the hemispheric field. Simpler, portable versions of the perimeter do not allow this. These consist only of a hemispheric arm along which stimuli may be moved by a simple mechanical system. Stationary, rather than moving, targets can be used for perimetry in the central fields, using special perimeters with targets of variable luminance.

Perimetry surveys the monocular field of vision, from which the limits of perception can be charted (Fig. 10.9). The centre point of the chart corresponds to the point of fixation. Around this point are arranged a series of more or less concentric lines, each of which denotes equal visual acuity: an *isopter*.

The fixation point is not exactly central so that the outer and inner parts of the field are unequally divided. Further, the boundary is delimited inwards and upwards by the nose and brow. With a 5 mm object the extent of the average field of vision is 100° outwards, 60° upwards and inwards and 75° downwards. The field charted with a 20 mm object is shown in Fig. 10.9; note the restriction of the lower nasal field by the bridge of the nose.

The binocular field extends 200° or more laterally and about 140° vertically, in the middle of which is a circular portion common to each eye with a diameter of about 120°. On each side of this paired area is a lateral semilunar area which is unpaired (monocular) and which accounts for the remainder of the field. This is called the temporal crescent. Since the visual acuity is much lower at the periphery than at the point of fixation, it is possible, by using a graduated series of objects, to plot out a series of isopters each of which corresponds to the field for a known size of object, used at a known distance from the eye and at a constant illumination.

The area within 30° from fixation is best examined either with a sophisticated perimeter, e.g. a Goldmann perimeter, having first corrected any refractive errors with lenses, or by presenting objects against a 2 m^2 wall-mounted black screen—*Bjerrum's screen*—at a distance from the patient of one, or two, metres.

The patient is seated comfortably at this distance, preferably with the head steadied by a chin and head rest, and a white object 1 cm in diameter is fixed to the screen on a level with the patient's eye. The blind spot is mapped first using a white object 10 mm in diameter. The peripheral field is then mapped with the same 10 mm object: at a distance of 2 m the field should be circular and extend to about 25°, that is, to the edge of the 2 m^2 screen. With a smaller white or red object areas of blindness or defective perception should be sought around the blind spot, especially between this area and the macula (the *centrocaecal* area), and in the horizontal meridian on the nasal side of the fixation spot. The findings are marked upon the screen with black pins, and subsequently transferred to a chart for recording in the patient's case notes.

Changes in the field of vision A zone of loss of vision confined to the centre of the field is called a *central scotoma*. A unilateral central scotoma is commonly

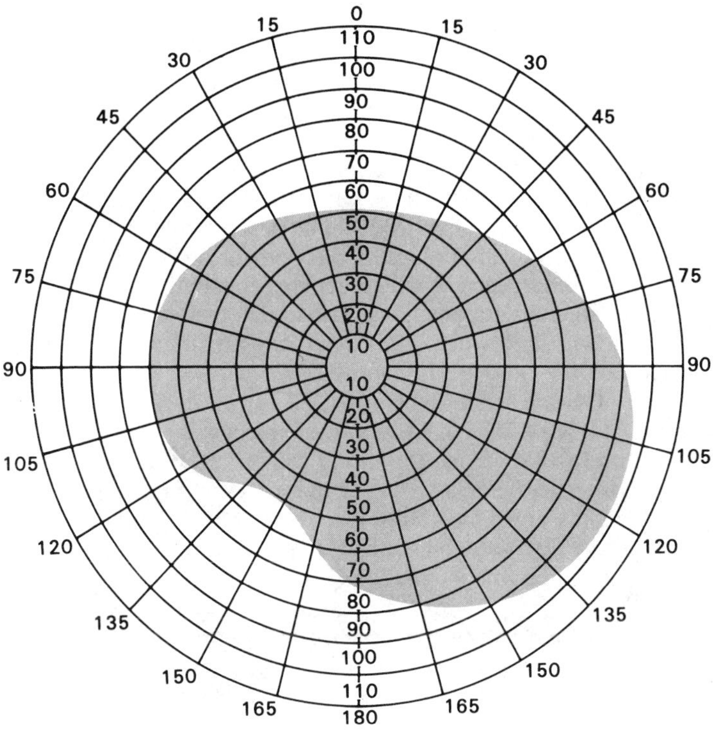

Fig. 10.9 The extent of the right field of vision with a white target of 20 mm diameter mapped on a perimeter at a distance of 330 mm.

due to demyelination in the optic nerve (retrobulbar neuritis), which in most cases in Britain is a symptom of multiple sclerosis. Sometimes it occurs from local disease of the choroid or of the retina in the neighbourhood of the macula, especially with vascular disease. In that case it often affects only one eye. Less commonly, it may be due to toxic causes, especially alcoholism, or to vitamin B_{12} deficiency, when it is generally bilateral. Pressure on the optic nerve is another cause. It may also result from a lesion of the posterior part of the visual cortex and is then bilateral, but this is very rare.

Hemianopia means loss of sight in one-half of the visual field. When the same half of both fields of vision is lost, the hemianopia is described as *homonymous*, e.g. right homonymous hemianopia when the right half of the field of each eye is affected (see Fig. 10.7). Blindness limited to one quadrant of a field is termed a *quadrantanopia*.

Superior and *inferior altitudinal hemianopia* means loss of the upper and lower halves of the visual field respectively. This may occur with damage to an

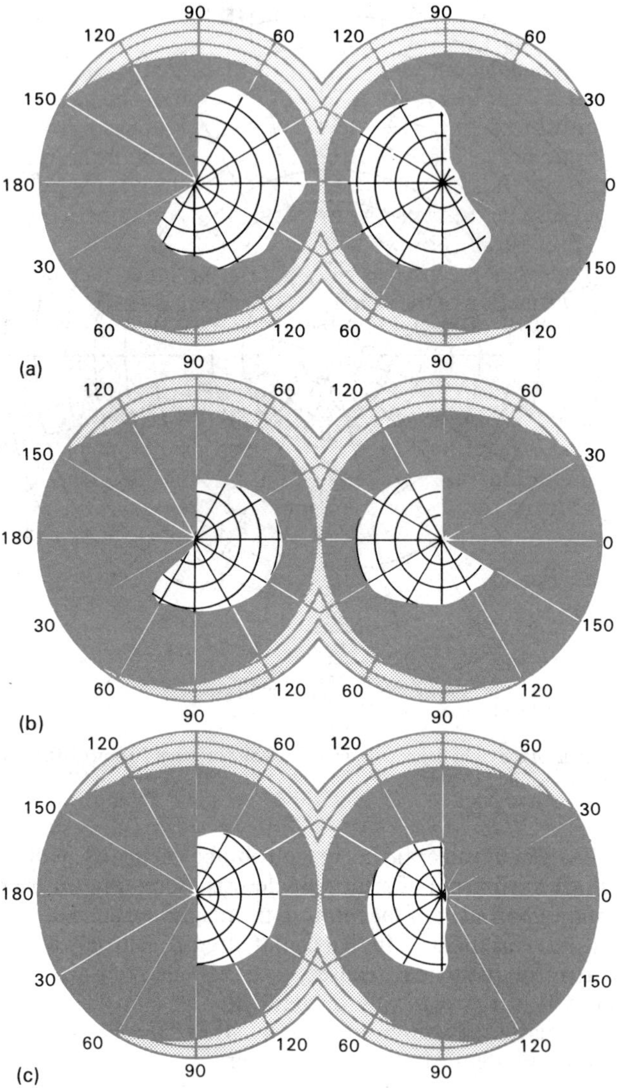

Fig. 10.10 Fields of vision in a case of pituitary tumour (chromophobe adenoma) showing the development of bitemporal hemianopia. (*a*) May: VA (visual acuity) Lt 6/12 Rt 6/18. (*b*) August: VA Lt 6/12 Rt 6/12. (*c*) October: VA Lt 6/12 Rt 6/12. The fields were plotted on a Bjerrum's screen at a distance of 2 m from the eye to the point of fixation at the centre of the screen, using a 10 mm white object. The coloured areas show the average normal field of vision and the white areas the patient's fields.

optic nerve by ischaemia or trauma. Bilateral altitudinal field defects are rare; they are usually due to occipital lesions.

Bitemporal hemianopia means loss of vision in the temporal (outer) halves of both fields, and is due, therefore, to loss of function of the nasal half of each retina. It can only be produced by a lesion of the optic chiasm, involving those fibres of the optic nerves, derived from the nasal parts of the retina, which decussate at this site. It is usually due to a tumour of the pituitary gland or sella turcica but may also be produced by inflammatory or traumatic lesions of the optic chiasm (Fig. 10.10).

Binasal hemianopia means loss of the nasal or inner half of each field, indicating loss of function of the temporal half of each retina. It is very rare but can result from bilateral lesions confined to the uncrossed optic fibres on each side of the optic chiasm, and it may also occur in open-angle glaucoma.

Concentric constriction of the visual fields sometimes occurs in long-standing papilloedema, in bilateral lesions of the striate (visual) cortex and in some retinal disorders, e.g. retinitis pigmentosa. It is also found in hysteria.

Bitemporal and binasal hemianopia are sometimes described as *heteronymous*, in contradistinction to the homonymous variety.

Colour vision For methods of testing, see p. 392.

Subjective visual sensations

Among the commonest subjective visual sensations are *muscae volitantes*—little grey specks seen floating before the eyes, especially on looking at a white surface or up to the sky. They are a normal phenomenon due to awareness of parts of the retinal blood vessels seen reflected from the posterior surface of the lens, or to vitreous opacities. In migraine, peculiar zigzag lines, known as 'fortification figures' or *teichopsiae*, are often seen at the beginning of the attack. *Visual hallucinations* occur in a number of neurological diseases, notably in delirium tremens and in temporal and occipito-parietal lobe disorders; they may also form part of the aura in epilepsy. *Photopsias*, tiny white flashes seen in the visual field, often particularly during ocular movement, may occur in acute retrobulbar neuritis.

Visual agnosia and cortical blindness

Complex disturbances of visual perception and of visually directed behaviour result from lesions in the parietal connections of the occipital cortex. In these visual agnosias the patient is unaware or uncomprehending of the visual deficit, but in cortical blindness, in which the lesions are in the striate cortex of both hemispheres, the patient is aware of his visual disorder. The pupillary light reflexes are normal in both these disorders.

The oculomotor (3rd), trochlear (4th) and abducent (6th) nerves

These three nerves and their central connections are usually considered together since they function as a physiological unit in the control of ocular movement.

Anatomy

The fibres of these nerves arise from a series of nuclei which begin in the floor of the sylvian aqueduct below the superior corpora quadrigemina, and extend as far caudally as the eminentia teres in the floor of the 4th ventricle. The nucleus of the oculomotor nerve is farthest forward; its most rostral nerve cells supply parasympathetic innervation to the ciliary muscle and iris (Edinger–Westphal nucleus), those for the extra-ocular muscles being located in the more caudal part of the nucleus. Caudal to this is the nucleus of the trochlear nerve. The abducent nerve nucleus is situated in the floor of the 4th ventricle at the level of the pons.

The trochlear nerve emerges on the inner aspect of the cerebral peduncles, between the superior cerebellar and posterior cerebral arteries, and passes forward in close relation to the posterior communicating artery before entering the lateral wall of the cavernous sinus. It is thus at risk in certain patients with brain herniation associated with cerebral mass lesions, and in aneurysms of the nearby arteries discussed above.

The trochlear nerves emerge on the rostral part of the roof of the 4th ventricle. They are unique in that they are the only cranial nerves which decussate between their nuclei and their point of emergence from the brain stem and that they emerge dorsally.

The abducent nerve emerges between the medulla and pons. Its long intracranial course renders it particularly vulnerable to the effects of pressure.

Functions

The abducent nerve innervates the external rectus muscle and the trochlear innervates the superior oblique muscle. All the other extra-ocular muscles, the sphincter pupillae, the muscle of accommodation, and the levator palpebrae superioris, are suppled by the oculomotor nerve.

Ocular movements

Horizontal movement outwards is termed *abduction*; inwards, *adduction*; vertical movement upwards, *elevation*; and downwards, *depression*. The eye is also capable of diagonal movements at any intermediate angle. Rotatory movements, the eye rolling like a wheel towards the nose (internal rotation) or away from the nose (external rotation), are not possible voluntarily, but occur

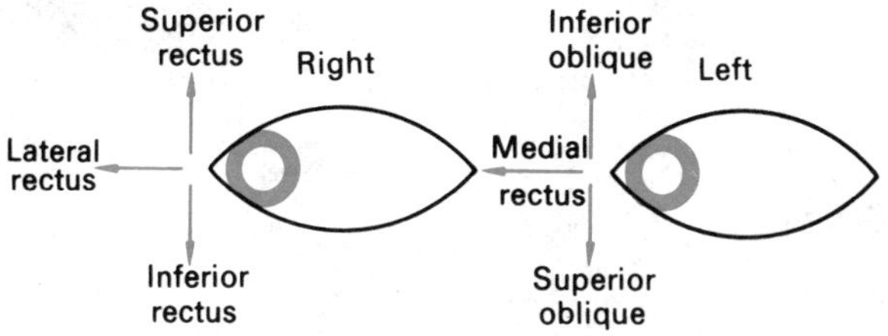

Fig. 10.11 The action of the external ocular muscles with the patient confronting the examiner.

normally as part of the reflex compensation necessary to adjust for slight degrees of head tilt during tasks involving macular fixation, e.g. when reading. Note that the *recti act as elevators and depressors alone when the eye is in abduction, and the obliques act similarly when the eye is in adduction* (Fig. 10.11). Their function may therefore be assessed by testing the movements of elevation and of depression in both full abduction and full adduction. This method of testing gaze movements is much more informative than simply testing elevation and depression in the mid-position of gaze. Lateral gaze must always be tested separately. Vertical and horizontal ocular movements made from the mid-position of gaze are called *cardinal movements*. The medial and lateral recti always act directly in a single plane, but all movements require the coordinated activity of the whole group of extra-ocular muscles. The eyes normally move 50° laterally, 50° medially, 33° upwards and 50° downwards.

Normally the movements of the two eyes are symmetrical, so that the visual axes meet at the point at which the eyes are directed. This is referred to as *conjugate* movement of the eyes; it is a result of the brain stem integrating the function of the oculomotor, trochlear and abducent nerves. Thus *infranuclear* (lower motor neurone) lesions of the oculomotor, trochlear and abducent nerves lead to paralysis of individual eye muscles or groups of muscles. *Supranuclear* (upper motor neurone) lesions lead to paralysis of conjugate movements of the eyes.

Lower motor neurone (infranuclear) lesions

Infranuclear lesions of these three nerves lead to the following abnormalities:

Abducent nerve Inability to move the eye outwards and diplopia on looking in that direction. Sometimes convergent squint because of the unopposed action of the medial rectus, innervated by the ipsilateral oculomotor nerve.

Trochlear nerve Impaired downward movement; on attempting to look downwards in the mid-position of gaze the eyeball is rotated inwards by the unopposed action of the inferior rectus (Fig. 10.11). Diplopia only below the

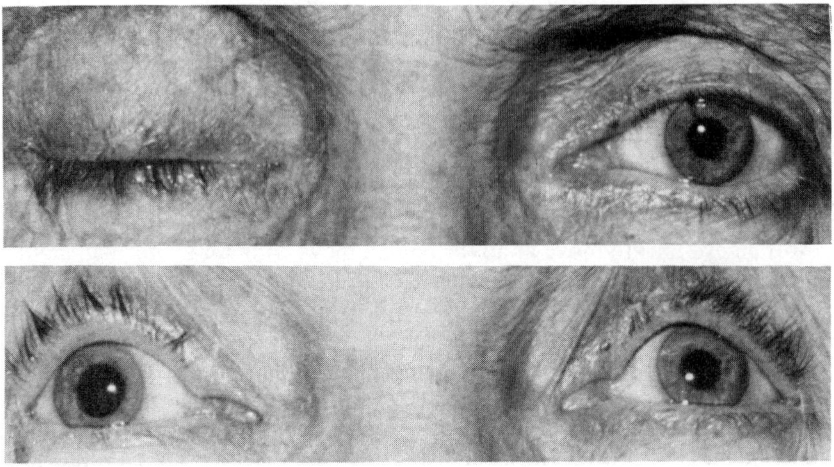

Fig. 10.12 Right third nerve palsy. Note the right ptosis, the dilated pupil, and the external strabismus.

horizontal plane, with the images uncrossed, but the false one tilted. There is rarely a visible squint.

Oculomotor nerve Ptosis: the eye is displaced downwards and outwards and further movement is only possible outwards and a little downwards. Pupil usually dilated and fixed; loss of accommodation. These are the features of a complete oculomotor nerve palsy (Fig. 10.12). However, paralysis of the oculomotor nerve is often partial, only one or a few of these functions being lost.

It must be remembered that smooth muscle in the upper lid is innervated by the cervical sympathetic and exerts a tonic elevating action. Slight ptosis therefore occurs after a lesion of the cervical sympathetic but the pupil is then small, rather than large (Horner's syndrome; see Fig. 13.3, p. 404).

Thus the signs of a lesion involving one or more of these three nerves may be: (*a*) defective movement of the eye; (*b*) the presence of a squint; (*c*) the presence of diplopia; and (*d*) pupillary abnormalities. Of these signs diplopia and pupillary abnormalities are the most reliable.

Strabismus

By *squint* or *strabismus* is meant an abnormality of ocular movement such that the visual axes do not meet at the point of fixation. There are two varieties: *paralytic* and *non-paralytic* (*concomitant*).

Paralytic strabismus Paralytic strabismus is due to weakness of one or more of the extra-ocular muscles.

Limitation of movement Since paralytic strabismus is due to weakness of one or more extra-ocular muscles, a prominent feature is impairment of ocular movement in the direction of action of the muscle(s) affected. Although this weakness is usually obvious it is sometimes so slight, or the unaffected muscles mask it so much, that the defective movement of the eye is hardly apparent.

If an eye fails to move at all, or fails to move through its normal angular excursion, the deviation of this eye in a direction opposite to the physiological action of the muscle is called the *primary deviation* or *squint*. It is measured by the angle which a line from the object to the nodal point of the eye makes with the visual axis. If the unaffected eye is covered, so that the patient fixates with the affected eye (cover test; p. 301), the covered normal eye will deviate still more than the primary deviation of the affected eye. This deviation of the healthy eye is called *secondary deviation*. The difference between the primary and secondary deviation in paralytic strabismus is the most important feature differentiating it from concomitant strabismus.

False orientation of the field of vision consists of erroneous judgement by the patient of the position of an object in that portion of the field of vision toward which the paralysed muscle should normally move the eye. Consider as an example a patient who has paralysis of the right lateral rectus muscle. If the patient closes the left eye and is asked to touch an object held in the horizontal plane on his right side, he will point wide of the object on his right hand side. This results from an error in the information reaching the brain from the retina due to the weakness of action of the affected lateral rectus muscle.

Dizziness is occasionally a symptom of paralytic strabismus when both eyes are opened. It is due partly to the confusion of double vision and partly to false orientation.

Double vision (diplopia) Patients with paralytic strabismus complain of double vision. This occurs because defective movement of one eye results in the images found by the two eyes falling upon non-identical points of the two retinae. Binocular fusion cannot therefore occur in the visual cortex and two separate or overlapping images are perceived. Further, in paralytic strabismus, the image falling upon the macula of the healthy eye is seen distinctly and is called the *true image*, whereas in the affected eye this image falls upon the retina outside the macula; since this image is indistinct and blurred, it is called the *false image*. Most patients can therefore clearly recognize which of the two images they perceive is the true image and which the false. The false image is projected into that part of the field of vision into which the paralysed muscle should move the eye if it were normal; it is perceived *in the direction of action of the weak muscle*. Doubt as to which is the false image can usually be resolved by covering one eye with a red glass and asking the patient whether the red or the normally coloured image is the real one.

In order to overcome diplopia the patient turns his head in the direction of action of the paralysed muscle. This *head tilt* gives information as to which muscle is involved.

The investigation of paralytic strabismus and the diagnostic value of diplopia First make certain that the diplopia is *binocular*, since certain conditions, for example lens opacities and astigmatism, may produce monocular diplopia. Diplopia should always be assessed in the nine cardinal directions of gaze (Fig. 10.11 and Table 10.3). This greatly simplifies its analysis and interpretation. The objective of this analysis is to decide to which eye the *furthest displaced of the two images belongs*. In testing, the test object is thus moved in the cardinal directions until the position of maximal displacement of the two images is ascertained.

Method of finding the direction of maximal diplopia The patient is seated with the head fixed in a head rest, with a red glass over the right eye and a green glass over the left. At a distance of about 5 m the observer moves a light in the directions indicated in Table 10.3. Each of the lateral squares corresponds to a pair of associated muscles: Thus a maximal vertical diplopia produced when the patient looks up and to the right, into the right superior square, shows that either the right superior rectus or the left inferior oblique muscle is the one affected. It is necessary only to find to which eye the false image belongs to decide which muscle is paralysed. The higher of the two images indicates the affected eye.

Table 10.3 Charting the diplopia in the nine cardinal directions of gaze in paralytic diplopia (see also Fig. 10.11).

	The patient looks	
Upwards to the left left SR right IO	*Upwards* left and right SR left and right IO	*Upwards to the right* right SR left IO
To the left left LR right MR	*Straight ahead* general contraction of all extra-ocular muscles	*To the right* right LR left MR
Downwards to the left right SO left IR	*Downwards* left and right IR left and right SO	*Downwards to the right* left SO right IR

Key SR: superior rectus; LR: lateral rectus; SO: superior oblique; IR: inferior rectus; MR: medial rectus; IO: inferior oblique.

Non-paralytic strabismus In paralytic strabismus the angular deviation of the two visual axes varies with different positions of the two eyes, and the secondary deviation is always greater than the primary deviation. In non-paralytic (concomitant) strabismus, as its name implies, the angular deviation of the visual axes is the same in whatever position the eyes may be; in other words, the primary and secondary deviations are always equal.

The *cover test* is performed as follows in order to assess the primary and secondary deviations. Ask the patient to look at an object immediately in front of him. Suddenly cover the apparently fixing eye. If the uncovered eye makes any movement in taking up fixation, it must have previously been deviating, indicating that a squint is present. If now the eye behind the cover (which was previously fixing) is observed, it will be seen to deviate in the same relative direction as was the other eye, and *to the same angular amount*, that is, the primary and secondary deviation are equal.

The *clinical features* of non-paralytic strabismus are characteristic:

1 It begins in early childhood, usually before the fifth year and almost always before 3 years of age.
2 The movements of the eyes, tested individually, are good in all directions.
3 Diplopia is practically never a symptom.
4 The primary and secondary deviations are equal.
5 The deviating eye usually has defective vision (amblyopia ex anopsia).

A squint may be *intermittent* or *constant* and, if constant, *monocular* when only one eye deviates whilst the other usually fixes, or *alternating* when either eye fixes independently.

Upper motor neurone (supranuclear) lesions

In addition to the defects of movement due to paralysis of the individual ocular muscles, impairment or paralysis of the movement of *both* eyes in one direction sometimes occurs (*conjugate gaze palsy*). Thus the patient may be unable to look to either side, or upwards or downwards; or convergence alone may be lost. Weakness of *lateral conjugate movement* may occur in hemiplegia due to cerebral lesions, especially in the acute stage. However, paralysis of lateral conjugate gaze is more characteristically found with lesions in the pons. The lesion is in the pontine paramedian reticular formation (PPRF) near the abducent and vestibular nuclei. Bilateral paralysis of lateral conjugate gaze may occur in centrally placed pontine lesions above the level of the abducent nuclei. Palsies of *conjugate upward gaze* are always associated with disease of the central parts of the mid-brain or inferior thalamic region, or in the neighbourhood of the oculomotor nuclei. Impaired downward gaze is very rare, but occurs with brain stem lesions at a lower level.

Tonic or maintained conjugate deviation of the eyes is an abnormality in which both eyes are kept persistently turned in one direction. It is usually either to the right or to the left. It may be due either to a lesion which produces paralysis or to one which causes irritation. In the former, the eyes (and usually also the head) are turned towards the side of the lesion if the lesion is in the cerebral hemisphere, i.e. the patient 'looks towards his lesion'. An irritative lesion in a similar situation causes deviation towards the healthy side, usually accompanied by nystagmoid jerks of the eye toward this side. This is a form of *focal epilepsy*. If, however, the lesion is in the pons, these rules are reversed, the deviation being towards the sound side in a paralytic lesion and towards the affected side in one which is irritative. Irritative lesions in the brain stem, it should be remembered, are very rare.

Assessment of *saccadic* (rapid, programmed, conjugate fixation movements) and *pursuit* (following) gaze movements can be performed separately by asking the patient to move his eyes rapidly from fixation on one finger to another held about 30° away in the horizontal plane, and by asking him to follow a slowly moving finger across visual space in the same, or in the vertical, plane. However, localization of abnormalities of these two systems of ocular movement is not yet well understood. In Huntington's chorea, pursuit movements are slowed or interrupted by slowed saccades, and a similar disturbance may occur in Parkinson's disease. In higher-level disturbances of visual perception, e.g. parieto-occipital lesions causing agnosia or misperceptions of visual space to one side, saccadic movements may be impaired toward the midline in the affected field.

Skew deviation of the eyes—in which one eye is directed upwards and the other downwards—occurs in lesions of the labyrinth and in cerebellar disease. Other abnormal ocular movements, such as *ocular bobbing*, *opsoclonus* and *ocular dysmetria*, also associated with acute cerebellar lesions, are rare.

Internuclear ophthalmoplegia is due to a lesion in one medial longitudinal fasciculus in the mid-brain or upper pons. On attempted lateral gaze there is pronounced rhythmic nystagmus of the abducting eye and impaired medial deviation of the adducting eye. The latter may cause diplopia. In addition the adducting eye moves more slowly than the contralateral abducting eye, especially during attempted saccadic movements. All other gaze movements, and the pupils, are normal. The lesion is on the side of the impaired adduction, not on the side of the nystagmus (Fig. 10.13). This sign is important because it is common in multiple sclerosis.

In the 'one and a half syndrome' a lesion in the parapontine region involves both the PPRF and the MLF (Fig 10.13) on the same side. There is failure of lateral conjugate gaze to the same side, together with impairment of adduction of the eye on that side and nystagmus in abduction of the opposite eye. Thus this is the only horizontal movement possible; one eye will not move at all horizontally and the other only in abduction—1½ movements are paralysed. The pupils and vertical movements are normal.

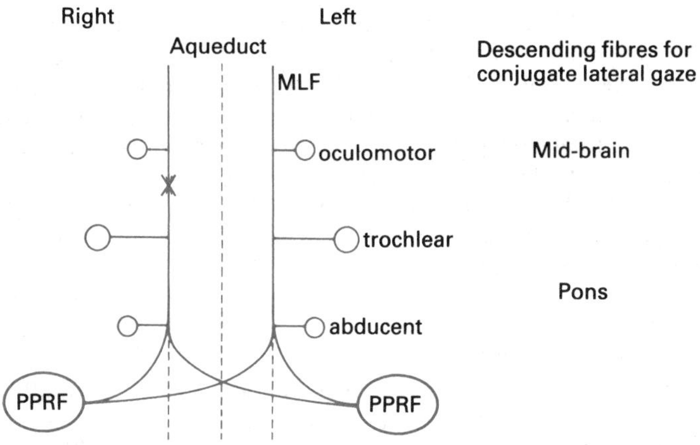

Fig. 10.13 Diagrammatic representation of interconnection of oculomotor, trochlear and abducent nerve nuclei with the parapontine reticular formation (PPFR) via the medial longitudinal fasciculus (MLF). A lesion (X) in the right MLF will cause impaired adduction of the right eye with nystagmus of the abducting left eye during attempted lateral gaze to the left. A lesion in or near the PPRF causes impaired conjugate lateral gaze to the same side.

Nystagmus

The term nystagmus is applied to a disturbance of ocular movement characterized by involuntary, conjugate, often rhythmical oscillations of the eyes. These movements may be horizontal, vertical or rotary. In any given direction of gaze the speed of the movement is usually quicker in one direction than the other; the *quicker movement* indicates the direction of the nystagmus. To examine for nystagmus, ask the patient to look straight in front of him and observe whether the eyes remain steady. Then ask him to look to his extreme right, then to the left, and then upwards and downwards. It is best to ask the patient to look at your finger in these positions. Observe the rate, amplitude and rhythm of any nystagmus in each direction and whether or not the nystagmus is sustained. Nystagmus can be conveniently graded; for example:

Grade 1 Nystagmus with fast phase to left, looking toward the left.
Grade 2 Nystagmus with fast phase to left, looking straight ahead.
Grade 3 Nystagmus with fast phase to left, looking toward the right.

Nystagmus is most commonly due to disorders of the vestibular system (either centrally or peripherally), to lesions affecting the central pathways concerned in ocular movements, e.g. the vestibulo-cerebellar connections in brain stem or cerebellum or the medial longitudinal fasciculus, or to weakness of the ocular muscles. Nystagmus is often induced by drugs, especially benzodiazepines, phenytoin and other anticonvulsant drugs, and barbiturates. Nystagmus of visual origin is pendular and often rotary on central fixation of the eyes. Congenital nystagmus also shows this pendular quality. Some forms of nystagmus, particularly that associated with benign epidemic vertigo, and with posterior fossa neoplasms, may be induced only by certain movements of the head (positional nystagmus); this nystagmus is of brief duration and can often be elicited only once.

A few irregular jerks of the eyes are often seen in full lateral deviation in normal subjects. The brief duration and irregularity of these movements distinguish them from true nystagmus.

Optokinetic nystagmus occurs when the patient follows a rapidly moving scene. The eyes fixate and follow the moving stimulus and then refixate by making a rapid saccade back to the primary position of gaze. There is thus a slow component in the direction of the moving stimulus and a fast phase in the opposite direction. This phenomenon may be used as a crude test of visual acuity by utilizing a striped drum or tape, but the test is used mainly to assess patients with hemianopia or brain stem lesions. In parietal hemianopia there may be neglect of the visual environment on the hemianopic side, even with a very mild degree of visual impairment (p. 295), and this is accompanied by suppression of the fast phase of optokinetic nystagmus when the stimulus is moved from this abnormal visual field toward the normal field. The fast phase is replaced by a slow tonic deviation of the eyes in the direction of movement of the stimulus. In brain stem lesions optokinetic testing is useful in establishing the presence of conjugate gaze palsies, internuclear ophthalmoplegia and abnormalities of the velocity of saccadic eye movements.

Examination of the pupils

The following points must be noted about the pupils in every patient:

Size Compare the size of the two pupils, first in a bright light and then in a dim light. Note whether the pupils are large or small and whether any irregularity is present. The size of the pupil in healthy subjects is very variable. As a rule, the pupils are larger in dark eyes than in light and they tend to be small in elderly subjects. Slight inequality of the pupils may be present in perfectly healthy subjects.

If one pupil is larger than the other, one must decide which is the normal. This is not always very easily answered, but the pupil which is less mobile is usually the abnormal one.

Shape Note whether the pupil is circular in outline, as it should be, or whether its contour is irregular. Such irregularities are due to adhesion of the iris to the lens, as a result of an old iritis.

Mobility: *Reaction to light* The pupillary reaction to light is a reflex. The afferent fibres involved travel in the optic nerve, leaving it before the lateral geniculate bodies to enter the brain stem in the pretectal region. These fibres synapse in the oculomotor nuclei, the efferent fibres reaching the pupillary sphincters in the oculomotor nerve and then through a synapse in the ciliary ganglia in the orbit.

Examine each eye separately with the patient in a shady, indirectly illuminated place. Ask him to look into the distance, e.g. across the room, to be sure his accommodation is relaxed. Shine a bright light into the eye to be tested. The pupil should contract almost immediately, then dilate again a little, and after undergoing a few slight oscillations, settle down to a smaller size. When the light is switched off the pupil will rapidly dilate to its previous diameter.

Swinging light test for afferent (optic nerve) pupillary abnormality Owing to the decussation of some of the fibres in the optic nerves at the optic chiasm, light shone into one eye stimulates the brain stem nuclei (oculomotor nerve) concerned with pupillary constriction bilaterally. As a consequence, if bright light is shone into one eye only, both pupils contract; and if light is shut off from one eye, both pupils dilate slightly. The former is the *consensual reaction* of the pupils. It should be tested by keeping one eye in the shade while shining a bright light into the other. The effect on the pupil of the unilluminated eye is then observed. The pupillary constriction may be brisk and well sustained in one eye, but when the light is shone immediately into the other eye, this pupil may slowly dilate a little, indicating that its consensually-mediated light reaction is more active than its direct reaction. On this second side there must therefore be an afferent defect (Gunn's pupil), i.e. a lesion in the optic nerve. This is a particularly useful sign in retrobulbar neuritis and in ischaemic or compressive lesions of the optic nerve.

In some patients with post-chiasmal, but pregeniculate hemianopia, the pupillary light reaction is less active when a narrow beam of light is shone from the hemianopic side than when shone from the normal side. However, this hemianopic pupillary reaction sign is difficult to elicit.

Reaction to accommodation The pupils become smaller on accommodating for a near object (*miosis*). Convergence of the eyes, accommodation and miosis are closely related reflexes.

Hold up one finger close to the patient's nose. Ask him to look away at a distant object. Then ask him to look quickly at your finger. As the eyes converge to accomplish this the pupils become smaller. If the patient is blind, the test may still be carried out by getting him to hold up his own finger about a foot in front of his face, and then asking him to 'look at the finger'. Accommodation is only rarely lost in brain stem lesions, but may be impaired with lesions of the oculomotor nerve and in certain neuropathies in which there is autonomic involvement.

The *Argyll Robertson pupil* is the classical pupillary abnormality in neurosyphilis. The pupil is small and irregular, reacts briskly to accommodation, but does not react to light directly or consensually. The pupil dilates slowly or imperfectly to atropine. The abnormality is typically bilateral but it is frequently more obvious on one side. The lesion is in the pretectal region of the mesencephalon.

Hippus is a rhythmic dilatation and constriction of the pupil, either in response to light or occurring spontaneously. It is rarely of clinical significance, although it may be unusually prominent in retrobulbar neuritis.

The *Adie pupil* is an abnormality characterized by absent or delayed pupillary constriction to light or to accommodation/convergence. Once constricted the pupil dilates only very slowly, either in response to darkness or to far gaze. The pupil may thus appear small or large and this sometimes leads to confusion with the Argyll Robertson syndrome. The pupil in Adie's syndrome varies in size from day to day but *never* reacts promptly to light. The abnormality is frequently unilateral so that it may cause unequal pupils (*anisocoria*). It is sometimes associated with absent tendon reflexes, often on the same side as the pupillary abnormality (Holmes–Adie syndrome). The distinction between the Argyll Robertson and Adie pupillary abnormalities is important since the latter, probably due to partial parasympathetic denervation, is usually of no clinical significance. The distinction may be made by instillation of sterile 2% methacholine into the conjunctival sac: the Adie pupil constricts but the Argyll Robertson pupil does not.

Horner's syndrome is due to paralysis of the cervical sympathetic. The sympathetic nerve fibres supplying the pupil originate in the lower cervical and upper thoracic regions of the spinal cord, from which they emerge in the first thoracic nerve roots and pass to the sympathetic ganglia by the rami communicantes. From the cervical sympathetic chain the sympathetic nerve fibres pass along the internal carotid to the cavernous plexus, and thence via the ophthalmic division of the trigeminal nerve to the eye. Sympathetic nervous activity causes pupillary dilatation and elevation of the upper lid; the latter through contraction of the smooth muscle fibres in the levator palpebrae superioris.

Horner's syndrome consists of: slight drooping of the upper lid (ptosis), pupillary constriction, absence of pupillary dilatation on shading the eye or on instillation of cocaine, abolition of the ciliospinal reflex, and, less commonly, absence of sweating on the corresponding half of the face and neck, both in front and behind, extending as low as the 3rd rib and 3rd thoracic spine, and over the whole of the upper limb on the same side. An apparent enophthalmos is often present, and is a useful clue to the diagnosis when the patient is first seen (see Fig. 13.3, p. 404).

Dilatation of the normal pupil when the skin of the neck is pinched (*ciliospinal reflex*) is due to reflex excitation of the pupil-dilating fibres in the cervical sympathetic; it is abolished by lesions of that nerve and by some medullary, cervical and upper thoracic cord lesions.

The trigeminal (5th) nerve

Anatomy

The *sensory root* takes origin from nerve cells in the trigeminal (gasserian) ganglion and enters the lateral surface of the pons at about its middle. The fibres which conduct impulses for light touch and postural sensibility terminate in a large nucleus in the pons, situated lateral to the motor nucleus near the floor of the 4th ventricle, while the fibres for pain and thermal sensibility enter the 'descending' or bulbospinal tract, which extends as low as the 2nd cervical segment of the cord before ascending in the medial lemniscus.

Immediately distal to the trigeminal ganglion the nerve separates into its three divisions (Fig. 10.14).

The *first* or *ophthalmic division* supplies the conjunctiva and the conjunctival surface of the upper but not of the lower lid, the lacrimal gland, the mesial

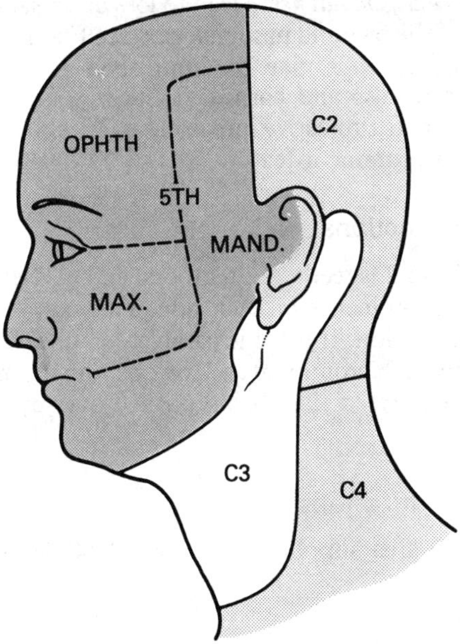

Fig. 10.14 Lateral view of the skin area supplied by the trigeminal (5th) nerve and the 2nd, 3rd and 4th cervical segments.

part of the skin of the nose as far as its tip, the upper eyelids, the forehead, and the scalp as far as the vertex. Lesions of the ophthalmic division result in loss of cutaneous and corneal sensibility in the areas described above. Trophic changes in the cornea, *neuropathic keratitis*, may occur. The corneal reflex is abolished; this must be tested with great care because of the risk of causing corneal ulceration.

The *second* or *maxillary division* supplies the cheek, the front of the temple, the lower eyelid and its conjunctival surface, the side of the nose, the upper lip, the upper teeth, the mucous membrane of the nose, the upper part of the pharynx, the roof of the mouth, part of the soft palate, the tonsils, and the medial inferior quadrant of the cornea. Lesions of the maxillary division lead to loss of sensation in the above areas and occasionally to loss of the palatal reflex.

The *third* or *mandibular division* supplies the lower part of the face, the lower lip, the ear, the tongue, and the lower teeth. It also supplies parasympathetic fibres to the salivary glands. The mandibular division is joined by the motor root and this innervates the muscles of mastication. The *motor root* originates from a small nucleus, medial to the main sensory nucleus, and partly also from nerve cells scattered around the cerebral aqueduct. It emerges at the side of the pons, just anterior to the sensory division, passes inferiorly to the trigeminal ganglion, and joins the mandibular division.

Lesions of the whole trigeminal nerve lead to loss of sensation in the skin and mucous membrane of the face and nasopharynx (see Fig. 10.14). The salivary, buccal and lacrimal secretions may be diminished and trophic ulcers may develop in the mouth, nose and cornea. Taste is spared, but lack of oral secretions may result in its subjective impairment. Weakness of the muscles of mastication is often a prominent feature.

Testing the motor functions

Ask the patient to clench his teeth: the temporal and masseter muscles should stand out with equal prominence on each side. This sign is better checked by palpation than by inspection. If there is paralysis on one side, the muscles on that side will fail to become prominent and, on opening the mouth, the jaw will deviate towards the paralysed side, being pushed over by the healthy lateral pterygoid muscles.

Testing the sensory functions

The sensibility of the area supplied (see Fig. 10.14) is tested in the usual way (p. 338).

Testing the corneal reflex

Twist a light wisp of cotton into a fine hair and lightly touch the lateral edge of the cornea at its conjunctival margin with the wisp, having asked the patient to gaze into the distance or at the ceiling. If the reflex is present the patient blinks. It is helpful to steady your hand by gently resting the little finger on the patient's cheek. The two sides should be compared. This can sometimes be done more easily by lightly blowing a puff of air into each cornea in turn. The cornea should *not* be wiped with the cotton and the central part of the cornea should never be touched, since to do so in the presence of corneal anaesthesia carries the risk of corneal ulceration and subsequent visual impairment.

The facial (7th) nerve

Anatomy

The course of the fibres from the cortex to the nucleus of this nerve has already been described (p. 265). The facial nucleus is situated in the pons lateral to that of the abducent nerve. On leaving the nucleus the fibres wind round the abducent nucleus and emerge medial to the vestibulocochlear nerve, between the olive and the restiform bodies.

The facial nerve then lies in close contact with the vestibulocochlear nerve and enters the internal auditory meatus with it, so that a lesion of one at this part often also affects the other. During its course through the temporal lobe, in close proximity to the aditus of the tympanic antrum, it gives off a branch to the stapedius muscle. It is joined by the chorda tympani, which contains taste fibres from the anterior two-thirds of the tongue, at the geniculate ganglion. In this part of its course the nerve is vulnerable to trauma and oedema, since it is enclosed in a bony tube. It emerges at a point opposite the junction of the anterior border of the mastoid process with the ear, and spreads out on the side of the face to supply the facial muscles.

The facial nerve is almost entirely a motor nerve. It supplies all the muscles of the face and scalp, except the levator palpebrae superioris. It also supplies the platysma. The chorda tympani travels with the facial nerve during part of its course and taste may therefore be lost on the anterior two-thirds of the tongue when the proximal part of the nerve is damaged. There is sometimes a small area of altered cutaneous sensation at the auricle in such cases, representing the somatic afferent component of the facial nerve.

Taste

The sense of taste should always be examined when a cranial nerve lesion is suspected. The nerve fibres subserving taste from the anterior two-thirds of the tongue pass from the lingual nerve into the chorda tympani and thence through the geniculate ganglion of the facial nerve and the nervus intermedius into the medulla oblongata. It has been suggested that these taste fibres sometimes enter the brain stem in the maxillary division of the trigeminal nerve, rather than through the chorda tympani and the facial nerve, but this is rare. The taste fibres from the posterior third of the tongue enter the brain stem in the glossopharyngeal nerve.

All the taste fibres enter the tractus solitarius and relay in the nucleus of this tract. The ascending fibres pass via the thalamus to the temporal part of the post-central gyrus and to the amygdala. *Ageusia* or loss of taste occurs with lesions of the peripheral pathways or with centrally placed pontine lesions, which may involve the gustatory lemnisci. Loss of taste may result from lesions in any part of the peripheral and central course of the taste fibres.

To test the sense of taste, use strong solutions of sugar and common salt, and weak solutions of citric acid and quinine, as tests of 'sweet', 'salt', 'sour', and 'bitter' respectively. These are applied by a wooden rod to the surface of the protruded tongue. The patient should be asked to indicate that he perceives the taste *before* he withdraws his tongue, in order to decide whether taste is disturbed anteriorly or posteriorly. After each test the mouth must be rinsed. The quinine test should be applied last, as its effect is more lasting than that of the others. Both the anterior and posterior parts of the tongue should be tested. Taste may also be assessed using a weak electrical stimulus.

In addition to loss of taste, one should always ask the patient whether he has any abnormal taste sensations or hallucinations of taste. These may form the aura of an epileptic fit, especially in temporal lobe epilepsy.

Motor effects of facial nerve lesions

These are usually obvious. The affected side of the face has lost its expression. The nasolabial fold is less pronounced, the furrows of the brow are smoothed out, the eye is *more* widely open than on the normal side, and when the patient smiles the mouth is drawn toward the normal side. The patient is unable to whistle and food is apt to collect between his teeth and his gums. Saliva, and any fluid he drinks, may escape from the affected angle of the mouth.

Testing the facial nerve

1 Ask the patient to shut his eyes as tightly as he can. Note that the affected eye is either not closed at all or, if the eye is closed, the eyelashes are not so deeply buried in the face as on the healthy side. Try also to open the eyes while the patient attempts to keep them closed. If the orbicularis oculi is acting normally, it should be almost impossible to open them against the patient's wish. The effect of screwing the eyes tightly shut causes the corners of the mouth to be drawn upwards. In paralysis of the lower part of the face, the corner on the affected side is either not drawn up at all, or not so much as on the healthy side.

Bell's phenomenon, in which the eyeball rolls upwards during attempted forced eye closure, is a normal phenomenon which is preserved in facial palsies of lower motor neurone type (p. 297). It is thus particularly obvious when eye closure is impossible in a patient with facial nerve palsy.

2 Ask the patient to whistle. He is unable to do so.

3 Ask him to smile or show his upper teeth. The mouth is then drawn to the healthy side.

4 Ask him to inflate his mouth with air and blow out his cheeks. Tap with the finger in turn on each inflated cheek. Air can be made to escape from the mouth more easily on the weak or paralysed side.

5 Test the sense of taste on the anterior part of the tongue.

Remember that *bilateral* facial weakness is difficult to recognize.

Signs of paralysis of the facial nerve in different parts of its course

Lesions situated above the facial nucleus, in the nucleus or distal to it result in different types of facial weakness. Lesions above the facial nucleus cause *upper motor neurone* or *supranuclear facial palsies*, lesions in the nucleus cause *nuclear facial palsy*, and lesions distal to the nucleus cause *lower motor neurone* or *infranuclear paralysis*.

In *supranuclear paralysis* the lower part of the face is chiefly affected. This is because the muscles of the upper part of the face are bilaterally innervated. A unilateral lesion, therefore, will cause only partial paralysis of the upper part of the face, including eye closure, on the one side, but movements of the mouth on that side will appear much more severely affected. Sometimes a supranuclear lesion affects only the fibres concerned in emotional movement and this function should be assessed separately from voluntary movement. Taste is not affected in supranuclear lesions.

In *infranuclear paralysis* both the upper and lower parts of the face are equally involved. Infranuclear facial paralysis may be produced by a lesion of the nucleus or of the facial nerve itself. A lesion inside the facial canal—unless it is towards the outer end—involves the fibres of the chorda tympani and therefore causes loss of taste sensation in the anterior two-thirds of the tongue. Because the stapedius muscle is paralysed, sounds on the side of the facial palsy may seem unusually loud (*hyperacusis*).

A lower motor neurone lesion, whether nuclear or infranuclear, causes atrophy of the facial muscles. Supranuclear lesions do not produce atrophy.

Abnormal facial movements

The muscles supplied by the facial nerve are frequently affected by spasmodic movements. These may involve all the facial muscles, or groups of them only. If present, the nature of the movements, their extent, the muscles affected by them, and any factors which modify them should be carefully noted. They are particularly characteristic of nuclear facial palsy, but occur most commonly as a result of aberrant regeneration of facial nerve fibres during partial recovery from an infranuclear (e.g. Bell's) palsy. Facial spasms of a different type occur in some patients with dystonia and in other extrapyramidal disorders, especially tardive dyskinesias following phenothiazine medication (p. 337).

The vestibulocochlear (8th) nerve

Anatomy

This nerve consists of two sets of fibres. One supplies the cochlea and subserves hearing; the other supplies the labyrinth and semicircular canals and subserves equilibration, balance and sensations of bodily displacement. The *auditory* fibres, which arise from the cochlear ganglion, enter the brain stem at the lower border of the pons and are distributed to the dorsal and ventral cochlear nuclei. The *vestibular* fibres originate in the vestibular ganglion, and terminate in a group of nuclei in the pons and medulla.

The secondary auditory tracts, after partial decussation, terminate in the inferior colliculi and the medial geniculate bodies, and another system, that takes origin from these, passes through the internal capsule to the cortical centre for hearing, in the first and second temporosphenoidal gyri. Sounds received in one ear reach the opposite hemisphere of the brain, but owing to the partial decussation of the secondary auditory tracts neither unilateral cerebral nor brain stem lesions produce unilateral deafness.

The vestibular nerve is closely connected with the cerebellum. It also has a cerebral projection to the temporal lobe.

Tests of hearing

See Chapter 12.

Abnormal auditory sensations

The patient may complain of 'ringing in the ears' (*tinnitus*). The precise character of the sound varies in different cases. It may be of a humming, buzzing, hammering or whistling character. This symptom, although common, is only rarely due to neurological disease.

Hyperacusis, a disorder in which even slight sounds are heard with painful intensity, sometimes occurs when there is paralysis of the stapedius muscle due to a facial nerve palsy. A similar phenomenon, *recruitment*, occurs in patients with sensorineural deafness due to damage to the cochlea, e.g. Ménière's syndrome (p. 374).

Auditory hallucinations and *delusions* of voices are common in the non-organic psychoses, e.g. schizophrenia, but may also occur in organic psychoses. Hallucinations of voices may also occur in normal people. Other auditory hallucinations, e.g. music, sometimes arise as epileptic auras when there is a lesion in the temporal lobe.

Vertigo

The patient will usually describe this as *giddiness* or *dizziness*. In vertigo, external objects seem to move round the patient. Ask if this is the case and, if so, in what direction the objects seem to move. Ask also whether the vertigo causes loss of balance. The distinction between vertigo and giddiness, although frequently discussed, is rarely of great importance. Both may occur in disease of the vestibular system, i.e. the ear, vestibulocochlear nerve, brain stem, or temporal lobe. The method of examination of this problem is described in Chapter 12.

Positional vertigo In some patients vertigo is induced by certain head postures, or by sudden changes in head posture. The subjective sensation of rotational disequilibrium is accompanied by a rotary nystagmus in the primary position, often enhanced by gaze to one or other side. If this posture is reproduced during examination, for example by suddenly laying the patient in the supine position, the nystagmus and vertigo will develop either after a short delay (*benign positional vertigo*, associated with labyrinthine disease) or immediately (an indication of brain stem disease). It usually continues for only a few seconds. Benign positional vertigo can often be reproduced only once or twice in an examination (p. 379).

The glossopharyngeal (9th), vagus (10th) and accessory (11th) nerves

Anatomy

The glossopharyngeal, vagus and accessory nerves arise, in order from above downwards, in an elongated nucleus in the floor of the 4th ventricle. They emerge by several roots along the lateral aspect of the medulla, beginning rostrally in the groove between the olive and restiform bodies. The spinal part of the accessory nerve emerges from the lateral column of the cord, perhaps beginning as low as the 6th cervical root. It passes up through the foramen magnum to join the medullary part, and emerges with it through the jugular foramen. After emerging, its two divisions separate, the medullary or accessory portion joining the vagus nerve and supplying motor fibres to the larynx and pharynx. The spinal portion supplies the sternomastoid and the upper part of the trapezius muscle.

The glossopharyngeal nerve

The glossopharyngeal nerve is sensory from the posterior third of the tongue and the mucous membrane of the pharynx. It innervates the middle pharyngeal sphincter and the stylopharyngeus muscle. It contains taste fibres from the posterior third of the tongue.

The glossopharyngeal nerve is rarely damaged alone, but damage can best be diagnosed by examining the nerve's sensory and reflex functions. Examine taste in the posterior part of the tongue. Loss of it may occur with a lesion of the trunk of the glossopharyngeal nerve.

Tickle the back of the pharynx, and note if reflex contraction occurs (*palatal reflex*). This is also a test of the vagus (below).

The vagus nerve

The vagus is motor for the soft palate (with the exception of the tensor palati), pharynx and larynx. It is sensory and motor for the respiratory passages, the heart and, through the parasympathetic ganglia, for most of the abdominal viscera. The fibres for the soft palate, pharynx and larynx take origin in the nucleus ambiguus, emerge in the upper roots of the accessory nerve, reach the pharyngeal plexus, and innervate the muscles of the palate, pharynx, and larynx. The visceromotor and the cardio-inhibitory fibres are derived from the dorsal nucleus of the vagus in the floor of the 4th ventricle. Damage to the vagus is obvious clinically only through its *palatine* and *laryngeal* branches.

The palate Ask the patient whether he notices regurgitation of fluids through his nose when he tries to swallow. This is a common symptom in total paralysis of the soft palate, owing to defective elevation during swallowing. For a similar reason the patient is unable to pronounce words which require complete closure of the nasopharynx. Thus 'egg' is sounded as 'eng', 'rub' becomes 'rum', and so on. In unilateral paralysis these symptoms are not observed. Difficulty in swallowing (*dysphagia*) particularly affects fluids in lower motor neurone lesions, but may be more marked for solids in upper motor neurone lesions.

For direct examination of the soft palate, place the patient facing the light with his mouth open and introduce a tongue depressor. The position of the uvula at rest is variable even in health. One must watch the movements of the palate during phonation. Ask the patient to say 'Ah!' and observe whether both sides of the palate arch upwards. If one side is paralysed, it will remain flat and immobile and the median raphe will be pulled towards the other side. In bilateral paralysis the whole palate remains motionless.

Remember that minor degrees of asymmetry of the palate and of the tongue occur as part of a hemiparesis due to an upper motor neurone lesion. This is not what is meant by palatal palsy since in the latter the lesion is invariably of lower motor neurone type.

The larynx The *superior laryngeal* branch of the vagus contains sensory nerve fibres from the larynx above the level of the true vocal cords, and motor fibres which innervate the cricothyroid muscle. Unilateral damage to the nerve does not produce any symptoms. Bilateral paralysis causes the vocal cords to be relaxed. The voice is therefore hoarse and deep and the utterance of high notes is impossible.

The *recurrent laryngeal* branch supplies sensation to the larynx below the level of the vocal cords and motor fibres to all the laryngeal muscles *except* the cricothyroid. Paralysis leads to appearances which can be recognized with the laryngoscope (see p. 387). *The speech is characteristically blurred and ineffectual* and the patient cannot cough clearly. Bilateral paralysis may cause serious stridor or even respiratory obstruction.

The accessory (11th) nerve

The accessory nerve is purely motor in function, contributing to the innervation of the larynx and pharynx as well as the sternomastoid and trapezius muscles. The spinal part of the nerve dips below the sternomastoid muscle about 2 cm below the tip of the mastoid process and re-emerges from underneath that muscle at about the middle of its posterior border.

Paralysis of the upper part of the trapezius is demonstrated by asking the patient to shrug his shoulders while the examiner presses downward on them. Paralysis of the sternomastoid causes weakness of rotation of the chin towards the opposite side.

The hypoglossal (12th) nerve

Anatomy

The hypoglossal nerve arises from a nucleus in the lower part of the floor of the 4th ventricle, close to the midline. It emerges between the anterior pyramid and the olive. It is a purely motor nerve, supplying the tongue and the depressors of the hyoid bone.

Test

Ask the patient to put out his tongue as far as possible. If the hypoglossal is paralysed, the tongue, instead of being protruded straight, is pushed over to the paralysed side. Be careful not to mistake an apparent deviation of the tongue, really due to the mouth being twisted to one side, for a real deviation. Such an apparent deviation occurs in facial paralysis. Ask the patient to move his tongue from side to side, and to lick each cheek with it; observe whether he can do so freely. Strength may also be assessed by pressing against the tongue with a finger as the patient protrudes it into each cheek in turn. Note whether there is any wasting of the tongue, and whether there is any tremor or fasciculation of it. The presence of wasting indicates that the lesion is either nuclear or infranuclear (lower motor neurone). *Fasciculation* must be assessed with the tongue relaxed in the mouth, not when protruded. Tremor of the tongue is common in Parkinson's disease, either when the tongue is at rest or protruded.

MOTOR FUNCTIONS

The motor system should be examined with the following aspects of motor function in mind:

1 Bulk of muscles
2 Tone of muscles
3 Strength of muscles
4 Reflexes
5 Coordination of movement
6 Gait
7 Involuntary movements

Bulk of muscles

The bulk of the muscles (Fig. 10.15) is most easily estimated by inspection and palpation. Wasted or atrophic muscles are not only smaller, but also softer and more flabby than normal when they are contracted. When muscular wasting is accompanied by fibrosis, as in muscular dystrophy or polymyositis, the muscles feel hard and inelastic. They may become shortened so it is difficult to stretch them passively to a normal degree—*contractures*. Contractures may also occur as a result of prolonged hypertonia in a group of muscles.

Muscular atrophy is not only caused by neurological disorders. Generalized muscular wasting is seen in cachexia of any cause. Localized muscle atrophy may be due to injury or disease of a joint; this occurs, for example, in the quadriceps in patients with diseases of the knee. In such instances strength is well preserved in relation to the degree of muscular wasting. Some patients with muscular dystrophy develop large muscles (*pseudo-hypertrophy*) due to pathological changes in the muscles themselves. The calves, buttocks and infraspinati are particularly affected. These enlarged muscles are strikingly weak in spite of their size. True hypertrophy of muscles occurs in response to continued excessive work loads as in certain occupations, or following athletic training. It may also occur in certain myotonic disorders.

Tone of muscles

Muscular tone is a state of tension or contraction found in healthy muscles. An increase in tone is called *hypertonia* and a diminution *hypotonia*. The degree of tone is estimated by handling the limbs and moving them passively at their various joints. The maintenance of tone is dependent on a spinal reflex arc. Afferent fibres from the primary and secondary endings of the muscle spindles enter the spinal cord and synapse with the anterior horn cells, from which

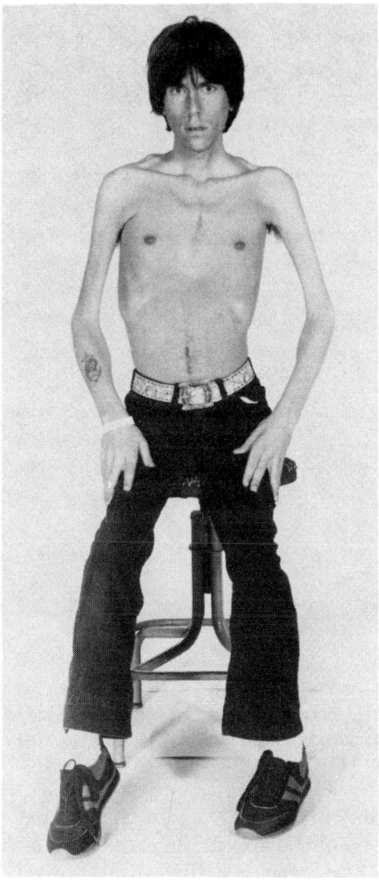

Fig. 10.15 Muscular atrophy due to facio-scapulo-humeral muscular dystrophy. Note the atrophy of the limb and shoulder muscles, especially the biceps and deltoids. Thinning of the thigh musculature can be recognized even through the trousers.

efferent fibres arise and pass to the muscles. Tone is diminished or lost if this reflex arc is damaged. *Hypotonia* therefore occurs in lower motor neurone lesions, in lesions of the afferent sensory pathways, as in tabes, and in cerebellar disease, in which suprasegmental mechanisms are abnormal. Tone may be reduced in sleep and by certain drugs.

Muscle tone is mainly regulated by corticospinal and extrapyramidal pathways. *Hypertonia* following lesions of the corticospinal system (upper motor neurone lesions) is termed *spasticity*. Spasticity is a term which should only be used to describe a state of increased tone which is of 'clasp-knife' type when the limb is fairly rapidly flexed or extended. These are the lengthening and shortenings reactions described by Sherrington. Spasticity is therefore a form of rigidity which is *stretch sensitive*. Moreover it can usually be shown that the

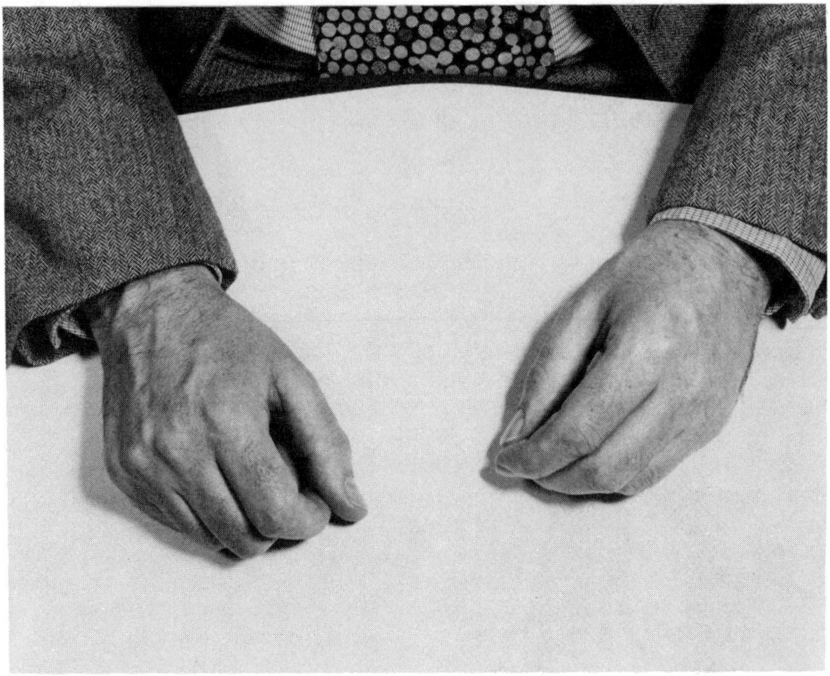

Fig. 10.16 Parkinson's disease. The left hand is held partially flexed and immobile. This has resulted in slight oedema of the skin of the hand causing the joints and tendons to appear indistinct. Since the hand is not used, its venous return is not as prominent as on the other side.

degree of increased tone developed during any given passive stretch is velocity-dependent, i.e. it is proportional to the speed of the applied stretch. Spasticity due to cerebral or brain stem lesions has a characteristic distribution shown by the typical posture of the limbs in such patients. The upper limbs are held in flexion and the lower limbs in extension with the feet in plantar flexion (physiological extension). Thus in the arms the flexor muscles are mainly involved, but in the legs the extensor muscles are predominantly affected. This distribution is most evident in the erect posture, and may even be reversed if the patient is placed head down.

Hypertonia resulting from disease of the basal ganglia is termed *extra-pyramidal rigidity*. The resistance to passive movement is regularly or irregularly variable and is aptly described as like a lever rubbing on the teeth of a cogwheel (*cogwheel rigidity*). It can usually be enhanced by asking the patient to contract another muscle, e.g. to clench his fist on the opposite side (Jendrassik's manoeuvre). In the commonest extrapyramidal disorder, Parkinson's disease, the hypertonia is accompanied by a general attitude of flexion of the limbs and trunk. This type of rigidity is often accompanied by *akinesia*, a tendency for the patient not to spontaneously move the affected limb or part of the body. Parkinson himself termed this 'a peculiar disinclination to move' (Fig. 10.16). Sometimes a plastic type of rigidity is found in which the resistance developed to passive movement is uniform during all phases of the applied movement. This is often referred to as *paratonic rigidity* or *'Gegenhalten'*. It is found in catatonic states and in patients with clouded or confused consciousness from any cause, especially dementia. It should not be regarded simply as evidence of 'lack of co-operation'. Its physiological basis is unknown. In *hysterical rigidity* the resistance to passive movement increases in proportion to the effort applied by the examiner. The increased resistance is usually developed in a characteristically jerky fashion.

When the muscles are *hypotonic*, there is little or no resistance to passive movement of the limb and when handled or shaken the unsupported part flops about inertly. Hypotonic muscles are abnormally soft to palpation. The outstretched hypotonic upper limb may assume an abnormal posture, as in cerebellar disease or chorea. It is hyperextended at the elbow, the forearm is overpronated, the wrist flexed, and the fingers hyperextended at the metacarpophalangeal joints.

Strength of muscles

Much the quickest and most reliable method of making a quick or preliminary assessment is to watch the patient walking, jumping, hopping, standing up from lying and sitting positions, and dressing or undressing. These movements require proximal and distal strength and coordination of a considerable degree and much can be learnt by observing them carefully. The strength of individual muscles can then be assessed more formally. Each movement made during this assessment is tested by comparison with the examiner's own strength or by comparison with what he judges to be normal in a person of comparable build to the patient. It therefore requires practice and experience. Very simple requests produce better results than long explanations: a demonstration or gesture is often more effective than any verbal explanation. Remember that most patients have no knowledge of anatomy.

Testing the muscles of the upper limb

Abductor pollicis brevis This is an important muscle (see Fig. 10.17) as it is supplied by the median nerve, which is commonly damaged by compression in the carpal tunnel at the wrist (carpal tunnel syndrome). The patient is asked to abduct his thumb in a plane at right angles to the palmar aspect of the index finger, against the resistance of the examiner's own thumb. The muscle can be seen and felt to contract.

Opponens pollicis Ask the patient to touch the tip of his little finger with the

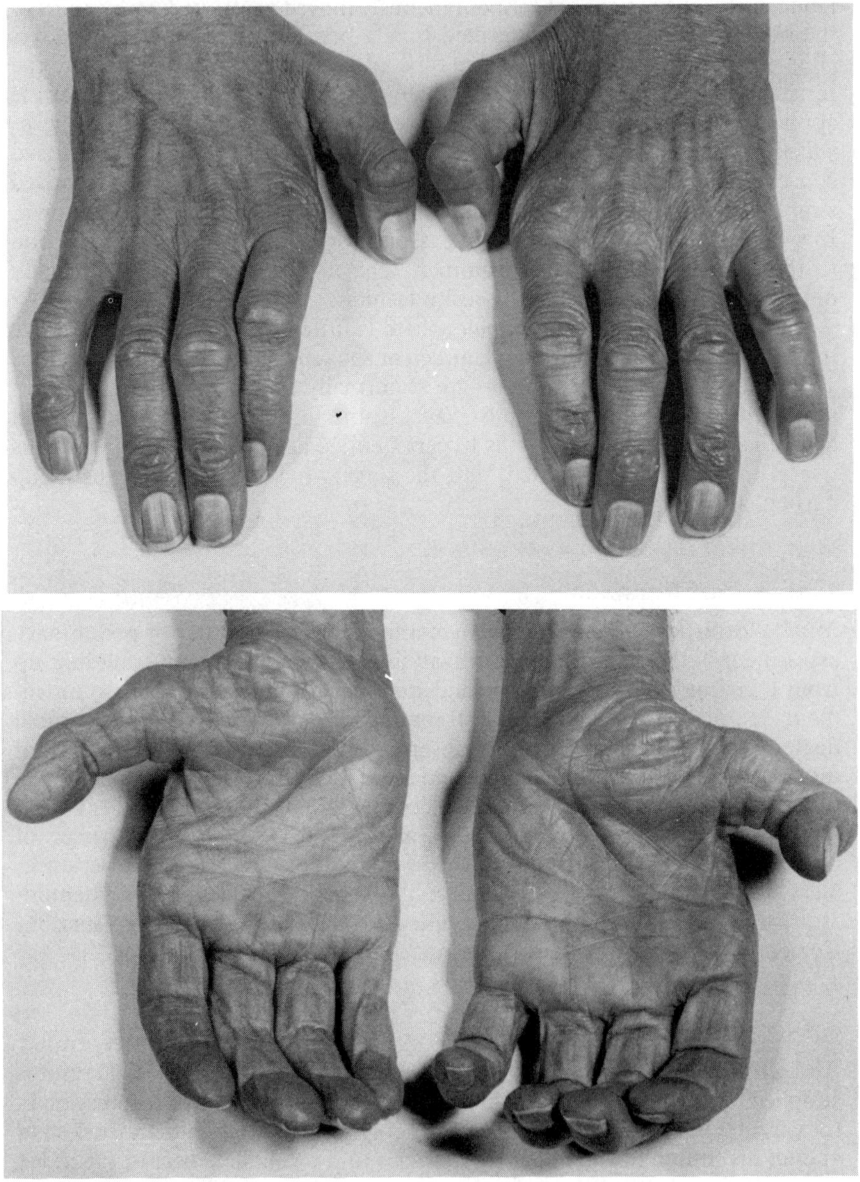

Fig. 10.17 Claw hands. In this patient with a long-standing, slowly progressive peripheral neuropathy there is wasting and weakness of all the intrinsic hand muscles with relative sparing of the long flexors and extensors, causing slight resting flexion and separation of the fingers. Note the flattening of the thenar eminences and hollowing of the dorsal web between thumb and index.

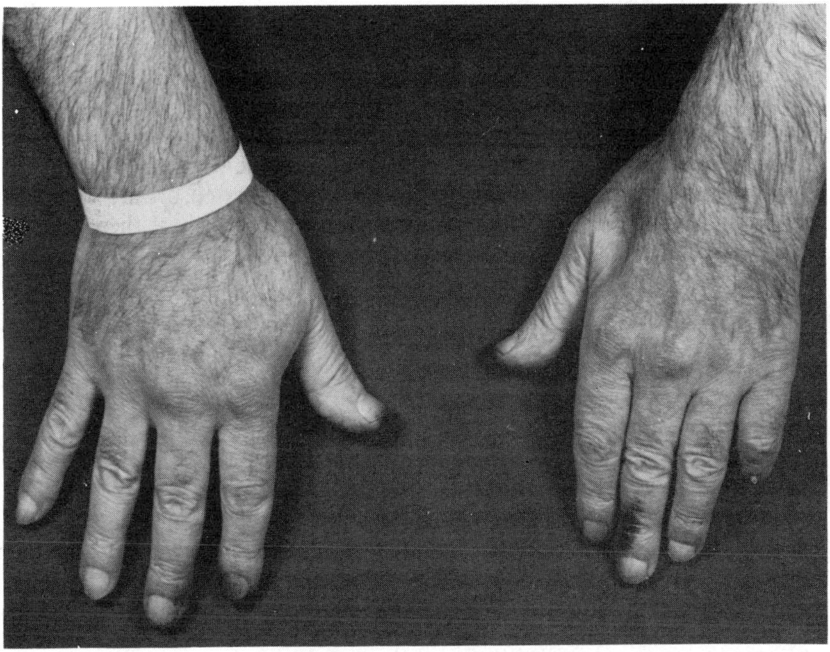

Fig. 10.18 Left ulnar nerve palsy showing marked atrophy of the left first dorsal interosseous muscles and flexion of the little finger. The right hand is normal.

point of his thumb. Oppose the movement with your thumb or index finger.

First dorsal interosseous (see Fig. 10.18) Ask the patient to abduct his index finger against your resistance.

Interossei and lumbricals Test the patient's ability to flex his metacarpophalangeal joints and to extend the distal interphalangeal joints. The interossei also adduct and abduct the fingers. When these muscles are paralysed and power is retained in the long flexors and extensors of the two fingers, as in ulnar nerve palsy, a 'claw-hand' deformity is produced. The first phalanges are overextended and the distal two are flexed. The fingers are slightly separated (Fig. 10.17).

Flexors of the fingers Ask the patient to squeeze your fingers. Allow him to squeeze only your index and middle fingers – this is sufficient to assess strength of grip without his painfully crushing your fingers.

Flexors of the wrist. Ask him to bring the tips of his fingers towards the front of the forearm.

Extensors of the wrist Ask the patient to make a fist, a movement which results in firm contraction of both the flexors and extensors of the wrists, and try to forcibly flex the wrist against his effort to maintain his posture. It should be almost impossible to overcome the wrist extensors of a healthy man or woman. The wrist flexors can be similarly tested.

Slight weakness of the extensors of the wrist may be elicited by asking the patient to grasp something firmly in his hand. If the extensors are weak the wrist becomes flexed as he does so, because the flexor muscles are then stronger than the extensors.

Weakness or paralysis of the extensors of the wrist as in radial nerve palsy leads to *wrist-drop*.

Brachioradialis Place the arm midway between the prone and supine positions; then ask the patient to bend up the forearm, whilst you oppose the movement by grasping the hand. The muscle, if healthy, will be seen and felt to stand out prominently at its upper part.

Biceps Ask the patient to bend up the forearm against resistance, with the forearm in full supination. The muscle will stand out clearly.

Triceps Ask the patient to straighten out his forearm against your resistance.

Supraspinatus Ask the patient to lift his arm straight out at right angles to his side. The first 30° of this movement is carried out by the supraspinatus. The remaining 60° is produced by the *deltoid*.

Deltoid The anterior and posterior fibres help to draw the abducted arm forwards and backwards respectively. The middle fibres abduct the shoulder (see 'Supraspinatus').

Infraspinatus The patient is asked to tuck his elbow into his side with the forearm flexed to a right angle. He is then asked to rotate the limb outwards against the examiner's resistance, the elbow being held against the side throughout. The muscle can be seen and felt to contract.

Pectorals Ask the patient to stretch his arms out in front of him, and then to clap his hands together while the observer endeavours to hold them apart.

Serratus anterior When this muscle is paralysed the scapula is 'winged', the vertebral border projecting. The patient is unable to elevate his arm above a right angle, the deformity becoming more apparent as he tries to do so. Pushing forwards with the hands against resistance, such as a wall, also brings out the deformity.

Latissimus dorsi The patient is asked to clasp his hands behind his back while the observer, standing behind the patient, offers passive resistance to the downward and backward movement; alternatively the two posterior axillary folds can be felt as the patient coughs.

Testing the muscles of the trunk

Weakness of the muscles of the abdomen is shown by the patient's inability to sit up in bed from the supine position without the aid of his arms. *Babinski's 'rising up sign'* consists in making the patient lie on his back with the legs extended and rise up without using his hands. In spastic paralysis of a leg the affected limb will rise first, but in hysterical paralysis this does not occur.

Paralysis of a portion of the anterior abdominal wall can be detected by the displacement of the umbilicus that occurs when the patient attempts to lift up his head from the pillow against resistance. With paralysis of the lower segment the umbilicus moves upwards, but when the upper segment is affected the umbilicus is pulled downwards. This is sometimes known as *Beevor*'s *sign*: it is a useful sign since it may indicate the level of a lesion in spinal cord disease.

To test the *erector spinae* and muscles of the back, make the patient lie on his face and try to raise his head from the bed by extending the neck and back. If the back muscles are healthy, they will be seen to stand out prominently during this effort.

The method of detecting paralysis of the *diaphragm* is described on p. 191. The upper part of the *trapezius* is tested by asking the patient to shrug his shoulders while the observer tries to press them down from behind. Its lower part can be tested by asking him to approximate the shoulder blades.

The cranial musculature is described on p. 296.

Testing the muscles of the lower limb

The intrinsic muscles of the foot cannot be easily examined. When the interossei are weakened or paralysed a 'claw-foot', analogous to the 'claw-hand', may develop. A similar deformity may develop in patients with spastic hemiparesis of very long duration; this is due to a form of dystonia and not to muscular weakness.

Dorsiflexion and *plantar flexion* of the feet and toes are tested by asking the patient to elevate or depress the part against resistance.

Extensors of the knee Bend up the patient's knee, and then, pressing with your hand on his shin, ask him to try to straighten it out again.

Flexors of the knee Raise the leg up from the bed, supporting the thigh with your left hand and holding the ankle with your right. Then ask the patient to bend his knee.

Extensors of the hip The knee being extended, lift the patient's foot off the bed, and ask him to push it down against your resistance. This is normally a very strong movement and should be impossible to overcome.

Flexors of the thigh With the leg extended ask the patient to raise his leg off the bed against resistance. Alternatively the related movement of flexion of the thigh, with the thigh already flexed to a right angle, can be tested.

Adductors of the thigh Abduct the limb and then ask the patient to bring it back to the midline against resistance.

Abductors of the thigh Place the patient's legs together and ask him to separate them against resistance.

Rotators of the thigh With the lower limb extended on the bed, ask the patient to roll it outwards or inwards against resistance.

Grading of weakness

The Medical Research Council Scale is usually used to grade muscle weakness:

Grade 0	Complete paralysis
Grade 1	A flicker of contraction only
Grade 2	Power detectable only when gravity is excluded by appropriate postural adjustment
Grade 3	The limb can be held against the force of gravity, but not against the examiner's resistance
Grade 4	There is some degree of weakness, usually described as poor, fair or moderate strength
Grade 5	Normal power is present

Patterns of weakness

The term *hemiplegia* is applied to a condition in which there is paralysis of one side of the body, especially of the arm and leg, and usually also of the face (*facio-brachio-crural hemiparesis*). The term *crossed paralysis* refers to paralysis of ipsilateral cranial musculature with a contralateral hemiparesis; it is a sign of brain stem disease. The term *paraplegia* is applied to a paralysis of both legs; the term *monoplegia* to a paralysis of one limb, which may be the arm (*brachial monoplegia*) or the leg (*crural monoplegia*). In *quadriplegia* all four limbs are weak.

In weakness due to a *corticospinal lesion*, as in spastic hemiparesis, weakness is usually particularly evident in the leg in hip flexion and in dorsiflexion of the foot; in the arm in shoulder abduction/extension and in dorsiflexion of the wrist; and in the face, in a supranuclear distribution. The face and arm, or the leg, may be particularly involved. Slowness and clumsiness of rapid, fine finger movement is often a feature. Antagonistic movements, such as hip extension, and plantar flexion of the foot, are strikingly less involved in the early stages of corticospinal weakness. The characteristic pattern of weakness in this clinical syndrome is thus of great value in diagnosis.

The detection of hemiplegia in a patient who is comatose may be difficult. However, if the paralysis is of recent onset, one can usually detect hypotonia in the paralysed limbs. If the arm, for example, is raised from the side and allowed to drop, it falls, if it is paralysed, as if it did not belong to the patient; the sound arm also falls, but not in such an utterly limp fashion. The face is asymmetrical, the angle of the mouth more open on the paralysed side, and the affected cheek moves loosely outwards and inwards with respiration. The abdominal and tendon reflexes may be absent on both sides, but an extensor plantar response can usually be obtained on the hemiplegic side (see 'Reflexes', p. 326).

Myasthenic weakness

In *myasthenia gravis*, weakness, which commonly affects the external ocular and bulbar muscles more than the rest of the skeletal musculature, is characteristically exacerbated or provoked by repeated contraction of the affected muscles. The degree of detectable weakness therefore varies during the course of the day. This is referred to as myasthenic weakness. In the myasthenic syndrome (Eaton–Lambert syndrome) there is weakness initially, but during contraction of a muscle or movement an increase in strength occurs at first, followed by weakness if exertion is continued.

Myotonia

In certain muscular disorders, of which *dystrophia myotonica* is the best known, relaxation following contraction of a muscle is impaired. The phenomenon is most evident when the muscles are cold and it is therefore often best demonstrated in the hand. Ask the patient to grip your hand firmly and then to let go suddenly. His grasp is maintained for a moment and then is slowly and gradually released. Myotonia can be demonstrated in the tongue and in other muscles, e.g. the thenar eminence, by lightly striking the muscle with a small patellar hammer. A dimple of contraction appears and relaxes only slowly.

Reflexes

Tendon reflexes

If the tendon of a lightly stretched muscle is struck a single, sharp blow with a soft rubber hammer (thus suddenly stretching the muscle and exciting a synchronous volley of afferent impulses from the primary sensory endings of the muscle spindles in the stretched muscle), the muscle contracts briefly. This is the monosynaptic stretch reflex. It is a test of the integrity of the afferent and efferent pathways, and of the excitability of the anterior horn cells in the spinal segment of the stretched muscle. Properly performed, examination of the tendon reflexes offers a reliable and reproducible method of assessment of this system of neurones and their higher connections; it is therefore very important to become skilled in the techniques for eliciting these reflexes.

Always use the same type of hammer; always examine these reflexes in the same manner, standing on the same side of the bed; always make sure the patient is warm and comfortable; and reassure him that the hammer is soft and not an offensive weapon. When examining the tendon reflexes in the legs, care taken to allow the patient's genitalia to be properly covered is repaid by more easily elicitable reflexes. The patient should be asked to relax or to 'let the muscles go to sleep'.

Knee jerk The patellar hammer derives its name from its invention as an instrument for eliciting this reflex, the first tendon reflex to become a regular part of the neurological examination. The knee jerk consists of a contraction of the quadriceps when the patellar tendon is tapped. The spinal segments concerned are the 2nd, 3rd and 4th lumbar. It is best tested with the patient supine. The examiner's hand is passed under the knee to be tested and placed upon the opposite knee; the knee to be tested rests on the dorsum of the observer's wrist. The patellar tendon is struck midway between its origin and insertion. Following the blow there will be a brief extension of the knee from contraction of the quadriceps. The reflex can sometimes be more easily elicited with the patient sitting up, his legs dangling freely over the edge of the bed.

The briskness of the knee jerk varies greatly in different individuals. In health it is hardly ever entirely absent. Sometimes, as in the case of the other tendon reflexes, it cannot be elicited without applying *reinforcement* (Jendrassik's manoeuvre). This is done by asking the patient to make some strong voluntary muscular effort with the upper limbs; for example to hook the fingers of the two hands together and then to pull them against one another as hard as possible, or to make a fist with the ipsilateral hand. While he is doing this, a further attempt is made to elicit the knee jerk. Reinforcement acts by increasing the excitability of the anterior horn cells and by increasing the sensitivity of the muscle spindle primary sensory endings to stretch (by increased gamma fusimotor drive).

Ankle jerk Place the lower limb on the bed so that it lies everted and slightly flexed. Then, with one hand, slightly dorsiflex the foot so as to stretch the Achilles tendon and, with the other hand, strike the tendon on its posterior surface. A sharp contraction of the calf muscles results. This reflex can also be conveniently elicited when the patient is kneeling on a chair. It depends upon the 1st and 2nd sacral segments.

Triceps jerk Flex the elbow and allow the forearm to rest across the patient's chest. Tap the triceps tendon just above the olecranon. The triceps contracts. The reflex depends upon the 6th and 7th cervical segments. Care must be taken to strike the triceps *tendon* and not the belly of the muscle itself. All muscles show a certain amount of irritability to direct mechanical stimuli; but this is a direct response, not a stretch reflex.

Biceps jerk The elbow is flexed to a right angle and the forearm placed in a semipronated position; the examiner then places his thumb or index finger on the biceps tendon and strikes it with the patellar hammer. The biceps contracts. The 5th and 6th cervical segments of the cord are concerned.

Supinator jerk A blow upon the styloid process of the radius stretches the supinator causing supination of the elbow. This reflex depends on the 5th and 6th cervical segments.

With lesions at this level the supinator reflex or biceps reflex may be lost but, when it is tested, brisk flexion of the fingers is seen. This phenomenon is known as *inversion* of the reflex and it is evidence of hyperexcitability of the anterior horn cells below the C5/6 level. The responsible lesion is in the C5/6 spinal segments.

Jaw jerk Ask the patient to open his mouth, but not too widely. Place one finger firmly on his chin and then tap it suddenly with the other hand as in percussion. A contraction of the muscles that close the jaw results. This jerk is sometimes absent in health and is increased in upper motor neurone lesions above the trigeminal nerve nuclei.

Clonus The phenomenon of clonus is often elicitable when the tendon reflexes are exaggerated as a result of a corticospinal lesion.

Ankle clonus: bend the patient's knee slightly and support it with one hand, grasp the forepart of the foot with the other hand and suddenly dorsiflex the foot. The sudden stretch causes a brief reflex contraction of the calf muscles, which then relax; continued stretch causes a regular oscillation of contraction and relaxation which is called *clonus*. *Sustained clonus* is abnormal, and is evidence of an upper motor neurone lesion. It is then always associated with increased tendon reflexes (hyperreflexia) and an extensor plantar response.

Unsustained clonus may occur in healthy persons, particularly in those who are very tense or anxious; in these subjects the plantar responses are flexor.

Grading the reflexes

The tendon reflexes may be graded:

0 Absent
1 Present (as a normal ankle jerk)
2 Brisk (as a normal knee jerk)
3 Very brisk
4 Clonus

Abnormal tendon reflexes

The tendon reflexes are *diminished* or absent with lesions affecting the afferent pathways, the anterior horn cells themselves, or the efferent pathways (lesions of the lower motor neurone). For example, in tabes dorsalis the posterior roots are affected; in poliomyelitis the anterior horn cells are diseased; and in most peripheral neuropathies both the efferent (motor) and afferent (sensory) nerve fibres are abnormal. In all these conditions tendon reflexes may be absent.

Hyperreflexia occurs with upper motor neurone lesions at all levels above the anterior horn cells. It may also occur with anxiety or nervousness, in thyrotoxicosis and as a manifestation of tetanus. Hyperreflexia is therefore only of pathological significance if it is asymmetrical or if it is associated with other signs of an upper motor neurone lesion.

In cerebellar disease the reflexes may have a characteristic *pendular* quality. This is clearly evident only when there is a severe cerebellar ataxia and it is not a sign of diagnostic importance. It may be considered a manifestation of hypotonia.

In myxoedema both the contraction and relaxation phases of the tendon reflex may be prolonged. This is sometimes called, somewhat confusingly, a *myotonic reflex*. It is also found in hypothermic patients. The relaxation time of the ankle jerk can be estimated by simple observation with surprising accuracy in relation to the normal, and is a sensitive and reliable clinical index of hypothyroidism.

Superficial reflexes (Table 10.4)

The plantar reflex Assessment of the plantar reflex is of great clinical importance; it is an objective response which can be easily compared by various observers. To elicit it the muscles of the lower limb should be relaxed. The *outer edge of the sole of the foot* is stimulated by gently scratching a key or a stick along it from the heel towards the little toe and then medially across the

Table 10.4 Chief superficial reflexes of spinal origin

Reflex	*How excited*	*Result*	*Level of cord concerned*
Anal	Stroking or scratching the skin near the anus	Contraction of anal sphincter	3rd and 4th sacral segments
Bulbocavernosus	Pinching dorsum of glans penis	Contraction of bulbocavernosus	3rd and 4th sacral segments
Plantar	Stroking sole of foot	Flexion of toes, of foot and toes, or leg	Lower part of lumbar enlargement (5th lumbar and 1st sacral segments)
Cremasteric	Stroking skin at upper and inner part of thigh*	Upwards movement of testicle	1st and 2nd lumbar segments
Abdominal	Stroking abdominal wall below costal margin, at level of umbilicus and in iliac fossa	Contraction of abdominal muscles	7th to 12th thoracic segments
Scapular	Stroking skin in interscapular region	Contraction of scapular muscles	5th cervical to 1st thoracic segment

* The cremasteric reflex can often be more easily elicited by pressing over the sartorius in the lower third of Hunter's canal.

metatarsus. In healthy adults even a slight stimulus produces a contraction of the tensor fascia lata, often accompanied by a slighter contraction of the adductors of the thigh and of the sartorius. With a slightly stronger stimulus, flexion of the four outer toes appears, which increases with the strength of the stimulus till all the toes are flexed on the metatarsus and drawn together, the ankle being dorsiflexed and inverted. This is called the *flexor plantar response*. With still stronger stimuli withdrawal of the limb occurs. The plantar reflex is never completely absent in healthy subjects.

An abnormality in the plantar response in lesions of the corticospinal system was first described by Babinski. This abnormal response, Babinski's *extensor plantar response*, replaces the normal flexor plantar response; it is found only in patients with corticospinal tract lesions and is thus a pathognomonic feature of an upper motor neurone lesion. In the extensor plantar response dorsiflexion (extension) of the great toe precedes all other movement. It is followed by spreading out and extension of the other toes, by dorsiflexion of the ankle, and by flexion of the hip and knee.

This abnormal response is called the *extensor* plantar response because the movement of the toes is in extension according to anatomical terminology. Nonetheless it is important to recognize that the extensor plantar response is, in reality, part of the nociceptive flexion withdrawal response described in the decerebrate preparation by Sherrington. Like the normal flexor plantar response, the extensor plantar response is best elicited from the outer edge of the sole of the foot; more medial stimuli usually elicit flexion as part of the grasp response, itself a different phenomenon. In major corticospinal lesions the area from which the extensor plantar reflex can be elicited (receptive field) enlarges, spreading first inwards and over the sole of the foot, and then upwards along the leg to the knee or even higher. For this reason extension of the great toe, generally associated with some dorsiflexion of the foot, can sometimes also be obtained by squeezing the calf or pressing heavily along the inner border of the tibia (*Oppenheim's sign*), or by pinching the calcaneus tendon (*Gordon's reflex*).

In adults, the extensor plantar response occurs with disease involving corticospinal pathways, but in children below the age of one year the extensor response is the normal response. The flexor response appears in the subsequent 6–12 months as myelination of the corticospinal pathways is completed.

Flexor spasms may occur during testing of the plantar reflex. These consist of an exaggerated extensor plantar response, the whole limb being suddenly drawn up into flexion and the large toe extended. This is the fully developed human counterpart of Sherrington's nociceptive flexion withdrawal response. It is common in spinal cord disease and in some patients with bilateral upper motor neurone lesions at a higher level. Flexor spasms are often particularly severe in the presence of posterior column disease (as in multiple sclerosis or subacute combined degeneration), or when there is a constant stimulation of small unmyelinated fibre input to the spinal cord, as in the presence of bedsores or urinary tract infection in a patient with a cord lesion. *Extensor spasms*, conversely, are more likely to occur in patients with corticospinal tract lesions when posterior column function is normal.

Superficial abdominal reflexes These are elicited with the patient lying relaxed and in a supine position, with the abdomen uncovered. A light stimulus, such as a key or a thin wooden stick, is passed across the abdominal skin in the plane of the dermatome from the outer aspect towards the midline. A ripple of contraction of the underlying abdominal musculature follows the stimulus. These reflexes are absent in upper motor neurone lesions above their spinal level. In disease of the thoracic spine they may indicate the segmental level of the lesion by their absence below this level.

It is often impossible to elicit abdominal reflexes in anxious patients, in the elderly or obese, and in multiparous women.

Corneal reflex See p. 308.

Palatal reflex See p. 314.

Sphincteric reflexes

These are the reflexes concerned with swallowing, micturition and defaecation. They depend upon complex muscular movements excited by increased tension in the wall of the viscus concerned, and involve both unstriated and striated muscles.

Ascertain from the patient whether there is any difficulty in swallowing (*dysphagia*), noting especially whether there is any regurgitation of food through the nose. As a rule patients with neurological disorders causing dysphagia complain of difficulty in swallowing liquids, whereas those with mechanical oesophageal obstruction complain they cannot swallow solids.

Defaecation The patient should be questioned as to any difficulty and as to the presence of rectal and anal sensation. Incontinence of faeces should be noted.

The reflex action of the voluntary anal sphincter may be tested by introducing the lubricated gloved finger into the anus and noting whether contraction of the sphincter occurs with normal force, whether it is weak or paralysed, or whether any spasm is excited. The activity of the reflex may also be tested by gently pricking the skin on either side near the anus. A brisk contraction of the sphincter should immediately occur—the *anal reflex*. In addition, the anal sphincter normally contracts briskly in response to a sudden cough—the *cough reflex*.

Micturition The patient should be asked whether there is any difficulty in controlling or initiating micturition and whether bladder and urethral sensation are normal. Retention and incontinence or urgency of micturition should be noted.

Incontinence in neurological disorders may be due to overflow from an atonic distended bladder in which sensation has been lost. In this case the bladder will be enlarged to palpation or percussion and suprapubic pressure may result in the expulsion of urine from the urethra. Incontinence may also be due to *reflex micturition*, occurring either at regular intervals as the bladder partially fills, or precipitately and unexpectedly in response to a sudden noise, to movement or to exposure to cold.

Coordination of movement

By coordination is meant the smooth recruitment, interaction and cooperation of separate muscles or groups of muscles in order to accomplish a definite motor act. If such coordination is imperfect, motor performance becomes difficult or impossible and *ataxia* is said to be present.

The coordination of groups of muscles is a function of various factors, among which are the afferent impulses coming from the muscle spindles and joint receptors, cerebellar function and the state of tone of the muscles. When ataxia is present it is not always easy to say which of these factors is at fault. The movements that constitute a motor act can be controlled and directed by vision, but sight itself is not concerned in the coordination of most normal movements. When, however, there is loss of the sense of position of a limb or joint, the sensory defect may be compensated for by vision, and the disturbance of movement may become apparent only when the eyes are closed or the patient is in the dark. Such ataxia occurs typically in tabes dorsalis, when position sense is diminished or lost in the legs. Before ataxia can be ascribed solely to cerebellar disease, therefore, it is important to ascertain whether joint position sense is impaired or not. Proximal weakness may mimic cerebellar ataxia, but this can usually be distinguished easily when muscular strength is tested.

How to test coordination

In the upper limbs Ask the patient to touch the point of his nose first with one forefinger and then with the other; or ask him to touch first his nose, then your forefinger with his index finger. If he performs these movements naturally and without making random errors, coordination is normal. He should then be asked to perform the same actions with his eyes closed; any additional irregularity indicates that there must be impairment of position sense in the limb.

A special and very useful sign of cerebellar ataxia is *dysdiadochokinesia*; it consists of impaired ability to execute rapidly repeated movements. The patient is asked to flex his elbows to a right angle and then alternately to supinate and pronate his forearms as rapidly as possible 'as though screwing in a light bulb'. All normal persons can do this very rapidly but usually slightly less rapidly with the non-dominant left than with the right arm. When dysdiadochokinesia is present the movements are slow, awkward and incomplete, and often become impossible after a few attempts. In addition, the rhythm of the movement is characteristically irregular. The sign can also be elicited by asking the patient to tap the examiner's palm with the tips of his fingers as fast as possible. Minor degrees of ataxia can then be both felt and heard.

It is often useful to watch the patient dressing or undressing, handling a book or picking up pins, since these more complex and more practised everyday movements offer a very sensitive way of assessing coordination.

In the lower limbs If the patient is able to walk, a good test of lower limb coordination consists of asking him to walk along a straight line. If incoordination is present he will soon deviate to one side or the other. Watch particularly for unsteadiness as he turns to walk back towards you. The test is made more difficult by asking the patient to 'tandem walk' along a line drawn on the floor, like a tightrope walker, placing the heel of one foot immediately adjacent to the toe of the one behind.

If he cannot walk, ask him, as he lies in bed, to lift one leg high in the air, to place the heel of this leg on the opposite knee and then to slide the heel down his shin towards the ankle. In cerebellar ataxia a characteristic, irregular, side to side series of errors in the speed and direction of movement occurs. The test should be performed *with the eyes open*. A similar test is to ask the patient to draw a large circle in the air with his toe or forefinger. The circles should be drawn smoothly and accurately.

Romberg's sign is a *test for loss of position sense* (sensory ataxia) in the legs; it is not a test of cerebellar function. The patient is asked to stand with his feet close together, and, if he can do this, he is then asked to close his eyes. If Romberg's sign is present, as soon as his eyes are closed he begins to sway about or may even fall. *The essential feature of the sign is therefore that the patient is more unsteady standing with his eyes closed than when they are open*. With defective position sense in the legs, as in tabes dorsalis or sensory neuropathy, the patient is unable to maintain his posture without the aid of vision. Patients with labyrinthine lesions or with cerebellar ataxia show little or no increase in instability in this test.

Gait

Analysis of a patient's gait is of major importance in diagnosis. The legs should be adequately exposed and free of constricting clothing such as a dressing gown. The feet should be bare. The patient is asked to walk away from the observer, to turn round at a given point and then to come towards him again. The points to be noted are:

1 Can the patient walk at all? If he can:

2 Does he walk in a straight line or does he tend to deviate to one side or the other? To bring out this point, ask him to walk along a straight line, e.g. a crack in the floor.
3 Does he tend to fall? In what direction?

The next point to be decided is whether the gait conforms to any of the well recognized abnormal types. Before deciding this, make sure that the abnormal gait is not due to some surgical cause or to local disease of a joint, e.g. osteoarthritis of the hip.

In a *spastic gait* the patient walks on a narrow base, has difficulty in bending his knees and drags his feet along as if they were glued to the floor. This can be heard as well as seen. The foot is raised from the ground by tilting the pelvis, and the leg is then swung forwards so that the foot tends to describe an arc, the toe scraping along the floor—*circumduction* of the leg. A spastic gait is a characteristic feature of patients with corticospinal lesions, especially in spinal cord disease. The *hemiplegic gait* is essentially a spastic gait in which only one leg is affected.

The gait in *sensory ataxia* may be described as 'stamping'. The patient raises his feet very suddenly, often abnormally high, and then jerks them forward, bringing them to the ground again with a stamp, and often heel first. If he watches the ground, he may be fairly steady, as he can use his eyes in place of his position sense, but he becomes severely ataxic when his eyes are closed or if he walks in the dark. This gait is best seen in tabes dorsalis. Other signs of loss of postural sensibility will be present.

The gait of *cerebellar ataxia* appears 'drunken' or 'reeling'. Patients with this gait disorder walk on a broad base, the feet being planted widely apart and placed irregularly. The ataxia is equally severe whether the eyes are open or closed. Other signs of cerebellar disease are usually present.

A *festinant gait* is characteristic of Parkinson's disease. The patient is bent forwards (flexion dystonia) and advances with rapid, short, shuffling steps, so that he appears as if he is trying to catch up with the centre of gravity, and his arms do not swing. In some cases, if he is suddenly pulled backwards, he begins to walk backwards, and is unable to stop himself (*retropulsion*). In bilateral corticospinal lesions in the deep cerebral white matter a rather similar, short-stepped but rapid tapping gait occurs, called *marche à petits pas* to describe its resemblance to the rapid steps of a ballet dancer on her points. In dystonia and chorea the involuntary movements are usually exaggerated during walking, and unusual foot placement responses may occur so that the toes may extend away from the floor (avoiding response) or the feet may appear glued to the floor (grasping response).

The *waddling gait* is like the gait of a duck. The body is usually tilted backwards, with an increase of lumbar lordosis; the feet are planted rather widely apart and the body sways from side to side as each step is taken. The heels and toes tend to be brought down simultaneously. This gait disorder is due to difficulty in maintaining truncal and pelvic posture because of proximal muscular weakness. It occurs, therefore, in the myopathies and the muscular dystrophies. A similar gait may occur with bilateral disease of the hip joints (Trendelenburg's sign).

A *high-stepping gait* is adopted in order to avoid tripping from the toes catching the ground. It occurs when there is weakness of the extensor muscles of the feet, for example in common peroneal nerve palsy.

Involuntary movements

In a number of different diseases of the nervous system, involuntary, unintended movements occur, either at rest or during voluntary movement. The different clinical varieties of involuntary movement are not specific disease entities, but represent clinical patterns of involuntary movement. Most are due to diseases of the basal ganglia and extrapyramidal system.

Epilepsy

The possibility should always be considered that an involuntary movement limited to one side of the body, or to one limb, might be due to focal epilepsy. Very rarely such an attack may continue for hours or even days (*epilepsia partialis continua*). The movement is usually complex and repetitive. It may be exacerbated by arousal or by handling or touching the limb and it will usually be relieved by anticonvulsant drugs. The movement differs from the involuntary movement disorders principally by its stereotyped repetitiveness.

Myoclonus

Myoclonus is a rapid, irregular jerking movement of the limb or of the whole body, often occurring in response to extraneous stimuli, such as a sudden loud noise. A sudden start when surprised, or bodily jerks on falling asleep or waking, are common varieties of myoclonus experienced by most normal people. In exaggerated form these jerks of *flexion myoclonus* may occur as a manifestation of major epilepsy or with degenerative disorders of the cerebellum. Generalized flexion myoclonus also occurs in certain types of encephalitis, when it often exhibits an obvious periodicity. Less commonly, irregular myoclonic jerks may occur in a single limb, or a ripple of jerky irregular contraction may pass through the muscles of a limb—*segmental myoclonus*. Myoclonus can occur with lesions at many levels in the nervous system and it does not, therefore, have localizing value.

Tremor

Regular or irregular distal movements having an oscillatory character are classified as tremors. The tremor of *anxiety* is usually fine and rapid, but it may be coarse and irregular. The tremor found in *thyrotoxicosis* is characteristically rapid. Coarser distal tremor, often exaggerated in awkward postures, as when the outstretched fingers are held pointing at each other in front of the patient's nose and usually relieved to some extent during movement, occurs as a familial disorder—*benign essential tremor*. This tremor is often coarse, but usually irregular, and it is present both at rest and during movement. It must therefore be distinguished from parkinsonian and cerebellar tremors. The latter is present only during movement (*intention tremor*) and the former is accompanied by signs of extrapyramidal disease. *Senile tremor* is similar to benign essential tremor. *Hysterical tremor* tends to involve a limb or the whole body and it is characteristically worsened by the examiner's attempt to control it.

The tremor of *parkinsonism* is usually easily recognizable. It consists of a rapid, rhythmic, alternating tremor, predominantly in flexion/extension but often with a prominent rotary component between finger and thumb (*pill-rolling tremor*). More proximal muscles may be involved, and the lips and tongue are frequently affected. The tremor is invariably more severe in the arm than in the leg. It is often strikingly unilateral and is associated with other symptoms and signs of extrapyramidal disease, such as hypokinesia, cogwheel rigidity, postural abnormalities and gait disorder.

Athetosis

Athetosis is a writhing movement, usually more pronounced in distal than in proximal muscles, in which the play of movement is very complex. It often seems to consist of a relatively constant interaction between two postures, those of *grasping and avoiding* (see p. 281). The fingers are alternately widely extended, the arm following into an extended, abducted and externally rotated posture, and then the fingers clench, often trapping the thumb in the palm, and the limb flexes slightly and rotates internally. In very severe forms of this disorder, as for example in *dystonia musculorum deformans* (torsion dystonia) the trunk and axial musculature is also affected and the patient may scarcely be able to stand.

Athetosis may be unilateral or generalized. The latter form is usually associated with degenerative disease of the basal ganglia. Very rarely it may occur as a paroxysmal phenomenon.

Chorea

The word means 'a dance'. The involuntary movements are brief, fluid and often difficult, at first, to discern. Ordinary voluntary movements, such as walking or picking up a cup and saucer, may be embellished with smooth, rapid extra little flourishes of movement. Muscular tone is often decreased. The outstretched upper limbs may assume a hyperpronated posture and little flicks of movement of the digits or wrist may occur. At rest the patient appears 'fidgety' and 'unable to sit still'. The movements often appear less obvious during voluntary movement, and are increased by agitation or nervousness. Chorea occurs as part of an inherited presenile dementia (*Huntington's chorea*), associated with rheumatic fever (*Sydenham's chorea*) and rarely in pregnancy and after certain *drugs* (phenothiazines). It may also occur with other systemic diseases, e.g. thyrotoxicosis and systemic lupus erythematosus, and in old age (*senile chorea*). Unilateral chorea may occur with deeply placed lesions in one hemisphere.

Dyskinesia

The word dyskinesia is particularly used to describe *phenothiazine-induced* involuntary movements, which predominantly affect the pharyngeal and facial peri-oral musculature, and *levodopa-induced* axial torsional movements, although similar movements occur in choreo-athetoid and dystonic patients not previously treated with these drugs.

Dystonia

This word is used to describe an *abnormally maintained posture*, often associated with a plastic rigidity. The dystonias are closely related to choreo-athetosis (dystonic movements), but the term can also be used to describe the flexed posture of Parkinson's disease (flexion dystonia) or the hemiplegic posture (hemiplegic dystonia). The abnormal posture varies in relation to different circumstances; for example, it is often relieved by lying or by standing in contact with a wall.

Hemiballismus

This is a characteristic involuntary movement, almost invariably unilateral and affecting the arm more than the leg, in which the limb is flung rapidly, and often with great force, from full extension into abduction and external or internal rotation. The movements may be so violent as to result in serious injury to the limb, and in loss of weight. The disorder is associated with lesions in the region of the subthalamic nucleus.

Torticollis

Spasmodic torticollis consists of a jerky or maintained rotational and abducted posture of the neck. It is a form of dystonia. It can often be partially controlled by the patient by certain postural adjustments, e.g. touching the chin with the index finger.

Tics

These are simple, normal movements which become repeated unnecessarily to the point that they become an embarrassment or a source of, or reaction to, psychiatric problems. In contrast to the other involuntary movement disorders, they can be readily imitated. Head nodding is a common example.

Myokymia

This is a persistent twitchy and often rhythmical movement of the peri-orbital muscles. It may occur as a benign phenomenon in fatigued or anxious people. It is sometimes due to lesions in the facial nerve or its nucleus.

Metabolic flap (asterixis)

An irregular, abrupt, brief loss of posture, especially evident in the outstretched hands or tongue occurs in decompensated hepatic failure (*hepatic flap*) and in other metabolic disorders, e.g. uraemia, poisoning with hypnotic drugs, and in respiratory failure.

Tetany

Tetany, commonly due to hypocalcaemia or alkalosis, can be recognized by the characteristic posture of the affected hand (see Fig. 2.3). The fingers and thumbs are held stiffly adducted and the hand is partially flexed at the metacarpophalangeal joints; the toes may be similarly affected (*carpopedal spasm*). Ischaemia of the affected limb, produced by a sphygmomanometer cuff inflated above the arterial pressure for 2 or 3 minutes, will augment this sign or produce it if it is not already present (*Trousseau's sign*). Another useful test is to tap lightly with a patellar hammer in the region of exit of the facial nerve from the skull, about 3–5 cm below and in front of the ear. The facial muscles twitch briefly with each tap (*Chvostek's sign*).

SENSATION

The following different forms of sensation are usually tested:

1 *Tactile sensibility*. This includes light touch and pressure, and tactile localization and discrimination

2 *Position sense*; the appreciation of passive movement

3 *Recognition of the size, shape, weight and form of objects*

4 *Appreciation of vibration*

5 *Pain*

6 *Temperature sense*

The presence or absence of any abnormal sensations should be noted.

These 'sensory modalities' do not necessarily represent different, discrete sensory functions, but rather are commonly experienced sensations in normal life. Perception depends on a complex physiological interaction of afferent input at many levels in the nervous system and, in some instances, as in the recognition and naming of objects, it depends also on the ability to manipulate the object felt. Perception of vibration, for example, does not depend on a special set of nerve fibres responsible only for transmitting vibration sense to the central nervous system, but rather is a form of sensation subjectively similar to light touch which, in clinical practice, is found to be disturbed when there is a lesion of the large diameter, afferent fibres in the peripheral nerves, posterior columns or, more rarely, at a higher level.

Begin testing sensation with touch and position sense. Use a pin later, when you have gained the patient's confidence. Always apply the sensory stimulus first to an area of impaired sensation and mark out its borders *from the abnormal to the normal*. The patient should readily note the sudden change to normality.

Areas of diminished sensation should be carefully, *but quickly*, mapped out so that their distribution in relation to root lesions, peripheral nerve lesions or lesions in the central nervous system can be studied. It is important to do this quickly, accurately and, as far as possible, without repetition. The longer the time spent on this the more confusing will be the result: it requires great concentration and co-operation from the patient and from the examiner.

Inconsistency in the patient's replies may be due to fatigue, poor co-operation, dementia or undue suggestibility. This can be checked by asking the patient to say 'now' whenever he feels the stimulus, his eyes being shut; by examining a related form of sensation such as temperature sense in the case of pinprick, or position or vibration sense in the case of light touch; or by exhorting the patient to be very careful to make the correct response. Never make much of small differences. Remember that many patients will experience changes in the acuteness or sharpness of a pin between the nail bed and the dorsum of the finger, or at about the level of the clavicle when the stimulus ascends the anterior chest wall. The pulp of the fingers is rather insensitive to pain but very sensitive to light touch and to discriminative tests such as two point discrimination. Vibration sense is best perceived over a bony prominence. On the whole it is better to test sensation with the patient's eyes open although it is, of course, necessary to prevent the patient seeing his fingers and toes when testing position sense. People are usually more alert and attentive with their eyes open than with them shut, and alertness is crucial in sensory testing. During most sensory testing it should not affect the result to have the patient actually watching the procedure. It can be a frightening experience to be suddenly pricked with a pin when one's eyes are closed. Such surprises, which destroy a patient's confidence in the examiner, should always be avoided.

Tactile sensibility

Use a wisp of cotton wool or the tip of your index finger. Ask the patient to indicate whether he feels the touch, and if it feels normal. If not, *how* is it abnormal? It may be abolished or reduced (*hypoaesthesia*), misperceived as a painful, irritating or tingling sensation (*hyperaesthesia*) or mislocalized. Very rarely there may be a delay between the stimulus and its recognition by the patient. Areas of diminished sensation should be carefully delineated and recorded.

The ability to discriminate between two points is tested by the use of blunt dividers. The patient is asked whether he is being touched with one or both points. Normally 2 mm of separation of the points can be recognized as two separate stimuli on the finger tips, and slightly wider separation on the pulps of the toes. This is an excellent objective sensory test which is particularly useful in cases of posterior column or parietal cortical lesions and in some peripheral nerve lesions (such as the carpal tunnel syndrome).

Position sense

Ask the patient to look away or shield his eyes. Explain that you will move his finger (or toe or elbow) up or down and ask him to tell you which way it has been moved. He should be able to recognize movements of only a few degrees at all joints, including knee, ankle, elbow and wrist, in addition to the more commonly tested fingers and toes. It is sometimes helpful to ask the patient to imitate with the opposite limb or digit the position of the limb or digit being tested. It is essential that the patient be relaxed and that he allows the limb to be moved *passively*.

When position sense is disturbed in the upper limbs, the outstretched fingers may twist, rise and fall when held with the eyes closed. These involuntary movements (*pseudo-athetosis*) occur unknown to the patient and disappear almost completely when the patient watches the position of his fingers. Patients with defective position sense may be unable to manipulate small objects, fasten buttons and so on without visually observing their movements (*sensory ataxia*).

The *appreciation of movement* is closely related to the sense of position and can be tested at the same time. Gradually move a digit or limb into a new position, with the patient's eyes closed, and ask him to say 'now' as soon as he recognizes the movement. Note the angle through which the limb was moved. If the appreciation of movement is diminished, this angle is many times greater than that in a normal limb. Movements of less than 10° can be appreciated at all normal joints.

Finally test that the patient can recognize the *direction* of the movement, that is, whether the joint is flexed or extended. Patients can sometimes recognize the occurrence of a movement but not its direction.

Recognition of size, shape, weight and form

These faculties can be tested most accurately in the hands with the eyes closed. To test size, place in the patient's palm objects of the same shape, but of different sizes, for example small rods or matches of different length. Ask him to say which is the larger. The objects should be applied consecutively.

To test recognition of shape familiar objects such as coins, a pencil, a penknife, scissors, etc., are placed in the hand, and the patient is asked to identify them or to describe their form. Loss of this faculty is known as *astereognosis*. It may occur, with parietal lesions, when position sense and light touch are normal, although there is usually some defect in these modalities. When astereognosis occurs with posterior column lesions, position sense, vibration sense and light touch are invariably profoundly disturbed.

Appreciation of vibration

If the foot of a vibrating tuning-fork is placed on the surface of the body the vibrations can be felt, provided they are sufficiently strong. This is a valuable test, as the ability to appreciate vibration may be lost in various diseases, as in tabes dorsalis, in peripheral neuritis and in posterior column disorders. A tuning fork of 128 Hz (middle C) should be used. Vibrations of higher frequency are more difficult to perceive. If the patient perceives the vibration, ask him to say when he ceases to feel it. If the examiner can then still perceive it, the patient's perception of vibration is impaired. There is often some loss of vibration sense in the feet and legs in old age.

Pain

Pain may be evoked either by a cutaneous stimulus, e.g. the prick of a pin, or by pressure on deeper structures, such as muscles or bones. Superficial and pressure pain should be tested separately.

Superficial pain The point of a pin should be used as the stimulus. Care must be taken that the patient distinguishes between the *sharpness* of the point (that is, its relative size) and the *pain* which the prick evokes; it often happens that, even when sensibility to pain is abolished, he can recognize that the stimulus is pointed, and thus confuse the observer by calling it 'sharp'. The pin used should be an ordinary domestic pin, rather than a hypodermic needle; the latter is designed to cut skin relatively painlessly and is thus not suitable for sensory testing.

Pressure pain is examined by squeezing the muscles or the Achilles tendon. Abolition of pressure pain is often the most prominent sensory disturbance in tabes dorsalis.

Absence of sensibility to pain is termed *analgesia*; partial loss of pain sensibility is called *hypoalgesia*; and an exaggerated sensibility, so that even a mild stimulus causes an unnatural degree of painful sensation, is known as *hyperalgesia*. This occurs in some patients with spinal cord disease, for example in tabes dorsalis, and in certain patients with deep-seated parietal or thalamic lesions (thalamic pain). The pain experienced has a peculiar, ill-localized and persistent character. It often has a burning quality and it may occur as an intractable spontaneous phenomenon or only in response to cutaneous stimuli.

Temperature sense

Temperature sense is conveniently examined by using test tubes containing warm and cold water. The part to be tested is touched with each in turn, and the patient says whether each tube feels hot or cold. At the bedside it is often sufficient to use the cold metallic sensation of the touch of the end of an ophthalmoscope or tuning-fork for rough assessment of temperature sensation.

Other disturbances of sensation

Sensory inattention is an important feature of lesions of the parietal lobe; it is demonstrated as follows. The patient is asked to close his eyes. Homologous points on opposite sides of the body are stimulated simultaneously by touch or with pins. The patient is asked to indicate which side, or sides, are touched. In sensory inattention the stimulus on the abnormal side is not perceived. This is also called *sensory extinction* or *sensory neglect*. *Bilateral simultaneous sensory stimuli* can also be used when testing vision and hearing; a similar defect may be found. In the presence of fixed hemisensory loss, of course, the sign is invalid.

Some patients with parietal lesions will also show *spatial summation*, a sensory abnormality in which a stimulus is perceived only if an area of skin larger than a certain critical area is stimulated, or *temporal summation* in which an ill-localized and often perverted or painful sensation is felt after rapidly repeated stimuli. Single stimuli will be missed. These abnormalities are part of a perceptual defect related to *agnosia*, a disorder in which the patient is unaware of the nature or the severity of his sensory disorder. In its most extreme form there may even be denial of illness (*anosognosia*). In patients with higher perceptual defects of this type a number of other bedside tests may be useful. These include *constructional tests* such as the patient's ability to draw a map of his surroundings, to copy a complex figure (for example, two interlocking irregular pentagons), to draw a clock face or a human face, or to draw more complex figures, for example a house. Visual and tactile memory can be tested by variations of these tests. Constructional ability is particularly impaired with right parietal lesions (*constructional apraxia*).

SIGNS OF MENINGEAL IRRITATION

Neck stiffness

The patient is asked to flex his neck as fully as he can to ascertain the degree of movement possible, and then to relax. The examiner then passively flexes the neck. The chin should normally touch the chest without pain.

In meningeal irritation neck flexion causes pain in the neck, sometimes radiating down the back, and the movement is resisted by spasm in the extensor muscles of the neck. Neck rigidity is also caused by diseases of the cervical spine. Head retraction represents an extensive degree of neck rigidity.

Kernig's sign

Kernig's sign is tested with the patient supine on the bed by passively extending the patient's knee when his hip is fully flexed. This movement causes pain

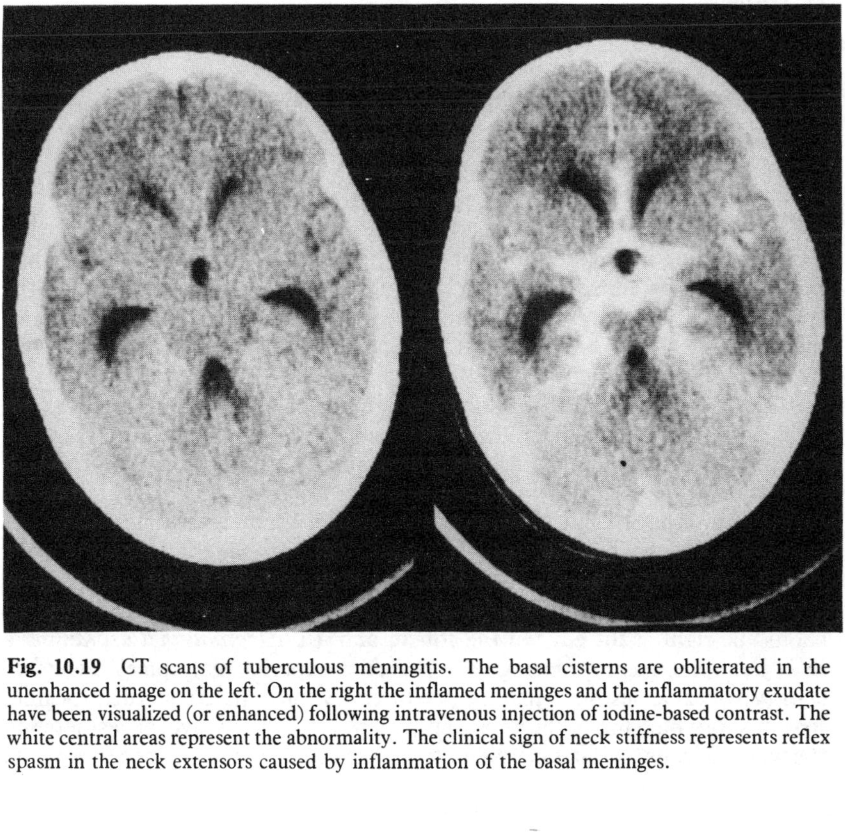

Fig. 10.19 CT scans of tuberculous meningitis. The basal cisterns are obliterated in the unenhanced image on the left. On the right the inflamed meninges and the inflammatory exudate have been visualized (or enhanced) following intravenous injection of iodine-based contrast. The white central areas represent the abnormality. The clinical sign of neck stiffness represents reflex spasm in the neck extensors caused by inflammation of the basal meninges.

and spasm of the hamstrings in meningeal irritation affecting the lower part of the spinal subarachnoid space. It is a less sensitive test than neck stiffness.

These two tests depend upon the fact that stretching the spinal nerve roots in meningeal irritation causes reflex muscular spasm in the paraspinal and sacral muscles. They are both positive in meningitis (Fig. 10.19) and subarachnoid haemorrhage, and also in patients with 'meningism', a state of irritation of the meninges seen most commonly in young children with acute fevers. In some patients with raised intracranial pressure in whom herniation of the cerebellar tonsils into the foramen magnum has occurred, neck stiffness may also be present.

Straight leg raising

This test is used in patients with sciatica. The sciatic nerve and its roots are stretched by passively elevating the patient's extended leg with the hand, which is placed behind the heel. The movement is restricted by sciatic pain when the spinal roots are entrapped as in lumbosacral intervertebral disc protrusion.

SPECIAL INVESTIGATIONS

The following special methods of investigation are in common use.

Lumbar puncture

This procedure is used for obtaining samples of cerebrospinal fluid (CSF) by puncturing the lumbar meninges with a long needle inserted between the spines of two lumbar vertebrae, below the level of the termination of the conus medullaris. It should be carried out under supervision in the first instance. It is performed as follows:

First, always examine the fundi to exclude raised intracranial pressure; lumbar puncture is contraindicated in the presence of raised intracranial pressure because of the risk of consequent transtentorial or tonsillar herniation.

Mark out the 3rd and 4th lumbar spines. The 4th lumbar spine usually lies in the plane of the iliac crests. The puncture may be made through either the 3rd or 4th interspace. The patient should be lying on his side on a firm couch, with the knees and chin as nearly approximated as possible; the patient's back should be right at the edge of the couch, and it is *important that its transverse axis*, i.e. a line passing through the posterior superior iliac spines, *should be vertical*. Local anaesthesia may be produced by injecting 2% sterile procaine, first raising a bleb under the skin, and, when this is insensitive, anaesthetizing the whole dermis. It is not necessary to inject procaine into the deep ligaments;

this procedure usually causes more pain than it relieves. A special needle, containing a withdrawable stylet about 8 cm in length should be used. The stylet should fit accurately and should not protrude through the bevelled cutting edge of the needle.

Push the needle firmly through the skin in the midline or just to one side of it and press it steadily *forwards and slightly towards the head*, the bevel pointing towards the side on which the patient is lying. When the needle is felt to enter the spinal cavity the stylet is withdrawn and the CSF which escapes is collected in 3 sterilized stoppered test tubes. If any blood is present, a marked difference in the amount in the first and subsequent tubes indicates that the blood is due to trauma from the puncture. The patient should lie flat for 8 to 24 hours afterwards, in order to reduce the chance of post-lumbar puncture headache developing.

It is often useful to have a manometer, connectable with the needle, so that the pressure of the fluid can be measured at the time of puncture. For this measurement, the patient's head must be on the same level as his sacrum and he must be breathing quietly and with his muscles relaxed. The neck and legs should *not* be too intensely flexed. The normal CSF pressure is 60 to 150 mm of CSF. The pressure rises and falls a centimetre or two with respiration, and the pulse is also reflected in pressure fluctuations.

Queckenstedt's test can be used to detect a block in the circulation of CSF in the spinal canal, for example in spinal tumours (although if spinal tumour is suspected it is preferable to proceed to myelography without previous lumbar puncture, since the latter may result in deterioration of the patient's signs). With the needle and manometer in position and the patient breathing quietly as described above, an assistant compresses one or other, but not both, jugular veins. This causes a sudden increase in intracranial pressure, which is immediately seen in the manometer as a sudden rise of cerebrospinal fluid pressure, followed by an equally rapid fall when the pressure on the vein is released. A similar sudden rise and fall is seen if the patient is asked to cough and this is a useful check that the needle tip is in free communication with the subarachnoid space. With slight degrees of block in the spinal canal there may be a rise of pressure in the manometer followed by a very slow fall when the pressure on the vein is released; and with more severe block no rise of pressure will be seen when the jugular vein is compressed.

This test should never be carried out in the presence of raised CSF pressure since it may then precipitate transtentorial or tonsillar herniation.

Difficulties with lumbar puncture

The commonest cause of a 'dry-tap', the failure to obtain CSF, is an incorrectly performed puncture, and this is usually due to the patient not being in the correct position. The needle will then not be introduced at right angles to the transverse axis of the back, and will miss the spinal canal.

A common error is to introduce the needle too deeply so that it traverses the spinal canal and wedges against the posterior margin of the intervertebral disc; if the needle is withdrawn slightly CSF will begin to flow. Occasionally, however, a 'dry-tap' is due to a complete block to the flow of CSF through the spinal canal. In this circumstance urgent myelography is required and for this procedure *cisternal puncture* or *lateral cervical puncture* may be required. This should be performed only by an experienced physician or surgeon. It is best undertaken under radiographic control.

Abnormalities of the CSF

Normal CSF is clear and colourless like water. Any yellowness is pathological and is due either to old haemorrhage, jaundice or excess of protein. In *Froin's syndrome* a pronounced yellow colour (xanthochromia) is associated with great excess of protein and the formation of a coagulum. It is a very rare phenomenon. Even slight increases in CSF protein, however, cause a noticeable increase in viscosity of the fluid and an excessive frothiness of its surface when it is gently shaken.

Turbidity of the fluid may be due to the presence of white blood cells, either as a result of infection or of subarachnoid haemorrhage. If it does not clear on standing it is due to micro-organisms.

The presence of *blood* may be due to injury to a vessel by the needle or to subarachnoid haemorrhage. In the latter case the blood is more uniformly mixed with the fluid, and the *supernatant fluid remains yellow after centrifugation*.

Cytological examination of a turbid fluid is of great importance. A centrifugal deposit should be examined with Leishman's stain in order to obtain an idea of the character of the cells present; and by Gram's and Ziehl–Neelsen's methods for bacteria. Cell counts are performed with a counting chamber and must be done immediately the fluid has been collected. Counts done some hours later give inaccurate results because the leucocytes stick together and to the sides of the tube, and endothelial cells break up in a short time. If any clot has formed, an accurate cell count cannot be obtained but the cells in the clot can be stained and examined. Normal fluid contains 2–5 lymphocytes/μl.

An increased cell count may consist of polymorphonuclear cells or lymphocytes. The increased cell count is termed *polymorphonuclear* if these cells are above 75% of the total, or *lymphocytic* if more than 90% are lymphocytes. Bacterial meningitis is associated with a polymorphonuclear pleocytosis, virus meningitis and syphilis with a lymphocytic one, and tuberculous meningitis with either a lymphocytic or a mixed type. The latter is termed *pleocytosis*.

The CSF should also be examined bacteriologically and chemically. Normal cerebrospinal fluid contains only a trace of albumin and hardly any globulin, the *total protein* being not more than 40 mg/dl. In some neurological diseases, particularly in multiple sclerosis and in many acute and subacute virus infections, the globulin fractions in the cerebrospinal fluid are increased.

Table 10.5 Typical changes in the cerebrospinal fluid in various diseases

Disease condition	Physical characteristics	Cytology (cells/μl)	Protein (g/l)	Glucose (mmol/l)	Tests for syphilis	Stained deposit	Culture	Lange curve
Normal	Clear and colourless	Lymphocytes 0–5	0.1–0.4	2.5–4.2	Negative	No organisms	Sterile	0000000000 0000110000
Meningitis								
Bacterial	Yellowish and turbid	Polymorphs 200–2000 Lymphocytes 5–50	0.5–2.0	<2.0	Negative	Bacteria	Positive	0001344310
Tuberculosis	Colourless sometimes viscous	Polymorphs 0–100 Lymphocytes 100–300	>0.5	<2.0*	Negative	Tubercle bacilli in films in some cases	Positive by special methods	0001344310
Viral (includes poliomyelitis)	Usually clear	10–100 mixed cells at first, becoming lymphocytic in 36 hours	0.1–0.6 Poliomyelitis 0.3–0.2, remaining high 6–8 weeks	2.5–4.2	Negative	No organisms	Sterile	0001344310
Multiple sclerosis	Clear and colourless	Rarely 5–15 lymphocytes	0.1–0.6 rarely higher IgG level raised with monoclonal bands	2.5–4.2	Negative	No organisms	Sterile	Paretic type of curve in 50% of cases
Syphilis								
GPI	Clear and colourless	5–100 lymphocytes	0.4–1.0	2.5–4.2	Positive	No organisms	Sterile	5555432100
Tabes	Clear and colourless	5–100 lymphocytes	0.3–0.6	2.5–4.2	20% negative by reagin tests†	No organisms	Sterile	0123210000
Meningeal	Clear and slightly turbid	10–50 polymorphs 50–500 lymphocytes	0.5–2.0	May be slightly low	Positive	No organisms	Sterile	0123210000

* CSF glucose is usually about half the blood glucose. Simultaneous blood and CSF glucose estimations should always be performed.
† Nearly all are positive by FTA-ABS or TPHA.

The *Lange test* takes advantage of this. Varying dilutions of cerebrospinal fluid are mixed in ten tubes with a colloidal gold suspension of constant strength. The degree of precipitation which results is expressed by arbitrary figures 0–5, 0 representing no change and 5 complete precipitation. The CSF IgG concentration can also be directly estimated by immunoelectrophoresis and in many laboratories this estimation has replaced the Lange test. It is often compared with the blood IgG and albumin levels in order to show whether a raised CSF IgG level is due to endogenous IgG synthesis within the central nervous system. Techniques are also available to study the various components of IgG found in the CSF; in multiple sclerosis the abnormal IgG may be oligoclonal.

Glucose is present in normal cerebrospinal fluid in a concentration of 2.5–4.2 mmol/l, which is about a half to a third of the blood glucose concentration. In purulent, tuberculous or fungal meningitis and rarely in carcinomatous meningitis the CSF sugar is *reduced to less than half of the blood glucose*. It is also low if the patient is hypoglycaemic.

One or more of the tests for syphilis are often performed on the cerebrospinal fluid.

The typical changes in the CSF in various neurological diseases are summarized in Table 10.5.

The electroencephalogram (EEG)

Electrodes applied to the patient's scalp pick up small changes of electrical potential, which after amplification are recorded on paper or displayed on a video monitor. The EEG is of particular value in the investigation of epilepsy; it is also used in the localization of cerebral tumours and other expanding intracranial lesions.

The electromyogram (EMG)

Electrical activity occurring in muscle during voluntary contraction, or in denervated muscle during rest, can be recorded with needle electrodes inserted percutaneously into the belly of the muscle, or with surface electrodes (silver discs attached to the skin overlying the muscle with a salty paste), amplified and displayed as an auditory signal through a suitable loudspeaker and as a visual signal on an oscilloscope. They may be recorded on magnetic tape or printed out on a paper recorder. Analysis of such electrical activity is useful in the diagnosis of primary diseases of muscle (*myopathies* and *dystrophies*) and of lower motor neurone lesions (*denervation*).

The speed of conduction of afferent impulses (*sensory nerve conduction velocity*) and efferent impulses (*motor nerve conduction velocity*) in peripheral nerves can be calculated using an electrical nerve stimulation technique and suitable recording electrodes and amplifying or digital averaging equipment.

These measurements are useful in the diagnosis of peripheral nerve disorders, particularly those due to local compressive lesions as, for example, carpal tunnel syndrome.

Neuroradiology

Apart from routine radiographs of the skull and spine a number of special techniques are useful.

Myelography

This is a method for demonstrating the subarachnoid space in the spinal canal. A lumbar or cisternal puncture is performed with the patient on the myelogram table in the X-ray department and 2–10 ml of a special radiopaque contrast medium are injected into the subarachnoid space. By tilting the table the contrast medium can be made to flow up and down the spinal canal under direct vision, preferably using TV amplification; and radiographs can be taken of regions of deformity or obstruction to the flow of contrast. This is a very useful method for accurate localization of tumours in the spinal canal.

Computerized axial tomography (CT scanning)

CT scanning provides tomographic sections of the brain of very high resolution, without the need for invasive procedures. A crystallographic X-ray detection device is used instead of conventional X-ray film and a photographic picture is produced by computerized averaging techniques. The resulting pictures are displayed as sections of the head in the coronal or basal plane (Figs. 10.20 and 10.21). Intravenous or subarachnoid iodine-based contrast may be used to enhance the vascular or CSF compartments respectively.

Similar computer-based tomographic techniques are being developed to image the brain using positron emission from isotopes, or signals derived from the nuclear magnetic resonance properties of protons in brain water.

Angiography

This is a method for studying the intracranial and extracranial vessels. A suitable radiopaque contrast medium is injected percutaneously into a carotid artery in the neck, or into a vertebral artery either by direct puncture or by catheterization of a major vessel such as the femoral, axillary, brachial or subclavian arteries. Radiographs are taken in various planes in the following few seconds as the contrast medium traverses the cerebral circulation. The arterial, capillary and venous circulations can be studied and abnormalities of the distribution, size, position and lumen of these vessels can be seen.

The technique is particularly useful for diagnosis of aneurysms, arterio-

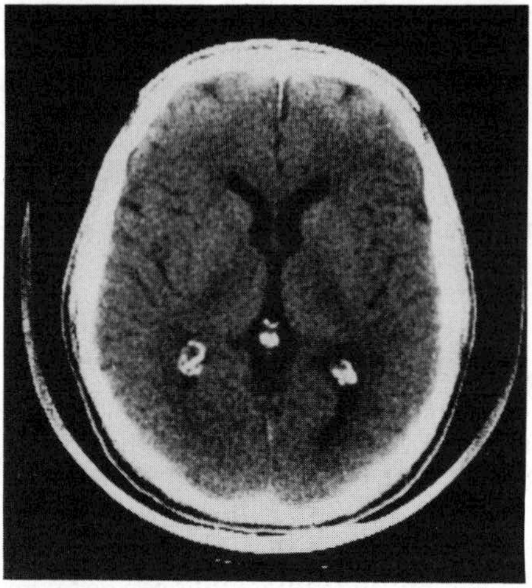

Fig. 10.20 Normal CT scan. The cerebral ventricles, the sulci at the surface of the brain, the central calcified pineal gland and the two calcified parts of the choroid plexus in the posterior parts of the ventricular system are symmetrical between the two sides of the brain. The thickness of the skull is an artefact resulting from the computer processing required to produce the image.

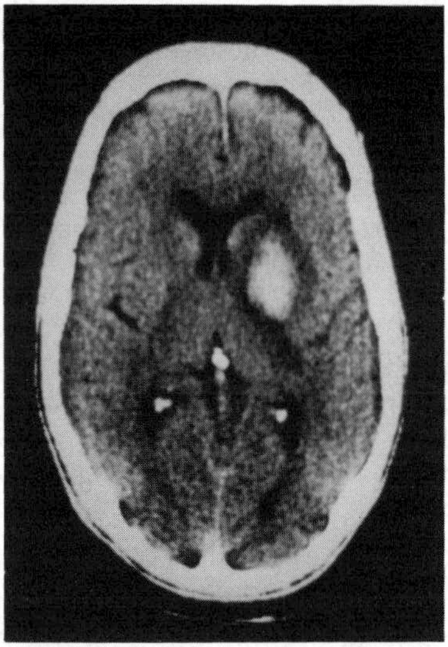

Fig. 10.21 CT scans illustrating lesions in the brain. (a) Left capsular haemorrhage. The haemorrhage appears relatively dense; it is surrounded by a zone of oedema, and has caused displacement of the midline structures to the opposite side. The haemorrhage is in the typical location associated with hypertensive cerebral haemorrhage.

venous malformations and cerebral tumours. It is also useful in cerebral vascular disease. General anaesthesia is usually preferred.

New angiographic techniques include the application of digital averaging so that intravenous contrast injections can be used to visualize circulating contrast in the cerebral and extracranial circulation, thus reducing the risk of the vascular complications of arterial catheterization or puncture.

Diagnostic ultrasound

A pulsed ultrasonic beam is directed through the head in a lateral direction from one temporal region to the other. Reflections are recorded by a second transducer on the same side of the head. The position of the ultrasonic midline can be compared with that of the 3rd ventricular walls and, occasionally, of the walls of the lateral ventricles themselves. A similar ultrasonic technique can be used in infants to produce tomographic scan pictures similar to those produced by X-ray CT scanning.

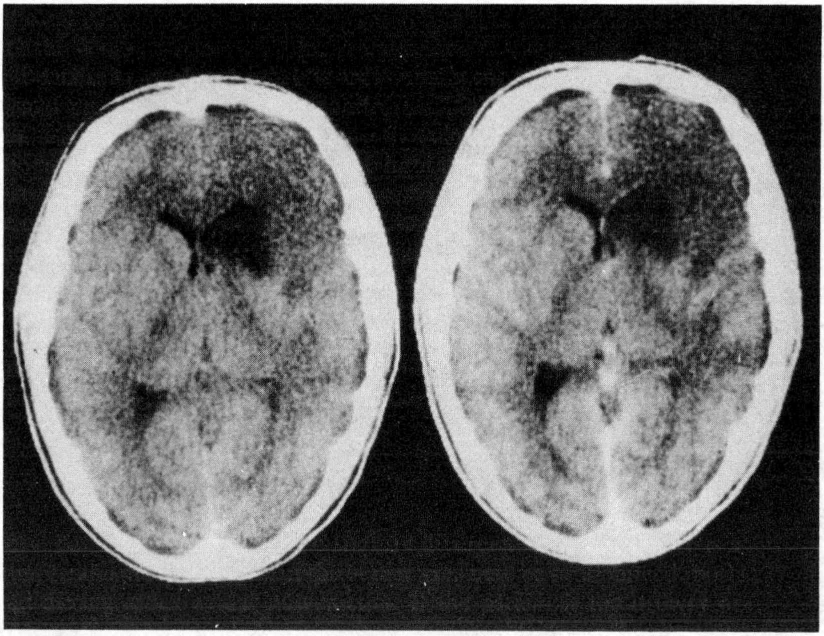

Fig. 10.21 (b) Left frontal infarction. There is a large zone of low density with shift of the midline to the opposite side in these two sequential tomographic images.

ROUTINE EXAMINATION OF THE NERVOUS SYSTEM

A detailed examination of the whole nervous system is time-consuming and something of an ordeal for the patient. A scheme for a quick routine examination is therefore useful in the examination of patients not suspected of neurological disease, in order to exclude major neurological disability.

Mental state

Much useful information can be obtained during history taking and physical examination; no specific questions need usually be asked.

Is the history given *accurately*, *concisely* and *with insight*? Or is the patient *concrete*, *circumlocutory* or *vague*?
Is his *memory* normal?
Is he *neatly dressed* and *well cared for*?
Is his *behaviour* normal?
Is he *aphasic* or *dysarthric*?

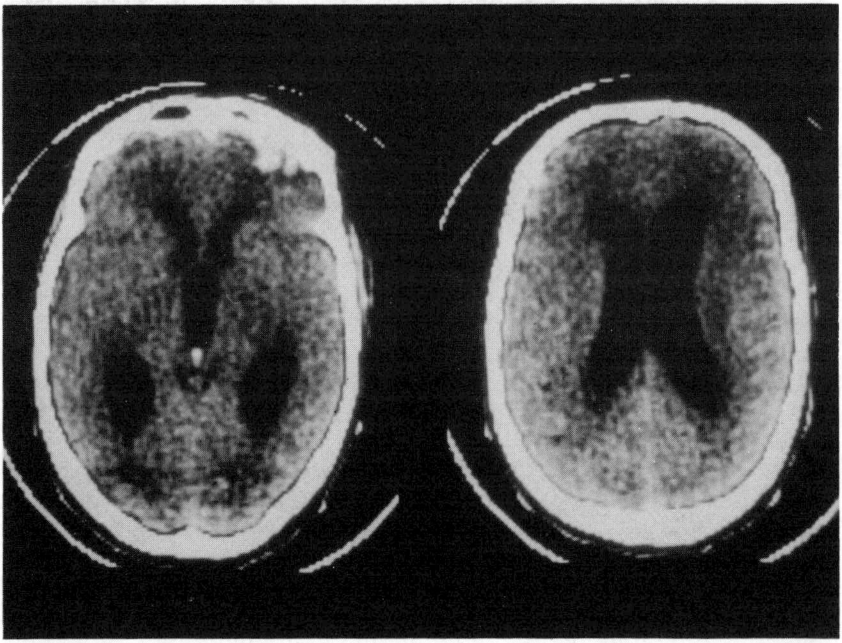

Fig. 10.21 (c) Hydrocephalus. The ventricular system is enlarged and there are periventricular lucent zones, due to oedema or seepage of CSF into the cerebral white matter in these regions, indicating that the hydrocephalus is progressing (decompensated hydrocephalus).

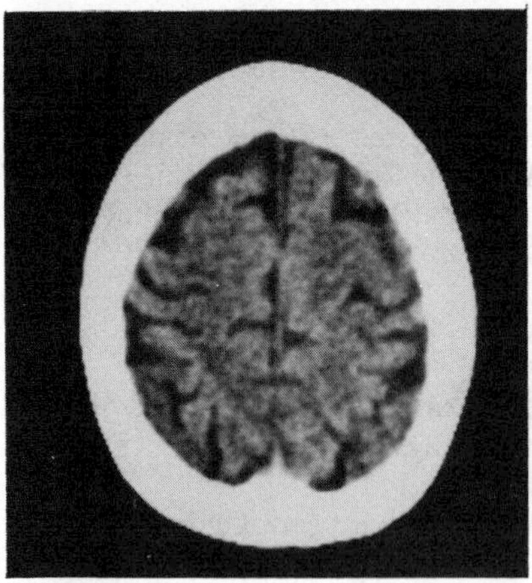

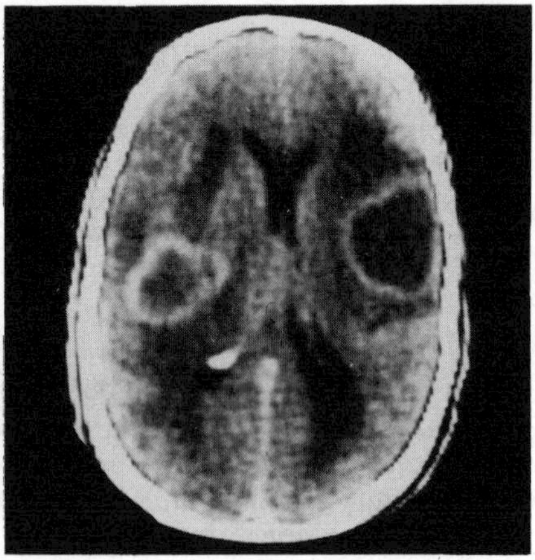

Fig. 10.21 (d) (left) Cerebral atrophy. The sulci are enlarged and prominent. This is a feature of dementia but occurs in many other disorders and may also be found in clinically normal elderly people.

Fig. 10.21 (e) (right) In this CT scan, taken after the intravenous administration of contrast, two metastases from carcinoma of the bronchus can be seen. There is oedema, shown by relatively low brain density, near the two lesions. Both metastases show ring-like enhancement in their periphery with relatively more lucent, perhaps necrotic, centres.

Is he *confused*?
Can he *find his way* in and out of the room?
Can he *dress* and *undress* himself?

Gait

Is it *spastic, hemiparetic, ataxic* or *parkinsonian*?
Is there a *foot drop*?

Cranial nerves

Test *ocular movements* and look for nystagmus.
Test *facial movements*.
Test *tongue protrusion* and *palatal movement*.

Visual fields

These, like aphasia, may provide absolute evidence of disease above the tentorium cerebelli.

Is there a *hemianopia*?
If so, is it *homonymous, bitemporal, unilateral* or something else?
Is *central vision* normal? This is crudely assessed by testing the visual acuity.
Can he read small print with or without glasses?

Fundi

Is *papilloedema* present?
Is *optic atrophy* present?
Are there *hypertensive, uraemic* or *diabetic* changes present?

Motor

Is there any *weakness* of the outstretched upper limbs?
Is there *distal or proximal weakness* or *wasting*?
Is *muscular tone* normal, spastic or extrapyramidal in type?
Look for *cerebellar ataxia* in the limbs.
Assess the *tendon reflexes* and *plantar responses*.

Sensory

Test *position sense* in the fingers and toes and vibration sense in the feet (posterior columns).

Test *pin-prick* in the four limbs and on the face (lateral spinothalamic tracts).

Light touch need only be tested if the patient complains of numbness.

General

Examine the *skull, spinal movements* and *posture*.
Look for *cutaneous naevi*.
Listen for *bruits in the neck*.

11
The unconscious patient

Coma is a common medical problem. Diagnosis can usually be accomplished at the bedside, provided attention is given to both the history and examination. In this chapter clinical methods relevant to diagnosis of the comatose patient will be described.

Consciousness is a state of normal cerebral activity in which the patient is aware of himself and of his environment and is able to respond to changes both within himself, for example hunger, and in his environment. *Sleep*, although a state of altered consciousness, is obviously a normal variation in consciousness. The sleeping patient can be roused, both spontaneously and in response to external stimuli, to a full state of wakefulness. Altered consciousness resulting from brain disease may take the form of a *confusional state*, in which the patient is alert but agitated, frightened, and disorientated in time, space and person. Such patients usually show evidence of misperception of their environment, and hallucinations and delusions may occur. Confusional states must be carefully distinguished from aphasia, in which a specific disorder of language is the characteristic feature, and from continuous temporal lobe epilepsy, a form of focal status epilepticus in which the behavioural disorder is often accompanied by aphasia if the epileptic focus is left-sided. Usually this can be recognized by the occurrence of frequent but slight myoclonic jerks of facial and especially, perioral muscles and by variability in the patient's confusion from moment to moment during the examination. *The examiner should always pause and observe an unconscious patient for a few moments before disturbing him.*

A state of abnormal drowsiness is often found in patients with space-occupying intracranial lesions or metabolic disorders before stupor or coma supervenes. The patient appears to be in normal sleep but cannot be easily wakened and, once awake, tends to fall asleep despite attempts to continue conversation or clinical examination. Further, while awake such patients can usually be shown to be disorientated; higher intellectual function, such as the ability to perform abstract tasks or to make judgements, is disturbed. By *stupor* is meant a state of disturbed consciousness from which only vigorous external stimuli can produce arousal. Arousal from stupor is invariably both brief and incomplete. In *coma* the patient is unrousable and unresponsive to all external stimuli. It is sometimes helpful to recognize states of light and deep coma to indicate the degree of abnormality in patients in whom coma is becoming progressively deeper, but this distinction is necessarily difficult to define.

The objective of examination of the unconscious patient is to achieve a diagnosis and so to plan management. Coma may be due either to metabolic or structural disease of the brain; it is only very rarely a psychogenic disorder. Coma results from lesions affecting the brain widely, diffusely or multifocally, and from lesions of deep centrally placed structures in the diencephalon or brain stem (Table 11.1). For example, supratentorial mass lesions, such as tumours, may damage deep diencephalic structures, while subtentorial neoplasms may directly damage the brain stem reticular formation. Metabolic disorders, for example hypoglycaemia, hypnotic drugs or hypoxia, widely depress brain function. It is important to distinguish supratentorial from subtentorial space-occupying lesions because coma due to the former has a better prognosis.

Table 11.1 Outline of causes of coma

Metabolic	*Structural*
drug overdosage (including alcohol)	meningitis
hypoglycaemia	encephalitis
diabetes mellitus	other infections (e.g. cerebral malaria)
renal failure	subarachnoid haemorrhage
hepatic failure	epilepsy
hypothermia	head injury
hypothyroidism	pituitary apoplexy
cardio-respiratory failure	hypertensive encephalopathy
hypoxic encephalopathy	

Supratentorial lesions	*Subtentorial lesions*
cerebral haemorrhage	cerebellar haemorrhage
cerebral infarction with oedema	pontine haemorrhage
subdural haematoma	brain stem infarction
extradural haematoma	tumour
tumour	cerebellar abscess
cerebral abscess	secondary effects of transtentorial herniation of brain due to cerebral mass lesions

HISTORY

The history is of very great importance and attempts should always be made to find family or other witnesses of the onset of the coma. Coma occurs suddenly in vascular disorders such as subarachnoid haemorrhage or stroke, especially with cerebral or cerebellar haemorrhage. A history of trauma with concussion followed a few days later by fluctuating drowsiness and stupor, suggesting subdural haematoma, should never be regarded lightly. Concussion followed by a brief lucid interval before rapidly deepening coma suggests extradural haematoma. A history of headache before coma supervenes is frequent in patients with intracranial space-occupying lesions of any cause. Seizures of recent onset, whether focal or generalized, strongly suggest cerebral disease, which may be due to tumour, encephalitis, abscess or trauma. Patients with drug-induced coma may be known by neighbours, family, medical attendants or the ambulance driver to have taken drugs by the presence of drug containers or alcohol in their homes. A history of depression might be known. A search of the patient's clothing may reveal hospital outpatient attendance cards, unfilled prescriptions, drugs or even syringes. Diabetic or epileptic patients sometimes carry some form of identification either in their clothing or as a wristband or necklace. *If there is any suspicion whatsoever that the patient might by hypoglycaemic, a blood sample should be taken for blood glucose estimation and then 20 g of 50% glucose given intravenously, before any diagnostic tests are undertaken.* Hypoglycaemia is characterized by a stupor or coma from which the patient can be roused to a resentful and aggressive state of partial awareness, with pallor and sweatiness, bounding pulse, and often focal or generalized seizures. It is important to try to discover whether the coma was of gradual or sudden onset; the latter clearly suggests vascular disease. Before examination commences the doctor must make sure that the patient is breathing adequately, that the pulse and blood pressure are satisfactory and that the patient is not bleeding rapidly. If oxygenation is not satisfactory, whatever the breathing pattern, oxygen should be administered. If the patient is clearly in status epilepticus this must be treated appropriately immediately, and clinical examination continued afterwards.

GENERAL EXAMINATION

Certain general features of the patient's clinical state are of great importance. Does the patient appear clean, well nourished and generally cared for, or are there signs of social decline such as a dishevelled appearance, lack of personal cleanliness, malnutrition or infestation? Is there evidence of trauma or exposure? A rapid search must be made for fractures and, especially, for signs of cranial trauma. Bruises in the scalp are difficult to recognize but scalp oedema or haematoma can usually be palpated and bruising of the skin behind the pinna, called a 'battle' sign, is a useful sign of basal or temporal skull fracture. Likewise, bleeding from the external auditory meati is a reliable sign of cranial trauma, with basal skull fracture. Pallor, circulatory failure and other evidence of shock must be recognized and a search made for external or internal haemorrhage, especially if trauma is suspected. In drug-induced coma there may be signs of repeated intravenous injections under conditions of imperfect sterility, causing venous thrombosis in forearm or antebrachial veins. The odours of alcohol, uraemia, diabetic acidosis and hepatic coma may be recognizable in rare instances. The stertorous, rapid respiration of acidotic coma (air hunger), usually due to diabetes, can be quickly recognized (see below). The presence of jaundice, liver palms, Dupuytren's contracture or spider naevi, even in the absence of hepatic enlargement, raises the suspicion of hepatic coma. Meningitis can usually be recognized by the presence of drowsiness, lethargy or stupor with fever and signs of meningeal irritation (p. 343). The pulse may be unexpectedly slow in relation to the fever in pyogenic meningitis, although the respirations are usually rapid. Seizures and focal neurological signs may develop and there is usually a history of headache and neck stiffness, perhaps with vomiting. Further, there may be a skin rash, or a primary site of infection such as otitis media or sinusitis may be apparent. The ocular fundi must always be examined by ophthalmoscopy for signs of papilloedema, retinal haemorrhages or exudates, or intra-arterial emboli, which appear as luminescent, highly refractile yellow or white plaque-like material occluding vessels.

Consciousness

Examination of the unconscious patient should be directed towards defining the state of consciousness, as described above, particularly noting any variation or tendency to improve or deteriorate during the period of observation. *Change in level of consciousness is the single most important piece of information which will indicate the need for a change of management* (see Table 11.2, p. 364). It is important to note exactly the *degree of responsiveness to external stimuli*, including conversation, calling the patient's first name, a sudden loud noise, a flash of light, contactual or painful stimulation, passive movement of the limbs and deep noxious stimuli such as squeezing the Achilles tendon, sternal pressure applied with a hard blunt object or supra-orbital pressure from the examiner's thumb. Special attention must also be directed to *pupillary reaction and ocular movements*, both volitional and reflex, to the *pattern of breathing* and to *motor responses*, either spontaneous or reflexly evoked.

Pupils

Pupillary size and responsiveness to light should be noted. If the pupils are unequal a decision as to which is the abnormal must be made. Usually the large pupil indicates the presence of an oculomotor nerve palsy, whether from damage to the oculomotor nerve from pressure and displacement, or from a lesion in the mesencephalon itself, but occasionally the smaller pupil may be the abnormal pupil from a Horner's syndrome. If the larger pupil does not react to light it is likely that there is a partial oculomotor nerve palsy on that side. If the smaller pupil also fails to react to light this may be the mid-position pupil of complete sympathetic and parasympathetic lesions, indicating very extensive brain stem damage. Pupillary dilation in response to neck flexion or to pinching the skin of the neck is not a reliable phenomenon.

In drug-induced coma and in most patients with metabolic coma the pupillary responses to light are normal. Exceptions to this rule are glutethimide poisoning and very deep metabolic coma, in which the pupils may become dilated and, rarely, may become unreactive to light. In pontine and in thalamic haemorrhage the pupils may be very small, like a pin point, and unreactive to light.

Ocular movements

In comatose patients the eyes become slightly divergent at rest. If there is a pre-existent strabismus, deviation of the ocular axes may be pronounced, both at rest and during reflex ocular movements. If the patient is too drowsy or stuporose to test voluntary or following eye movements *'doll's head' movements* should be tested. If possible the patient should be placed on his back, although the test can be carried out in any position. The examiner grasps the patient's head with both hands, using the thumbs to gently hold the eyelids open, and firmly rocks the patient's head from side to side through about 70°, and then from passive neck flexion to passive neck extension. The patient's eyes tend to remain in the straight ahead position despite these passive movements of the head, a phenomenon like that found in some children's dolls. The patient's eyes tend to deviate in the opposite direction to the induced head movement. This movement depends on intact vestibular reflex mechanisms, and is thus a test of the peripheral sense organs involved, the labyrinths and otoliths, and their central connections in the brain stem, including the vestibular nuclei, the medial longitudinal fasciculi and the oculomotor, trochlear and abducent nerves and their nuclei. Sometimes lesions in these structures can be recognized during the doll's head test by the presence of disturbances in ocular movements consistent, for example, with an abducent or oculomotor nerve palsy. Absence of the reflex on one side indicates an ipsilateral pontine lesion, but complete absence of doll's head movements may be found with both extensive structural lesion in the brain stem and in deep metabolic coma. In most patients with drug-induced coma, however, doll's-head ocular movements are intact.

Caloric reflexes may similarly be used as a test of brain stem function. Irrigation of the external auditory meatus on one side with at least 20 ml of ice-cold water induces slow conjugate deviation of the eyes towards the irrigated side after a few seconds' delay. In the awake or drowsy patient this slow, tonic, deviation is masked by a fast, coarse nystagmus towards the opposite side. Normal caloric nystagmus is characteristically also found in cases of psychogenic coma. After a few minutes' delay the opposite ear should also be tested. It is important to inspect the tympanic membrane on each side *before* irrigating the external auditory meatus since it is unwise to perform this test in the presence of a large perforation, or if there is an active otitis media.

Occasionally, in patients with infarction or other structural lesions in the posterior fossa *spontaneous ocular movements* may be observed. These may be accompanied by marked ocular divergence, sometimes with elevation of one eye and depression of the other. Rarely there may be a spontaneous 'see-saw' nystagmus in which one eye rotates up and the other down, the movements alternating at a very slow rate. Rapid ocular oscillations may occur especially after poisoning with tricyclic antidepressant drugs, and a slow, once or twice a second, conjugate downward bobbing movement is sometimes a sign of cerebellar haemorrhage or tumour. In thalamic haemorrhage the pupils are pin point, and the eyes seem to be looking downward as if at the patient's own nose. Rapid conjugate lateral movement, at a rhythm and rate reminiscent of cerebellar nystagmus, occurring in an unconscious patient should suggest focal motor seizures originating in the contralateral frontal lobe. Such seizures are often accompanied by deviation of the head and eyes in the direction of the 'nystagmoid movement', but not necessarily by a fully developed focal seizure involving face and limbs on the same side. Nystagmus itself cannot occur in the comatose patient because it requires ocular fixation to develop the fast, corrective phase.

Pattern of breathing

Depressed, but regular breathing at a normal rate occurs in most drug-induced comas, but Cheyne–Stokes respiration can occur in coma of any cause, especially if there is coincidental chronic pulmonary disease. In Cheyne–Stokes respiration, breathing varies in regular cycles. A phase of gradually deepening respiration is followed, after a period of very deep rapid breaths, by a phase of slowly decreasing respiratory excursion and rate. Respiration gradually becomes quieter and may cease for several seconds before the cycle is repeated (see Chapter 8). Deep sighing, rapid breathing at a regular rate should immediately suggest metabolic acidosis. Diabetic ketoacidosis or uraemia are the commonest causes of this acidotic (Kussmaul) breathing pattern, but a similar pattern may occur in some patients with respiratory failure, and in deep metabolic coma, especially hepatic coma. Deep, regular breathing may also occur with rostral brain stem damage, whether due to reticular pontine infarction or to central brain stem dysfunction secondary to transtentorial herniation associated with an intra- or extracerebral space-occupying lesion. This breathing pattern is called *central neurogenic (pontine) hyperventilation*. Interspersed deep sighs or yawns may precede the development of this respiratory pattern. Rapid shallow breathing occurs if central brain stem dysfunction extends more caudally to the lower pons. When medullary respiratory neurones are damaged, for example by progressive transtentorial herniation, irregular breathing (*ataxic respiration*) may develop. Irregular, slow, deep, gasping respirations, sometimes associated with hiccups, suggest terminal medullary failure. In patients with raised intracranial pressure, these abnormal breathing patterns are often associated with other evidence of brain stem dysfunction, including a rising blood pressure, a slow pulse, flaccid limbs, absence of reflex ocular movements and dilation of the pupils.

It should be apparent from the foregoing descriptions that changing patterns of respiration in an unconscious patient, particularly the development of central neurogenic hyperventilation, provide important and relatively objective evidence of deterioration. It must be recognized, however, that these changes in respiratory pattern may occur in structural lesions with raised intracranial pressure, in brain stem infarction and in some varieties of metabolic coma, especially hepatic coma. They are thus indicative of brain stem dysfunction, but not of its causation.

Motor responses

It is often difficult to elicit signs of focal cerebral disease in the unconscious patient. If progressive brain stem dysfunction from raised intracranial pressure with transtentorial herniation has occurred, focal signs indicative of the causative lesion may no longer be recognizable. However, papilloedema is usually present in such cases. In the drowsy or stuporose patient it may be possibly to recognize a hemianopia by testing to menace or, sometimes, by testing for optokinetic nystagmus (p. 304). Visual threat, or menace, consists of testing the patient's face, in first the left, and then the right field. Normally this threat induces rapid eye closure or a flinch. It is necessary to obtain the patient's attention transiently to assess any meaningful response and the test is, unfortunately, only rarely useful. Hemiplegia may be evident either from abnormal flaccidity of the arm and leg on the affected side or, in the stuporose or lightly comatose patient, by absence of spontaneous movements on that side. Noxious stimuli, for example pinching the skin of the forearms and thighs, deep rubbing pressure with a hard object applied to the sternum or, often most effective, lightly pricking the skin and mucous membranes near the nasal orifices on both sides will fail to induce movement of the paralysed limbs. Sometimes in a patient with a dense hemiplegia the cheek blows flaccidly in and out with each breath on the side of the hemiplegia. The tendon reflexes may be asymmetrical, but in most comatose patients both plantar responses are extensor (see p. 330). It should be noted that *asymmetry* of these motor responses is the important feature to assess.

In both structural lesions and metabolic disorders coma may be accompanied in its terminal stages by decorticate or decerebrate postures. These may occur asymmetrically and may be apparent, at first, only when induced by noxious external stimuli, such as deep sternal pressure or pinching the skin or Achilles tendon. Decorticate and decerebrate postures are features of severe upper brain stem dysfunction and are thus usually found in association with pupillary abnormalities, absence of doll's head and caloric reflexes and a disturbed breathing pattern. Decerebrate and decorticate postures are found much more commonly with structural coma than with metabolic coma, and thus do not usually occur in patients with drug-induced coma unless there has been additional hypoxic or ischaemic brain injury.

DIAGNOSIS OF BRAIN DEATH

With the advent of improved methods of intensive care, and especially of positive pressure ventilation in patients in whom spontaneous respirations have ceased, it has become important to define new criteria for the diagnosis of death. This has become important not only because of general recognition that brain death may have occurred in certain patients whose respiration has been maintained with a ventilator, although both the body temperature and the systemic circulation continue to be maintained spontaneously, but also because it has become possible to transplant organs, for example the kidney, from such patients to others. In both these situations the *diagnosis of brain death must be certain* before any decision is made to cease attempts to keep the patient alive. A conference of the Royal Colleges and Faculties of the United Kingdom considered this problem in 1976 in the light of previous attempts to define brain death, the changing needs of medical practice, and public concern about the issue, and agreed the following guidelines.

A Conditions under which the diagnosis of brain death should be considered.

- **1** The patient is deeply comatose.
  - **a** There should be no suspicion that this state is due to depressant drugs.
  - **b** Primary hypothermia as a cause of coma should have been excluded.
  - **c** Metabolic & endocrine disturbances that can be responsible for or can contribute to coma should have been excluded.
- **2** The patient is being maintained on a ventilator because spontaneous respiration had previously become inadequate or had ceased altogether.
  - **a** Relaxants . . . & other drugs should have been excluded as a cause of respiratory failure.
- **3** There should be no doubt that the patient's condition is due to irremediable structural brain damage. The diagnosis of a disorder that can lead to brain death should have been fully established.

B Diagnostic tests for confirmation of brain death

ALL BRAIN STEM REFLEXES ARE ABSENT

1. The pupils are fixed in diameter & do not respond to sharp changes in the intensity of incident light.
2. There is no corneal reflex.
3. The vestibulo-ocular reflexes are absent.
4. No motor responses within the cranial-nerve distribution can be elicited by adequate stimulation of a somatic area.
5. There is no gag reflex or reflex response to bronchial stimulation by a suction catheter passed down the trachea.
6. No respiratory movements occur when the patient is disconnected from the mechanical ventilator for long enough to ensure that the arterial carbon dioxide tension rises above the threshold for stimulation of respiration. In practice this is best achieved by ventilating the patient with 5% CO_2 in oxygen for five minutes before disconnection. This ensures a $PaCO_2$ of 8.0 kPa (60 mm Hg). A period of 10 minutes' observation for respiratory movement should then be carried out.

C Other considerations

1. Repetition of testing
   The interval between tests must depend upon the primary pathology & the clinical course of the disease . . . In some conditions the outcome is not so clearcut, and in these cases it is recommended that the tests should be repeated. The interval between tests depends upon the progress of the patient & might be as long as 24 hours . . .
2. Integrity of spinal reflexes
   It is well established that spinal-cord function can persist after insults that irretrievably destroy brain stem functions . . .
3. Confirmatory investigation
   It is now widely accepted that electroencephalography is not necessary for the diagnosis of brain death . . . Other investigations such as cerebral angiography or cerebral blood-flow measurements are not required for the diagnosis of brain death.
4. Body temperature
   . . . it is recommended that it should be not less than 35°C before the diagnostic tests are carried out.
5. Specialist opinion & the status of the doctors concerned.
   Only when the primary diagnosis is in doubt is it necessary to consult with a neurologist or neurosurgeon.
   Decision to withdraw artificial support should be made after all the criteria presented above have been fulfilled & can be made by any of the following combination of doctors:
   - **a** a consultant who is in charge of the case & one other doctor;
   - **b** in the absence of a consultant, his deputy, who should have been registered for 5 years or more & who should have had adequate experience in the care of such cases, & one other doctor.

(From The Lancet 1976, 2, 1069–1070)

These recommendations fall into three groups, parts A, B and C. The patient must be deeply comatose and on a ventilator, and it must be clearly established that the patient's coma is due to *irremediable structural brain damage* (part A). Drug-induced coma, hypothermia and metabolic causes of coma and relaxant drugs must have been clearly excluded as a cause of ventilatory failure. If these conditions are fulfilled brain death may be diagnosed if no brain stem reflexes can be demonstrated (part B). Repeated tests are necessary but the interval between such tests depends on the pathology and the course of the disease. Purely spinal reflexes can persist after total brain stem destruction but it must always be remembered that decorticate and decerebrate postures are far from necessarily irreversible phenomena and therefore that their presence does not inevitably indicate that brain death has occurred. Indeed, many authorities would not allow a diagnosis of brain death if such reflexes persisted. All these tests should be carried out at a body temperature not less than 35°C.

Electroencephalographic and other studies, such as angiography, are not necessary for diagnosis of brain death but absence of brain electrical activity in an electroencephalogram, recorded for not less than 20 minutes at an amplification of 5 μV/cm provides very strong confirmatory evidence of cerebral death, provided that depressant drugs have not been given. In the past, it has been recommended that such an isoelectric electroencephalogram should be recorded twice not less than six hours apart before brain death is diagnosed, but this is no longer regarded as necessary in the United Kingdom. It is recommended that at least two doctors, one registered for not less than five years, should be concerned in the diagnosis of brain death before a decision to withdraw artificial support is made.

Table 11.2 The Glasgow coma scale

Eye opening	Verbal response	Motor response
Spontaneous	Orientated	Obeying
To speech	Confused	Localizing
To pain	Inappropriate	Flexing
None	Incomprehensible	Extending
	None	None

The three categories of information required in this assessment require no special skills and are thus particularly suited for observations to be carried out serially in a patient after a head injury, for example by relatively untrained staff.

12
The ear, nose and throat

As a description of the examination of the ears, nose and throat must necessarily consider each of these areas in isolation, it is important to appreciate that these structures are closely interrelated and that disease in one area may be due, in part, to pathology elsewhere. For example, a patient with discharge from the ear and a perforation of the tympanic membrane may have underlying nasal or sinus disease or a persistent upper respiratory tract infection. Failure to appreciate this may lead to a less than comprehensive examination and thus prejudice successful treatment.

THE EAR

There are five major symptoms of ear disease. These are deafness, a sensation of inappropriate noise in the ear (tinnitus), aural pain (otalgia), aural discharge (otorrhoea), and a sensation of abnormal movement (vertigo). Often these symptoms overlap but, for descriptive purposes, it is convenient to consider them individually.

Deafness is a serious social handicap. The history should record whether one or both ears are affected and whether the loss is progressive, constant or fluctuant. The mode of onset of the hearing loss and the rate of progression should also be noted. Usually, deafness is insidious and slowly progressive, but occasionally the patient describes an acute onset and rapid progression of symptoms, which demands urgent investigation if the hearing is to be preserved. Fluctuations in deafness occur in many disorders, e.g. wax impaction, serous otitis media and endolymphatic hydrops.

Useful clues to the site of dysfunction may be obtained by noting the characteristics of the remaining hearing. For instance, the patient with a pure conductive loss will retain good discrimination and will hear well provided the intensity of sound received in the ear is raised. Such patients typically do well with a hearing aid. On the other hand, the patient with a cochlear hearing loss may complain of distortion of sound even amounting to pain in the ear, a phenomenon called *recruitment*, which results from damage to the specialized neuroepithelium of the organ of Corti.

Any hearing loss may be accompanied by *tinnitus*. This is defined as a sensation of sound in the absence of an appropriate auditory stimulus, and may be a feature of pathology at any level within the auditory mechanism. Characteristically, tinnitus is particularly severe in the absence of background noise and may so disturb the patient at night that he finds sleep difficult.

Otorrhoea is a symptom of inflammatory disease within the ear. Common causes of inflammation include infection in the external ear (otitis externa) or middle ear cleft (otitis media). The nature of the discharge may give a clue to the correct diagnosis. A discharge offensive to the patient or his relatives suggests chronic infection.

Since inflammatory changes cause pain, *otalgia* is commonly associated with otorrhoea. Severe otalgia accompanies infection of the pinna (perichrondritis) or localized infection of the external meatus due to furunculosis, because in these conditions pus or fluid is present under tension. Similar severe pain also accompanies acute suppurative otitis media, although infants may present with high fever and malaise without pain. In addition to these local causes, it is important to remember that otalgia may equally well be a referred symptom, e.g. from abnormalities of the teeth, temporomandibular joints, laryngopharynx or cervical spine.

Vertigo is the cardinal symptom of a vestibular disorder. It is important to appreciate that true vertigo involves an hallucination of movement, especially rotation, swaying or tilting. The examiner should seek to separate vertigo from the more common but less disabling complaint of 'light headedness', which may be due to a variety of unrelated causes, e.g. anaemia, hypoglycaemia, fever, cardiac insufficiency and anxiety. It is also important to realize that vertigo is usually due to a peripheral lesion, i.e. of the semicircular canals, labyrinth, Scarpa's ganglion or vestibular nerve. Cerebral lesions, i.e. of the vestibular nuclei and their central connecting tracts, usually cause loss of balance or ataxia (see pp. 313 and 332).

Past history

The past medical history is always important. The obstetric history is relevant when deafness is suspected in early infancy. It is particularly important to elicit a history of maternal contact with infectious diseases such as rubella, mumps or measles, or of administration of ototoxic drugs to the mother during the first trimester. Postnatal jaundice may also cause deafness due to the deposition of conjugated bilirubin in brain stem nuclei, and deafness may follow birth trauma or anoxic episodes in the neonatal period.

In adults the past history should include details of any previous inflammatory conditions and otological operations. Any history of previous head injury is also relevant since trauma may have damaged the middle ear structures and the vestibular apparatus.

Other important causes of deafness include blast injuries, excessive noise exposure or ototoxic drugs. Excessive noise exposure may consist of either excess impulse or steady state noise. Factory workers, engineers, gunners and pop musicians are particularly at risk. Ototoxic drugs include salicylates, quinine, cytotoxic drugs and some diuretics and antibiotics (especially aminoglycosides).

Finally, the family history may reveal a hereditary cause for deafness, and this is best recorded by drawing a family tree. The commonest example is conductive hearing loss caused by fixation of the stapedial footplate in *otosclerosis*, which is inherited as an autosomal dominant trait with varying penetrance. Dominantly inherited sensorineural deafness presenting in adult life, due to degeneration of the stria vascularis, is also common. Congenital deafness, affecting one per thousand livebirths, is also frequently hereditary. Numerous syndromes have been described, some associated with obvious congenital malformations of the ear.

Examination

Start with a careful inspection of the pinna (cartilaginous auricle) and the surrounding scalp. Then examine the external meatus and tympanic membranes. Good illumination and some degree of magnification are essential. These may be provided either by using a head mirror (with reflected light) and an aural speculum with an attached magnifying lens (Siegel's speculum: Fig. 12.1), or by using an auriscope (Fig. 12.2). Either method is acceptable, although the former system does require greater dexterity.

Trauma to the ear canal is avoided by straightening the contours of the meatus by gently pulling the pinna. In adults the pinna should be pulled upwards and backwards towards the occiput; in young children the different obliquity of the canal requires that the pinna is pulled in a horizontal and backward direction to achieve the same effect. The auriscope should be held like a pen between thumb and index finger with the ulnar border of the hand resting gently against the side of the patient's head (Fig. 12.2). Used in this way, any sudden movement will cause equal movement of the instrument, so the speculum is less likely to dig into the meatal skin and cause pain.

After insertion of the largest speculum that the ear will comfortably take, the external meatus and tympanic membranes can be inspected. The normal tympanic membrane has a translucent greyish appearance. Its structure is shown in Fig. 12.3. As the membrane lies obliquely to the ear canal and the curvature of the bony meatus is variable, it may be difficult to see all of the membrane; the antero-inferior margin may be hidden from view. If the examiner is in any doubt, the annulus is most easily identified by following the

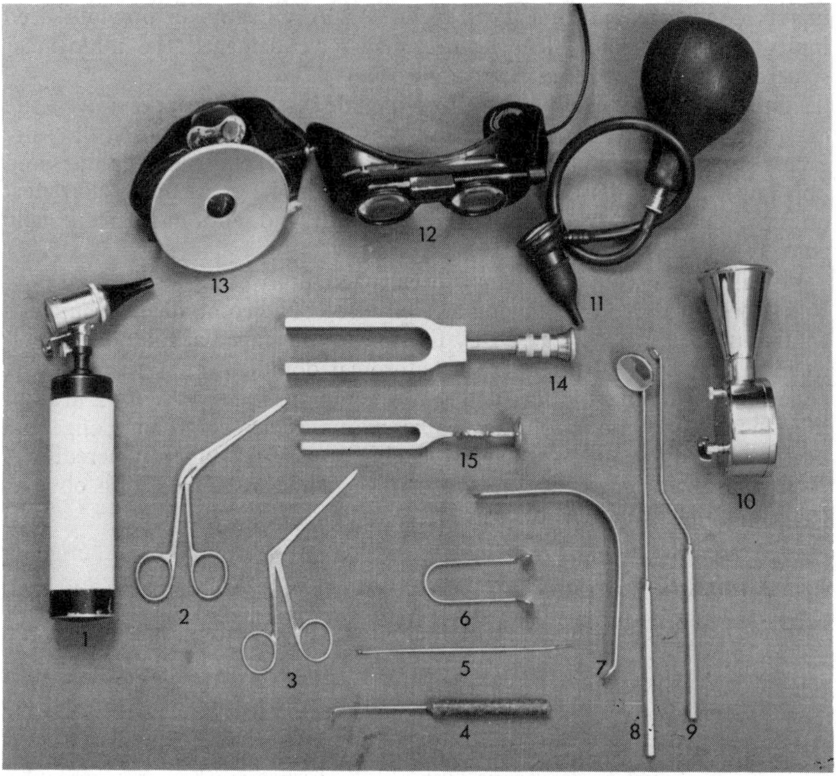

Fig. 12.1 Instruments used in examination of the ear, nose and throat. Key 1: Auriscope; 2: Dressing forceps; 3: Crocodile forceps; 4: Cerumen hook; 5: Jobson Horne probe; 6: Thudichum's nasal speculum; 7: Lack's tongue depressor; 8: Laryngeal mirror; 9: St Clair Thomson postnasal mirror; 10: Bárány noise box; 11: Siegel's speculum; 12: Frenzel's glasses; 13: Head mirror; 14, 15: Tuning forks.

floor of the meatus and identifying the membrane and its margin at this point.

Finally, membrane mobility should be assessed by observing the drum whilst blowing air into the meatus from the bellows of a Siegel's speculum or by a similar pneumatic device attached to an electric auriscope. Mobility may also be observed following alteration of middle ear volume in response to a Valsalva manoeuvre (forced expiration against a closed glottis) or a Toynbee manoeuvre (swallowing with the nasal airway occluded between thumb and forefinger). These tests also give information concerning eustachian tube patency.

Aural toilet and syringing

Examination of the external meatus may reveal wax, debris or pus, which must

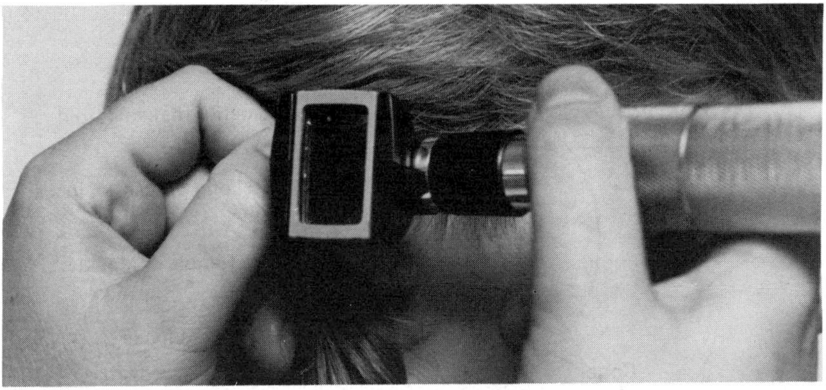

Fig. 12.2 Examination of the ear using the auriscope. Note the left hand applying gentle traction to the pinna. The fingers of the right hand rest on the patient's cheek.

be removed to ensure a good view of the tympanic membrane. Wax may be cleared by syringing, using water at body temperature, or by instrumentation using a wax hook or ringed end of a Jobson Horne probe (Fig. 12.1). Syringing involves direction of a stream of water along the superior meatal wall so that it is deflected by the tympanic membrane and accumulates behind the wax, forcing it out of the meatus. However, only slight deviations from 37°C will cause caloric-induced nystagmus and vertigo. Furthermore, this method is contraindicated by any previous history of infective ear disease that may have resulted in a chronic perforation or a thinned tympanic membrane. For these reasons, many otologists prefer instrumental removal under direct vision. An alternative method of cleaning the ear is by the use of vacuum suction and the binocular operating microscope. This method, if available, allows the most meticulous aural toilet to be performed. In all cases with otorrhoea it is, of course, essential that swabs of the discharge are taken and submitted for culture and antibiotic sensitivity before treatment is started.

Some common abnormalities

Minor congenital abnormalities are not uncommon. These include accessory auricles, which are seen as small, firm tubercles near the tragus or crus of the helix; bat ears, where there is undue prominence of the cartilaginous auricle; and pre-auricular sinus, opening just anterior to the ascending limb of the helix. The more severe congenital abnormalities such as microtia (small grossly deformed auricles), anotia (absence of the auricle) or melotia (displacement of the auricle to an abnormal site) are immediately obvious on examination, and are commonly associated with other abnormalities of the first branchial arch.

Injuries of the external ear are mostly the result of domestic or road traffic

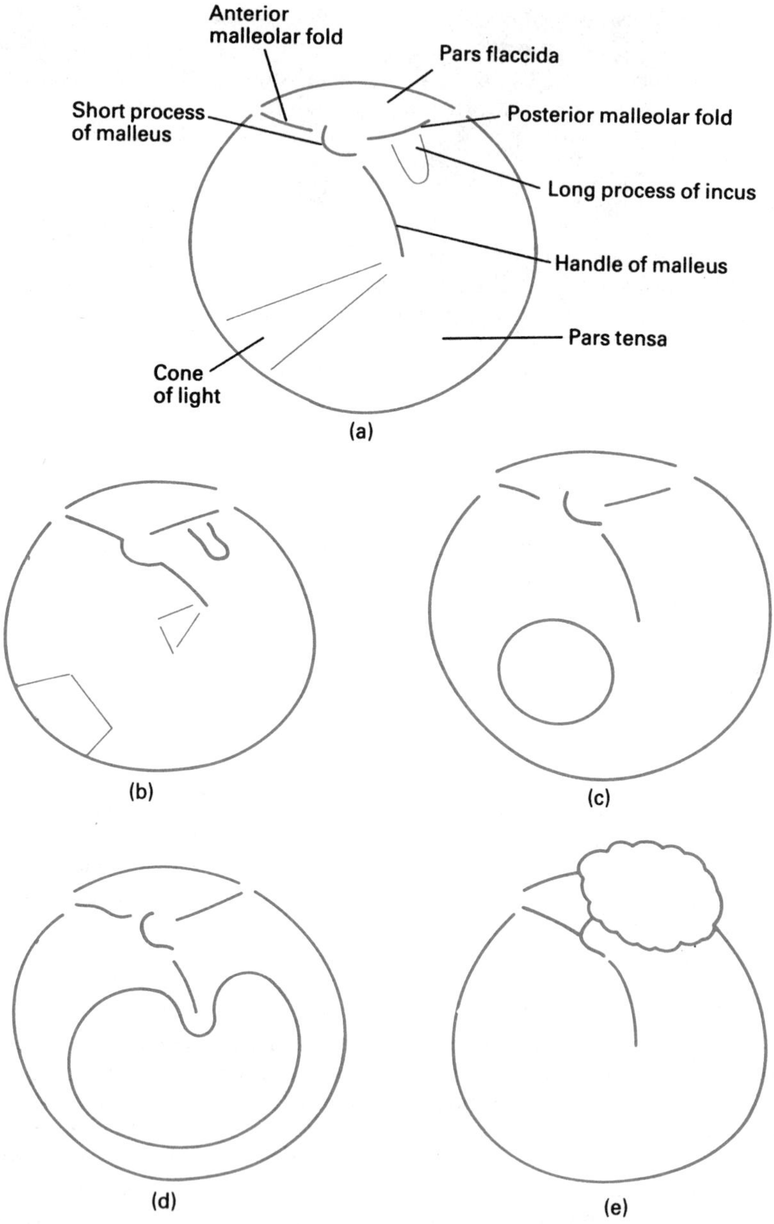

Fig. 12.3 The tympanic membrane: (a) normal, (b) retraction, (c) antero-inferior perforation, (d) subtotal perforation, (e) attic perforation.

accidents. Bruising with extravasation of blood between the perichondrium and the underlying cartilage is a common injury, especially in those engaging in contact sports (e.g. rugby football players and boxers). The skin of the auricle is stretched over a smooth doughy swelling and, if not aspirated, results in a permanent deformity of the pinna (cauliflower ear).

The external auditory meatus

The external meatus may be narrowed due to bony overgrowth in the deep meatus (exostosis). A single exostosis may be differentiated from a cyst or a foreign body by gentle palpation with a probe. Multiple exostoses are much more common and occur spontaneously in swimmers as they are due to prolonged stimulation of the external canal with cold water. Exostoses may cause wax impaction or stasis leading to otitis externa; very occasionally they may totally occlude the meatus and cause deafness.

Foreign bodies in the external meatus are often found in children, usually under the age of three. Wax and desquamated epithelium may form hard plugs of debris which totally occlude the meatus. This condition, called keratosis obturans, is sometimes associated with bronchiectasis, chronic sinusitis and chronic eustachian malfunction.

The tympanic membrane

Having examined the meatus, the tympanic membrane should be scrutinized, and it should be appreciated that relatively minor and subtle changes in appearance may have diagnostic significance. Thus a loss of the normal glistening appearance of the membrane accompanies thickening due to proliferation of the outler layer in otitis externa or the inner layer in otitis media. Similarly, in early otitis media the only abnormalities may be retraction with dilatation of the circumferential and manubrial blood vessels, and a slight pinkish hue.

Scarring of the membrane is common and takes on one of two appearances that are sometimes seen in the same ear. There may be an atrophic scar, which is thin and excessively translucent, due to loss of the middle fibrous layer, or there may be chalky white patches, called tympanosclerosis, which results from deposition of thickened hyalinized collagen in the fibrous layer.

The colour of the drum is also important. Occasionally the membrane is blue due to blood or blood-stained fluid within the middle ear; if seen after head injury, a temporal bone fracture is likely. In contrast, a fiery red appearance with bulging and loss of normal features may result from acute otitis media.

The position of the membrane should be assessed. Obstruction of the eustachian tube prevents replacement of the air in the middle ear cleft and, when this happens, the air becomes absorbed by the lining mucosa and a negative pressure develops. In turn, this results in retraction of the membrane, which, to the examining eye, appears as a foreshortening of the malleus handle and undue prominence of its short process (see Fig. 12.3). If retraction is very marked, especially if the drum is atrophic, the appearances may suggest perforation.

Reduction in middle ear pressure not only causes retraction but may also cause serous exudation into the middle ear. If this occurs then a fluid level may be seen and, if eustachian tube obstruction is incomplete, bubbles of air may be visible within the fluid.

The integrity of the membrane should now be assessed. Perforations of the pars tensa are classified as marginal or central according to whether the rim of the membrane forms, or does not form, part of the defect. Marginal or central perforations should be described by their position—anterior, posterior or inferior—and by their size—small, medium or large. If very large, central perforations warrant the description subtotal. In contrast, perforations of the pars flaccida are described as attic perforations or as erosions if involving the surrounding outer attic wall.

Finally, chronic negative intratympanic pressure may cause the posterior portion of the pars flaccida or posterior superior portion of the pars tensa to become indrawn to form a retraction pocket (see Fig. 12.3). If this pocket fills with infected keratin debris to form a cholesteatoma, it will expand and erode into the middle ear cleft and may damage vital structures such as the facial nerve, labyrinth and sigmoid venous sinus. Subsequent abscess formation in or around the brain may well endanger the patient's life.

The investigation of hearing and hearing loss

The simplest method of testing for hearing loss is by the use of the *human voice*. A conversational voice should be heard at 3.6 m (12 ft) in each ear separately and if this facility extends to 6 m (20 ft) it can be presumed that the patient has normal hearing. Lists of 'spondee' (phonetically balanced) words are used for this test, which should be repeated using the whispered voice. With practice the examiner can soon learn to relate the hearing distances to the likely hearing level in decibels, but technique is important and, in particular, the non-test ear must be adequately blocked or masked by noise.

Further important information may be obtained by the use of *tuning fork tests*. The most widely used are forks vibrating at 256 or 512 Hz (see Fig. 12.1). The Rinne test compares the hearing by air and bone conduction (with the base of the fork on the mastoid process). In the normal ear, air conduction is better than bone conduction (Rinne positive). This also applies to patients who have a sensorineural deafness (deafness due to abnormality in the cochlea or vestibulocochlear nerve), whereas patients with a conductive deafness will show the opposite response (bone conduction better than air conduction—Rinne negative). However, care must be taken to avoid eliciting a false negative response when, in the presence of a severe sensorineural deafness, the tuning fork is

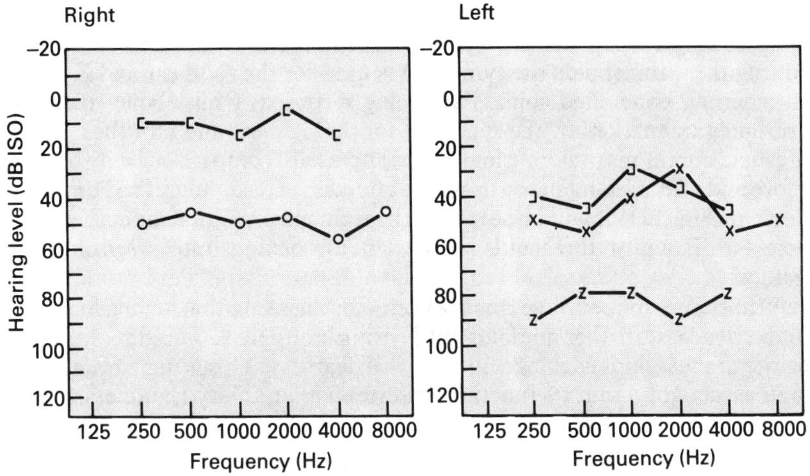

Fig. 12.4 Pure tone audiogram showing a right conductive deafness and a left sensorineural deafness with recruitment. *Right ear:* O, air conduction; [, bone conduction. *Left ear:* X, air conduction;], bone conduction; Z, acoustic reflex threshold (p. 377).

falsely perceived in the cochlea of the good ear when applied to the mastoid process on the deaf side. For this reason a Rinne-negative response should always be confirmed by masking the other ear with noise using a Bárány box (see Fig. 12.1).

The second test commonly used is the Weber test, in which the base of the tuning fork is placed anywhere on the midline of the skull or mandible. In the patient with a conductive deafness, this is perceived in the deaf or deafer ear whilst, in cases of sensorineural loss, it is referred to the better hearing ear.

Audiometric tests

Broadly speaking, hearing tests with electronic equipment can be divided into two main groups. Those that rely on judgements made by the patient are described as 'subjective', whereas tests that record responses over which the patient has no control are called 'objective'.

Subjective hearing tests

Pure tone audiometry The pure tone audiogram (Fig. 12.4) is one of the most generally used techniques for assessing hearing. Pure tones are delivered to the ear under test through a suitable earphone (for air conduction) or by a vibrator attached to the mastoid process (for bone conduction), and the hearing level in decibels above the normal threshold plotted. The frequencies tested usually range from 250 to 8000 Hz in octave or half octave steps. In plotting these thresholds the symbol O is used for the right ear and X for the left when air-conducted sounds are being recorded, whilst bone-conducted thresholds are marked by the symbols [for the right ear and] for the left. The threshold curves may take various forms and useful comparisons may be made before and after treatment, or from one attendance to another. In the example shown in Fig. 12.4 it will be seen that the right ear shows a conductive loss of some 50 dB whilst thresholds in the left ear demonstrate a sensorineural deafness.

Whilst pure tone audiograms are useful for the recognition or exclusion of a conductive loss, further audiological investigations are required to determine the site of the lesions causing sensorineural deafness. This is done by assessing three aspects of auditory function; discrimination ability, loudness recruitment and abnormal adaptation.

Speech audiometry (discrimination ability) This measures the patient's ability to recognize and to repeat correctly lists of words that are presented to him. Phonetically balanced words arranged in groups of 25 are delivered at different intensities to the patient's ear from a tape recording, and the percentage of the presented speech sounds correctly repeated by the subject are noted.

A person with normal hearing will score 100% discrimination with a sound intensity of 45–55 dB. A patient with a pure conductive deafness may also manage to achieve 100% discrimination but only at much higher intensity levels (Fig. 12.5). In contrast, patients with sensorineural deafness are unable to attain good scores. Subjects with sensory deafness classically show improving discrimination at low intensities but, at 50–70% of the maximal score, there is a fall off due to recruitment (see below). Neural deafness causes an even more severe impairment of discrimination, and, in an extreme instance, the score may be as low as 0–20%; this impairment may be seen in spite of a reasonably good pure tone threshold.

Alternate binaural loudness balance test (loudness recruitment) The phenomenon of recruitment is due to lesions of the cochlear end organ. As such, it is almost diagnostic of a sensory hearing disorder, although approximately 10% of retrocochlear lesions will also exhibit this phenomenon.

To ears showing recruitment a pure tone will be just audible when the intensity is slightly greater than the hearing threshold, but intense sounds (80–100 dB) create a sensation of loudness at least as great as that experienced by a normal ear at that intensity. In other words the dynamic range of the ear is compressed.

The alternate binaural loudness balance test attempts to uncover this phenomenon by comparing stimulus intensities that give an equal sensation of

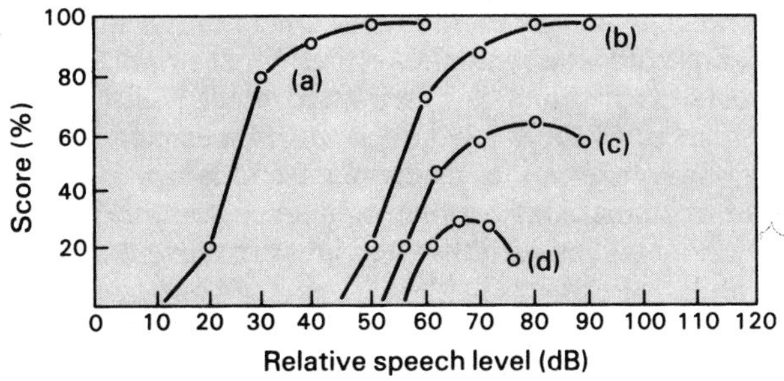

Fig. 12.5 Speech audiogram. (a) Normal, (b) conductive deafness, (c) sensory loss, (d) neural lesion.

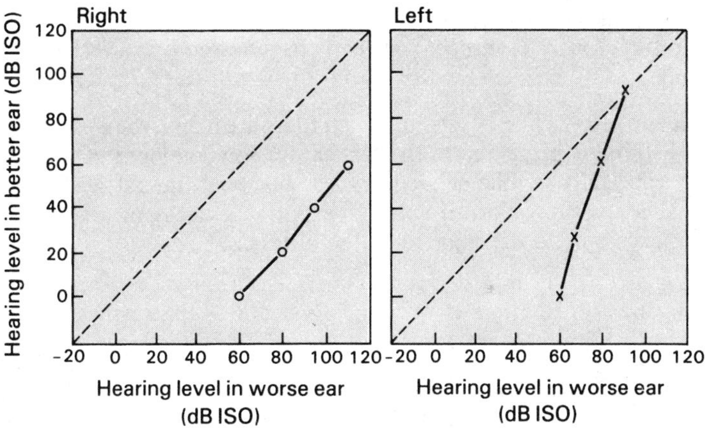

Fig. 12.6 Alternate binaural loudness balance. The right ear (O) shows recruitment indicating a cochlear (sensory) deafness; the left ear (X) shows a non-recruiting deafness.

loudness in both the normal and deafened ear. The results can be plotted graphically (Fig. 12.6).

Loudness discomfort level This simple test is also based on the phenomenon of recruitment. Normal subjects can readily identify an intensity level (90–105 dB above their threshold) at which sounds feel unpleasant. When recruitment is present discomfort is experienced at lower intensity levels than normal, despite the threshold hearing loss. In contrast, in the absence of recruitment, discomfort may not be experienced even at the maximal output of the audiometer (usually 125 dB).

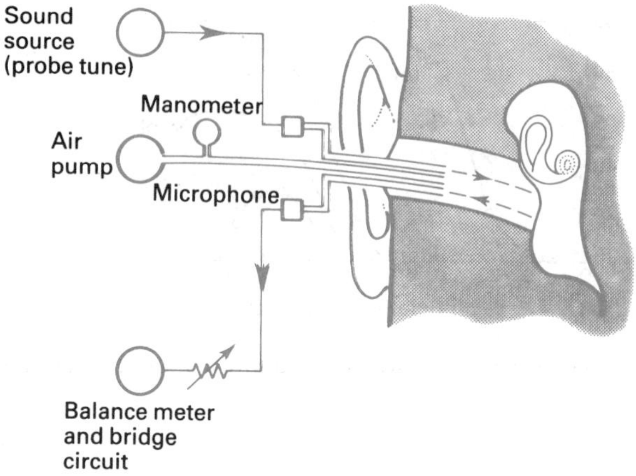

Fig. 12.7 Components of the acoustic impedance bridge.
(*After S.R. Mawson and H. Ludman (1979) in Diseases of the Ear, 4th edn. London: Edward Arnold.*)

Tone decay tests These tests, of which there are many, measure decay of an auditory stimulus presented to the test ear. A small amount of tone decay is normal, especially at higher frequencies, but with neural lesions there is abnormal adaptation. Normal subjects experience decay of less than 15 dB; decay in excess of 20 dB suggests a neural lesion.

Objective hearing tests

Impedance measurements The impedance (the reciprocal of the resistance) of the tympanic membrane is estimated by measuring the amount of sound reflected from the membrane under various applied external pressures. An impedance bridge is used (Fig. 12.7). The probe is fitted into the external meatus of the test ear so that it makes an air-tight seal. It conveys three tubes. The first delivers a continuous pure tone (the probe tone) into the external meatus. The second is connected to a manometer so that the external meatal pressure can be altered. The third is a means of transmitting sound, which is reflected from the meatus to a microphone and thence to an impedance bridge, where this sound is balanced against a reference tone.

(a) Tympanometry The tympanic membrane is stiffened artificially by changing the pressure in the meatus over the range from +200 to − 200 mm H_20 using the manometer. When subjected to extremes of pressure, most of the sound introduced into the system is reflected and only low intensities are required to balance the impedance bridge. Conversely, when the tympanic membrane is mobile and the middle and external canal pressures equate, a

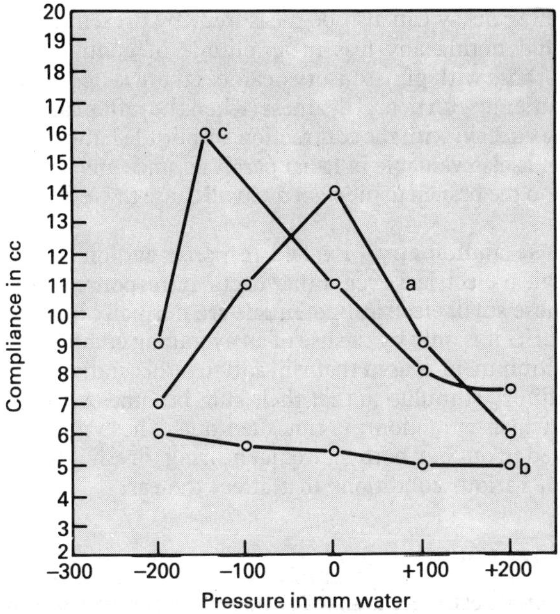

Fig. 12.8 The 3 types of tympanometry curve. a, Normal; b, tympanic effusion or adhesive otitis; c, negative middle ear pressure (eustachian tube dysfunction).

greater percentage of the sound introduced is now transmitted. The changes can be plotted graphically as a tympanogram (Fig. 12.8), and characteristic changes will be seen in a range of common conditions such as eustachian tube dysfunction, ossicular fixation or alterations in the structure of the drum.

(b) Intra-aural reflex measurements Contractions of the intra-aural muscles cause a stiffening of the tympanic membrane, and the resulting changes in compliance may be recorded by the use of the impedance meter. The stapedius muscles will normally contract in response to a pure tone stimulus of 70–100 dB. In practice the minimal intensity of sound required to evoke this response is measured. This is termed the Acoustic Reflex Threshold (ART) and is recorded by the symbol Z (see Fig. 12.4).

Whilst in normal ears the ART for pure tones (500–4000 Hz) lies between 70 and 100 dB above the subjective pure tone threshold, in conductive deafness the reflex may be unobtainable at any level owing to middle ear pathology. In sensory deafness the ART often occurs at levels less than 70 dB above the pure tone threshold due to the phenomenon of recruitment. Conversely, in neural deafness the ART is usually absent or occurs at levels in excess of 70 dB above the subjective threshold provided sufficient neurones are intact.

Acoustic reflex decay can also be measured, by presenting the pure tone continuously and noting any loss in amplitude of contraction. In normal subjects and in those with pure sensory deafness there is no decay at 500 Hz or 1000 Hz, but patients with neural deafness (when the reflex can be elicited) will often show reflex decay, with the contraction amplitude halved in 2–3 seconds.

This system is also valuable in facial paralysis since any lesion of the facial nerve proximal to the branch to the stapedius will cause the reflex to be abolished.

Evoked response audiometry Evoked response audiometry measures the small physiological electrical events that occur in response to sound stimuli. However, as these small electrical potentials are normally buried in the background of the EEG it is only by the use of an averaging computer that they can be displayed. Equipment is used that will add together individual responses to a repetitive auditory stimulus so that their sum becomes visible whilst background noise, which is random, is cancelled out. These methods have been increasingly used in otology both to predict hearing thresholds and as an aid to the diagnosis of various conditions that affect the ear.

Vestibular investigation

In the normal ear at rest there is a steady neural discharge from the vestibular labyrinth. These impulses, together with information from the eyes and the muscle, joint and skin sense receptors, are centrally integrated to provide an overall appreciation of spatial orientation.

Vestibular nerve discharge is normally equal on both sides, and is composed of information from the utricular maculae and the cristae of the semicircular canals. The utricular maculae, which are situated in the horizontal plane, are quiescent as long as the head is horizontal and stationary, but they respond both to changes in gravity and to linear acceleration. The semicircular canals respond to changes in angular acceleration. Either or these movements causes changes in the respective end organs, which results in enhanced impulses from one side of the system and inhibition of the impulses from the other. Movement thus causes equal and opposite effects in the two parts of the system. When deprived of vestibular information from one side the brain stem is swamped by unbalanced neural impulses from the normal side. Vertigo and nystagmus result, and during the acute phase (before compensation occurs) there is a sensation of objects moving to the opposite side and a tendency to fall towards the side of the lesion.

Vestibular nystagmus is characterized by rotational movements of the eyes which are alternately slow in one direction and quick in the opposite direction. The slow component is labyrinthine in origin whilst the quick adjustment movement is central (see p. 303).

Start by looking for nystagmus with the patient sitting in a chair. During this time, and whilst otoscopy is being undertaken, particular attention should be paid to jerk nystagmus resulting from changes in air pressure in the external acoustic meatus. Such changes can be induced by the use of a Siegel's pneumatic speculum (Fig. 12.1) or by pressing the tragus into the canal. If nystagmus results then a 'fistula sign' is said to be present, suggesting that the outer bony labyrinthine wall has been breached so that pressure changes are transmitted directly to the membranous labyrinth.

Positional vertigo

With disease in the ear itself, and sometimes with tumours of the 4th ventricle, brain stem or cerebellum, vertigo or disequilibrium can sometimes be induced by sudden movement of the head. The patient may be able to reproduce this and it may then be possible to observe lateralized nystagmus during the period of vertigo. However, it is often necessary to use a *provocative test* for positional vertigo and nystagmus. The patient should be asked to sit quietly on the edge of a couch for several minutes before the test is begun. Suddenly lay the patient down on his back on the couch, having removed the pillow from the couch. Encourage the patient *not* to shut his eyes, even if vertigo develops, by asking him to look closely at your finger. During the 30 seconds after laying the patient supine, look for nystagmus on gaze to the left or right. In patients with positional vertigo due to a labyrinthine lesion, nystagmus will develop after an interval of 5 to 15 seconds and will disappear in a few more seconds (*benign positional vertigo*). The nystagmus is directed toward the side of the lesion. In some patients with cerebellar, brain stem or 4th ventricle tumours, a similar nystagmus develops but without the characteristic delay of benign positional vertigo. Further, in benign positional vertigo it is usually possible to reproduce the sign only after several minutes' rest in the sitting position, whereas in posterior fossa tumours the vertigo and nystagmus can be readily reproduced on repeated testing.

Following recovery from a recent lesion or less severe vestibular insult, peripheral nystagmus may become masked by optic fixation. This suppression may be uncovered by abolishing fixation with Frenzel's glasses (Fig. 12.1) which have 20 dioptre lenses and internal illumination. The patient wearing these glasses can see very little but the observer has an excellent magnified and illuminated view of the eyes. Alternatively, latent nystagmus may be demonstrated by observing the eyes in the dark with a special infra-red viewer. Measurements of nystagmus can also be made by electronystagmography (ENG), which monitors changes in electrical potentials recorded from two electrodes near the eyes; changing potentials resulting from eye movement are transmitted on to a moving paper strip for later analysis, or the data may be digitally presented with suitable equipment.

The principle of abolition of fixation is important for differentiating peripheral from central nystagmus. Peripheral nystagmus is enhanced by abolition of fixation, whereas nystagmus of central origin may be diminished or abolished.

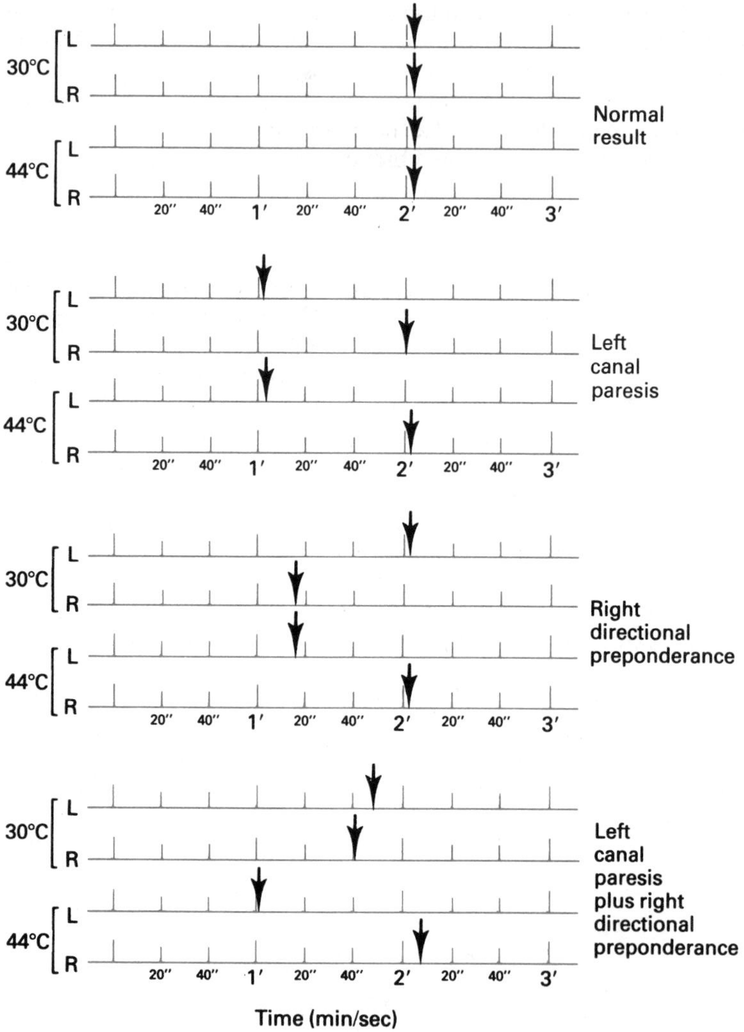

Fig. 12.9 Bithermal caloric tests.

Caloric tests

These are performed by introducing water at 30°C or 44°C (7°C above and below normal body temperature) into each ear with the head raised 30° (to bring the lateral semicircular canals into the vertical plane). These manoeuvres induce convection currents in the semicircular canal which, by causing movement of the cristae in the ampulla, induce nystagmus. In each test approximately 250 ml of water from thermostatically controlled tanks is used, and each ear is irrigated at each temperature for 40 seconds. The nystagmus may be timed for each of the four tests or alternatively movement may be analysed using electronystagmography. As with spontaneous nystagmus of peripheral origin, caloric-induced nystagmus can be significantly enhanced by the abolition of optic fixation.

Peripheral lesions tend to cause a diminished response on one side (*canal paresis*) but *directional preponderance* to the opposite side may also result (Fig. 12.9). Directional preponderance, however, is more likely to occur with central lesions, especially brain stem disorders but also occasionally in temporal lobe lesions.

Radiological examination

Radiology of the temporal bones can give the clinician invaluable additional information. In acute and chronic middle ear and mastoid infection, the extent of mastoid cellular involvement or of bone erosion can be determined from plain X-rays. Linear tomography shows more detail. To visualize the ossicles and cavities of the inner ear and internal auditory canals in detail, hypocycloidal or spiral tomography is desirable. Ossicular abnormalities, hairline fractures, osteolytic or sclerotic bone pathology, or early evidence of tumour erosion may be seen. Neuroradiological techniques are necessary to confirm the presence of space-occupying lesions which affect the facial or vestibulocochlear nerves, and computerized axial tomography has both diminished the morbidity associated with these investigations and improved the diagnostic yield; with high-definition images from modern scanners it is now possible to demonstrate much of the detailed anatomy of the cavities and structures within the temporal bone.

THE NOSE AND PARANASAL SINUSES

Diseases of the nose and paranasal sinuses may produce a plethora of symptoms. These are conveniently considered in two major groups: nasal and regional.

Nasal symptoms are immediately recognized as originating in the upper airway. They include complaints of nasal obstruction, nasal discharge (rhinorrhoea or post-nasal drip), disturbances of smell, nose bleed (epistaxis), nasal irritation and itching, and recurrent sneezing. *Regional* symptoms, on the other hand, are not so obviously related to the nose and sinuses, and indeed may equally well have their origin elsewhere. They include headache, facial pain (which can easily mimic dental pain) and numerous symptoms referable to the eye including epiphora, diplopia, proptosis and orbital pain. Furthermore, severe nasal obstruction may present with symptoms that are solely due to mouth breathing such as dryness of the mouth, soreness of the throat, coughing or snoring.

Specific questions are valuable in diagnosis. Thus the patient with rhinorrhoea should be asked whether the discharge is bloody, purulent, watery or mucoid, and the amount and duration of the discharge should be recorded. It is also important to establish whether the discharge is unilateral or bilateral, and particular attention should be paid to unilateral obstruction with blood-stained discharge in an older person, since this may be the presenting symptom of malignancy.

In cases of *airway obstruction*, some estimate of the severity of the disability should be made and it is again relevant to enquire whether the problem is unilateral or bilateral; occasionally nasal obstruction appears to alternate but it should be appreciated that this may be no more than an enhanced 'nasal cycle', which is a normal physiological phenomenon occurring in approximately 80% of the population.

Sneezing accompanies excessive secretion in the nasal airway. Patients with allergic rhinitis (seasonal or perennial) often sneeze in staccato-like repetitive patterns with up to half a dozen or more sneezes in a row. Associated itching or watering of the eyes is also suggestive of an allergic diathesis and, in these circumstances, any previous history of asthma or eczema or a family history of an allergic phenomenon is relevant.

Epistaxis (bleeding from the nose) may be arterial or venous in origin and may vary from an annoying and disturbing symptom to one that is life threatening. Common sites of arterial bleeding are from Little's area on the anterior nasal septum or from the inferior turbinate. Venous bleeding usually emanates from a small preseptal vein which lies anteriorly on the medial wall of the nasal vestibule. As with bleeding elsewhere, the duration and severity should be accurately assessed. Any history of blood dyscrasia or clotting disorder should prompt the examiner to perform an immediate clotting screen and this may also be relevant after prolonged ingestion of drugs such as phenylbutazone, aspirin or anticoagulants.

Examination

First inspect the outside of the nose. The base (columella) should lie in the midline. On each side are the nostrils, which normally have an oval or pear-shaped contour, whose lateral walls are formed by the alar cartilages covered with skin. Gentle occlusion of each nostril by compression of the ala with the thumb gives some indication of airway patency. Alternatively, the airway can be assessed by holding a laryngeal mirror under the nostril; moist expired air will cause surface misting and direct comparison between the two sides can readily be made.

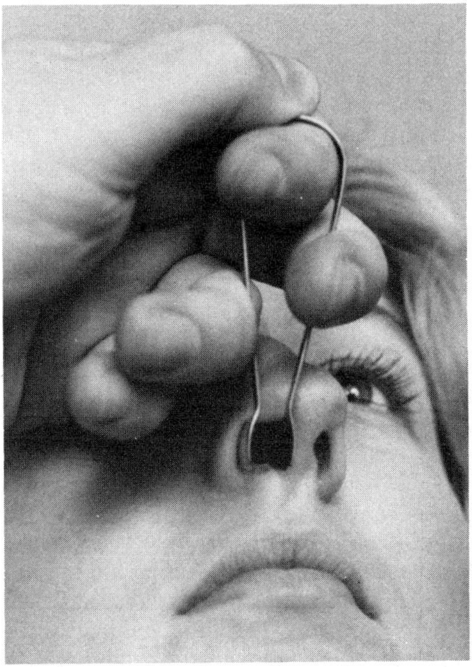

Fig. 12.10 Examination of the nose using the nasal speculum.

Then the nasal vestibule and anterior part of the lateral wall and septum are examined. In children, often alarmed by instrumentation, the vestibule may be adequately assessed by using an auriscope with a wide speculum attached. Alternatively, simple upward pressure on the tip of the nose with a finger will normally allow a reasonable view of the remainder of the airway provided good illumination is available.

In adults, however, a Thudichum's nasal speculum is required (Fig. 12.1). This is held suspended over the crooked index finger of the left hand and is closed by compression between the extensor surface of the middle phalanx of the ring finger and the flexor surface of the middle finger. Light is provided by a beam directed from a head mirror and the speculum is closed, inserted into the nostril and then gently opened to give a view of the anterior airway (Fig. 12.10).

The skin of the vestibule, which is heir to all common skin conditions, extends inwards for about 1 cm and is separated by a clear line of demarcation from the pink moist mucous membrane of the interior of the nose. Medially lies the nasal septum and on the lateral wall the inferior nasal turbinates may be seen with the anterior part of the middle turbinate lying immediately above.

The superior turbinate and meatus and olfactory mucosa are not seen on routine examination, but the nasal floor should be inspected; it becomes visible after gentle flexion of the head with the speculum in situ.

The posterior choanae and postnasal space can be inspected by means of a small mirror inserted into the mouth and oropharynx so that it lies just behind the soft palate. This manoeuvre is difficult and is best performed with the patient leaning forward, his mouth open (dentures having been removed) and the tongue firmly depressed with a Lack's tongue depressor (Fig. 12.1) held in the left hand. A St Clair Thomson postnasal mirror (Fig. 12.1) is then warmed in a spirit lamp until, when tested on the hand, the back of the mirror feels hot (but not uncomfortably hot). The mirror, held in the right hand, is passed into the mouth over the upper surface of the tongue until it lies in the space between uvula, tongue and pillars of the fauces. If movement is clumsy or hurried the patient will almost certainly gag. Inspection should be made rapidly since even the most cooperative patient cannot for long resist the desire to swallow.

There will be no view if the palate lies against the posterior pharyngeal wall; in these circumstances the palate may fall away anteriorly if the patient sniffs gently through his nose.

The view of the nasopharynx is often fleeting but in a cooperative patient the posterior end of the nasal septum will be seen as a sharp white dividing line in the middle of the field. On either side of the septum, the posterior end of the inferior turbinates can be seen and directly behind the turbinates are the openings of the eustachian tubes. The fossa of Rosenmüller lies directly above and behind the auditory tubes and these areas should be inspected with particular care as it is here that disease may cause compression of the tube or referred pain to the ear.

To examine the sinuses the bony walls should be palpated, paying particular attention to the infra-orbital margins; any tenderness, swelling, expansion or depression of bone may be significant. The palate and alveoli must also be inspected and should be palpated from inside the mouth, using the gloved finger.

Transillumination of the sinuses by placing a strong light in the centre of the hard palate (maxillary sinuses) or under the frontal ridge of the orbit (frontal sinuses) has limited clinical use and is often misleading; it has been superseded by radiological investigation, which should include a lateral as well as occipitomental and occipitovertical views. Further information may be given by films taken with the head tilted (to demonstrate fluid levels) and, where a sinus tumour is suspected, by the use of linear and computerized axial tomography.

Some common abnormalities

Examination of the outside of the nose may reveal old scars or recent cuts and bruises. Trauma may also cause a displacement of the nasal bones; the septum should be inspected in case there is a septal haematoma.

Chronic infection will cause redness and fissuring around the nostrils and within the nasal vestibule, where furunculosis is commonly seen.

Dislocation of the anterior end of the septal cartilage from its groove in the maxillary crest may cause it to project into one or other vestibule, causing nasal obstruction; since the skin overlying the projecting cartilage is easily damaged and infected, this predisposes the patient to vestibulitis. In addition to anterior dislocation, the septum may be distorted and deviated. C- or S-shaped deviations involve both the bony and cartilaginous septum and are associated with deviations in the external nasal pyramid. Nasal obstruction and turbulence of the inspired air flow causes excessive drying of the mucosa with crusting and possible ulceration.

Epistaxis may result from crusting but more commonly comes from arterial bleeding over Little's area or venous bleeding from a preseptal vein; there is usually no obvious primary cause for this.

The normal nasal mucosa is pale-pink and moist. Excessive pallor of a blue–violaceous colouring suggests vasomotor instability or allergic rhinitis; a hypertrophied, thickened mucosa is characteristic of patients who over-use nasal sprays (rhinitis medicamentosa). Atrophy of the mucosa accompanies ageing but may also result from trauma, including surgery.

Nasal secretions may in themselves help diagnosis. The normal secretion is mucoid, but profuse watery discharge is common and accompanies upper respiratory tract infection, vasomotor reactions or an allergic rhinitis. Mucopus may be seen along the floor of the nose and the presence of pus leaking into the nasal cavities from the middle meatus strongly suggests purulent sinusitis, since most of the paranasal sinuses open under the middle turbinate.

Nasal polypi are another common finding. These appear as moist greyish swellings in the nasal airway and they commonly originate from the ethmoidal air cells. Consequently growth into the nose is from under the middle turbinate; if confusion exists, they can be differentiated from the turbinate by palpation with a probe. An antro-choanal polyp has a similar appearance but has its origin in a maxillary sinus. After growing through the ostium of the sinus, it appears as a pedunculated mass obstructing the nose and hanging down into the nasopharynx.

THE THROAT

Examination of the throat includes inspection of the mouth, oropharynx, nasopharynx, larynx and laryngopharynx. The mouth and oropharynx are considered in Chapter 5 and examination of the nasopharynx has already been described; this account is therefore devoted almost entirely to the larynx and laryngopharynx.

Laryngeal disorders commonly present with either sore throat, difficulty in swallowing (dysphagia), hoarseness or a lump in the neck. Less commonly, there is respiratory difficulty with stridor and examination is required to assess the adequacy of the upper airway. Unfortunately, evaluation of symptoms may often prove difficult since minor complaints such as throat clearing or an annoying cough may herald severe disease (e.g. carcinoma of the supraglottis) whereas dramatic symptoms such as a sudden onset of aphonia may have no organic basis. In some cases, mirror examination may be inconclusive and direct examination under anaesthesia is then necessary.

Nonetheless, a *sore throat* is one of the commonest symptoms in clinical medicine. Acute infections of the upper respiratory tract are particularly common in children and young adults and the patient usually makes a full and rapid recovery with no sequelae. Unfortunately, not all acute infections are so benign and, in particular, acute epiglottitis (caused by *Haemophilus influenzae*) or acute laryngotracheobronchitis (caused by parainfluenza virus type I, respiratory syncytial virus or the virus of measles) may present with rapidly increasing airway obstruction necessitating intubation or tracheostomy.

Recurrent sore throat is also a common complaint. It is the major presenting symptom of chronic tonsillitis and may vary considerably in severity. The degree of disability may bear no relation to tonsillar size, shape or appearance. Acute tonsillar infection may also cause *dysphagia*, especially if there is peritonsillar involvement. However, painful dysphagia may accompany any inflammatory changes within the pharynx and is also a feature of swallowed foreign bodies, parapharyngeal inflammation and abscess formation. The pain may be so severe that protective muscle spasm (trismus) is a feature of the presentation and the patient may be unable to swallow saliva, which drools from the corner of the mouth.

Alternatively, dysphagia may accompany mechanical obstruction or neuromuscular abnormality within the pharynx or upper oesophagus. Again the history is very important. Both types of dysphagia are painless but, whereas mechanical obstruction commonly presents with dysphagia that starts as difficulty with solids and progresses to liquids, neuromuscular abnormalities result in dysphagia for liquids at the outset. This is because paralysis or incoordination affecting the complex movements associated with deglutition easily allows fluid to escape into the nasopharynx or to overspill into an incompetent larynx. Attempts to swallow liquids therefore result in choking and coughing attacks which may ultimately lead to secondary pneumonia.

Hoarseness may accompany many different laryngeal pathologies. As in other sites, the mode of onset of the disability and rate of progression of the symptom are important in establishing the correct diagnosis. Thus an acute onset of self-limiting dysphonia is common, especially following voice abuse or simple laryngitis. Constant over-use or incorrect use of the voice by straining causes chronic changes in the larynx and characteristically, in these cases, the history is of dysphonia that is mild on waking but which becomes progressively more severe during the day.

Conversely, paralysis or carcinoma of a vocal cord shows no diurnal variation. The voice progressively weakens over a short period and once the symptom is established there is no spontaneous recovery. Most of these patients have been heavy cigarette smokers or have abused alcohol in the past.

Examination

To perform indirect laryngoscopy the examiner seats himself facing the patient with his legs nearest to the source of light. Normally illumination is provided by a bull's-eye lamp placed on the patient's left, on a level with his mouth, and its beam is adjusted so that it is reflected and focused by the head mirror worn by the examiner.

A head mirror (Fig. 12.1) is concave and has a hole in the centre through which the examiner's right eye will inspect the image seen in the laryngeal mirror. It is fastened to the head by means of a band and can be adjusted easily because it is fitted with a ball-and-socket joint.

A suitably sized laryngeal mirror (Fig. 12.1) is selected and moved gently in a spirit flame (or hot water) to prevent misting when the patient exhales. The mirror is then tested to ensure it is not too hot by holding it firmly against the ventral surface of the examiner's wrist.

The patient (with dentures removed) is asked to lean forward, to open his mouth and to put out his tongue. With a small square of clean gauze in the left hand, the examiner takes hold of the tip of the patient's tongue between his thumb and second finger whilst the index finger of the same hand gently lifts the upper lip. With the light from the head mirror directed at the patient's mouth the mirror is then introduced and placed against the soft palate near the base of the uvula (Fig. 12.11). Gentle pressure on the uvula is usually well tolerated and no surface analgesia is required for the great majority of patients. Hurried movement or contact with the tongue or posterior pharyngeal wall is, however, liable to induce gagging and, once the patient's confidence is lost, further examination may be prejudiced. A calm unhurried approach is therefore essential and examination may be easier if the patient is encouraged to concentrate on regular mouth breathing throughout the procedure.

The larynx and laryngopharynx (Fig. 12.12) should be inspected methodically and with great care. The epiglottis lies anteriorly and is easily identified by its upper curved margin and characteristic yellowish colour. Anterior to the epiglottis lies the base of the tongue and, between the two, the valleculae. Running posteriorly and inferiorly from the epiglottis are the aryepiglottic folds and lateral to these are the piriform fossae. Pooled saliva in a piriform fossa or excessive mucus or saliva posteriorly should be noted, since either of these abnormalities is indicative of upper oesophageal obstruction or paralysis.

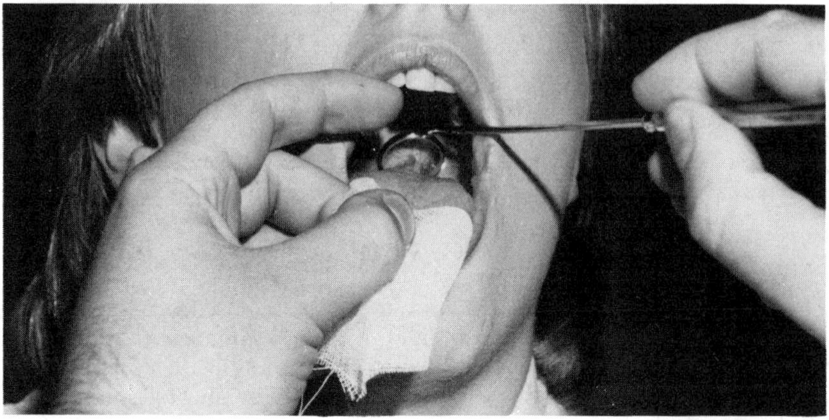

Fig. 12.11 Examination of the larynx and laryngopharynx by indirect laryngoscopy.

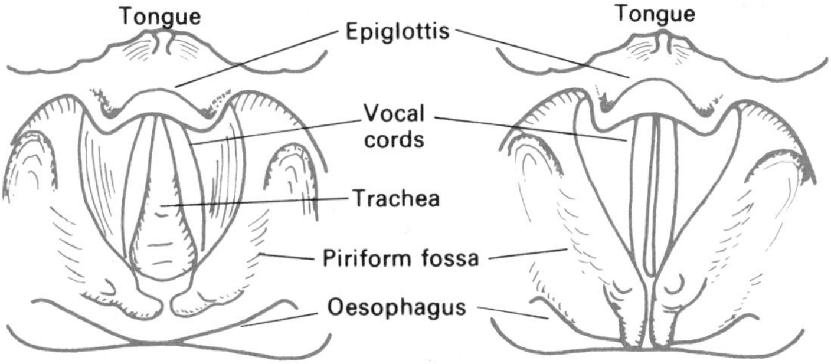

Fig. 12.12 The larynx seen in the laryngeal mirror with the vocal cords in abduction (left) and adduction (right).

Medial to the aryepiglottic folds is the laryngeal vestibule. This leads to the glottis at the vocal cords. The true cords are normally clear-cut and are pale yellow, in contrast to the remaining laryngeal mucosa which is a pinkish red in colour. Between the vocal cords the lumen of the cervical trachea can be seen, and above lie the laryngeal ventricle and false cords.

After inspection, and with the mirror still in situ, the patient is asked to phonate by singing a sustained vowel (commonly 'ee' or 'aay'). This manoeuvre serves a double purpose since it allows the mobility of the vocal cords to be assessed and improves visualization of important structures by elevation of the larynx.

Examination of the neck

No evaluation is complete without an external examination of the neck. The position of the thyroid cartilage and gland and the position of the trachea should be established with care and any associated masses or enlarged nodes palpated. The larynx should normally be mobile from side to side and crepitus should be elicited; a pharyngeal mass displacing it away from the vertebral column will diminish the sensation. The thyroid isthmus, lying in front of the cervical trachea, and the lateral lobes under cover of the strap muscles are best examined by light palpation during swallowing and this manoeuvre may even draw a small retrosternal extension up towards the examining fingers. Cervical lymph nodes, which mostly lie under the sternomastoid muscle in the line of the jugular vein, can best be assessed by gentle flexion and rotation of the head to the contralateral side, since it is only by this movement that muscle tension is relaxed sufficiently to allow proper palpation.

Finally, it is important to realize that not every patient can co-operate sufficiently to provide the examiner with an adequate view of the larynx. Recent advances with flexible fibreoptic endoscopy seem certain to reduce the number of patients who fall into this category since it seems to be well tolerated in nearly all subjects.

Some common abnormalities

The epithelium should be inspected for irregularity, ulceration, change of colour or oedema. Raised irregular epithelium suggests malignant change. Ulceration with oedema in the inter-arytenoid area suggests tuberculosis. Oedema alone indicates non-specific inflammation or trauma and diffuse redness suggests acute laryngitis. Whenever the epithelium of the larynx is ulcerated or irregular an X-ray of the lung fields and serological tests for syphilis should be performed before biopsy. If there is purulent sputum this should also be examined.

The movement of the larynx should be symmetrical. When normal movement is absent the examiner must consider whether some local condition such as fixation due to malignant change or myopathy is responsible, or whether there is a lesion along the course of the recurrent laryngeal nerve which is causing the abnormality. If local change is responsible there will usually be swelling, obstruction or ulceration.

Common sites for disruption of the recurrent laryngeal nerves are behind the thyroid (due to neoplasm or as the result of thyroid surgery), the cervical oesophagus, the apices of the lungs, and the structures related to the undersurface of the aorta on the left side and the subclavian artery on the right. Absence of movement of one or both cords should always suggest a lesion at one of these named sites. An enlarged left atrium or disease of the aortic arch may also cause paralysis of the recurrent nerve.

Chronic laryngitis may produce a variety of appearances. Polypoid thickening at the junction of the anterior and middle thirds of the cords is common and may be unilateral or bilateral. Nodules due to vocal strain may also be seen and may take a variety of different forms macroscopically.

Since squamous cell carcinoma arising on the surface of a vocal cord is one of the commonest malignancies in men, hoarseness of more than 4–6 weeks' duration should always be investigated. All such cases, and all cases of chronic laryngitis, must be subjected to direct laryngoscopy with biopsy or excision of the lesion. In clinical practice today microlaryngoscopy (using specially constructed instruments and an operating microscope) is commonly used.

13
The eye

Before examining the various parts of the eye, one should test the visual acuity, the extent of the visual fields and, when relevant, colour vision.

VISUAL ACUITY

Test for distant vision

Visual acuity is measured with Snellen's test types, a series of letters of varying sizes constructed so that the top letter is visible to the normal eye at 60 metres, and the subsequent lines at 36, 24, 18, 12, 9, 6 and 5 metres respectively. Visual acuity (V) is recorded according to the formula $V = d/D$, where d is the distance at which the letters are read, and D that at which they should be read. The patient is normally placed at a distance of 6 metres from the test types ($d = 6$) and each eye is tested separately. The patient reads down the chart as far as he can. If only the top letter of the chart is visible, the visual acuity is 6/60. A normal person should read at least the seventh line, i.e. a visual acuity of 6/6. If the visual acuity is less than 6/60, the patient is moved towards the test types until he can read the top letter. If the top letter is visible at 2 metres, the visual acuity is 2/60. Visual acuities of less than 1/60 are recorded as *'counting fingers'* (CF), *'hand movements'* (HM), *'perception of light'* (PL) or *'no perception of light'* (no PL). A person with an uncorrected refractive error may have reduced visual acuity, and a rough estimate of his corrected visual acuity may be obtained by asking him to view the chart through a pin-hole aperture.

If the patient wears glasses, the type of lens he is wearing should be determined. Hold the lens up and look at an object through it. Then move the lens from side to side and watch the object. If the object seems to move in the opposite direction to the lens, the lens is convex; if in the same direction, it is concave. Patients with *myopia* i.e. short sight, use concave (diverging) lenses and those with *hypermetropia* i.e. long sight, convex (converging) ones.

In order to tell whether a lens is spherical or cylindrical, look at a straight object through it and then slowly twist the lens round. If the lens is cylindrical, the object will appear to take up an oblique position. Patients who are *astigmatic* need cylindrical lenses.

Test for near vision

Visual acuity at the ordinary reading distance is assessed by using reading test types of varying sizes, the notation being based on the printers' 'point' system. The smallest print used is N5. The near vision is recorded as the smallest type which the patient can read comfortably.

COLOUR SENSE

Colour sense is most easily tested by the use of pseudo-isochromatic plates, the best known being those of Ishihara. People with defective colour vision confuse certain colours. Ishihara pseudo-isochromatic plates are so constructed that a person with abnormal colour vision will read a different number to a normal person on the same plate.

The most common anomalies of colour vision are various types of red–green deficiency, inherited as sex-linked recessive conditions, which occur in about 8% of males and 0.5% of females in this country. People with congenital blue–yellow deficiencies and with total colour-blindness are rare. Acquired defects of colour vision occur in macular and optic nerve disease.

VISUAL FIELDS

The methods for testing the visual fields are described on p. 290.

EXAMINATION OF THE EYE

After the vision has been tested, the eyes should be examined systematically.

The eyelids

The shape and position of the eyelids should be noted. People of Asiatic origin have a long narrow palpebral aperture with an upward and outward obliquity and a characteristic fold of skin along the upper lid. The highest point of the aperture is at the junction of its middle and inner thirds. In Down's syndrome the palpebral fissure is also oblique. However, in addition it is short and wide with its highest point at the centre of the lid.

Ptosis or drooping of the upper lid, may be congenital or acquired. A congenital ptosis may be unilateral or bilateral, whereas an acquired ptosis is usually unilateral if due to paralysis of the oculomotor nerve or of the cervical sympathetic, and usually bilateral if due to ocular myopathy.

Lid retraction If the upper lid is abnormally retracted, a band of white sclera is visible above the iris when the eyes are looking straight ahead. Lid retraction, which is usually due to thyrotoxicosis (Plate IV), is often associated with infrequent blinking and with lid-lag, i.e. the upper lid seems to lag behind the eyeball when the patient looks downwards. Patients with thyrotoxicosis frequently also have a slight degree of forward displacement of the eyeball (*exophthalmos* or *proptosis*). Some patients with thyrotoxicosis and some whose thyrotoxicosis has been successfully treated medically or surgically develop a more severe and progressive form of exophthalmos, which may be associated with optic nerve dysfunction and corneal ulceration. Exophthalmos also results from space-occupying lesions in the orbit, and an apparent exophthalmos may be present when the eye is longer than normal, as in myopia.

The presence of any inflammation of the margins of the lids (marginal blepharitis) should be noted, together with any abnormality in the position of the lid margins, i.e. eversion (ectropion) or inversion (entropion) of the lashes.

The lacrimal gland

The lacrimal gland is examined by pulling up the outer part of the upper lid while asking the patient to look downwards and inwards. Acute inflammation (dacryoadenitis) results in a tender swollen gland, with oedema of the upper lid and localized conjunctival injection. Chronic dacryoadenitis, a painless enlargement of the lacrimal gland which is frequently bilateral, occurs in the reticuloses, sarcoidosis and tuberculosis. Tumours of the lacrimal gland produce a hard swelling of the gland associated with proptosis.

The conjunctiva

The conjunctiva lining the eyeball (bulbar conjunctiva) and that lining the inner surface of the eyelids (palpebral conjunctiva) should be examined. To examine the palpebral conjunctiva of the lower lid, the lower lid should be pulled down while asking the patient to look upwards. To expose the palpebral conjunctiva of the upper lid, ask the patient to look downwards, then place the right thumb at the upper part of the upper lid and pull it upwards so as to evert the eyelashes. Grasp the lashes between the forefinger and thumb of the left hand and evert the lid by rotating it round the right thumb.

The conjunctiva may be pale in anaemia, jaundiced, or injected in conjunctivitis. Marked injection of the bulbar conjunctiva with a mucopurulent discharge suggests a severe bacterial inflammation; marked injection with a little serous discharge is indicative of a viral infection; slight oedema of the conjunctiva with a milky hue suggests an allergic condition. Follicles on the upper palpebral conjunctiva occur in trachoma, whereas their presence on the lower palpebral conjunctiva suggests an allergic condition or a conjunctivitis of viral origin.

Conjunctivitis In conjunctivitis the injection is maximal in the fornices (the junction of bulbar and palpebral conjunctiva). This appearance must be distinguished from the circumcorneal injection that occurs in keratitis, anterior uveitis (see below) and acute glaucoma. In circumcorneal injection there is a narrow band of dilated blood vessel around the limbus, and the injection is minimal in the fornices.

The cornea

Inflammation of the cornea (keratitis) This may be superficial or deep; it is accompanied by circumcorneal injection. Superficial keratitis and corneal ulcers result in breaches in the corneal epithelium; these lesions can be shown with fluorescein. A drop of fluorescein is instilled into the conjunctival sac and the excess dye is then washed out with normal saline. Corneal ulcers are stained green.

Deep keratitis results in a hazy cornea, often with an intact epithelium; it is usually caused by a viral infection but can also occur in syphilis. Both keratitis and trauma to the cornea may result in corneal opacities; small opacities are described as *nebulae*, larger ones as *leucomata*.

Arcus senilis Arcus senilis is a crescentic opacity near the periphery of the cornea. It usually starts at the lower part of the cornea, extending to form a complete circle. It is common in old people, but may occur in the young (arcus juvenilis). It is sometimes associated with type IV hypolipoproteinaemia but frequently is of no significance.

The iris

Anterior uveitis In anterior uveitis (iridocyclitis) circumcorneal injection also occurs. In addition, white specks may be visible on the posterior surface of the cornea (keratitic precipitates), there may be an exudate in the anterior chamber, and the pupil may be constricted and irregular due to the formation of adhesions between the edge of the pupil and the anterior surface of the lens.

The latter are called *posterior synechiae*. Other abnormalities of the pupils are described on pp. 305 and 403.

Ocular tension

The ocular tension may be roughly assessed by palpating the eyeball, although only gross variations from normal can be appreciated. The sclera is palpated with the two forefingers through the upper lid with the patient looking downwards, the other fingers resting on the patient's forehead. The degree of fluctuation gives an indication of the ocular tension. More accurate measurements of ocular tension can be made with Schiøtz or applanation tonometers. A diminished tension occurs in diabetic coma and in severe dehydration from any cause. A myopic eye frequently feels softer than a normal one. An increased ocular tension is a characteristic feature of glaucoma.

The fundus (Plate II)

Examination of the fundus of the eye, i.e. the retina and its associated structures, with an ophthalmoscope is an essential part of every complete medical examination. Valuable information may be obtained about the state of the optic nerve head (papilla) and of the arteries and veins of the retina, in addition to the detection of local ophthalmic disorders.

In routine medical examinations it is usually possible, with practice, to examine the optic disc and surrounding retina without dilating the pupil but for a complete examination of the fundus the pupils should be dilated by instilling a few drops of 1% cyclopentolate (Mydrilate) or 1% tropicamide (Mydriacyl) into the conjunctival sacs. In patients with a predisposition to closed-angle glaucoma an acute attack of glaucoma may be precipitated when the pupils are dilated. Before a mydriatic is instilled, the patient should therefore be asked whether he has ever seen haloes (coloured rings) around lights, and, if he has, this, or the presence of a shallow anterior chamber, is a contraindication to the use of a mydriatic. After the examination of the fundus has been completed, the effects of the mydriatic should be counteracted by the instillation of a few drops of 2% pilocarpine.

The patient should be examined either sitting or lying down in a darkened room. He is asked to look straight ahead and to keep his eyes as still as possible. The ophthalmoscope is held a few centimetres from the patient's eyes, and a suitable plus lens is used in the ophthalmoscope so that the iris is in focus. Opacities in the media of the eye (cornea, anterior chamber, lens, vitreous) will appear as black specks or lines against the red reflex of the fundus.

The ophthalmoscope should then be brought as close as possible to the patient's eye and the light directed slightly nasally. In this way the optic disc can be found and, in addition, the light will not shine directly on the macula. If the patient's pupils are not dilated, shining a light on to the macula will make the pupils contract and may make the examination of the fundus difficult or impossible. If the optic disc is not in focus, the strength of the lenses of the ophthalmoscope should be gradually reduced until the disc becomes sharply focused. If the observer's eye is emmetropic and his accommodation is relaxed, the strength of the lens necessary to bring the fundus into focus gives an indication of the refractive error of the patient's eye. Plus lenses indicate hypermetropia, and minus ones myopia. The optic disc, the retinal blood vessels, the macular region and the periphery of the fundus should be examined in turn.

The optic disc: *Shape* The normal disc is round or slightly oval. If astigmatism is present, the disc may appear more oval than normal.

Colour The normal disc has a pale-pink colour, distinctly paler than the surrounding fundus. The temporal side of the disc is usually paler than the nasal side.

In atrophy of the optic nerve, the disc becomes pale and may even become white or greyish-white in colour. In oedema of the optic nerve head, resulting from raised intracranial pressure (papilloedema) or from inflammation (papillitis), the disc is pinker than normal and may approach the colour of the surrounding retina. In pseudopapilloedema, a congenital anomaly sometimes associated with hypermetropia, the disc may appear swollen and pinker than normal, but the retinal blood vessels are normal in appearance, corrected vision is normal and the condition is stationary.

Physiological cup In its central part there is usually a depression in the disc: the physiological cup. The cup is paler than the surrounding disc, and from it the retinal vessels enter and leave the eye. In glaucoma the cup may be greatly increased in size and the retinal vessels will kink as they cross the edge of the disc. When the cup is deep, as in advanced glaucoma, retinal vessels disappear as they climb from the floor to the rim, and reappear again as they bend sharply over the cup; in less advanced cases a vertically oval cup extending to the edge of the disc may be seen.

Edge of the disc This is normally well defined. In normal eyes there is sometimes a white scleral ring, a dark-pigmented ring, or a stippled choroidal ring surrounding the optic disc.

The retinal blood vessels These radiate from the disc, dividing dichotomously into many branches as they pass towards the periphery of the retina. The retinal arteries are narrower than the veins, are a brighter red in colour, and have a brighter longitudinal streak where light is reflected from their convex walls. *Spontaneous retinal artery pulsation* is an abnormal finding, and occurs in some cases of glaucoma and aortic regurgitation. *Spontaneous venous pulsation* is frequently seen in normal eyes; it never occurs in papilloedema. It is important to study the points where arteries and veins cross. Most frequently it is the artery that crosses the vein, and in normal eyes neither vessel shows any change in colour, diameter or direction.

The macular region This is situated about 1·5 disc diameters from the temporal border of the optic disc. It is recognized by being darker in colour than the surrounding fundus, and is frequently surrounded by a halo of annular light reflex. It is devoid of blood vessels. At the centre of the macular region is a small depression, the fovea, which is lighter in colour and often glistens. Pathological changes in the macular region are important, as they produce a greater reduction of vision than similar changes in any other part of the fundus.

The periphery of the fundus This area can be examined only if the pupil is dilated with a mydriatic. Certain disease processes start in this region, for example retinal tears and retinitis pigmentosa.

The abnormal fundus

Papilloedema (Plate II) This is a passive oedema of the optic nerve head, most commonly due to raised intracranial pressure. There is an absence of inflammatory changes and little or no disturbance of visual function. In severe papilloedema the patient may notice transient loss of vision for a second or two (visual obscurations). In the initial stages of papilloedema there is an increased redness of the disc with blurring of its margins, the blurring appearing first at the upper and lower margins, particularly in the upper nasal quadrant. The physiological cup becomes filled in and disappears, and the retinal veins are slightly distended. Spontaneous pulsation of the retinal veins is absent.

As the condition progresses the disc becomes definitely swollen (Fig. 13.1). In order to measure the degree of swelling of the disc, start with a high plus lens in the ophthalmoscope and reduce the power of the lens until the centre of the disc is just in focus. The retina, a short distance from the disc, is then brought into focus by further reduction of the power of the lens. This further reduction indicates the degree of swelling of the disc (3 dioptres is equivalent to 1 mm of swelling).

If papilloedema develops rapidly, there will be marked engorgement of the retinal veins with haemorrhages and exudates on and around the disc, but with papilloedema of slow onset there may be little or no vascular change, even though the disc may become very swollen. The retinal vessels will, however, bend sharply as they dip down from the swollen disc to the surrounding retina. The oedema may extend to the adjacent retina, producing greyish-white

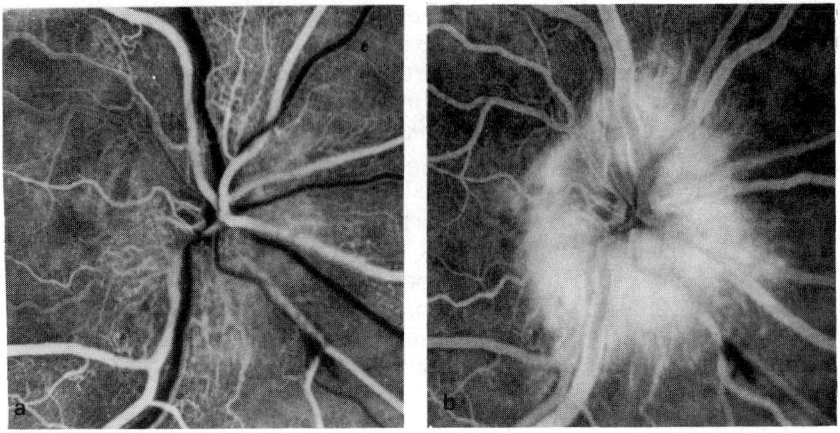

Fig. 13.1 Fluorescein retinal angiogram of fundus in papilloedema. The disc is swollen and there is marked leakage of fluorescein from the capillary circulation at the disc. (a) Early arterial phase. The (white) arteries are filled with fluorescein. The disc margin is slightly swollen and this is out of the plane of focus. There is dilatation of the capillary beds with early leakage of fluorescein. (b) Late phase. Both arteries and veins are filled with fluorescein. There is a dense white halo of capillary leakage of fluorescein at the disc. (See also Fig. 13.2.)

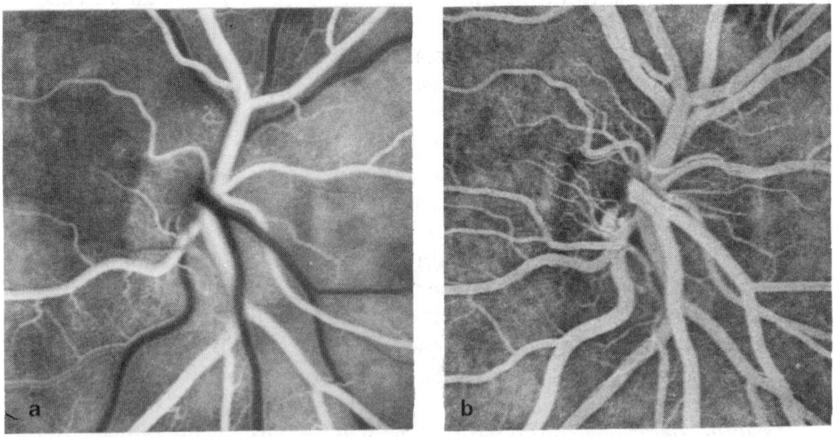

Fig. 13.2 Fluorescein retinal angiogram of fundus in pseudopapilloedema, a congenital anomoly of disc development that resembles papilloedema. The disc is normal. There is no capillary leakage of fluorescein. (a) Early arterial phase. The (white) arteries are filled with fluorescein, and normal early filling of the capillary bed near the disc itself can be seen. The veins, unfilled with fluorescein, appear black. (b) Late phase. There is filling both of arteries and veins, and peripapillary arteries are also visible. Note there is no leakage of dye.

striations near the disc, and a white macular fan between the fovea and disc may develop in some cases. These appearances result from swelling of the nerve axons in the nerve and retina as a result of interference with axoplasmic flow.

Papilloedema occurs frequently in patients with brain tumour, but is particularly liable to occur in children with tumours of the cerebellum and 4th ventricle. It is rare in patients with pituitary tumours. An acute form of papilloedema with haemorrhage extending into the vitreous is characteristic of subarachnoid haemorrhage. A subdural haematoma may produce a similar clinical picture to that of a cerebral tumour. Papilloedema is uncommon in acute meningitis, but is a feature in subacute and chronic meningitis and in patients with brain abscess. It may be the only physical sign in benign intracranial hypertension. Papilloedema occurring in malignant hypertension is accompanied by arterial changes characteristic of this condition and the haemorrhages and exudates extend far beyond the region of the disc.

Optic neuritis Inflammatory, demyelinating, or vascular disease may affect any part of the optic nerve, producing an optic neuritis, the characteristic symptom of which is loss of vision, which presents as either a central scotoma or complete blindness. There is often pain on moving the eye, and the pupil on the affected side shows an ill-sustained contraction to a bright light (see p. 305).

When the disease affects the optic nerve head (papillitis) there is hyperaemia and some swelling of the optic disc. It must not be confused with papilloedema, in spite of their similar ophthalmoscopic appearances. The two conditions can usually be distinguished by the severe visual impairment that occurs with optic neuritis, as compared with the minimal loss in papilloedema. In optic neuritis the swelling of the optic disc is usually slight, the distension of the retinal veins is less marked than in papilloedema, and there may be signs of inflammation, e.g. hazy vitreous and retinal exudates.

Retrobulbar neuritis This is a form of optic neuritis in which the disease process affects the optic nerve behind the eye. The same severe visual loss occurs as in patients with optic neuritis in whom there is papillitis, but the optic disc appears normal in the acute stage of the disease. Optic neuritis and retrobulbar neuritis may be followed by optic atrophy, with residual reduction in visual acuity and, often, central scotoma.

Optic atrophy In this condition the optic disc is paler than normal and may even be white (Plate II). Because of the wide variation in colour of the normal disc, a useful sign of optic atrophy is the reduction in the number of capillaries on the disc. In optic atrophy the number of capillaries that cross the disc margin is reduced from the normal of 10 to 7 or less (Kestenbaum's sign). From the appearance of the disc it is customary, although not always very useful, to divide optic atrophy into primary and secondary types. In the *primary* type the disc is flat and white with clear-cut edges. *Secondary* optic atrophy follows swelling of the optic disc, due to papilloedema. The disc is greyish-white in colour and its edges are indistinct.

Optic atrophy may occur in a number of disorders, of which the following are a few.

1 Interference with the blood supply to the optic nerve, as in occlusion of one of the ciliary vessels supplying the optic nerve head (*ischaemic optic neuropathy*).
2 Pressure on the nerve, whether in its intra-ocular, intra-orbital, intra-canalicular or intracranial portions.
3 Following optic neuritis.
4 Following trauma, where the optic nerve or its blood supply is involved.
5 In toxic conditions due to substances such as tobacco, alcohol, lead, etc.
6 In certain congenital disorders, when it is frequently associated with other neurological signs.
7 Following widespread chorioretinal inflammation or degeneration.

Opaque or medullated nerve fibres These usually present as one or more bright white patches radiating for a short distance from the optic disc (Plate II). The patch has a characteristic feathered edge and retinal vessels may disappear for a short distance within it. This condition is a harmless and non-progressive congenital anomaly.

A myopic crescent This is a ring of exposed white sclera, usually on the temporal side of the optic disc (Plate II) but in some cases extending all round it. When marked it may be associated with other degenerative changes in the fundus, which, if they involve the macula, will result in reduction of central vision.

Retinal haemorrhages These occur in a number of different conditions and are due to one or more of the following factors.
1 Increased blood pressure within the retinal vessels, as in hypertension.
2 Abnormalities in the walls of the retinal vessels, as in arteriosclerosis, diabetes mellitus and occlusion of the retinal veins.
3 Abnormalities in the circulating blood, as in severe anaemia, leukaemias, and bleeding diatheses.
4 Sudden reduction in intra-ocular pressure, following a penetrating wound (surgical or traumatic) of the eye.

When superficial, within the nerve fibre layer of the retina, the haemorrhages are elongated and 'flame-shaped', whereas when deep they are round blotches or spots. Subhyaloid haemorrhages, situated in front of the retina, are occasionally seen as very large round haemorrhages with a straight, horizontal upper border; they sometimes occur in diabetic retinopathy and after a subarachnoid haemorrhage.

Retinal arteriosclerosis This occurs either as an exaggeration of the general ageing process of the body or in association with hypertension. It is characterized by (*a*) broadening of the arterial light reflex, producing a 'copper wire' or 'silver wire' appearance; (*b*) tortuosity of the vessels; (*c*) nipping, indentation or deflection of the veins where they are crossed by the arteries; (*d*) white plaques on the arteries; and (*e*) in hypertension, 'flame-shaped' haemorrhages and 'cotton-wool' exudates in the region of the macula.

Hypertensive retinopathy (Plate IV) This is characterized by a generalized narrowing of the retinal arteries, particularly in the young patient. In older patients these changes are masked by the accompanying arteriosclerosis. If the hypertension is severe, fullness of the retinal veins and 'flame-shaped' haemorrhages occur around the optic disc, and there is retinal oedema extending towards the macula, sometimes accompanied by a star-shaped collection of white exudates around the macula. In malignant hypertension, papilloedema is also present. The retinopathy seen in some cases of acute and chronic nephritis is due to the associated hypertension.

Diabetic retinopathy (Plate IV) The fundamental change in this condition is the formation of capillary micro-aneurysms, seen as tiny red spots around the macula. Micro-aneurysms are not seen in such abundance in any other condition. Retinal haemorrhages and exudates may occur; the haemorrhages are punctate or round, and the exudates have a waxy yellow–white appearance. In the more severe form of diabetic retinopathy—proliferative retinopathy—new vessels extend into the vitreous and bleed. The resulting glial proliferation may destroy vision by covering the macula or by producing a retinal detachment. Patients with diabetic retinopathy often have associated arteriosclerotic or hypertensive changes in their fundi.

Retinopathies in disorders of the haemopoietic system In severe anaemias the fundus may be paler than normal and a few small 'flame-shaped' haemorrhages and small woolly exudates may be present.

In polycythaemia the retinal vessels are dark, tortuous and dilated. There may be oedema of the optic disc, and a few retinal haemorrhages may be observed.

In the leukaemias the retinal veins may be tortuous and dilated. In the later stages of these diseases the arteries and veins may be yellowish in colour, and the fundus may have a generalized pallor. Retinal haemorrhages of various types may occur, the characteristic ones in leukaemia being round with a pale centre.

Occlusion of the central artery of the retina The optic disc and surrounding retina are pale, and there is a cherry-red spot at the macula which contrasts with the milky pallor of the adjacent retina. The retinal arteries are narrow or even thread-like.

Occlusion of the central vein of the retina There is intense swelling of the optic disc, with gross venous dilatation, and numerous retinal haemorrhages extend from the disc in all directions.

Choroiditis In acute choroiditis there are one or more round or oval whitish patches in the fundus, lying deep to the retinal vessels. These patches have ill-defined edges and the vitreous may be hazy. When the acute phase subsides, flat white scars with pigment around their edges are left. The numerous causes of choroiditis include tuberculosis, syphilis (which may cause a disseminated choroiditis), and toxoplasmosis (which characteristically produces lesions at the maculae).

Examination of the eye in children

The points made in Chapter 16, on the examination of children in general, also apply to the examination of children's eyes. In particular, children may object strongly to lights and instruments, particularly when they are wielded by white-coated strangers. Allow the child to get used to the surroundings whilst taking a history from the parent. At the same time, constantly observe the child, noting the child's visual behaviour, the position and movements of the eyes, and the general appearance of each eye.

The assessment of visual acuity should then be made. Babies should rapidly fix a large object and follow it. The examiner's face is the best visual target. In infants, the visual acuity can be assessed by the ability to follow rolling white balls of varying sizes. From the age of 2½ years a more accurate estimate of acuity can be made using the Sheridan–Gardiner test. In this test the child, or the child's mother, holds a card with a number of letters on it. The examiner then shows the child one of the letters on an identical card and asks the child to point to the same letter on his own card. When the child has understood the test the examiner moves to a distance of 6 metres and shows the child a series of letters of decreasing size, until the child fails to make a match. This test is also useful for assessing visual acuity in patients with whom the examiner has no common language, in illiterate patients, and in patients with dysphasia.

Next, the position and movements of the eyes should be assessed. The least disturbing method is to observe the corneal light reflex; a light held at about one metre should produce a reflection in the centre of the pupil of each eye. If the reflection in one eye is at a different location to that in the other, there is probably a squint. If squint is suspected, a cover test should be performed (see p. 301). The range of movement of the eyes should then be assessed and the pupillary responses to light, and to accommodation, should be observed. Finally, the media and fundi are examined with the ophthalmoscope. It is best to carry out ophthalmoscopy without touching the child as this can produce resistance and tight closure of the eye. Begin with a relatively dim light and gradually increase the brightness.

SOME CLINICAL PROBLEMS

The painful red eye

Three conditions have to be differentiated:

1 Conjunctivitis
2 Anterior uveitis
3 Acute glaucoma

Whilst the character of the red injection of the conjunctiva, the nature of the discharge, if any, and the state of the patient's vision are helpful in diagnosis, the simplest way to differentiate between these three disorders is to examine the pupils. In conjunctivitis, the pupil appears normal and reacts briskly to light. In anterior uveitis, the pupil is small and reacts poorly to light; it may be irregular as a residuum from previous episodes of uveitis. In acute glaucoma the pupil is moderately dilated and may be unreactive to light.

Sudden loss of vision

It is important to decide whether the patient's vision was lost suddenly or if the patient suddenly became aware of relatively long-standing or slowly progressive loss of vision in one eye, for example by accidentally covering the other eye. Sudden visual loss is usually unilateral and very often results from vascular disease. Sudden transient loss of vision, sometimes described as coming on like a curtain falling over the eye, and resolving gradually or like the lifting of a curtain after a few seconds or a minute or so, is usually due to transient embolic ischaemia of the retinal vessels. Sudden permanent loss of vision in one eye occurs from central retinal artery occlusion, or from optic nerve ischaemia, due to involvement of the ciliary circulation. The ciliary vessels are often involved also in giant cell arteritis. When a retinal detachment involves the macula, it may cause sudden loss of vision.

In all cases of sudden loss of vision, it is essential to test the pupillary light response. When there is disease in the retina, or in the optic tract, there will be an afferent pupillary defect (p. 305). Sudden blindness with normal pupillary responses to light strongly suggests a functional cause for the loss of vision. Bilateral sudden loss of vision may also be psychogenic in origin, but it can result from acute compression of the optic chiasm and optic nerves, for example in untreated hydrocephalus or in pituitary apoplexy, i.e. infarction of a pituitary tumour. Infarction of both occipital lobes, from vertebro-basilar disease or due to embolism from the heart, similarly may produce bilateral loss of vision but in this disorder the pupillary light responses are normal.

Unequal pupils (anisocoria)

Approximately 12% of normal individuals have a slight, but clinically evident, pupillary inequality. Such physiologically unequal pupils react normally. *Pathological pupils dilate and constrict abnormally*.

In the absence of local disease of the eye, a small pupil may be due to paralysis of the dilator pupillae muscle, which is supplied by sympathetic nerve fibres. The sympathetic nerve fibres also supply part of levator palpebrae superioris. Damage to these sympathetic nerve fibres, derived from the stellate cervical sympathetic ganglion, produces slight drooping of the lid on the affected side (*ptosis*). The small pupil, together with slight ptosis, constitutes *Horner's syndrome* (Fig. 13.3). The easiest way to confirm a diagnosis of Horner's syndrome is to put the patient into a semi-darkened room for a minute or two. If Horner's syndrome is present, the pupil will dilate very poorly; the normal contralateral pupil dilates fully.

An abnormally dilated pupil suggests a partial *oculomotor palsy*. The internal ophthalmoplegia in partial oculomotor palsy results from damage to the parasympathetic fibres, which arise in the Edinger–Westphal nucleus of the oculomotor nerve. This may be associated with partial or complete weakness of the external ocular muscles supplied by the oculomotor nerve (p. 298). In internal ophthalmoplegia due to partial oculomotor nerve palsy, the enlarged pupil reacts very poorly to light and to accommodation. A *tonic pupil* (Holmes–Adie pupil), which is usually smaller than normal, reacts very slowly to light, but better to accommodation. The tonic pupil reacts in a supersen-

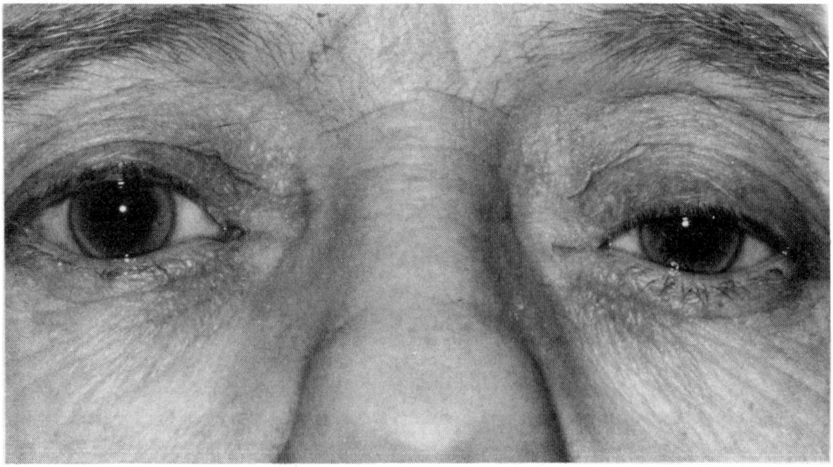

Fig. 13.3 Left Horner's syndrome. On the affected side there is ptosis, which may be very slight, and a small pupil (miosis), which reacts to light and to accommodation.

sitive manner to weak cholinergic drugs instilled into the conjunctival sac, e g. pilocarpine 0.125% solution. After accidental medication with mydriatics, there is no reaction either to light or to accommodation.

14
The locomotor system

Musculoskeletal symptoms are common and occasionally may be the first manifestation of systemic disease. The aim of examination is to determine, wherever possible, whether symptoms are derived from bone, muscle, joint or other structures. It is important to appreciate that pain may often be due to nerve root compression, for example in cervical spondylosis or lumbar disc protrusion. A common presenting feature of hip joint disease in children is pain referred to the knee. This stresses the importance of a full examination and not one limited to the apparent site of symptoms.

Examination should begin by observing the patient as he enters. Abnormalities of *gait* and *posture* may provide important information that can be pursued in history taking. Observation of any difficulty in undressing and getting onto the examination couch will further help in assessing the patient. The locomotor system includes the muscles, bones, joints and soft tissue structures, such as tendons and ligaments. The examination of the muscles has been considered on p. 319, but it should be noted that although muscle wasting in the rheumatic diseases may be due to primary muscle involvement (e.g. myositis), it is more commonly secondary to disuse, nerve root or peripheral nerve problems (Fig. 14.1).

THE BONES

In examining the *long bones* of the limbs, look for any alterations in shape or outline and measure any shortening. In osteitis deformans (Paget's disease) bowing of the long bones, particularly the tibia and femur, is associated with bony enlargement and usually increased local temperature. The skull is commonly involved but clinically this may not be apparent until advanced. Pain may be due to the bony changes or, if these extend to the end of a long bone, to damage to the adjoining joint. Alteration in the shape of bones also occurs in

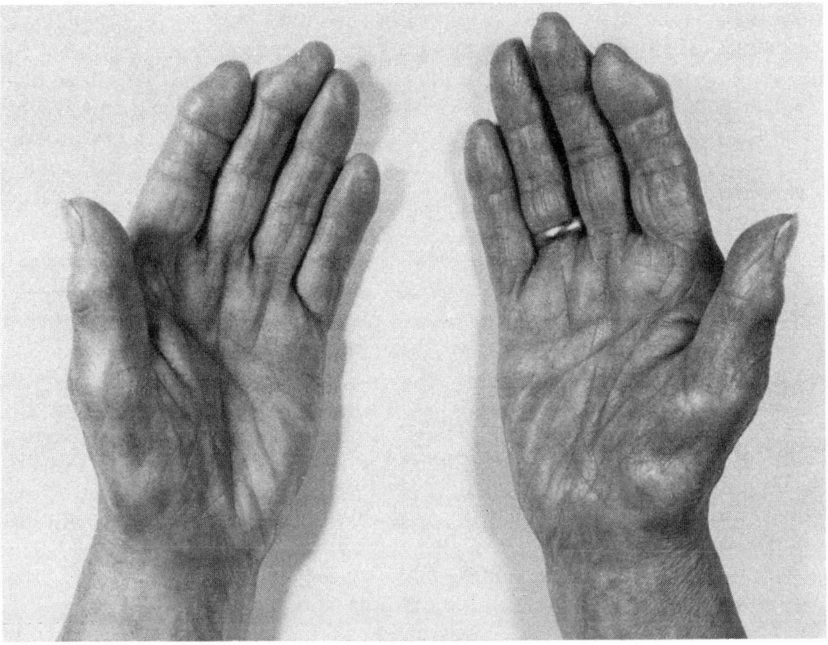

Fig. 14.1 Bilateral thenar muscle wasting due to carpal tunnel compression. Note the osteoarthritic change in the terminal phalanges.

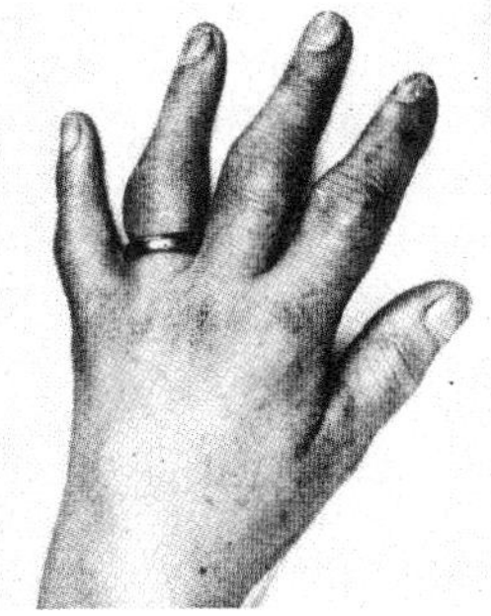

Fig. 14.2 Rheumatoid arthritis.

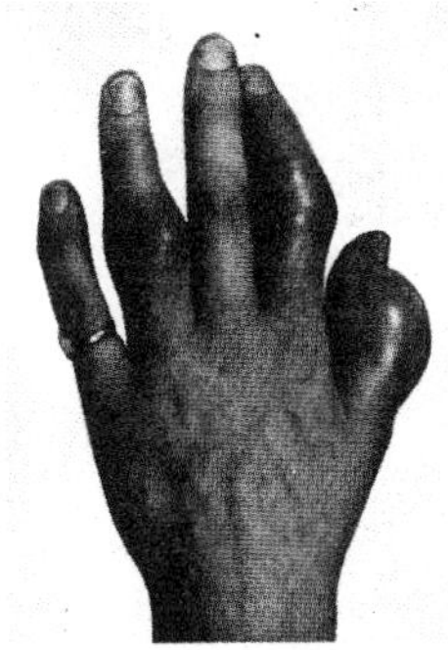

Fig. 14.3 Gout.

rickets, with costochondral enlargement (rickety rosary) and epiphyseal enlargement. Localized swellings may be caused by infections, cysts or tumours. Spontaneous fractures may occasionally assist in the diagnosis of secondary carcinoma, generalized osteitis fibrosa (hyperparathyroidism), osteogenesis imperfecta or multiple myeloma. Undue tenderness of the bones is found with osteomalacia, in generalized osteitis fibrosa, myelomatosis, occasionally in carcinomatosis of bones, and very rarely in leukaemia.

In the *vertebral column* note the presence of any local projections or angular deformity of the vertebral spines, which vertebrae are involved and at what level the projection is most prominent. Landmarks are C7 (vertebra prominens) and the last rib, articulating with the 12th thoracic vertebra. In many cases, however, the last rib cannot be distinctly felt and is therefore rather untrustworthy as a guide.

THE JOINTS

General principles

These should be examined by *inspection* and *palpation*, and by tests for their range of *movement*. It is best to proceed in a routine manner, e.g. the jaw, cervical spine, shoulder girdle and upper limb, thoracic and lumbar spine, pelvis and lower limb, so that inconspicuous but important joints like the temporomandibular, sternoclavicular and sacroiliac will not be overlooked. Always compare the corresponding joints on the two sides of the body. Great care must be taken to avoid undue discomfort.

The overall pattern of joint involvement should be assessed. Note whether the distribution is *symmetrical*, as is usual in rheumatoid arthritis (Fig. 14.2), or *asymmetrical*, as in psoriatic arthropathy or gout (Fig. 14.3). The seronegative spondyloarthropathies (e.g. Reiter's disease) tend to involve the lower limb joints predominantly. It is also important to decide whether the joint involvement is *inflammatory* or not. In the history, inflammatory joint disease is almost always associated with *early morning stiffness* of more than thirty minutes; it takes some time for the joints to loosen up after waking.

On inspection and palpation look for enlargement or irregularity of the joint. Determine whether this is due to bony enlargement, to osteophytes (e.g. Heberden's nodes, Fig. 14.4), to thickening of synovial tissues, such as occurs in inflammatory arthritis, or to effusion into the joint space, when it usually has a characteristic shape and fluctuation can often be elicited. Enlargement of the ends of the bones, particularly the radius and ulna, can be found due to hypertrophic pulmonary osteoarthropathy, and complete disorganization of a joint with absence of deep pain sensation occurs in neuropathic (Charcot's) joints.

In addition to enlargement, look for *other signs of inflammation*, *redness*, *tenderness* and *warmth*, and note whether the overlying skin is dry or moist. Tenderness may be recorded in four grades, depending upon the patient's reaction to firm pressure of the joint between finger and thumb. Grade 1 tenderness: the patient says the joint is tender. Grade 2: the patient winces. Grade 3: the patient winces and withdraws the affected part. Grade 4: the

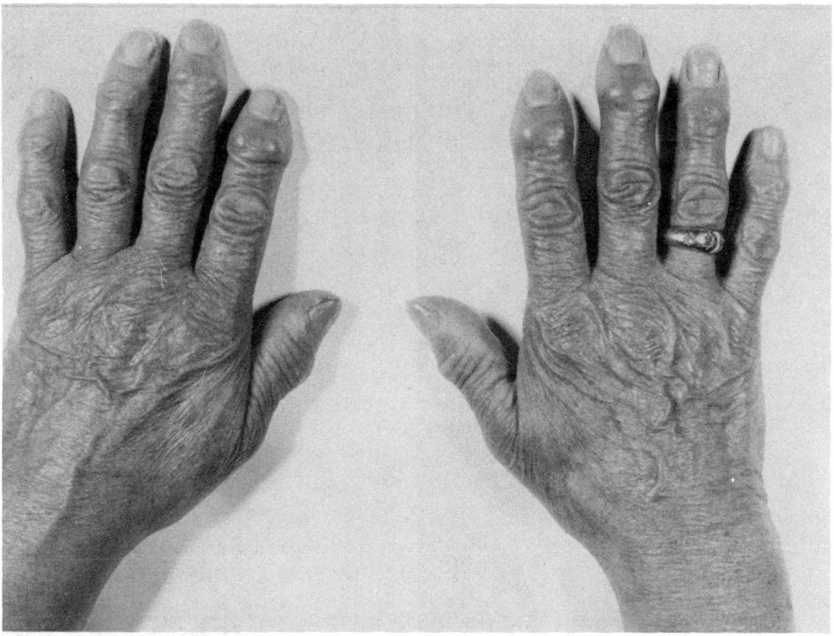

Fig. 14.4 Heberden's nodes: bony enlargement of the distal interphalangeal joints in osteoarthritis.

patient will not allow the joint to be touched. Grade 4 tenderness occurs only in crystal arthritis, rheumatic fever and septic arthritis. In gout the skin overlying the affected joint is dry, whereas in septic arthritis or rheumatic fever it is moist.

If *tenderness* is present localize it as accurately as possible and determine whether it arises in the joint or in neighbouring structures, e.g. in the supraspinatus or bicipital tendon rather than the shoulder joint. Tendon sheath *crepitus*, a grating or creaking sensation, may be felt, particularly if there is a tenosynovitis of the long flexor tendons in the palm. Crepitus may also be derived from a joint and can be detected by feeling the joint with one hand while it is moved passively with the other. This often indicates osteoarthritis, but not invariably so, for crepitus is commonly felt in the shoulder joints of older people, whereas osteoarthritis of these joints is rare.

In examining joints for the range of movement it may often be sufficient to estimate the degree of limitation based on previous experience or in comparison with the normal side, but for accurate description the actual range of movement should be measured with a protractor (goniometer). Testing the range of *passive* movement is generally more informative than observing *active* movement, although it is sometimes useful to test the latter as well. Gentleness

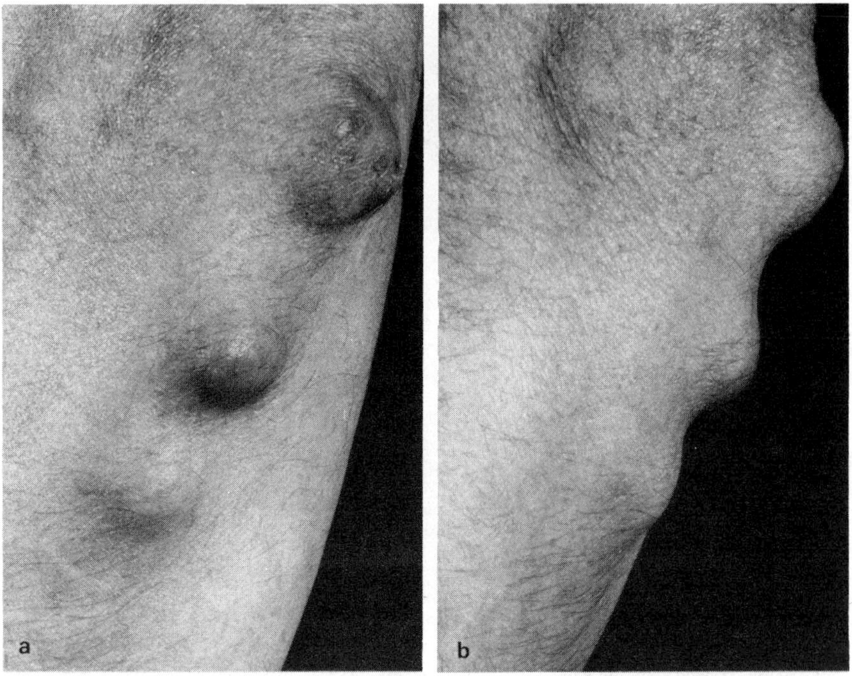

Fig. 14.5 Subcutaneous nodules at the elbow in rheumatoid arthritis.

must be exercised, particularly in the case of painful joints. Limitation of movement in a joint may be due to pain, muscle spasm, contracture, inflammation or thickening of the capsules or peri-articular structures, effusion into the joint space, bony overgrowths, bony ankylosis, or to painful conditions quite unconnected with the joint.

In general examination look for other signs associated with joint disease. Rheumatoid *subcutaneous nodules* are firm and non-tender; they may be detected by running the examining thumb from the point of the elbow down the proximal portion of the ulna (Fig. 14.5). They can also be found at other pressure sites, such as bony prominences, including the sacrum. Rheumatoid *vasculitic lesions* are typically seen at the nail fold (cutaneous infarcts), but also occur at pressure sites. Look for gouty *tophi* on the helix of the ear as well as over joints. *Lymphadenopathy* may be found proximal to an inflamed joint, not only in septic arthritis but also in rheumatoid arthritis. *Pitting oedema* is sometimes seen over inflamed joints (Fig. 14.6), but other causes of oedema must of course be excluded. Look also for other systemic associations, particularly in the eyes and skin.

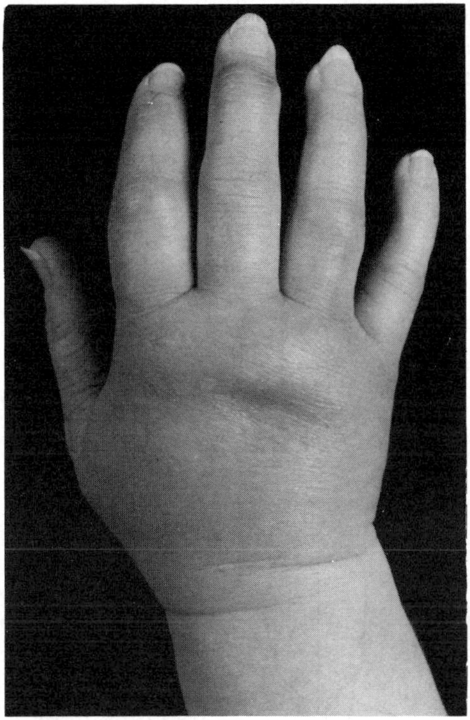

Fig. 14.6 Pitting oedema of the dorsum of the hand: note also synovitis of several interphalangeal joints.

Examination of individual joints

In describing the range of movement of joints the scheme shown in the following pages will be found useful.* All motion should be measured in degrees from a neutral or zero position, which must be defined whenever possible.

Spinal examination

Neutral position is a normal upright stance with head erect and chin drawn in. Note any curvature of the spinal column as a whole or of part of it. The curvature may be in an anterior, posterior or lateral direction. Anterior curvature (extension deformity) is termed *lordosis* and is commonest in the lumbar region. General posterior curvature (flexion deformity) is spoken of as *kyphosis*. It occurs most typically in the thoracic region in old persons and must

* Modified by permission of the authors and publishers, from E.F. Cave & M.R. Sumner (1936) *Journal of Bone and Joint Surgery*, *18*, 455.

be distinguished from the localized angular deformity (*gibbus*) of Pott's disease (spinal tuberculosis). Lateral curvature is termed *scoliosis*, and may be towards either side. It is always accompanied by a rotation of the bodies of the vertebrae in such a way that the spines come to point towards the concavity of the curve, i.e. the curvature is greater than it appears from inspection of the posterior spinous processes. Kyphosis and scoliosis may often be combined.

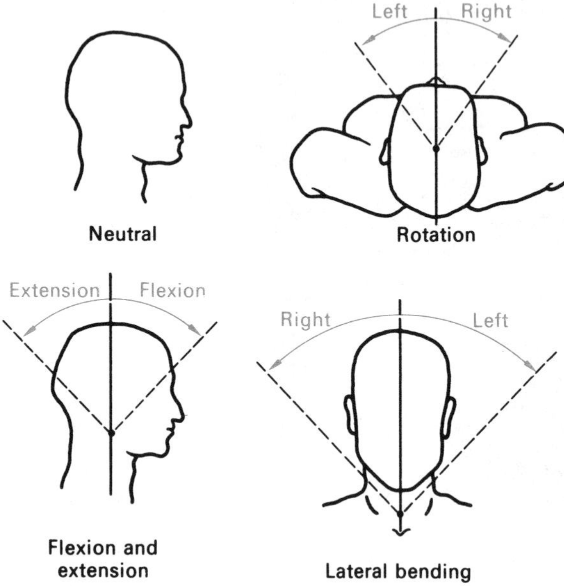

Fig. 14.7 Movements of the neck.

Cervical spine (Fig. 14.7)

Test:
1 Rotation
2 Flexion
3 Extension
4 Lateral bending

Note any pain or paraesthesia in the arm reproduced by neck movement, suggesting nerve root involvement, and look for any neurological deficit. Particular care is essential in examining the neck in rheumatoid arthritis as atlanto-axial instability may cause a myelopathy.

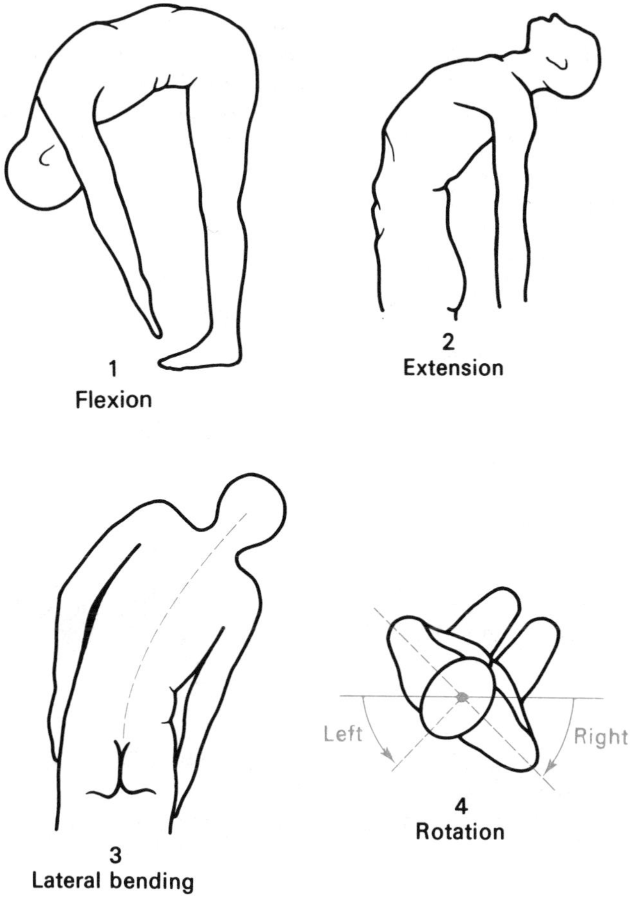

Fig. 14.8 Movements of the lumbar and dorsal spine.

Thoracic and lumbar spine (Fig. 14.8)

The thoracic spine permits mainly rotation, while the lumbar spine can flex, extend and bend laterally. Test:

1 Flexion
2 Extension
3 Lateral bending
4 Thoracic rotation (patient seated)

The normal lumbar lordosis should be abolished in flexion. The extent of lumbar flexion can be more accurately assessed by marking a 10 cm gap on the skin overlying the lumbar spinous processes and measuring the increase in the gap on flexion (Schober test). Painful restriction of spinal movement is an important sign of *cervical and lumbar spondylosis*, but may also be found in disc or other mechanical disorders of the back or neck. The spine may be fixed in *ankylosing spondylitis*, but in the early stages of this condition lumbar lateral flexion is typically reduced first, whereas in mechanical back problems flexion and extension are reduced.

Chest expansion is a measure of costovertebral movement and should be recorded using a tape measure. Reduced expansion characteristically occurs early in ankylosing spondylitis, but is also a feature of pulmonary disease.

Sacroiliac joints

Their surface markings are two dimples low in the lumbar region. Test for *irritability* in three ways:

1 Direct pressure over each sacroiliac joint
2 Firm pressure with the *side* of the hand over the sacrum
3 Inward pressure over both iliac bones in an attempt to distort the pelvis

In the second and third a positive test is indicated by the patient localizing discomfort to the sacroiliac joint.

Shoulder (Fig. 14.9)

Neutral position is arm to side, elbow flexed to 90° with forearm pointing forwards. Because the scapula is mobile, true shoulder (glenohumeral) movement can be assessed only by the examiner anchoring the scapula. Test:

1 Flexion
2 Extension
3 Abduction
4 Rotation in abduction
5 Rotation in neutral: in practice internal rotation can best be compared by recording the height reached by each thumb up the back (combined glenohumeral and scapular movement)
6 Elevation (also involving scapular movement)

Note any pain during the range of movement. In supraspinatus tendonitis a full passive range is found, but there is a painful arc on abduction and pain on resisted abduction.

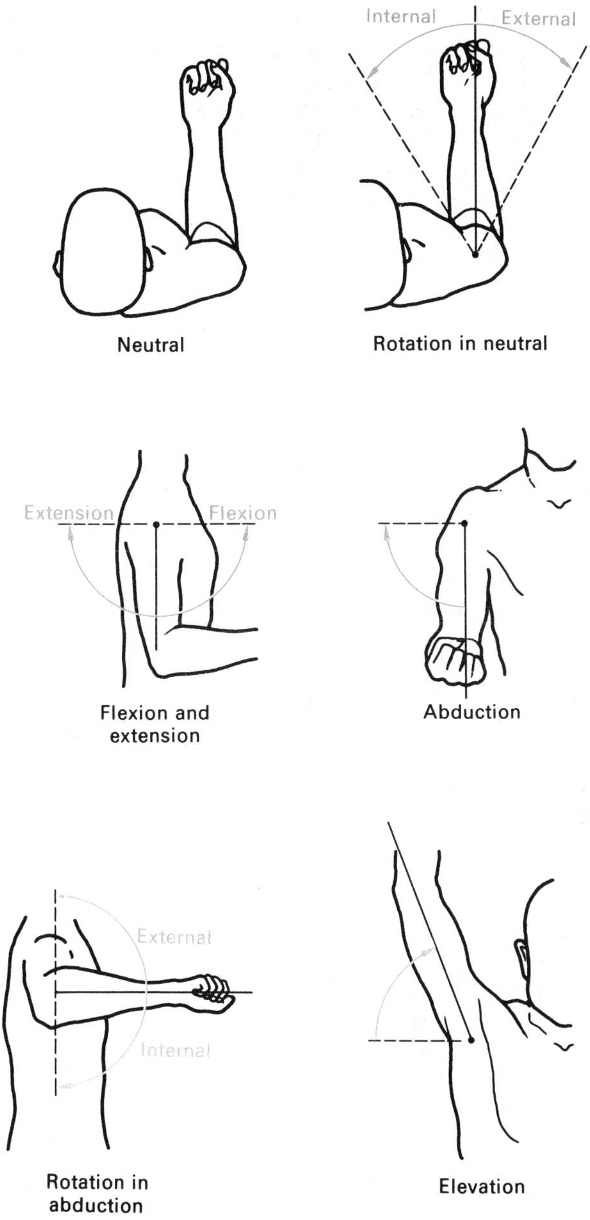

Fig. 14.9 Movements of the shoulder.

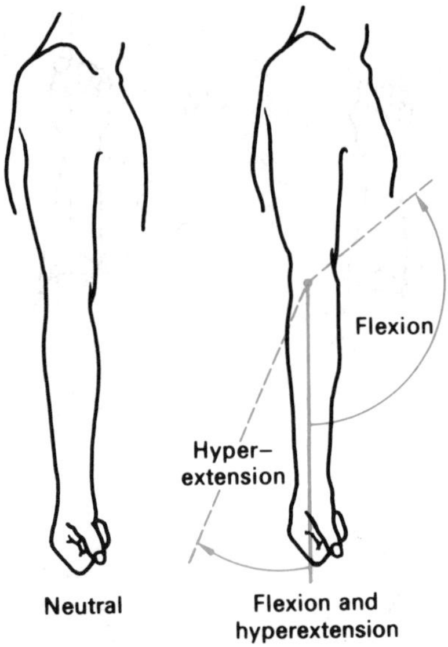

Fig. 14.10 Movements of the elbow.

Elbow (Fig. 14.10)

Neutral position is with forearm in extension. Test:
1 Flexion
2 Hyperextension

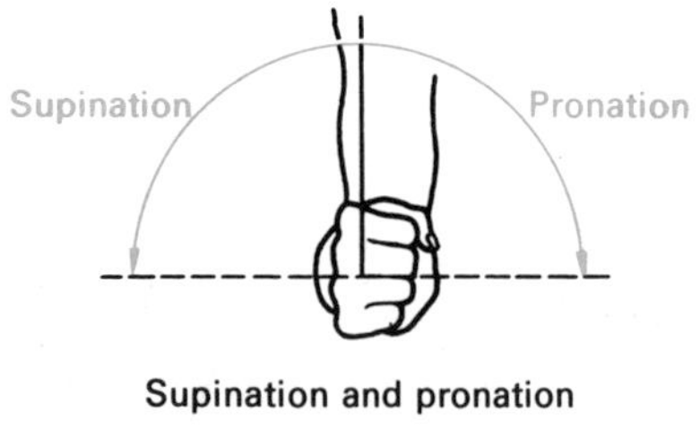

Fig. 14.11 Movements of the forearm.

Forearm (Fig 14.11)

Neutral position is with arm by side, elbow flexed to 90°, thumb uppermost Test:
1 Supination
2 Pronation

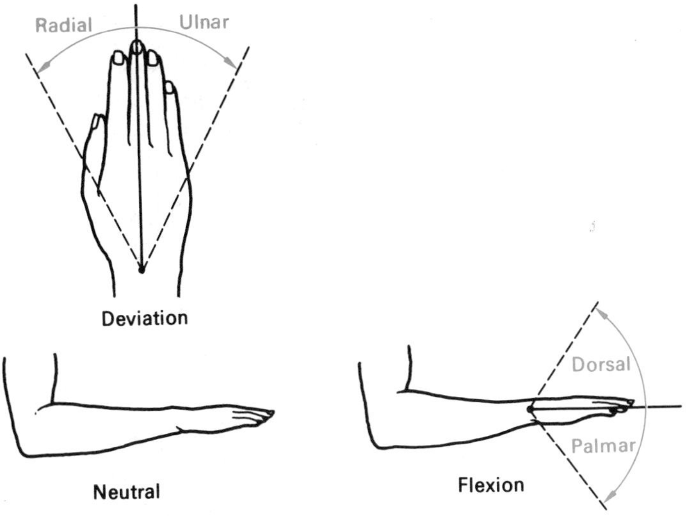

Fig. 14.12 Movements of the wrist.

Wrist (Fig. 14.12)

Neutral position is with hand in line with forearm and palm down. Test:
1 Dorsiflexion (extension)
2 Palmar flexion
3 Ulnar deviation
4 Radial deviation

Even minor limitation of wrist flexion or extension can be detected by comparing both wrists at the same time (Fig. 14.13). Wrist joint arthritis is almost invariably due to an inflammatory arthritis, as primary osteoarthritis of this joint is rare.

Fingers (Fig. 14.14)

Neutral position is with fingers in extension. Test the flexion at metacarpophalangeal, proximal interphalangeal and distal interphalangeal joints.

Thumb (carpometacarpal joint) (Fig. 14.15)

Neutral position is with thumb alongside forefinger and extended. Test:
1 Extension
2 Flexion, measured as for the fingers
3 Opposition
4 Abduction (not illustrated) is movement at right angles to plane of palm.

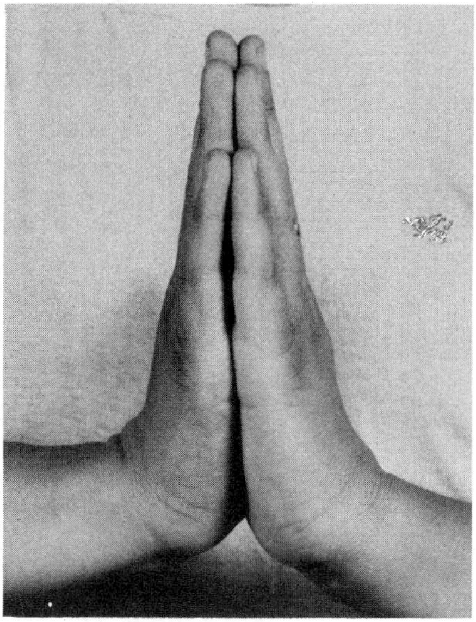

Fig. 14.13 Minor limitation of the left wrist extension compared with the right. Note the slightly different angulation of the left forearm.

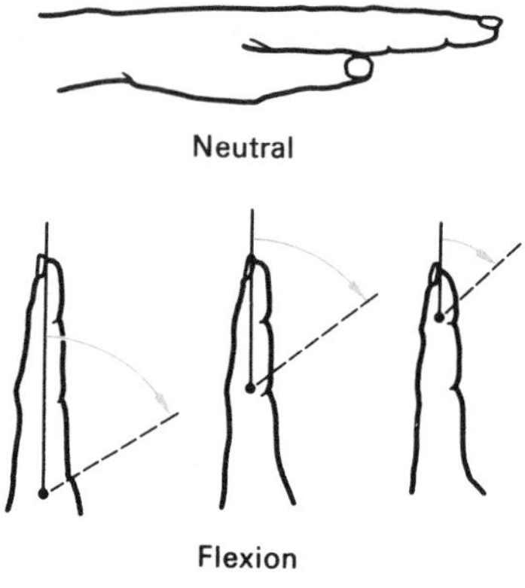

Fig. 14.14 Movements of the fingers.

Hand deformities

Examination of the individual joints of the hand may be less informative than inspection of the hand as a whole. The combination of Heberden's nodes (see above) and thumb carpometacarpal arthritis occurs in osteoarthritis (Fig. 14.4), while a variety of deformity patterns are characteristic of rheumatoid arthritis: metacarpophalangeal joint subluxations, ulnar deviation of the

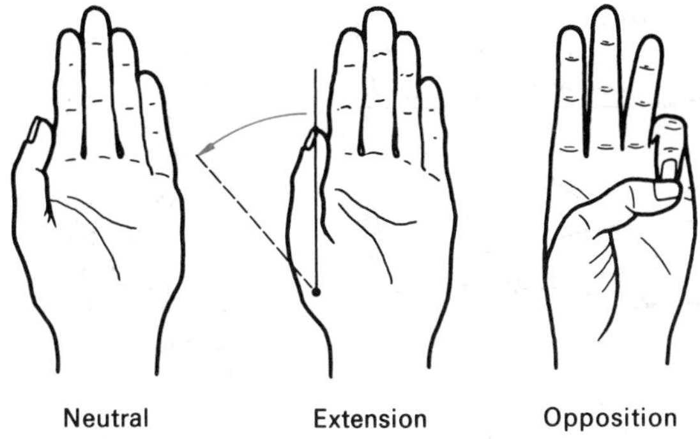

Fig. 14.15 Movements of the thumb.

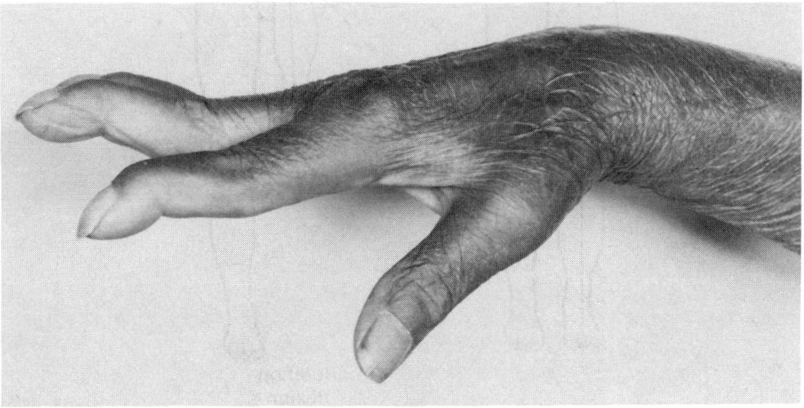

Fig. 14.16 'Swan-neck' deformity: hyperextended proximal and flexed distal interphalangeal joints.

fingers at these joints, 'swan-neck' fingers (Fig. 14.16), and 'boutonnière' deformities (flexed proximal and hyperextended distal interphalangeal joints). In psoriatic arthritis, terminal interphalangeal joint swelling may occur with psoriatic deformity of the nail on that digit.

Assessment of hand function should include testing grip and pinch grip (between index and thumb).

Hip (Fig. 14.17)

Neutral position is with hip in extension, patella pointing forwards. Ensure the pelvis does not tilt by placing one hand over the pelvis, while examining the hip with the other. Test:

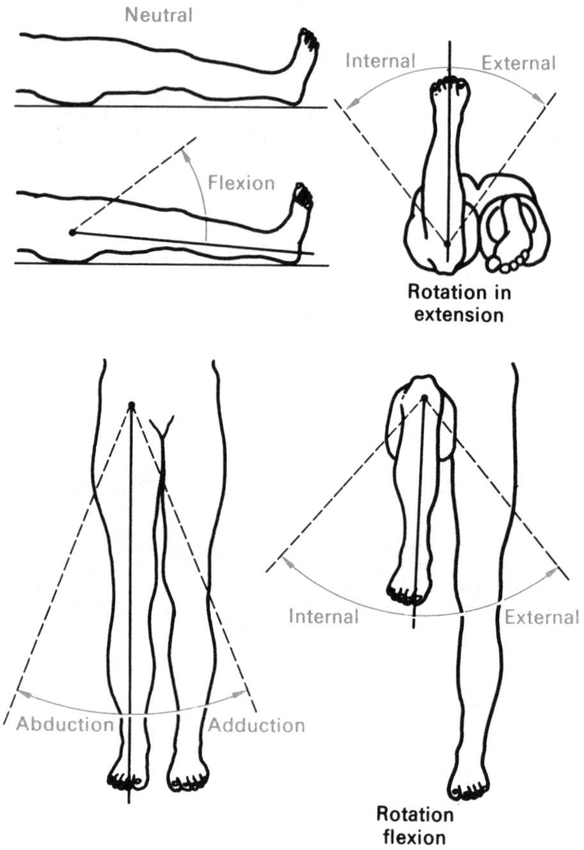

Fig. 14.17 Movements of the hip.

1 Flexion measured with knee bent. Opposite thigh must remain in neutral position. Flex the knee as the hip flexes
2 Abduction, measured from a line which forms an angle of 90° with a line joining the anterior superior iliac spines
3 Adduction, measured in the same manner
4 Rotation in flexion
5 Rotation in extension
6 Extension: attempt to extend the hip with the patient lying in the lateral position

Additional examinations of the hip joint:
1 Test for *flexion deformity*. With one hand flat between lumbar spine and the

couch, flex the hip fully to the point of abolishing the lumbar lordosis. If there is a flexion deformity on the opposite side, the leg on that side will move into a flexed position.

2 *Trendelenburg test*. Observe from behind the patient and ask him to stand on one leg. The pelvis in health tilts upwards on the side with the leg raised. When the weight bearing hip is abnormal, or there is muscular weakness on that side, the pelvis sags downwards.

3 Measurement of 'true' and 'apparent' shortening. If the length of the legs is measured from the anterior superior iliac spine to the medial malleolus on the same side, any difference is referred to as 'true' shortening, and almost invariably indicates disease of the hip joint or the neck of the femur on the shorter side. If the length of the legs is measured from the umbilicus to the medial malleoli, any difference is referred to as 'apparent' shortening and may be due either to disease, as mentioned above, or to tilting of the pelvis, usually due to an adduction deformity of the hip.

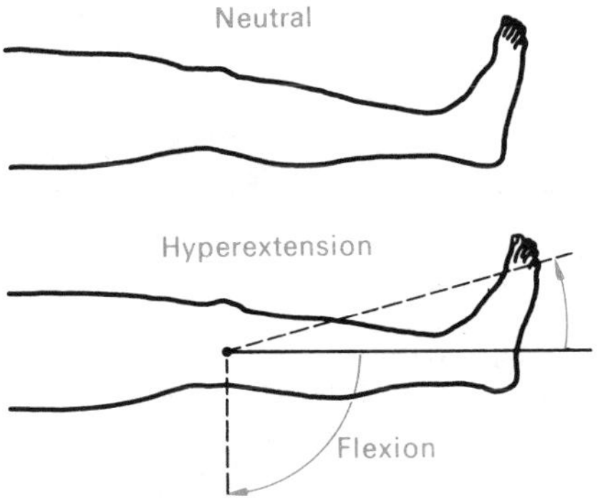

Fig. 14.18 Movements of the knee.

Knee (Fig. 14.18)

Neutral position is complete extension. Observe any *valgus* (lateral angulation of the tibia) or *varus* deformity on the couch and on standing. Test:

1 Flexion
2 Hyperextension

Test for instability by examining the laxity of the cruciate (anterior and posterior) and collateral ligaments.

Pain may be derived from the patellofemoral compartment or from the main tibiofemoral joint. Swelling may be obvious, particularly if distending the suprapatellar pouch, or may be elicited by the patellar tap test or, for small effusions, by the bulge test. Posterior knee joint cysts, particularly in rheumatoid arthritis, may be palpable in the popliteal fossa and they sometimes rupture producing calf pain (see below). They may therefore mimic a deep vein thrombosis and can produce venous obstruction in their own right.

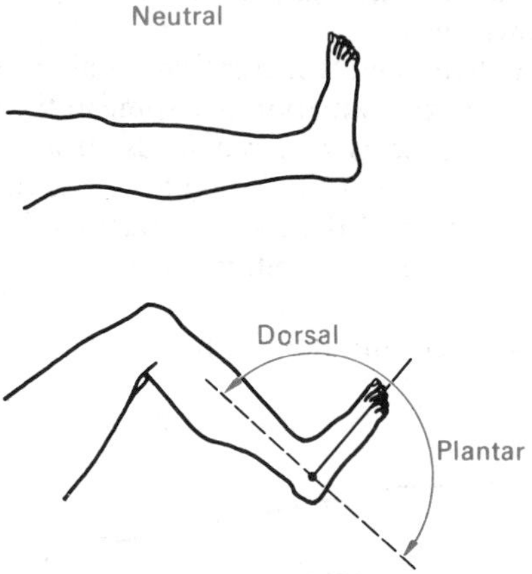

Fig. 14.19 Movements of the ankle.

Ankle (Fig. 14.19)

Neutral position is with the outer border of foot at an angle of 90° with the leg, and midway between inversion and eversion. Observe from behind the foot position with the patient standing. Subtalar joint damage or flattening of the longitudinal arches of the feet produces *valgus deformity*. Test:

1 Dorsiflexion. Test with knee in flexion and extension to exclude tight calf muscles

2 Plantar flexion

Foot (Fig. 14.20)

Neutral position cannot be defined. Test:

1 Subtalar inversion and eversion

2 Midtarsal inversion/eversion and adduction/abduction, with the os calcis held in neutral

3 Metatarsophalangeal and interphalangeal flexion/extension

Look also for tenderness at the Achilles tendon insertion on the back of the calcaneum and for plantar tenderness at the site of plantar fascial insertion. Inflammatory involvement of these attachments (enthesopathy) is common in *ankylosing spondylitis* and *Reiter's syndrome*.

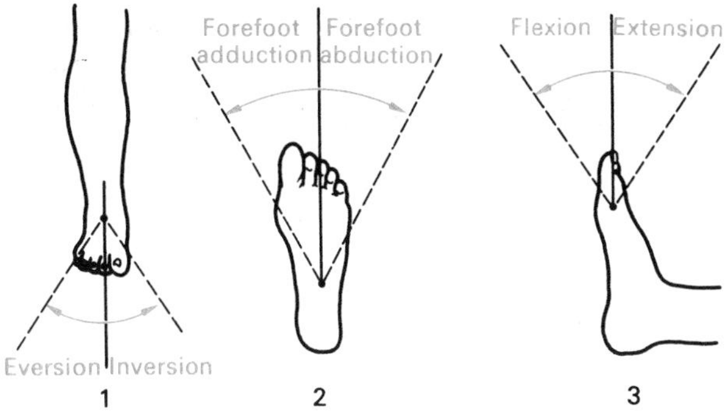

Fig. 14.20 Movements of the foot.

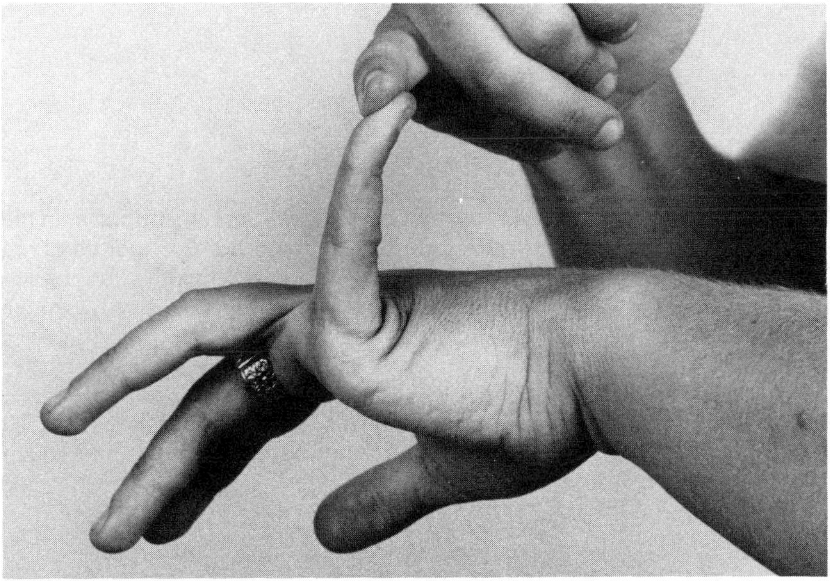

Fig. 14.21 Hyperextension of the little finger: one of the tests for hypermobility.

The gait

It is best to study gait with the legs and feet fully exposed. Ask the patient to walk away from you, to turn around at a given point and then to walk towards you.

Abnormalities of the gait are usually due either to local lesions in the lower limbs or to neurological disorder, though intoxication, hysteria or malingering may occasionally cause difficulty. A full examination of the legs and feet should reveal any local cause, which may range from a painful corn to osteoarthritis of the hip. Abnormalities due to neurological disorder are described in Chapter 10.

Hypermobility

There is a wide variation in the range of joint movement in a population, with age, sex and ethnic differences. However, excessive laxity or hypermobility of joints (Fig. 14.21) can be defined in about 10% of healthy subjects and is frequently familial. It is also a feature of two inherited connective tissue disorders, Marfan's syndrome and Ehlers–Danlos syndrome. Repeated trauma, haemarthrosis or dislocation may produce permanent joint damage.

SOME INVESTIGATIONS USED IN RHEUMATIC DISEASES

Rheumatoid factors

Most patients with rheumatoid arthritis have in their sera autoantibodies in the IgM, IgG, or IgA classes that are directed against other IgG molecules. In routine investigation IgM 'rheumatoid factor' can be detected by its ability to clump either polystyrene particles coated with human IgG (*latex test*, positive in about 80% of patients with rheumatoid arthritis) or sheep erythrocytes coated with rabbit IgG (*Rose–Waaler, DAT* or *SCAT tests*). A significant titre in the latex test is 1/80, in the sheep tests 1/32. The former is more sensitive, the latter more specific for rheumatoid arthritis, but positive tests may also be obtained in the elderly, in patients with subacute bacterial endocarditis, and in hepatic and other diseases.

Antinuclear antibody test (ANA)

Frozen sections of normal tissue (e.g. rat liver) are incubated with the patient's serum. After washing, a fluorescent antiserum to human gammaglobulin is used to detect human antibody adhering to rat nuclear antigens. The significance increases with the titre and adequate standardization is important.

This test is virtually always positive in active systemic lupus erythematosus (SLE), but positive tests, usually in lower titre, are found in many other diseases including progressive systemic sclerosis, Sjögren's syndrome and rheumatoid arthritis. In juvenile arthritis, a positive ANA is particularly associated with chronic iridocyclitis, which is frequently asymptomatic until advanced; slit lamp examination of the eye is essential.

DNA binding test

This is a radioisotope immunochemical technique detecting antibodies to native (double-stranded) DNA. If expressed as units/ml (Amersham), results over 25 are positive. This is the most specific laboratory test for active SLE.

Serum complement

Low levels of complement may reflect activation following immune complex formation, which is the result of disease activity in conditions such as SLE.

HLA typing

There is a strong association of the tissue antigen HLA-B27 with ankylosing spondylitis. However, the presence of this antigen is of limited value as a diagnostic test, because although 95% of patients in the United Kingdom who suffer from ankylosing spondylitis possess HLA-B27, it also occurs in about 8% of the normal population. It is of some value in the differential diagnosis of seronegative (latex-negative) arthritis, particularly in childhood.

Antistreptolysin-O (ASO) test

The presence in the serum of this antibody in a titre greater than 1/200 (reported as the divisor, i.e. '200') or, more significantly, a rising titre indicates a recent haemolytic streptococcal infection. A positive test does not establish a diagnosis of rheumatic fever, but a negative test makes this diagnosis unlikely.

Uric acid determinations

A consistently normal plasma uric acid level (below 375 μmol/l in women, 425 μmol/l in men) effectively excludes the diagnosis of (untreated) gout. Raised levels occur in a wide variety of circumstances and, in themselves, do not establish the diagnosis of gout (see below). On a low purine diet, the 24-hour urinary urate excretion should not exceed 600 mg. Higher levels indicate 'overproducers' of urate who may be at risk of renal stone formation.

Synovial fluid examination

Synovial fluid may be obtained for examination from any joint in which it is clinically detectable. The knee is the most convenient source: after infiltration with 1% local anaesthetic, a 21 gauge needle is inserted on the medial aspect between the patella and the femoral condyle. The aspirated fluid should be placed in a plain sterile container; if a cell count is required, some should also be mixed with EDTA anticoagulant.

Synovial fluid examination is diagnostic in two conditions: bacterial infections and crystal synovitis, and every effort should be made to obtain fluid when either of these is suspected. Polarized light microscopy can differentiate between the crystals of urate in gout and those of calcium pyrophosphate dihydrate in pseudogout. Outside these conditions synovial fluid examination is unlikely to be diagnostic: frank blood may point to trauma, haemophilia or villonodular synovitis, while inflammatory (as opposed to degenerative) arthritis is suggested by an opaque fluid of low viscocity, with a total white cell count over 1000/μl, neutrophils over 50%, protein content over 35 g/l, and the presence of a firm clot.

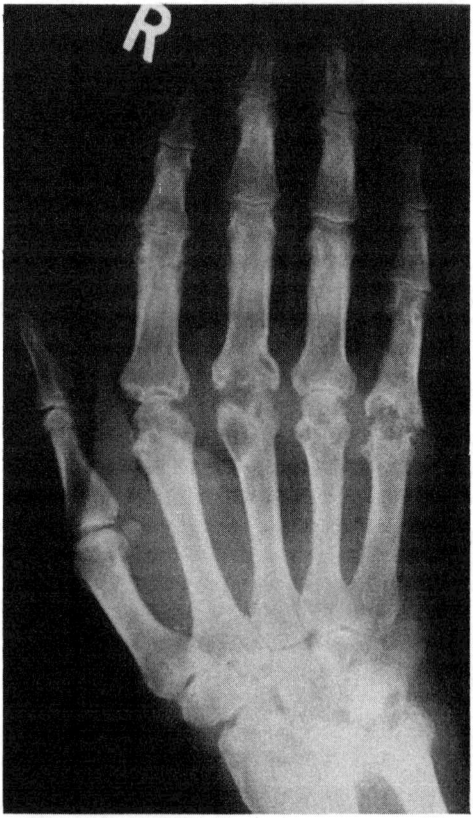

Fig. 14.22 Rheumatoid arthritis. There are small radiolucent erosions in the heads of the metacarpals and phalanges at the metacarpophalangeal and interphalangeal joints.

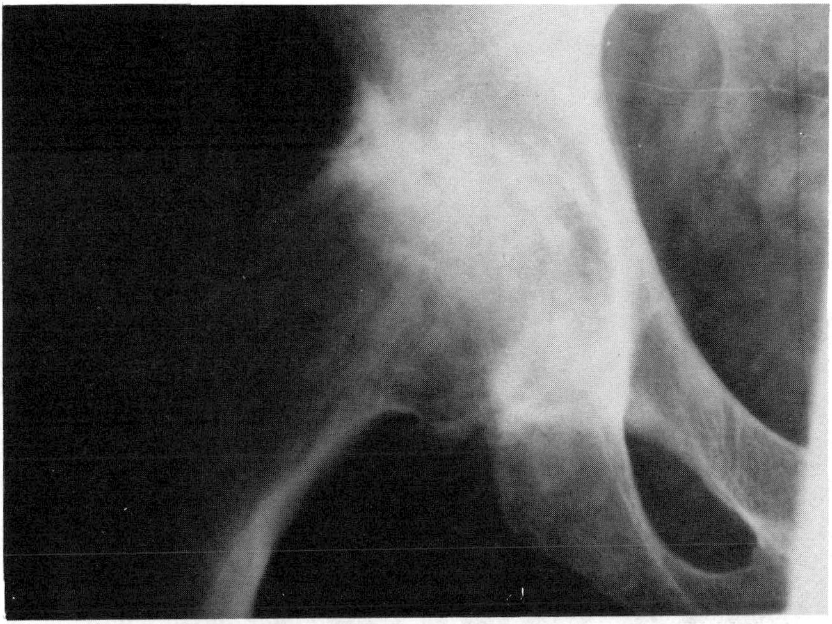

Fig. 14.23 Osteoarthritis of the hip. Note the gross narrowing of the joint space, and the dense bone in the region of the joint.

Radiological examination

Only X-rays likely to yield specific information should be ordered. However, in unilateral disease it is best to X-ray both sides for comparison. In patients with inflammatory polyarthritis three routine films are helpful in the diagnosis and assessment of progression: both hands and wrists on one plate, both feet on another, to compare bone density and to look for periosteal reaction or erosive change, and one of the full pelvis, to show the sacroiliac and hip joints (Figs. 14.22, 14.23, 14.24).

Arthrography

Injection of contrast medium into the knee joint can be used to confirm the diagnosis of ruptured popliteal cyst (Fig. 14.25). A double contrast technique is useful in demonstrating abnormalities of the menisci in the knee.

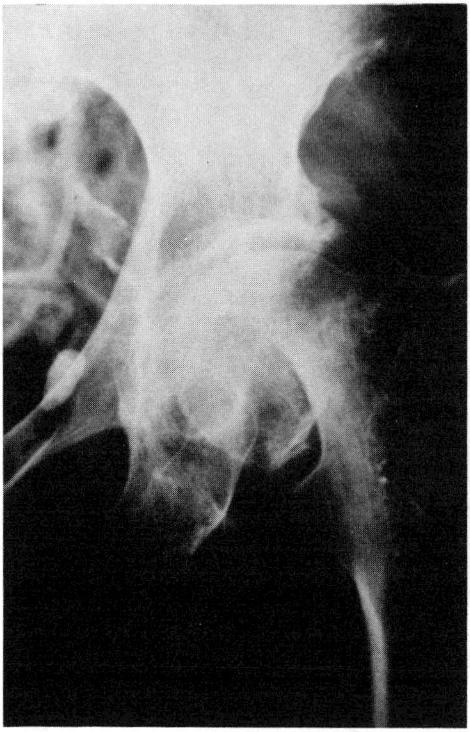

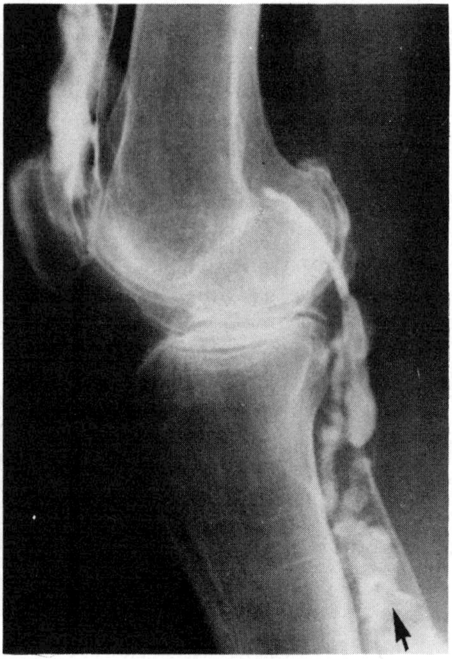

Fig. 14.25 Posterior rupture of the knee joint demonstrated by arthrography (arrow).

Fig. 14.24 Fracture of the neck of the femur. The fracture is displaced resulting in shortening of the leg.

15 The blood

The investigation of a patient with a blood disorder includes a history and clinical examination as well as the examination of the blood in the laboratory

CLINICAL EXAMINATION

Symptoms and signs in blood disease are due to:

1 Anaemia (lack of haemoglobin) and polycythaemia (excess haemoglobin)
2 Leucopenia, leucocytosis and functional disorders of white cells
3 Failure of haemostasis

It is particularly important to take a careful past history, family history and drug history as many blood disorders are chronic, inherited or drug induced. Details of history taking will be found in the various sections of this chapter. Physical examination is often concentrated on the lymphoreticular system (i.e. lymph nodes, liver and spleen) and the skin gives valuable information on anaemia, infection and bleeding tendencies. A full physical examination cannot be neglected as many blood disorders have general effects and many illnesses in the field of general medicine affect the blood.

The lymph nodes

Figure 15.1 shows the distribution of the principal lymph node groups which may be felt. These areas should be examined and if lymph nodes are found the following points should be considered.

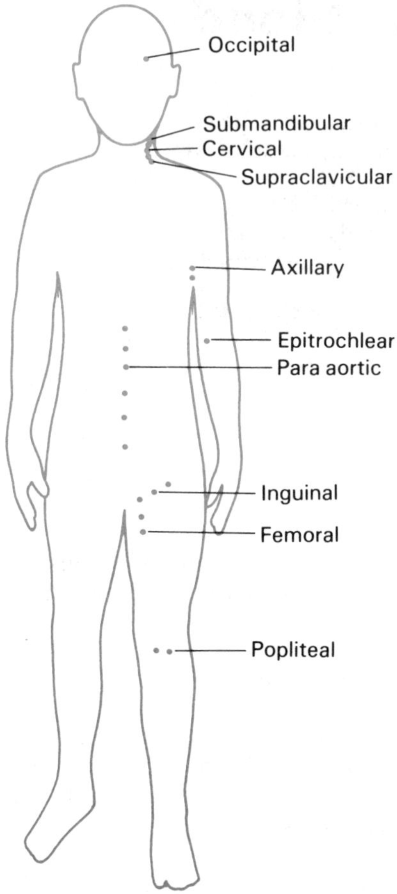

Fig. 15.1 The lymph nodes: clinical examination.

1 How many nodes are palpable?
2 What is their approximate diameter in centimetres?
3 What is their consistency?
4 Are they discrete or confluent?
5 Are they mobile or fixed?
6 Is the skin in the vicinity of the nodes abnormal?

The liver and spleen

Blood disorders often cause very marked enlargement of the liver and spleen.

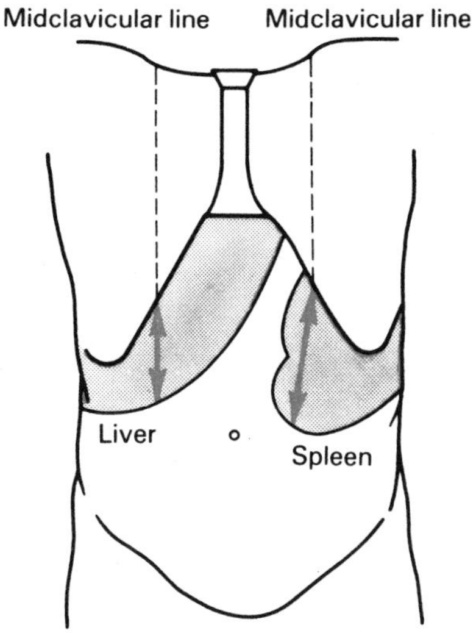

Fig. 15.2 The liver and spleen: clinical examination.

The examination should begin in the iliac fossae to avoid missing the edge of an organ which has reached the level of the pelvic inlet. If the liver and spleen are palpable (see pp. 91, 94) they should be measured in centimetres during natural expiration. A suitable landmark on the costal margin is the midclavicular line and the measurement should be from this point to the furthest extent of the organ (Fig. 15.2).

The skin

The skin surface may be infected or ulcerated and various forms of haemorrhage into the skin may occur. Haemorrhages are classified as follows:

1 *Purpura and petechial haemorrhages*: tiny pinpoint haemorrhages into the skin which do not blanch on compression with a glass slide

2 *Ecchymoses*: haemorrhages which are larger than petechiae and with more obvious confluence

3 *Bruises*

Telangiectasia are small dilated blood vessels which may be visible on the skin surface, particularly the lips. They blanch on compression and are sometimes a source of severe haemorrhage when the nose, gastrointestinal tract or bladder is affected.

Skin infiltration occurs in some malignant conditions of the blood, e.g. Hodgkin's disease.

The conjunctivae should be inspected for pallor or jaundice and the mouth may show evidence of haemorrhage, ulceration or infection. The tongue may be smooth or red, and cracking may be noted at the corners of the mouth (angular cheilosis).

The fundus oculi

Fundal haemorrhages are often visible in disorders of haemostasis, especially thrombocytopenia. When blood viscosity is increased (e.g. in macroglobulinaemia or chronic granulocytic leukaemia with a high white cell count) there may be engorgement of retinal vessels with papilloedema and retinal haemorrhage.

LABORATORY EXAMINATION

Sampling

Blood should be collected by venepuncture, usually from the antecubital fossa. Venous occlusion by a cuff is permissible in most haematological investigations but should not be severe or prolonged. A medium-sized needle should be used; undue suction should not be applied to the syringe as this may cause haemolysis. The patient should be resting comfortably during venepuncture and the procedure should be explained clearly before starting.

The treatment of many blood disorders is by the intravenous route and every effort should be made to avoid laceration of veins or haemorrhage around the vein punctured. At the end of the procedure the arm can be held up in the air while the venepuncture site is pressed.

Blood clots when removed from the body and this occurs more rapidly in glass than in plastic tubes. If clotted blood is required, e.g. for blood grouping, it should be taken into a new plain glass tube and allowed to stand at room temperature for 10 minutes before separation of clot from serum. Most other samples are taken into plastic tubes to which some anticoagulant has been added. Anticoagulants commonly used include:

1 *Sequestrene (EDTA)*, which binds calcium by chelation and is used for routine blood counts.

2 *Citrate*, which also removes calcium and is used in coagulation work.

3 *Heparin*, which inhibits many parts of the coagulation mechanism and is useful for chemical estimations, e.g. plasma iron.

The peripheral blood film

If blood is required only for making a stained film then the patient's finger may be pricked with a lance and the blood spread directly onto a slide. Unfortunately this causes platelet clumping and films are best made from freshly collected blood placed in a sequestrene tube, spread expertly and stained correctly with a Romanowsky method.

Examination The high power of the microscope is generally used to examine blood films except where the presence of large blood parasites (e.g. microfilaria) is suspected. Each element of the peripheral blood should be examined systematically, i.e.

red cells	size, shape, colour, presence of nucleated cells, rouleaux
white cells	distribution of various types, maturity, morphology
platelets	numbers (normal, reduced or increased), morphology

A more detailed account of the peripheral blood will be found in the various sections below.

The bone marrow

In the adult, blood production is confined to the skull, spine, pelvis, and upper ends of the long bones. It is often necessary to examine the bone marrow in disorders of the blood and this can be done either by aspiration with a syringe and a specially designed needle or by removing a core of bone marrow tissue (trephine biopsy). Aspirates may be taken from the manubrium or body of the sternum or from the anterior or posterior iliac crest, but trephine samples must be obtained from the iliac crest.

Bone marrow aspirates can be spread on slides and stained in the same way as peripheral blood, or they may be examined histologically after formalin fixation. Trephine samples are fixed in formalin and processed before examination.

Examination The principles of examination of bone marrow aspirates are the same as those for the peripheral blood, but the slide must be examined under the low power of the microscope to assess cellularity in the fragments at the ends of the trails and to assess megakaryocyte numbers. Erythropoiesis, granulopoiesis, lymphocytes and plasma cells are examined under the high power of the microscope and a search is made for any evidence of infiltration by cells not usually found in the bone marrow (e.g. carcinoma cells). It is important to stain the aspirate by Perls' ferrocyanide Prussian blue method to assess iron (haemosiderin) in fragments and erythroblasts.

Bone marrow appearances are considered in more detail in the various sections, as are the more complex investigations associated with particular disorders. Photomicrographs of normoblastic and megaloblastic marrow are shown in Plates VIII and X.

ANAEMIA

Common symptoms of anaemia are usually the result of deficient oxygen supply to the tissues:

Dyspnoea appears at first only on exertion but, with progressive anaemia, cardiac function becomes affected and shortness of breath occurs also at rest.

Ankle oedema also occurs in severe anaemia and is associated with cardiac dysfunction.

Palpitations occur when anaemia is severe and the cardiovascular dynamics are affected.

Lassitude is variable, but tends to become more pronounced as the haemoglobin level falls.

Anaemia will also accentuate features of vascular insufficiency, such as *angina, claudication* and *cerebral ischaemic symptoms*.

Clinical evidence of anaemia can be assessed only by examination of the mucous membranes of the mouth, conjunctivae, nails and skin creases. Because of variation in the thickness and depth of pigmentation, skin colour is an unsuitable clinical index of anaemia.

Examination of the peripheral blood

Sampling The initial screening for anaemia is best carried out on a small (4.0 ml) sample of venous blood taken into a container prepared with dipotassium ethylenediamino tetra-acetic acid (EDTA: sequestrene). A sample of this size is necessary for the requirements of the automatic counting machines, which are much more accurate than the older manual methods; furthermore, additional tests can be carried out on the same specimen should preliminary tests indicate they are necessary.

Red cell indices Estimation of the red cell indices (Tables 15.1 and 15.2) provides invaluable information for the basic differentiation of the type of anaemia. The *haemoglobin* and the *haematocrit* or *packed cell volume* (PCV) are the basic values revealing the degree of anaemia. A simple calculation relating these two estimations produces the *mean corpuscular haemoglobin concentration (MCHC)*; this is a useful index of the average haemoglobin concentration of the red cells. The accuracy of the *total red cell count* is considerably greater when an automatic counter is used because a very large number of cells can be enumerated in a short time. A reliable red cell count enables the computation of other useful indices such as the *mean corpuscular haemoglobin (MCH)* and the *mean corpuscular volume (MCV)*, which can be derived by relating the red cell count to the haemoglobin and PCV values respectively. The MCH indicates the average weight of haemoglobin per red cell and the MCV provides an estimate of the mean cell size. In some machines the MCV is obtained automatically by sizing the individual cells and the PCV can then be produced

Table 15.1 Normal red cell values

	Men	Women
Red cell count × 10^{12}/l	4.4–6.1	4.2–5.4
Haemoglobin g/dl	13.0–18.0	11.5–16.5
Haematocrit (PCV)	0.40–0.54	0.37–0.47
Mean corpuscular volume fl	75–99	75–99
Mean corpuscular haemoglobin pg	27–31	27–31
Mean corpuscular haemoglobin concentration g/dl	32–36	32–36

Table 15.2 Typical red cell values in anaemia

	Iron deficiency	Macrocytic anaemia
Red cell count × 10^{12}/l	4.9	2.7
Haemoglobin g/dl	10.4	10.4
Haematocrit (PCV)	0.35	0.32
Mean corpuscular volume fl	72	119
Mean corpuscular haemoglobin pg	21	38
Mean corpuscular haemoglobin concentration g/dl	29	32

In these two examples there is a similar degree of anaemia (haemoglobin 10.4 g/dl). Note the differences in size (MCV) and haemoglobinization (MCHC) of the red cells in the two types of anaemia. The MCH is increased in the macrocytic anaemia because the red cells are *larger* than normal.

In iron deficiency, on the other hand, the MCH is reduced because the red cells are smaller than usual, and also because they are poorly haemoglobinized. Generally, in iron deficiency anaemia the red cell count is well maintained, but in macrocytic anaemia the red cell count is lower.

without the need for direct measurement.

Confirmatory information on the size and haemoglobin content of the red cells can be obtained in the course of examining a blood film.

The blood film The morphological features of individual red cells often provide clues to the nature of the anaemia.

Normocytic red cells are found in acute blood loss, bone marrow failure and the anaemia of chronic disorders.

Anisocytosis, or variation in cell size, is an observation almost valueless in small degree; in marked degree it is much more important to know the types of cell involved, such as microspherocytes or macrocytes.

Macrocytosis may be due to the presence of large *polychromatic* (grey–blue staining) immature red cells (Plate IX) produced by increased erythropoietic stimulation, or from megaloblastic red cell precursors.

Microcytosis and *hypochromia* are usually associated with iron deficiency (Plate IX), thalassaemia and other haemoglobinopathies.

Poikilocytosis or variation in cell shape is found with significant ineffective erythropoiesis as in megaloblastic anaemia, myelofibrosis or when the cells are damaged in their circulation.

Spherocytosis occurs whenever the red cell membrane is damaged; it is characteristic of hereditary spherocytosis and autoimmune haemolytic anaemia (Plate XII).

Bone marrow examination Frequently it is necessary to study an aspirate of marrow tissue to identify the underlying disorder more exactly.

Iron deficiency

Clinically the patient with iron deficiency shows symptoms and signs of anaemia. More specific evidence in long-standing iron lack is indicated by *glossitis* with atrophy of papillae and *angular stomatitis (cheilosis)*. These may be associated with *dysphagia* to form the *Plummer–Vinson* or *Paterson–Kelly* syndrome. The nails may be brittle and spoon-shaped (koilonychia; Fig. 2.5).

The history may reveal evidence of dietary lack or a cause of chronic blood loss such as menorrhagia, aspirin ingestion, symptoms of gastrointestinal neoplasm, peptic ulcer, hookworm or haemorrhoids. The diagnosis of iron deficiency is not complete without an indication of its cause.

Peripheral blood Table 15.2 shows the features of reduced haemoglobin content (low MCH and MCHC) and reduction in mean cell size (low MCV). The hypochromic microcytic state of the red cells is confirmed on examination of the blood film, in which the central pallor of the cells is considerably enlarged.

Estimation of plasma iron is essential to confirm the deficiency; the plasma iron binding capacity is typically increased.

Hypochromic anaemia without iron deficiency is a feature of 'anaemia of chronic disorders', thalassaemia syndromes, sideroblastic anaemias and occasionally renal failure.

Bone marrow Though not usually necessary, bone marrow aspirates show erythroblasts in increased numbers in the later stages of maturation, with deficient haemoglobin formation. Staining the film to determine its iron content reveals a deficiency of storage iron (haemosiderin).

Deficiency of vitamin B_{12} and folic acid

In addition to the symptoms and signs of anaemia, the history may reveal a primary cause such as dietary deficiency or total or partial gastrectomy. Pregnancy, or any condition that increases the body's demand for folate, may cause folate deficiency. Other important clinically related conditions include pernicious anaemia and malabsorption syndrome.

Deficiency of vitamin B_{12} and of folate can be confirmed by serum assays of these vitamins; malabsorption of vitamin B_{12} is best demonstrated by the radioactive B_{12} urinary excretion (Schilling) test.

Pernicious anaemia is the most common cause of vitamin B_{12} deficiency in the United Kingdom. It is rare in Africa and Asia. It commonly presents after the age of 30. A sore tongue is a usual symptom and the features of subacute combined degeneration of the nervous system may precede or succeed the symptoms of anaemia. Indigestion and diarrhoea may occur. In addition to the anaemia, mild jaundice is common and the tongue becomes reddened, smooth and shiny. The spleen is often moderately enlarged.

Additional and more specific tests for pernicious anaemia include *gastric analysis* following pentagastrin stimulation to demonstrate achlorhydria. This is not usually done when the other tests are available. Autoantibody studies in the serum are positive for *parietal cell antibodies* in 95% of cases and for *intrinsic factor antibodies* in 60%.

Malabsorption syndromes produce folic acid deficiency more readily than vitamin B_{12} deficiency and are found in association with tropical sprue, adult coeliac disease and other small bowel pathology such as blind loops, fistulae, ileitis and jejunal diverticulosis. Sprue and coeliac disease may be accompanied by steatorrhoea and features due to lack of absorption of other important dietary components such as protein and calcium.

Peripheral blood The total red cell count is reduced in number but each cell is well haemoglobinized (normal MCH and MCHC) and larger than normal (high MCV). In the blood film the macrocytes are typically oval in outline and a number of 'tear-drop' poikilocytes are seen. They are normochromic unless there is a complicating iron deficiency also. The polymorph leucocytes tend to be reduced in number and have hypersegmented nuclei. Platelets are also reduced in severe cases.

Bone marrow Bone marrow films show a marked increase in cellularity due to proliferative (but ineffective) erythropoiesis with defective maturation of the cell nuclei, resulting in the formation of megaloblastic red cell precursors and giant metamyelocytes. Iron stores are increased due to the excessive breakdown of the abnormal red cell series.

Haemolytic anaemias

Anaemia due to premature destruction of the cells may be congenital or acquired. The congenital forms have a history of anaemia and usually hyperbilirubinaemia dating from early life, often accompanied by a family history. They are usually due to intrinsic abnormalities of the red cell membrane (e.g. congenital spherocytosis), metabolism (e.g. enzyme deficiencies) or haemoglobin structure. Acquired haemolysis is usually of recent onset and results from the cells being exposed to the destructive effects of, for example, antibodies and poisons. A rare form of acquired red cell membrane abnormality is *paroxysmal nocturnal haemoglobinuria*.

The patient presents with a variable degree of anaemia and jaundice, though in mild cases the latter may be absent. The spleen is usually palpable. In severe long-standing haemolysis of congenital origin the increased red cell production tends to produce stunted growth with distortion of the bones of the skull due to the marrow hyperplasia. Typically, this results in mongoloid facies and radiological thickening of the diploe. There is a tendency for skin ulceration to occur particularly on the lower legs.

The laboratory findings, in addition to a degree of anaemia, are:

1 Abnormal red cell morphology, e.g. spherocytes
2 Reticulocytosis
3 Erythroid hyperplasia of the bone marrow
4 Increased indirect plasma bilirubin
5 Increased urinary urobilinogen
6 Shortened survival of isotope-labelled red cells
7 Typically, the urine contains no bilirubin

Extravascular and intravascular haemolysis

In many cases of haemolysis, the damaged red cells are removed from the circulation by the reticuloendothelial tissues, particularly the spleen. When red cell destruction is acute they are broken down in the circulation. This is the intravascular haemolysis which results in loss of serum *haptoglobins*, the presence of *methaemalbumin* in the serum, *haemosiderinuria* and *haemoglobinuria*.

Congenital haemolytic anaemia

Membrane defects Hereditary spherocytic anaemia is an autosomal dominant abnormality of membrane structure. Removal of red cell membrane by the spleen results in the circulation of small spherocytic red cells (Plate XII). The saline osmotic fragility test is used for diagnosis.

The saline osmotic fragility test This test measures the ability of the red cell to increase its volume under an osmotic load before it bursts, releasing its haemoglobin. Spherocytes are more fragile and thin cells, such as target cells, are less fragile than normal. The increased fragility of a red cell sample is proportional to its spherocyte population. The test is therefore also positive in autoimmune haemolytic anaemia or in any condition in which the number of spherocytes is increased.

Red cell enzyme deficiences

A breakdown in the mechanism of red cell carbohydrate metabolism may occur either in the pentose phosphate pathway, when deficiency of glucose-6-phosphate dehydrogenase (G6PD) is the more common defect, or in the Emden–Meyerhof glycolytic pathway, which is particularly affected by a lack of pyruvate kinase. These enzymes can be quantified by fairly simple methods. G6PD deficiency may be recognized by a simple qualitative dye screening test.

Each of these important inherited enzyme deficiencies may be associated with forms of non-spherocytic congenital haemolytic anaemia. Severe G6PD deficiency occurs particularly in Mediterranean peoples. An additional factor in some of these individuals, which may produce severe haemolysis, is an associated sensitivity to the fava bean or its plant pollen. A less severe variety of G6PD deficiency occurs in some 10% of African males and less frequently in African females, the character being sex linked. Such deficient individuals show no adverse effects except after treatment with certain drugs such as primaquine.

Family studies should always be carried out.

Abnormal haemoglobin formation

Abnormal haemoglobin may arise as a result of substitution of abnormal variants of haemoglobin for the normal adult (A) type, or it may occur when normal adult haemoglobin formation is inhibited as in the thalassaemia syndromes.

A prominent example of a substituted abnormal variant is haemoglobin S, which produces *sickle cell disease* (Plate XI). If sickle cell haemoglobin is deoxygenated, it becomes insoluble and crystallizes out in the red cell. Such red cells take on a characteristic sickle shape and may obstruct the blood flow in nutrient vessels and cause infarction. When sickle formation is not obvious, as is likely to be the case in the heterozygous form, sickling may be provoked in vitro by incubating a wet preparation of the erythrocytes under conditions of reduced oxygen tension. Alternatively the haemoglobin S component can be detected by a simple tube test which depends upon the fact that sickle haemoglobin is less soluble than the normal form. Sickle cell disease is common in African and New World negroes. Other qualitatively abnormal haemoglobins of note are C (in West African and New World negroes), D punjab (in northern Indians) and E (in south east Asians). These abnormal components can be identified by electrophoretic techniques.

Of the *thalassaemias*, the common variety is β-thalassaemia, in which the production of β-polypeptide chains of the globin is lacking. It is distinguished by an increase in the minor normal haemoglobin components A_2 and F. In α-thalassaemia, where α chains are deficient, there is no increase in A_2 or F but

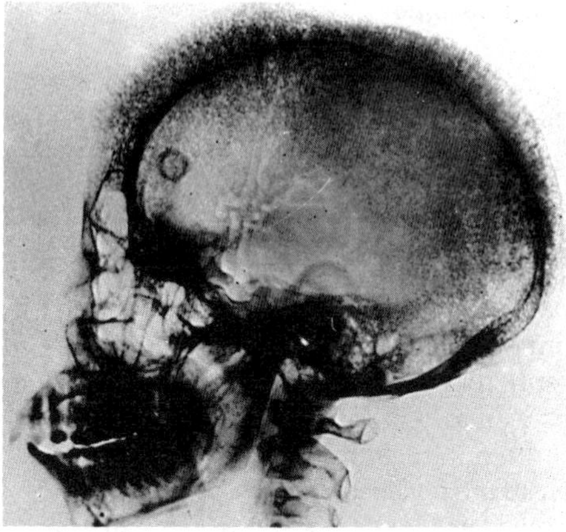

Fig. 15.3 'Hair-on-end' appearance in the calvarium in thalassaemia.

the formation of haemoglobin Barts ($\gamma 4$) and haemoglobin H ($\beta 4$) may occur.

The overall picture of thalassaemia is that of hypochromia resulting from the genetically determined deficiency of haemoglobin A production. The abnormally thin red cells that are produced frequently appear as *target cells* (Plate XI). The *leptocyte* has an increased resistance to more dilute solutions of saline compared with normal cells when the osmotic fragility test is applied. The level of iron in the plasma is high in these conditions and the iron-binding capacity is greater than normal. In the marrow there are abundant iron stores and the metabolic defect in haemoglobin synthesis results in the presence of iron granules in the developing red cells. A characteristic abnormality may occur in the skull X-ray (Fig. 15.3).

Acquired haemolytic anaemia

Acquired haemolytic anaemia results from red cell damage caused by auto-antibodies or toxic chemicals, poisons and therapeutic agents or by red cell trauma.

The direct antiglobulin (Coombs') test Red cells which have been sensitized by antibodies are coated with immunoglobulin (IgG, IgA or IgM) and sometimes components of complement also. An anti-human globulin (Coombs') serum, obtained by deliberately immunizing an animal (e.g. rabbit) to human globulin, will agglutinate cells sensitized in this way and so demonstrate the presence of the antibody. The affected cells in *haemolytic disease of the newborn* due to Rhesus fetal–maternal incompatibility can be detected by the same technique.

POLYCYTHAEMIA

If the red cell count is in excess of normal, polycythaemia is present. This is usually associated with increases in the haemoglobin level and PCV. The condition may be due to a primary bone marrow disorder—polycythaemia rubra vera—or may be secondary, for example in congenital heart disease, chronic lung disease, and some renal conditions.

Polycythaemia causes headache, plethora and tinnitus. Patients with the primary condition often complain of pruritus and the spleen is usually palpable.

In polycythaemia rubra vera the neutrophil and platelet counts are typically increased and the neutrophil alkaline phosphatase and plasma uric acid levels are elevated. The red cell mass is increased in all forms of polycythaemia except when the plasma volume is reduced, e.g. dehydration.

BLOOD TRANSFUSION

Collection of donor blood

In the United Kingdom a highly organized blood collection service is available on a nationwide basis. Donors are selected from healthy adults of either sex between the ages of 18 and 65, except for pregnant and lactating women. Usually about 500 ml of blood is taken into a special plastic bag containing 75 ml of a citrate anticoagulant. Donors are safeguarded by a routine haemoglobin estimation prior to donation using a simple finger prick method and estimating the specific gravity of a drop of blood in copper sulphate solution. Males are accepted if their haemoglobin equivalent is over 13.5 g/dl; for females the minimum level is 12.5 g/dl. Usually donors give only two donations in a year. Care must be taken to avoid air embolism during donation.

Processing of donor blood

In order to protect the recipient, the possibility of *transmitting disease* in the transfused blood must be avoided (p. 443). An attempt to avoid *hepatitis* is made by testing all donor samples for hepatitis-associated antigen (HAA). The serum of all donors is also tested for *syphilis*. The ABO and Rh(D) blood groups are determined routinely before transfusion. If the donor is group O, the serum should be tested for high titre anti-A and anti-B and, if present, the blood should be reserved for group O recipients only.

Storage of whole donor blood in acid–citrate–dextrose (ACD) or citrate–phosphate–dextrose (CPD) must be maintained at a constant temperature of 4°C. Optimally this should be for a maximum period of three weeks.

Blood components

Individual components of donor blood are available for specific therapeutic requirements. Transfusion thus becomes both more economical and more specifically effective. Such components include packed red cells, platelets, leucocytes (occasionally), whole plasma (fresh frozen at −20°C) and factor VIII (as cryoprecipitate at −20°C). Dried preparations of whole plasma, fibrinogen and factor VIII and IX concentrates are also available.

Compatibility testing of blood for transfusion

When a patient requires a transfusion, blood of the same ABO and Rh(D) group must be selected. The red cells of each donor sample must be tested with the recipient's serum by several methods at different temperatures. Agglutination by complete cold antibodies in saline is tested for at room temperature and at 37°C. Tests for incomplete warm antibodies should be done in bovine albumin at 37°C and by the indirect antiglobulin (Coombs') test using 'broad spectrum' antiglobulin serum that will detect both IgG antibody and complement. Treatment of the donor red cells with proteolytic enzymes may also be used as a technique for discovering potentially incompatible antibodies in the recipient's serum.

Indications for blood transfusion

It is important to confine blood transfusion to clinical conditions in which there is a clear indication; there are very real hazards which may occur as a direct consequence of transfusion.

Acute blood loss must be rectified by giving whole blood sufficient to restore blood volume. *Trauma* may additionally involve excessive loss of plasma, which may require proportionately more plasma to restore equilibrium. *Burns*, when extensive, need almost exclusively plasma replacement to rectify the marked haemoconcentration following severe plasma loss.

Most *chronic anaemias* of nutritional type can be corrected by giving the appropriate replacement therapy such as iron, folic acid or vitamin B_{12}. Transfusion of packed red cells may be necessary if rapid restoration is required in iron deficiency of pregnancy or if anaemia is severe in B_{12} or folate deficiency. Chronic *bone marrow failure* due to aplasia, fibrosis or leukaemic infiltration requires correction at intervals with donor red cells.

Transfusion of *platelet concentrate* is indicated when spontaneous bleeding is due to thrombocytopenia.

In cases of leucopenia with severe infection resistant to antibiotics, *granulocyte transfusion* may be accomplished by separating neutrophils from the fresh blood of normal donors. Patients with chronic granulocytic leukaemia have also been used as a source of cells.

Complications of blood transfusion

Incompatibility Incompatibility is the most serious hazard associated with blood transfusion. Acute haemolysis arises from ABO blood group incompatibility. Massive red cell agglutination and destruction is followed by intense haemoglobinaemia, jaundice and acute renal failure due to tubular necrosis. The renal lesion is partly due to circulatory shock and hypotension and partly to the presence of haemoglobin casts and red cell debris. Careful documentation and sample labelling are required to avoid this potentially fatal consequence.

Pyrogen reaction The pyrogen reaction is probably due to the presence of antibodies to transfused leucocytes and platelets in the patient.

Allergic reactions Urticaria and asthma may occur during transfusion if the donor blood contains material to which the patient is sensitive.

Toxic effects due to excess of citrate may occur following multiple transfusion and symptoms of hypocalcaemia develop.

Air embolism is much less likely to occur with the use of plastic bags, which collapse down as they empty of blood.

Circulatory overload is more likely to occur in elderly patients with chronic anaemia. The use of packed cells for transfusion and potent diuretics help to prevent its occurrence.

Iron overload occurs in patients who have been sustained over a long time with numerous blood transfusions.

Thrombophlebitis tends to occur when the same infusion needle remains in the same site for over 12 hours.

Transmission of disease *Malaria* parasites survive for about three weeks at 4°C and can easily be transmitted. In non-malarious countries, potentially infected donors are rejected. In malarious areas the simultaneous administration of anti-malarials may be necessary.

Hepatitis due to hepatitis-associated antigen (HAA) should be avoided by screening the serum of all donors. Some anicteric cases have sera positive for the antigen and are capable of giving the recipient hepatitis. Furthermore, hepatitis may result even when no HAA has been identified in the donor sample.

Syphilis is due to *treponema pallidum*, which may survive for six days at 4°C. All donors in the UK are screened serologically.

Brucellosis and *cytomegalovirus* may also be transmitted.

Faulty storage Storing blood at freezing temperatures or over-heating it prior to transfusion may result in massive haemolysis of donor red cells with dangerous consequences if transfused into a patient. Grossly infected blood may result from storage at temperatures above 4°C.

DISORDERS OF WHITE CELLS

The clinical effects of white cell disorders arise from lack of white cells, disturbances in white cell function and the effects of white cell proliferation. When taking a history the following points should be considered.

Has the patient noticed a reduced resistance to infection, e.g. frequent colds or influenza, sore throats, chest infections, earache, boils, pustules, dysuria and fever or sweats?

Does the patient complain of mouth ulceration, skin rash or irritation (pruritus)? Has the patient noticed any enlargement of lymph nodes or the sensation of dragging or pain in the left hypochondrium which can arise from an enlarged spleen?

In practice it is remarkable how few symptoms may arise from very enlarged lymph nodes, liver and spleen. One may see a patient whose spleen is enormous presenting with an entirely different complaint.

Symptoms may be related to invasion and displacement of normal tissues by tumour. Thus patients with acute leukaemia also suffer from symptoms of anaemia and thrombocytopenia and may develop bone pain. When the meninges are invaded, symptoms of headache and neck stiffness may be prominent and deposits may damage the spinal cord causing paraplegia. If lymph nodes in the mediastinum become sufficiently large as a result of lymphoma they may cause mediastinal obstruction with venous engorgement of the head and respiratory embarrassment, whilst in the abdomen large nodes may cause lymphatic and/or venous obstruction in the lower limbs. Bone pain is also a prominent symptom of the plasma cell tumour myelomatosis, in which pathological fractures also occur.

A variety of symptoms may be caused by the systemic effects of white cell tumours. These include fever without evidence of infection, weight loss, pruritus, polyneuropathy, myopathy and renal failure from a variety of causes. In myelomatosis an abnormal globulin may circulate in the blood and contribute to renal failure and may cause visual and circulatory disturbances. Characteristic 'lytic' lesions may be seen in X-rays of the skeleton and of the skull (Fig. 15.4). Autoimmune haemolytic anaemia may occur in some lymphomas.

When the white cell count is very high, i.e. greater than $300 \times 10^9/l$, this alone may cause symptoms due to failure of the peripheral circulation. Thus in chronic granulocytic leukaemia patients may present with priapism, visual loss or dyspnoea.

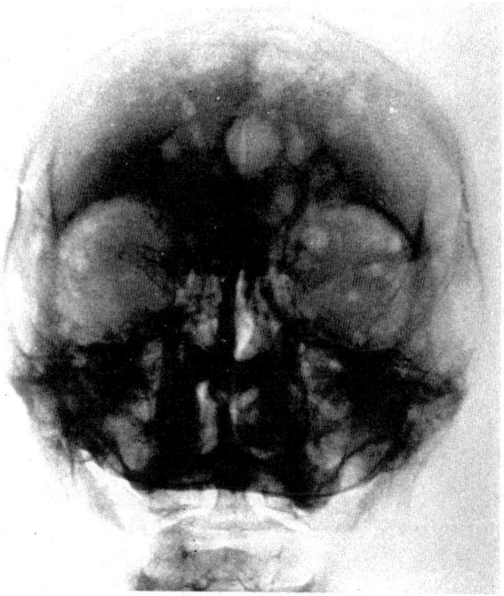

Fig. 15.4 Multiple osteolytic lesions in the skull in myelomatosis.

Physical examination is mainly concentrated on the mouth, skin and lymphoreticular system; neutropenic mouth ulceration may be very severe. The lymph nodes are usually enlarged in the lymphoid malignancies but many viral illnesses (e.g. glandular fever) may cause lymphadenopathy. The liver and spleen are also often enlarged in lymphoid diseases.

In the *laboratory*, investigation centres on the *peripheral blood* and the *bone marrow*.

The peripheral blood

The white cell count ranges from $4{\cdot}5-11 \times 10^9$/l in the normal adult. With modern apparatus the white cell count is usually measured automatically at the same time as the haemoglobin and other red cell values. The differential white cell count is usually calculated by examination of the stained film and in health a typical result would be:

Neutrophils	60%
Lymphocytes	30%
Monocytes	6%
Eosinophils	3%
Basophils	1%

Variations of normality are very wide and values are different for infants and young children. Differential counting using the microscope is very inaccurate so one should not put too much emphasis on individual results. Trends in serial counts are easily seen by charting figures. Automatic differential counters are much more accurate than manual methods and will allow valid calculation of absolute white cell numbers which are derived from the total white cell count and the differential count.

An abnormality in the number and/or distribution of white cells does not necessarily imply a white cell disorder as almost any illness may alter the total or differential white cell counts. The typical response to bacterial infection or any stress is a neutrophil leucocytosis, though in children a lymphocytosis often occurs, especially in whooping cough. Sometimes the reaction may be so marked as to mimic a leukaemic process, and is termed a leukaemoid reaction. Glandular fever is an infectious illness which causes a non-specific lymphocytosis in which the lymphocytes are morphologically abnormal and in some respects resemble leukaemic cells, but the illness is self-limiting (Plate X).

The white cell count is also increased in most types of leukaemia due to the presence of abnormal white cells in the peripheral blood. In acute leukaemia these will be lymphoblasts or myeloblasts (see below). In chronic lymphocytic leukaemia mature lymphocytes (Plate XIII) form the majority of the white cells and in chronic granulocytic (myeloid) leukaemia a spectrum of maturing granulocytes is found (Plate XIII).

The white cell count may be reduced by:

1 Aplasia—idiopathic or due to drugs, chemicals or irradiation
2 Infiltration, e.g. myelofibrosis
3 Vitamin B_{12} or folic acid deficiency
4 Sequestration and/or destruction due to an enlarged spleen, e.g. Felty's syndrome
5 Overwhelming infection
6 Inherited conditions

Inherited defects may also lead to disorders of neutrophil function as in the sex-linked chronic granulomatous disease of childhood. Both inherited and acquired disorders of lymphocytes are described but the acquired defects are more common and are often found in patients with Hodgkin's disease, lymphoma or myeloma.

The lymphoid series Many morphological alterations are non-specific but malignant lymphoid cells are often larger than normal and contain a prominent nucleolus (lymphoblasts). Morphological abnormalities may also be seen in the more 'mature' lymphocytic and plasmacytic malignancies.

The myeloid series More primitive white cells may appear in the peripheral blood in various forms of myeloid leukaemia and also in infection (see above). The most primitive myeloid cells (myeloblasts) are large cells with more plentiful cytoplasm than lymphoblasts and the nuclei often contain multiple nucleoli. In the cytoplasm, rod-like structures (Auer rods) may sometimes be seen. Abnormal myeloid cells often resemble monocytes morphologically. Some forms of myeloid leukaemia are specifically monocytic.

The bone marrow

It is difficult to give precise indications for examination of the bone marrow and details of interpretation are outside the scope of this chapter. However, bone marrow aspiration is indicated in the investigation of disorders associated with diffuse marrow infiltration, e.g. leukaemias and myelomatosis (Plate XII), whilst a combination of aspiration and trephine biopsy is to be preferred in those conditions associated with patchy marrow involvement, e.g. lymphomas. A bone marrow trephine may be necessary to confirm the diagnosis of aplastic anaemia. In myelofibrosis the 'solidification' of the marrow makes aspiration impossible and a trephine sample must be obtained. It is important to note that bone marrow infiltration in acute leukaemia does not always spill over into the peripheral blood though there is usually a clue to be found in the associated pancytopenia.

HAEMOSTASIS

The haemostatic mechanism involves the following:

1 The properties of the vessel wall
2 The platelets
3 The coagulation mechanism
4 The fibrinolytic mechanism

These mechanisms are closely interrelated and are separated conventionally only for ease of description.

The majority of haemostatic defects result in a tendency to bleed excessively. Hypercoagulable states are comparatively rare. Different defects produce different clinical syndromes and in defects of haemostasis the history is often more important than the physical examination.

First it is important to establish whether excessive bleeding has taken place or not. This may be very difficult as 'a little blood goes a long way'. A history often has to be taken from the anxious mother of a child who has bled after dental extraction or tonsillectomy and it is useful to have some objective evidence of excessive haemorrhage from another source, such as the need for blood transfusion.

The history should include the following questions:

Does spontaneous bleeding occur (e.g. epistaxis, joint or muscle haemorrhage)? Is haemorrhage excessive after trivial trauma (e.g. easy bruising or haematoma formation during everyday life or gentle sports)? Is haemorrhage excessive only after severe trauma, e.g. has there been severe haemorrhage after tonsillectomy, dental extraction or appendicectomy?

Has there been any blood in the vomit (haematemesis), altered blood in the stools (melaena) or blood in the urine (haematuria)? Has the patient noticed any small red blood spots (purpura) on the skin or in the mouth? Do the gums bleed? In women, has menstruation been excessive? Does the patient enjoy good general health? Follow up any specific points.

Can the patient remember any previous incident involving excessive haemorrhage at any time? Is there a family history of excessive haemorrhage and if so what is the pattern of inheritance?

What drugs is the patient taking and what drugs have been taken in the recent past? Aspirin is the most common drug to consider because of its various effects on the haemostatic mechanism and because it is often included in proprietary preparations which the patient may not regard as 'drugs'. It is also important to make sure that the patient is not taking oral anticoagulants.

What is the patient's occupation? Does he come into contact with any dangerous chemicals? These questions are obviously important in the analysis of the cause of any defect. If a defect is found it may influence the choice of occupation for the patient in the future; a patient with haemophilia makes a poor security guard.

Physical examination will demonstrate whether or not there is any damage from previous excessive haemorrhage: large untidy scars may be due to previous wound haematomata and recurrent haemarthroses may cause degenerative joint disease. The skin, mucous membranes and fundi should be examined for purpura, petechial haemorrhages and bruises. Examination of the lymph nodes, liver and spleen may reveal a white cell abnormality.

Haemorrhage due to vessel wall and platelet defects tends to be from the mucous membranes and into the skin. In patients with hereditary telangiectasia, bleeding occurs from the nose, mouth and gastrointestinal tract and also sometimes from the urinary tract. Patients with reduced numbers of platelets (thrombocytopenia) also suffer from nose bleeds and purpura, and bleed excessively at surgery. The degree of haemostatic defect depends on the number of circulating platelets (see below). In patients with a coagulation defect primary haemostasis, which relies on platelet function, may be normal but haemorrhage occurs after surgery, often after a short delay. In severe coagulation defects spontaneous haemorrhage may occur, especially into joints and muscles but intra-abdominal and intracranial haemorrhage are also well described. In von Willebrand's disease both platelet function and the coagulation mechanism are abnormal and there is a mixed clinical picture though the platelet functional defect predominates.

The bleeding time

The bleeding time test is an in vivo test of platelet function. It involves making a small wound and measuring the time taken for bleeding to cease. The two methods commonly used are Ivy's method and Duke's method.

Ivy's method A cuff is placed round the upper arm and is inflated to 40 mmHg. The forearm is cleaned and two cuts or puncture marks are made with a standard lance taking care to avoid damaging veins. Every 15 seconds the blood is gently removed with a filter paper, without pressing on the arm, until bleeding ceases. This usually takes less than six minutes but varies with the method used. The average of the readings is taken, ignoring wounds that fail to bleed and wounds that have obviously damaged veins. This test is not easy to reproduce or standardize. It should be avoided when a patient is known to be thrombocytopenic as it is then unnecessary and may cause severe bleeding into the forearm.

Duke's method The ear lobe is stabbed by a standard lance and the blood removed as for the Ivy method. This technique is even more difficult to standardize than the Ivy method but it may be less traumatic, especially in young children.

Laboratory tests of haemostasis

A peripheral film should always be examined and particular attention paid to platelet numbers and morphology.

The standard tests are the platelet count and the tests which measure the various parts of the coagulation mechanism (Fig. 15.5).

Platelet count The normal range of platelet count is 150–400 $\times$ 10^9/l. Platelet numbers can be estimated roughly from the peripheral film and this examination is usually enough for emergencies. Platelets can also be counted visually but automatic machines are usually used.

The platelet count is reduced in bone marrow failure from any cause and in conditions where peripheral destruction of platelets takes place for immunological reasons (e.g. idiopathic thrombocytopenic purpura) or because of trapping and/or destruction by an enlarged spleen (e.g. myelofibrosis). Thrombocytopenia also takes place after massive blood transfusion as stored blood does not contain viable platelets. When the platelet count is above 100 $\times$ 10^9/l no clinical symptoms arise; between 50 and 100 $\times$ 10^9/l bleeding may occur after major surgery or trauma and between 20 and 50 $\times$ 10^9/l after minor trauma. Below 20 $\times$ 10^9/l spontaneous haemorrhage may occur and purpura is very likely. At very low platelet counts there is a risk of fatal cerebral haemorrhage.

The platelet count is increased in many myeloproliferative diseases and thrombocytosis may occur in Hodgkin's disease or after chronic haemorrhage. Sometimes thrombosis or bleeding may occur as a result.

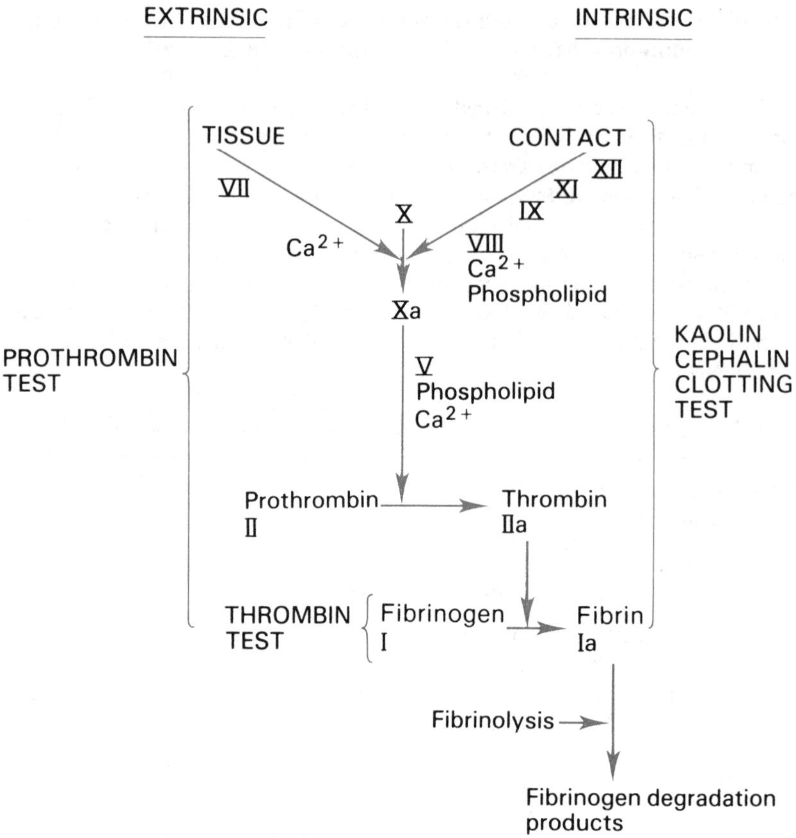

Fig. 15.5 The coagulation and fibrinolytic mechanisms.

Many qualitative platelet defects are described. Apart from the effects of aspirin ingestion most of these are very rare and their investigation requires sophisticated tests of platelet function such as platelet adhesion and aggregation, which cannot be described here.

The prothrombin test and ratio (PTR) The PTR is the most commonly performed coagulation test and measures the extrinsic coagulation pathway (factors VII, X, V, II and I) (Fig. 15.5). Citrate is used as an anticoagulant in a volume of one part citrate to nine parts blood. Platelet-poor plasma is obtained by centrifugation and is added to an equal volume of human brain extract at 37°C (tissue thromboplastin). After recalcification with 0·025 M calcium chloride a clot forms in approximately 13 seconds using normal plasma. The test is performed in duplicate and the result is compared with that obtained from a pooled normal control. The result is expressed as a ratio of the control sample, i.e. if the test sample takes 26 seconds to clot the ratio is 2·0. Human brain thromboplastin is now standardized in the United Kingdom so prothrombin ratios should be comparable in different parts of the country.

Situations in which the PTR is abnormal include:

1 The use of oral anticoagulants (therapeutic range 2·0–4·0) and heparin
2 Hepatic failure
3 Haemorrhagic disease of the newborn
4 Intravascular coagulation
5 Malabsorption of vitamin K

In practice the test is usually performed to control the dose of oral anticoagulants (e.g. warfarin). These vitamin K antagonists inhibit the formation of factors II, VII, IX and X. The prothrombin ratio is chosen mainly because it is easy and rapid to perform.

A commercial test (Thrombotest) is also available for the control of oral anticoagulants and works on the same basic principle as the prothrombin test. It can be performed on plasma or capillary blood but is not as popular as the prothrombin test.

The kaolin cephalin clotting test (KCCT) The KCCT, also known as the partial thromboplastin test (PTT), again uses citrated platelet-poor plasma and measures the intrinsic coagulation pathway (factors XII, XI, IX, VIII, X, V, II, I) (Fig. 15.5). Plasma is added to a mixture of kaolin (surface contact) and cephalin (phospholipid) and is incubated at 37°C. After recalcification with 0·025 M calcium chloride a clot forms in approximately 40 seconds. The result is not usually expressed as a ratio and the test is more difficult to standardize than the PTR.

Situations in which the KCCT is abnormal include:

1 Haemophilia (factor VIII or IX deficiency)
2 Von Willebrand's disease (factor VIII deficiency with associated factor VIII-related platelet defect)
3 Contact factor deficiency (factor XII or XI deficiency)
4 Anticoagulant therapy
5 Hepatic failure
6 Intravascular coagulation

Factor VIII and IX deficiency (haemophilia) make up over 90% of inherited coagulation defects and the test is used to screen for these conditions. It has also been used for the laboratory control of heparin treatment (see below).

The thrombin test (TT) An equal volume of thrombin (or a calcium and thrombin mixture) is added to citrated platelet-poor plasma. A clot forms in about 10 seconds. Only the final reaction of fibrin formation from fibrinogen is measured (see Fig. 15.5). The test is abnormal in the presence of hypofibrinogenaemia, dysfibrinogenaemia, heparin or fibrinogen degradation products (FDPs). It is used to monitor heparin therapy and may be preferable to the KCCT for this purpose as the clot takes a shorter time to form. It is also used in the diagnosis of intravascular coagulation.

PARASITES IN THE BLOOD

In fresh blood viewed under a cover slip, some parasites, such as microfilariae and trypanosomes, may be seen and moving; others may be seen in thick or thin, fixed and stained films. The important parasites of the blood are those of malaria, microfilariae of several varieties, trypanosomes, Leishman–Donovan bodies and the spirochaetes of relapsing fever.

Malaria

For the diagnosis of malaria, thick films should be used for the detection of parasites and thin films for their identification. Films should preferably be taken when the patient's temperature is raised. Thick films should be examined systematically for 10–15 minutes before concluding that no parasites are present. The recognition of parasites in thick films requires practice. Parasites have definite morphological and staining properties and objects which do not show these are not parasites.

For details of the identification of the different types of parasite in thin films, larger works must be consulted. The main distinguishing points are as follows (Plate XVI).

In infection with *Plasmodium falciparum*, which produces malignant tertian malaria, schizogony generally takes place in the tissues, so that except in rare cases in moribund patients, only ring forms and a few crescent-shaped gametocytes are seen in the peripheral red blood cells. Ring forms of any species consist of a rim of cytoplasm which stains blue and a small nucleus or chromatin dot which stains red. The rings of *Plasmodium falciparum* are usually, though not invariably, small and delicate, and the red cells are not enlarged. More than one ring may appear in a single red cell and some rings may have two chromatin dots. Marginal forms or *formes appliquées* with the parasite lying along the edge of the cell may be seen. A few crescent-shaped gametocytes, which are easily recognized (Plate XIV), may have been seen in films from untreated patients, but if absent at this time they may appear some 7–10 days after the beginning of treatment.

In the remaining three species, schizogony takes place in the peripheral blood, so that ring forms, large trophozoites and schizonts will be present together in films.

In infections with *Plasmodium vivax*, which produces benign tertian malaria, the rings are large and stout and often measure one-third of the diameter of the red cell. The red cells may be enlarged, and if properly stained may show well marked Schüffner's dots (Plate XVI). Large irregular trophozoites containing brown pigment, and mature schizonts with 12–24 merozoites, may be seen (Plate XVI).

In infections with *Plasmodium malariae*, which produces quartan malaria, the ring forms are also large and stout, but the larger trophozoites are more compact and dense-looking and frequently take a characteristic band form (Plate XVI). Mature schizonts contain some 8 merozoites arranged in a rosette form around a mass of golden yellow pigment. Schüffner's dots are not seen and the red cells are not enlarged.

In infection with *Plasmodium ovale*, which is much the rarest of the four species, the parasites have some of the characteristics of *Plasmodium vivax* (e.g. large and prominent Schüffner's dots) and others of *Plasmodium malariae* (e.g. compact large trophozoites and occasional band forms). The most characteristic feature is the distortion in shape of the red cells, which become oval or fimbriated, and the schizonts contain only 8–10 merozoits (Plate XVI).

In some cases, mixed infections may be present.

Trypanosomiasis

In the diagnosis of trypanosomiasis, examination of the blood is generally less efficient than the examination of fluid obtained by lymph node puncture. An enlarged node, usually in the posterior triangle of the neck, is held firmly between the thumb and fingers of the left hand, while a moderate-sized hypodermic needle is plunged through the skin and into the substance of the node. A small amount of fluid passes into the needle and suction is neither necessary nor desirable. The needle is withdrawn and its contents ejected on to clean glass slides. The fluid should be examined fresh and unstained as described for fresh blood films; thin films should be stained with Leishman's stain.

Trypanosomes (Plate XVI) may also be found in thick or thin blood films and, in advanced cases, in films made from the deposit of centrifuged cerebrospinal fluid.

The important trypanosomes of man are *Trypanosoma gambiense* and *T. rhodesiense*, which cause African sleeping sickness, and, as seen in human blood, are usually morphologically indistinguishable; and *Trypanosoma cruzi*, which causes Brazilian trypanosomiasis (Chagas' disease). The latter exists chiefly in a non-flagellated form in the organs and muscles and only occasionally appears in the blood as a flagellate trypanosome (Plate XVI).

In a suspected case of trypanosomiasis, several specimens of node fluid and of blood should be examined, both fresh and unstained and in stained films. Trypanosomes may be seen 'lashing' their way amongst the cells and are often first detected by the commotion they produce in the latter. This movement must not be confused with that produced by the organisms of relapsing fever (*Borrelia recurrentis*) (Plate XVI).

In stained films, typical trypanosomes are seen as elongated fusiform structures some 14–30 μm long and 1–3 μm broad with a longitudinal undulating membrane and a terminal flagellum projecting from the anterior end (Plate XVI). There is a centrally placed nucleus, and at the posterior end a smaller black-staining kinetoplast. The shorter forms are more stumpy and may have little or no free flagellum.

Kala-azar

In the diagnosis of kala-azar, Leishman–Donovan bodies may be looked for in the blood or in material obtained by aspiration of bone marrow, lymph node, spleen or liver. Of these, examination of marrow obtained by sternal puncture (p. 433) is probably the simplest and safest method, but in occasional cases the parasites may be found by the examination of stained blood films, when they are seen in the cytoplasm of large mononuclear cells. When direct microscopic examination fails, culture methods are frequently successful.

The bodies may be seen in thick or thin stained blood films, which should be searched systematically. The parasites are round or oval bodies from 2 to 5 μm in diameter, containing a large round or oval solid-looking nucleus and a smaller more deeply stained and usually rod-shaped kinetoplast. In Leishman-stained films the cytoplasm is blue and the nucleus and kinetoplast are red (Plate XVI). Giemsa staining is preferable.

While the term Leishman–Donovan bodies strictly applies to the Indian form of kala-azar, the similar *Leishmania* may be found in the blood or tissues in cases of Mediterranean kala-azar, from fluid obtained by puncture at the margin of the lesion in the various forms of cutaneous leishmaniasis or 'tropical sore', and from the mucous membranes of the mouth, nose or throat in espundia or South American leishmaniasis.

Microfilariae

Adult filarial worms or microfilariae are parasites of the lymphatic system or connective tissues. Their presence is diagnosed by the finding of their larvae or microfilariae in the blood stream. Three main varieties of microfilariae are found in the blood of man:

1 *Wuchereria bancrofti* is found in the blood stream in any numbers only at night and causes filariasis, characterized by irregular fever, lymphangitis and various forms of elephantitis.

2 *Loa loa* is found in the blood stream only by day, and causes loaisis, characterized by transient red painful swellings known as calabar swellings.

3 *Dipetalonema perstans* is non-periodic, appearing equally by day and night, and has no recognized pathogenic effects.

If filariasis is suspected, blood should be examined say at 8 a.m., noon and 4 p.m., and again at 8 p.m., midnight and 4 a.m. Fresh unstained films should be used for the detection of the filariae, and stained ones, thick if the larvae are scanty and thin if they are plentiful, for their identification.

In fresh unstained films microfilariae are easily seen as actively moving linear objects. In stained films they are seen as wormlike objects with a round head and a pointed tail, from 5 to 8 μm broad (i.e. about the diameter of a red cell) and from 100 to 300 μm long (Plate XVI). The main differentiating features of the three species, apart from their periodicity, are as follows. *W. bancrofti* and *L. loa* have a delicate sheath, which can be seen where it projects beyond the rounded head and pointed tail of the larva, whereas *D. perstans* is unsheathed. All larvae have a central column of nuclei extending from the head more or less to the tail. In *L. loa* and *D. perstans* the nuclei extend to the extreme tip of the tail, whereas in *W. bancrofti* the column ends short of the tip.

Microfilariae do not stain well by Leishman's stain. Thick films should be dehaemoglobinized and stained by Giemsa. Microfilariae are readily recognized by the intense staining of their nuclei, and the sheath, if present, is easily seen.

Relapsing fever

The *Borrelia recurrentis* of relapsing fever should be sought in fresh unstained films of blood and in thin films stained by Leishman's method under the oil-immersion lens. Fresh unstained films should be examined with the light well cut down. Agitation of the red cells usually calls attention to the presence of parasites, which may otherwise be difficult to detect (Plate XV).

In thin stained films the spirochaete is seen as a linear object with tapering ends, 0·4 μm in breadth and 10–30 μm in length (Plate XV). The spiral shape which it possesses in life is lost and the body lies in irregular curves. In searching for the organism, it is important to direct the eyes deliberately to the spaces between the red cells rather than to the red cells, or the parasite may be missed.

16
Examination of children

The clinical examination of young children is a skill which must be learnt by experience. However, since children who object very strongly to being examined usually do so because they are afraid, the beginner can often achieve an adequate examination by patience and a gentle approach. The child and his mother should be greeted in a friendly manner and the child offered a selection of toys suitable to his age. The *history* is then taken from the mother incorporating the special questions set out on p. 17. While talking to the mother, the examiner should observe the patient and take note of certain points. Does the child look well or ill? Is he apathetic or alert, anxious or relaxed? Is there anything unusual about the facies? Are there any obvious physical deformities? Is the child well nourished or wasted? Is there any difficulty in breathing?

GENERAL EXAMINATION

The child should now be at ease and getting used to the strange surroundings. This is the time to record the respiration and pulse rates. The average respiratory rate in a normal newborn child is 40/minute; by the second year it has fallen to 25 or so, and by the fifth year to about 20. A raised respiratory rate in a child at rest usually indicates some disorder of the respiratory or cardiovascular systems. The normal pulse–respiration ratio is 3 or 4 to 1.

The pulse rate is counted in young infants by palpation or auscultation of the chest, in older children by palpation at the wrist. The average pulse rate at birth is about 130/minute, at 1 year 110, at 3 years 100, at 8 years 90, and at 12 years 80. During sleep the pulse rate falls about 10–20 beats/minute. The normal range for pulse rates is wide. Tachycardia is common and may be due to crying, excitement, exercise or fever as well as to various diseases. Bradycardia is rare and usually indicates some cardiac abnormality. Sinus arrhythmia (see p. 201) is present in almost all children, but other irregularities of rhythm are uncommon even in the presence of cardiac disease. Always feel for the femoral pulses; they are either absent or weak in coarctation of the aorta.

Examination should now proceed by the usual methods of inspection, palpation, percussion and auscultation; but no set routine can be followed and the examination is by regions rather than by systems. Each child will, by his reaction to the various procedures, dictate the order of examination and even the position in which he will be examined. Young infants are usually examined on the mother's lap; older children who may not be prepared to lie down on a couch can be examined standing at the mother's side. Most children are prepared to have some of their clothes removed, although they are often modest and should be allowed to keep their pants on.

It is important to be gentle and to have warm hands. Begin by looking at and feeling the child all over. Observe the general state of development and nutrition. Is the skin dry or moist, and is there the normal degree of elasticity? Is there a rash present? Are there any bruises? Multiple bruises of different ages in children under the age of 3 suggest the possibility of non-accidental injury. The shape of the chest and abdomen should be noted. The abdomen is normally rather protuberant in young children.

Feel the head and the *anterior fontanelle*: this closes normally between 15 months and 2 years and delayed closure may be due to rickets or hydrocephalus. The *posterior fontanelle* is always small and closes by the second month. The degree of tension of the anterior fontanelle is important. In health it pulsates and is in the same plane as the rest of the surrounding skull. A depressed fontanelle is a sign of dehydration, and a tense bulging fontanelle indicates raised intracranial pressure. The fontanelle is normally tense when the child is crying. The *shape of the head* should be noted. It may be abnormally shaped, owing to premature fusion of the sutures. It is globular in hydrocephalus and is often asymmetrical in normal infants, who tend to lie persistently on one side (plagiocephaly).

Inspect the *eyes* for cataracts and conjunctivitis. In infants a squint may be detected by shining a light in front of the face. The light reflex should be at the same position on each cornea.

Examine the *limbs*. Look for wasting, swelling and tenderness, and for limitation of movement of joints. A painful limb may be immobile in infants (pseudo-paralysis) or cause a limp in older children. Feel the wrists for widening of the epiphyses of the radius and ulna, which is a sign of rickets. Note the presence of deformities such as knock-knee, bow-legs and flat feet.

The *lymphatic glands* should be palpated. Small glands can normally be felt in the anterior and posterior triangles of the neck, the axillae and the inguinal regions. Lymph glands enlarge readily in children as a result of local conditions such as tonsillitis or generalized diseases such as rubella.

The *abdomen* cannot be palpated satisfactorily in a child who is crying or resisting. Small infants can be given a feed to stop them crying, but with an older child one must wait until he settles down before attempting examination. Children from about 1 to 3 years old will often refuse to be examined lying down, but in this age group the abdomen can be palpated from behind when the child is standing on the mother's lap and looking over her shoulder. Palpation should be gentle and light. The liver edge can be felt quite easily and in young children normally extends down to 2 cm below the costal margin. The spleen when enlarged can be felt below the left costal margin. Slight enlargement of the spleen is common in children with infections of all types. Faecal masses can be felt in constipated children and a full or distended bladder presents as a firm mass arising out of the pelvis. Abdominal tenderness is best detected by watching the child's facial expression during palpation. Feel for testes in the scrotum but remember that an active cremasteric reflex may retract them into the abdomen.

The *thorax* should be inspected for deformity of the chest wall and for intercostal or subcostal recession, which indicates respiratory obstruction, chronic lung disease or a cardiac abnormality. Listen for the grunting respirations of the child with pneumonia. This is due to a reversal of the normal respiratory rhythm. The grunting expiration is followed by inspiration and then a pause. The thickening of the costochondral junctions which occurs in rickets can be seen and felt. Palpate the anterior chest wall for the cardiac impulse and for thrills. In children under the age of 6 or 7 years the cardiac impulse is normally in the fourth intercostal space, just to the left of the midclavicular line. In older children it is usually in the fifth space in the midclavicular line. Vocal fremitus is not a sign of great value in children.

Percussion of the chest should be light and in small children can be direct, that is to say the chest wall is tapped directly with the percussing finger without the use of a pleximeter finger. The chest is much more resonant in children than in adults.

A stethoscope with a small bell chest-piece is suitable for general auscultation of a child's chest. Listen for the breath sounds and for adventitious sounds. Because of the thin chest wall, breath sounds are louder in children than in adults, and their character is more like the bronchial breathing of adults (puerile breathing). Upper respiratory infections frequently give rise to loud coarse rhonchi, which may be conducted down the trachea and main bronchi.

The normal splitting of first and second heart sounds is easier to hear in children than in adults. Venous hums and functional systolic flow murmurs are often heard in normal children.

In older children examination of the *nervous system* can be carried out in the usual manner. In young children the extent of the neurological examination depends on their age and willingness to cooperate. If the child can walk, look for abnormalities of gait and the presence of a limp or ataxia. Note any abnormal movements. Tics or habit spasms are repetitive but purposeful movements, such as turning of the head or shrugging of the shoulders. Choreiform movements are coarse, involuntary, purposeless jerks which follow no particular pattern. These are best demonstrated by asking the child to hold out his arms in front of him. In this position the child with chorea adopts a characteristic posture, with the wrists in flexion and the fingers in hyperextension. Coordination is tested by some modification of the finger–nose test, for example reaching out to touch a toy held in the examiner's hand.

Muscle tone and muscle power should be assessed. The child with marked hypotonia will slip through one's hands when picked up under the armpits. Meningeal irritation or spasm of the spinal muscles is detected more readily by resistance to passive flexion of the head and neck (neck stiffness) than by testing for Kernig's sign.

Tendon reflexes are often difficult to elicit in normal children, and some time may be needed to find the correct position of the limb for this purpose. Only gentle percussion of tendons is required and this is often better done with the examiner's finger than with an adult-sized patellar hammer. The plantar responses are extensor in normal infants up to the age of about 18 months, but the persistence of an extensor response after the age of 2 years indicates an upper motor neurone lesion.

With a little ingenuity, most of the cranial nerves can be tested. For example, by getting a baby to follow a bright object moving in various directions the eye movements can be studied and the presence of nystagmus noted. Examination of the fundi is particularly difficult in infants, as they cannot be instructed to fix their gaze appropriately. Infinite patience is needed for this manoeuvre, as it entails waiting with the ophthalmoscope in position for fleeting glimpses of the optic disc. Forcible attempts to keep the eyes open only make the procedure more difficult. Older children will often fix their eyes on a toy held up behind the examiner by an assistant.

The testing of vision, hearing and certain motor functions in young children is included in the developmental screening examination described on p. 469.

For the child the most unpleasant examinations are those of the *ears*, *nose*, *mouth* and *throat* and these should be left until last. With skill, gentleness and patience, even these procedures can usually be carried out without making the child cry. Start with the nose, which need only be examined superficially. By placing a shiny surface, such as a mirror, under the nostrils, patency of the nasal airways can be judged by the size of the area of clouding. With a good light, the appearance of the mucous membrane of the anterior nares can be inspected. Look for the pale swollen inferior turbinates which are characteristic of allergic rhinitis. Proceed next to examine the external auditory meati and tympanic membranes. Allow the child to see and handle the auriscope and speculum, using the instruments as a toy in a simple game for a few moments. If, in spite of these preparations, the child still resists, he will have to be held by his mother. Sit the child on her lap facing to one or other side, and get her to

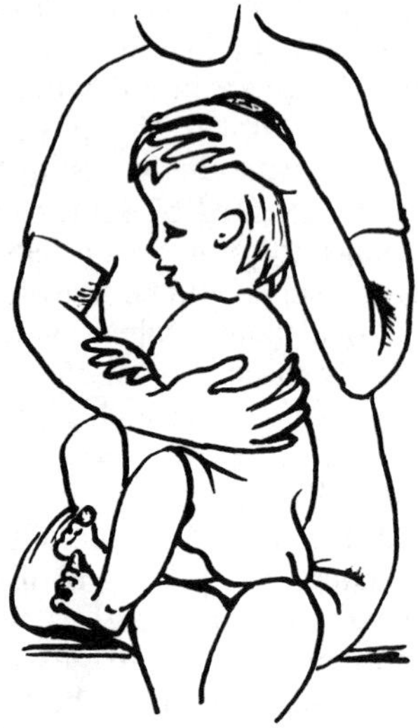

Fig. 16.1 Position for examination of the ear in infants.

hold the child firmly with one arm around his head and the other around his upper arms and shoulders (Fig. 16.1). Held in this way, the child can be kept still long enough for the ear drums to be inspected.

The mouth and throat are examined in similar fashion. A cooperative child can be encouraged to 'show his teeth' and thus open his mouth without the use of a spatula, which so many children dread. The uncooperative or very young child must be held by the mother, as for the examination of the ears, but in this case the child sits facing the examiner. The use of a spatula may be unavoidable. Force it gently between the teeth and on to the tongue, which is then depressed. Note the state of the teeth, the tongue, and the mucous membrane of the mouth. Look for Koplik's spots (in measles), the pharyngeal lesions of chicken pox, and the white patches of thrush. Inspect the tonsils and the pharynx. Look for streaks of mucopus on the posterior pharyngeal wall (post-nasal drip). Examine the frenulum of the upper lip, which may be torn in non-accidental injury.

SPECIAL EXAMINATIONS

The following examinations need special mention.

Measurements

Measurements of weight and height are important in the examination of children. Height can be measured only in children over the age of about two years. Below this age supine length can be measured roughly with a tape measure or more accurately with a special measuring board. All measurements should be made under standard conditions, and children should be weighed unclothed. One of the particular features of childhood is that it is a period of growth, the pattern of which may be adversely affected by many disturbances of health. Heights and weights should be compared with those of healthy children of similar sex, age and build, and for this purpose the percentile charts (Figs. 16.2–16.7) are invaluable. Serial measurements over a period are essential in assessing changes in growth rates. As a rough guide, the average weight of children can be taken as 3 kg (7 lb) at birth, 6·5 kg (14 lb) at 1 year, 13 kg (28 lb) at 2 years and 22·5 kg (49 lb) at 7 years (the 'rule of seven' when using the old Imperial measure). However, it can be seen from the percentile charts that there is a wide range above and below the average.

In infants under the age of 2 years the head circumference should be measured. The standard measurement is the occipito-frontal circumference, which is the largest circumference of the head. The average head circumference at birth is 35 cm, at 3 months 41 cm, at 6 months 43 cm, at 1 year 46 cm and at 2 years 49 cm (Fig. 16.8). Hydrocephalus should be suspected when the rate of growth of the head is greater than is normal for the sex, age and size of the infant.

Figs. 16.2–16.7 show standard heights and weights for boys and girls aged up to 3 years, 2 to 10 years and 9 to 18 years.

Figs. 16.8 and 16.9 show head circumference and skeletal maturity (or bone age), assessed by the state of fusion of the epiphyses on radiographs.

The range of normal is expressed in percentiles and each chart shows the third, tenth, twenty-fifth, fiftieth, seventy-fifth, ninetieth and ninety-seventh percentiles. The meaning of the tenth percentile for height is that 10% of all normal children are shorter than this height at the age concerned. As a rough guide, it can be said that children who fall outside the area between the tenth and ninetieth percentiles should be regarded with slight suspicion, and those outside the area between the third and ninety-seventh percentiles should be regarded as unhealthy unless proved otherwise.

Blood pressure

Abnormalities of blood pressure are uncommon in childhood, and measurement of blood pressure is a distressing examination for some young children. Consequently this procedure is sometimes omitted from the general examination, but it must be carried out in all cases of suspected cardiovascular or renal disease. Blood pressure readings are best obtained in most children after the main examination is over and the child is partially dressed. Allow the child to see and play with the cuff and give some simple explanation of what is going to happen. The size of cuff is most important if accurate readings are to be

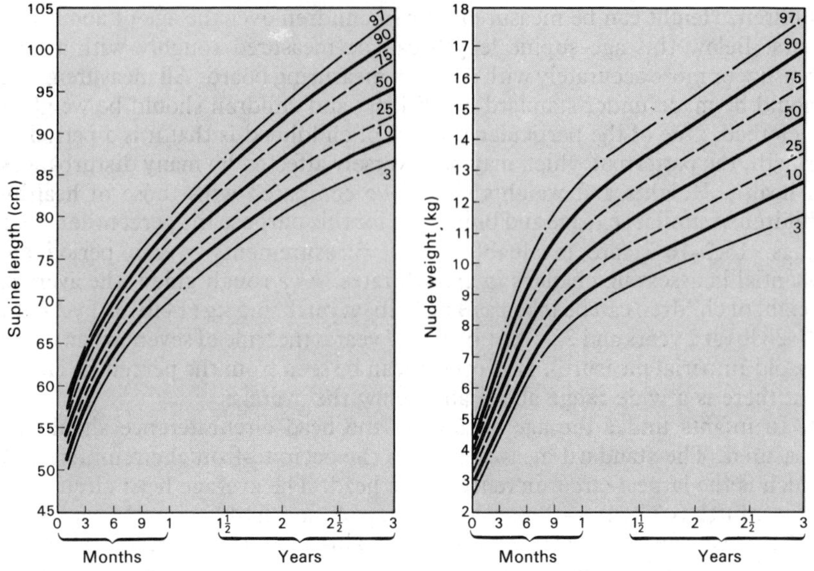

Fig. 16.2 Supine length and nude weight in boys up to 3 years.
(These and the following charts are modified from those developed at the Institute of Child Health and the Hospital for Sick Children, Great Ormond Street, London.)

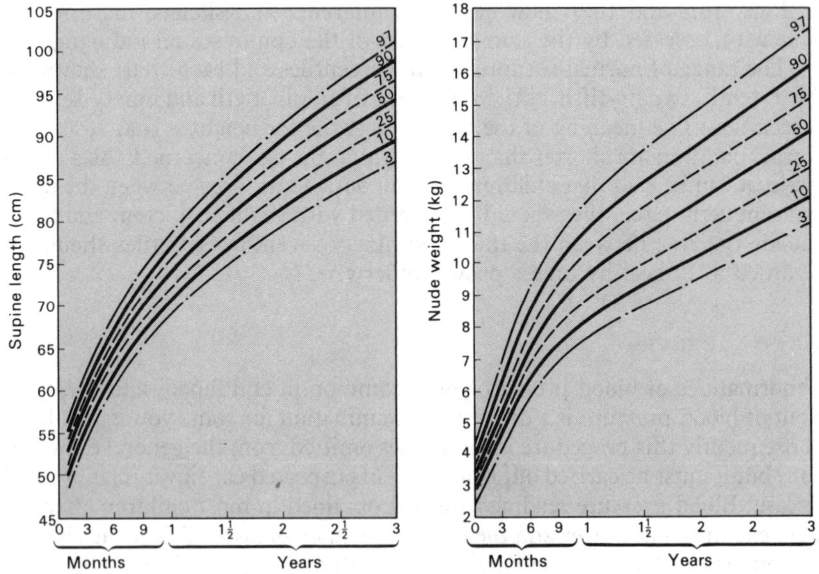

Fig. 16.3 Supine length and nude weight in girls up to 3 years.

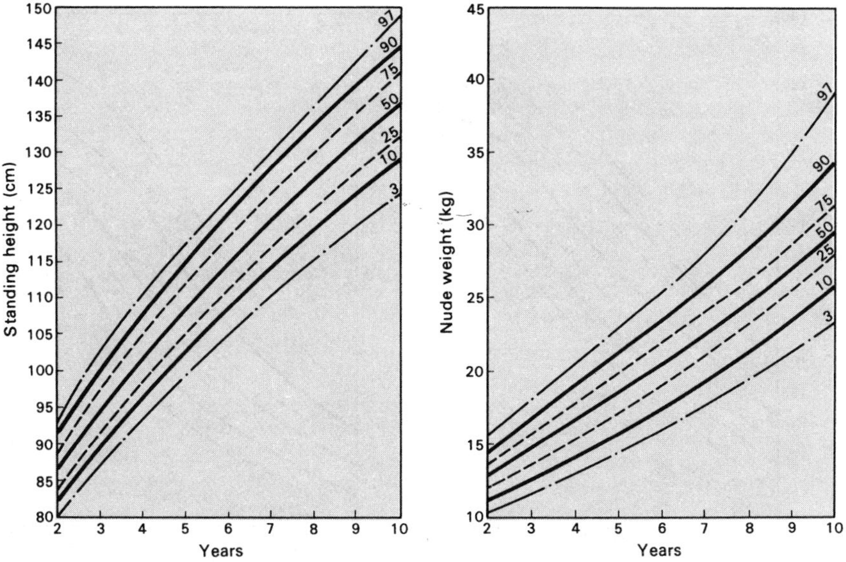

Fig. 16.4 Standing height and nude weight in boys aged 2 to 10 years.

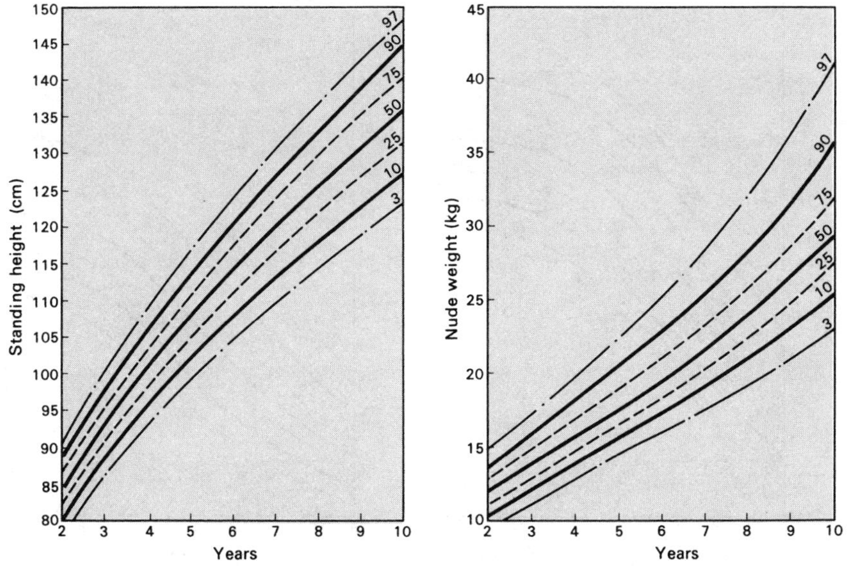

Fig. 16.5 Standing height and nude weight in girls aged 2 to 10 years.

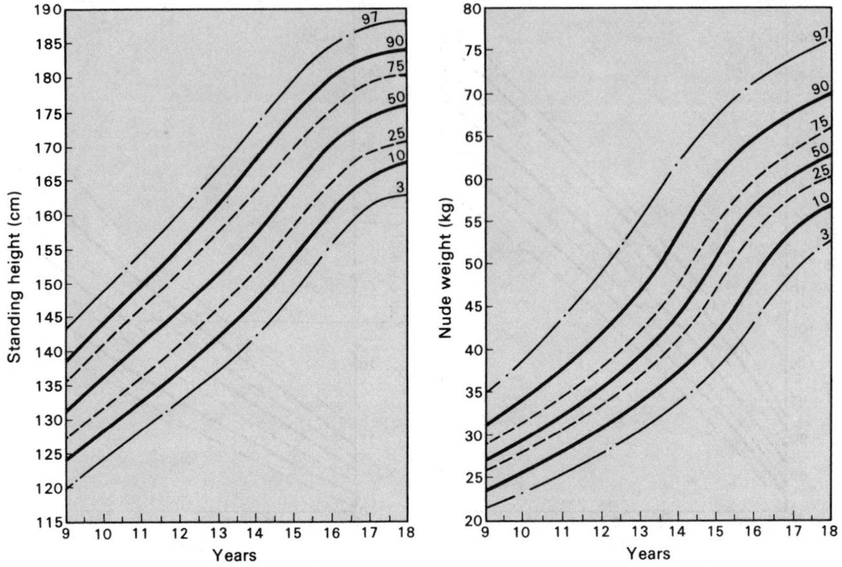

Fig. 16.6 Standing height and nude weight in boys aged 9 to 18 years.

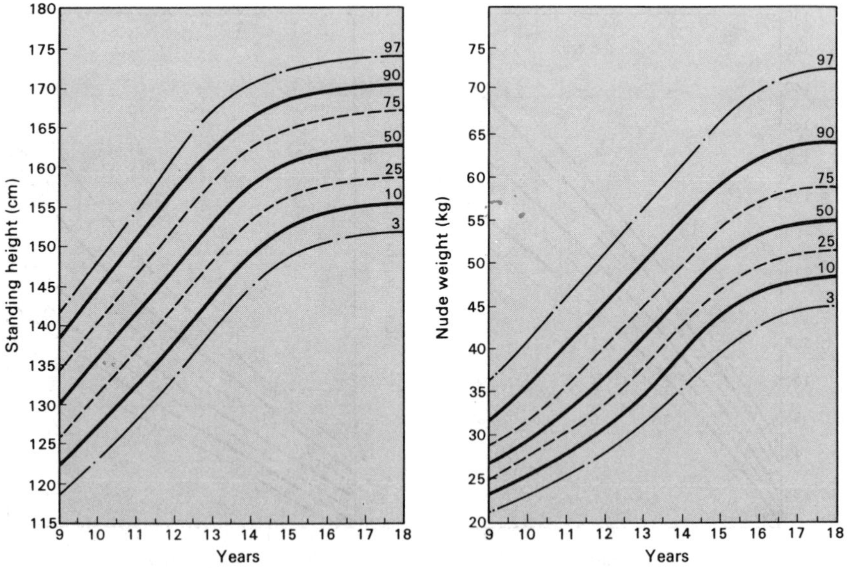

Fig. 16.7 Standing height and nude weight in girls aged 9 to 18 years.

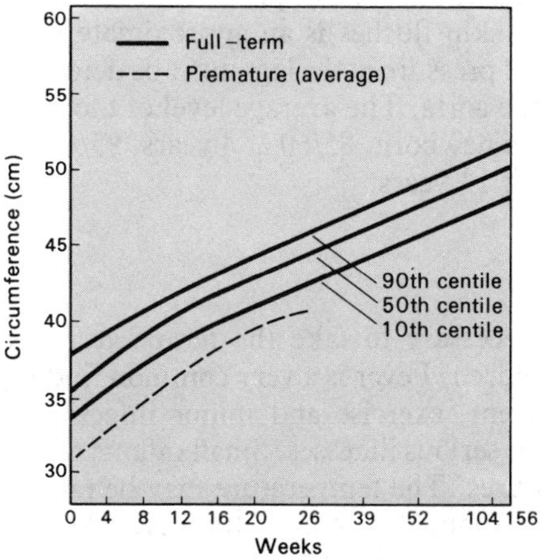

Fig. 16.8 Head circumference.

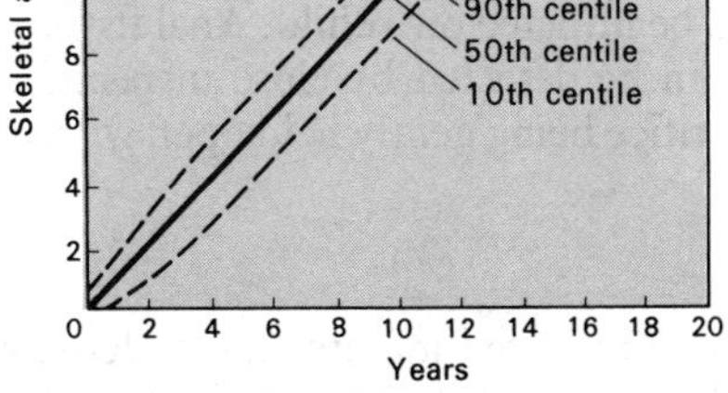

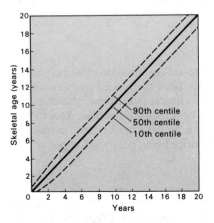

Fig. 16.9 Skeletal maturity.

obtained, and a variety of sizes are available. The inflatable bag should be long enough to encircle the full circumference of the arm and should be of a width roughly equal to half the length of the upper arm. In small children and infants it may not be possible to determine the blood pressure by auscultation, and the pulse can be palpated to obtain the systolic pressure. In babies the flush method may be used. The arm is held up and tightly bandaged to exclude the blood to the level of the cuff, which is then inflated. The bandage is then removed to reveal a white limb. The pressure in the cuff is slowly reduced. The point at which the skin flushes is an approximate indication of the systolic pressure. The blood pressure in the legs must be determined in suspected cases of coarctation of the aorta. The average level of blood pressure in the arms is 80/50 mmHg in the newborn, 85/60 at 4 years, 95/65 at 8 years, 100/70 at 10 years and 110/75 at 13 years.

Temperature

It is not always necessary to take the temperature as part of the routine examination of children. Fever is a very common finding in children and may be due to excitement, exercise and minor infections as well as to severe infections and other serious illnesses. Small infants often respond to infections with low temperatures. The temperature may be taken either before or after the physical examination. Oral temperatures are taken in children over the age of about 6 years. In smaller children, between 2 and 6 years, the thermometer can be placed in the axilla or groin. Rectal temperatures are taken in infants. The temperature in the axilla or groin is about 0·5°C lower and in the rectum about 0·5°C higher than the oral temperature. The temperature of normal children varies between 36·5 and 37·5°C and is about 1°C higher in infants than in older children. Rapid rises of temperature to 39·5 or 40°C are sometimes associated with febrile convulsions in young children.

Rectal examination

Most children find rectal examination extremely unpleasant and small infants experience some pain from the procedure even when the little finger is used. One must use one's clinical judgement, therefore, in deciding whether this examination should be inflicted on a child. Anal fissure is a common condition in childhood and can be detected by close inspection of the anal canal, the buttocks and anal orifice being gently held open with one hand on either side.

Stools

The stools of normal breast-fed infants may be loose and green or pasty and yellow. Infants fed on cow's milk preparations pass stools of a paler yellow colour and of a much firmer consistency. The character of the stool in older children is more variable than in adults. *Toddler's diarrhoea* occurs in otherwise healthy infants who pass frequent loose stools containing undigested vegetable matter.

Urine

Special techniques are required for the collection of urine specimens in infants who have not yet acquired sphincter control. It may be possible to 'catch' a specimen by holding the infant over a sterile container. Alternatively specially made sterile plastic containers with an adhesive opening can be applied to the washed genitalia. In the last resort bladder urine may be obtained by careful suprapubic aspiration.

DEVELOPMENTAL SCREENING EXAMINATION

Development is the normal process of maturation of function which takes place in the early years of life. It may be delayed by disease or adverse environment and the delay can be detected by developmental examination. A simple developmental screening examination should be carried out at regular intervals on all normal infants and as part of the clinical examination of infants presenting with symptoms.

It is usual to consider development under four main headings:

1 Movement and posture
2 Vision and manipulation
3 Hearing and speech
4 Social behaviour

Screening for developmental delay involves testing the child's performance of a few skills in each of the four fields of development and comparing his achievements with the average for children of the same age. Children who appear to have delayed development on screening should be referred to an appropriate specialist for more detailed assessment.

Movement and posture

Head control By 4 months a baby will bring his head up in line with the trunk when pulled from supine to sitting, and when held in the sitting position will keep his head upright (Fig. 16.10). Before this age the head lags behind the trunk.

Sitting At 7 months a baby begins to sit unsupported.

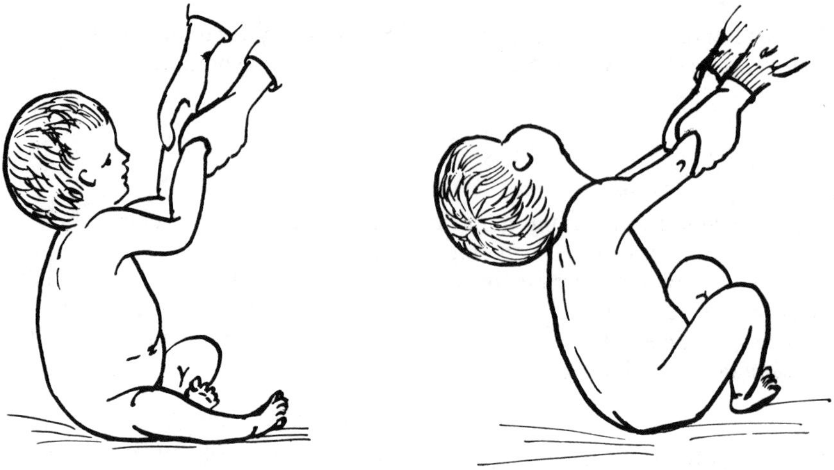

Fig. 16.10 Head control. *Left*. At 4 months the head is in line with the trunk when the baby is pulled to sitting. *Right*. Before the age of 4 months, the head lags.

Standing and walking At 9 months a baby can stand with support; at 10 months he takes a few steps with support and can crawl on hands and knees; at 13 months he begins to walk unsupported.

Vision and manipulation

Vision At 8 weeks a baby lying supine will fix his gaze on a bright object dangling on a string 20 cm from his face and will move his head to follow it briefly. At 6 months he will follow a rolling ball at a distance of 3 m.

Manipulation At 6 months a baby will reach out for an object and grasp it in the palm of his hand (palmar grasp) and will transfer it from one hand to the other. At 10 months he develops a pincer grasp and can pick up a small sweet between index finger and thumb.

Hearing and speech

Hearing Hearing should be tested first at 6 months. The baby is seated on his mother's lap facing forward. The examiner makes a series of soft sounds to one or other side but behind the mother and baby and out of the baby's vision (Fig. 16.11). The sounds used are a rattle, a spoon in a cup, a bell and the rustle of tissue paper. At 6 months the baby should turn to the source of sound when it is about 45 cm from his ear. At 9 months he reacts more quickly and localizes the sound at a distance of 90 cm.

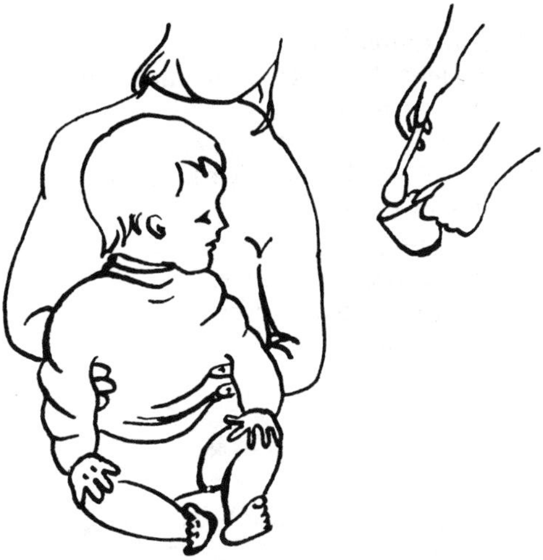

Fig. 16.11 Testing hearing at 6 months.

Speech By the age of 9 months the infant is babbling with a series of syllables and at 1 year the first words used with meaning appear. By about 2 years three-word sentences are used. The variation in speech development among normal children is particularly wide.

Social behaviour

One of the first social skills to be developed is smiling in response to a pleasurable stimulus, which can be observed from about 6 weeks. At 9 months a baby can hold and chew a biscuit. At 18 months he can drink from a cup, no longer puts objects into his mouth, and can build a tower of three cubes. At 3 years he can feed himself with a spoon and fork and makes a good attempt at dressing himself.

The range of normal developmental progress is wide and the milestones described above are achieved at the ages given by an average normal baby. Delay in all fields of development is more significant than delay in only one and severe delay is much more significant than slight delay. Allowance must always be made for those babies who were born prematurely, at least up to the age of 1 year, by which time they should have caught up. The following is a list of some of the important milestones of development:

6 weeks	Smiles
3 months	Holds head steady
4 months	Turns head to sound
5 months	Reaches out and grasps object

7 months	Sits unsupported
7 months	Transfers objects from one hand to the other
9 months	Stands with support
11 months	Crawls
12 months	Says 2–3 single words with meaning
13 months	Walks unsupported
15 months	Holds cup and drinks
18 months	Builds a tower of 3 cubes
2 years	Says 2–3 word sentences
3 years	Dresses himself

EXAMINATION OF THE NEWBORN

The routine examination of the newborn baby is designed to assess his general state of health and to detect congenital abnormalities. It is usual to carry out one examination immediately after birth and another before discharge from hospital or on about the seventh day.

The routine measurements—weight, length and head circumference (occipito-frontal)—will usually have been taken by the midwife. Note the time of passing of the first urine and meconium, which is the dark green sticky stool of the newborn baby in the first few days of life.

General inspection of the baby will indicate whether or not he is in good general condition, i.e. active and with a strong cry. Look for *abnormal facial features* such as those of Down's syndrome and for *external abnormalities* such as cleft lip, neural tube defects along the length of the spine, and abnormalities of the genitalia such as hypospadias and hydrocoele. The testes can usually be felt in the scrotum at birth. Remember to examine the *palate* for clefts, and the *anus*, which may be imperforate.

Examine the *eyes* with an assistant who will gently hold the lids apart, and look for conjunctivitis, clouding of the cornea, which suggests glaucoma, and for lens opacities (cataract).

Observe the colour of the *skin*. Peripheral cyanosis is a common finding in normal newborns but central cyanosis indicates cardiac or respiratory disease. So-called physiological jaundice is present after 48 hours in most preterm and some fullterm babies but severe jaundice on the first or second day is usually due to some haemolytic disorder. Look for birth marks, which are either pigmented lesions or haemangiomata. Most babies have a collection of dilated capillaries on the upper eyelids or at the nape of the neck which fade after a few weeks. Some babies develop crops of small papules on the trunk during the first week (erythema toxicum) but these fade quickly and are of no significance. 'Mongolian blue spot' is the name given to dark blue areas of racial pigmentation seen over the sacral area or on the back or legs in babies of African, Asian or Oriental origin.

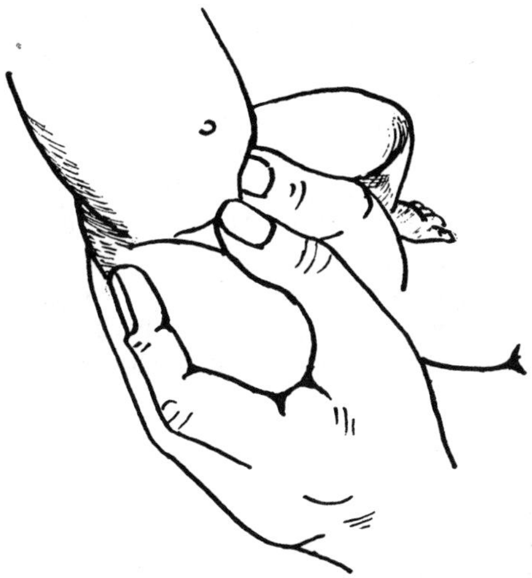

Fig. 16.12 Examination of the hips in the newborn.

Breast enlargement with exudation of a milky fluid from the nipples is sometimes seen in newborn babies of both sexes. This is due to the effect of transferred maternal hormones and disappears in a few days without causing problems.

The *head* should be inspected and palpated. There is considerable normal variation in the size of the fontanelles and in the width of the sutures. A cephalohaematoma is a subperiosteal haematoma which appears a few days after birth as a large cystic swelling limited to the area of one of the bones of the skull vault. The caput succedaneum is an area of oedema of the scalp over the presenting part of the head. It pits on pressure and is not fluctuant.

It is essential to examine the *hips* of all newborn infants in order to detect actual or potential dislocation. The infant is laid on his back with hips and knees flexed. The examiner grasps the thighs with the middle fingers over the greater trochanters and the thumbs over the lesser trochanters (Fig. 16.12). Pressure with the fingers will replace a dislocated femoral head and pressure with the thumbs will dislocate an unstable joint. Both abnormal movements will be associated with a pronounced and palpable click.

Soft *systolic murmurs* are heard in many newborn infants. They are usually of no significance and disappear after a few weeks but may, if they persist, indicate a congenital abnormality of the heart.

Examine the *hands* for abnormalities such as extra digits and for the single transverse palmar crease associated with Down's syndrome. Look for deformities of the *feet*. Talipes equinovarus is the common type of 'club foot', in which the foot is plantar flexed and rotated inwards.

Gently feel the *abdomen* for abnormal masses such as an enlarged kidney or bladder. The umbilical cord begins to shrivel up soon after birth and normally drops off at about the seventh day to leave a moist, slightly infected stump, but redness and oedema of the skin around the stump indicate more serious infection.

In the neurological examination note the muscle tone and observe the posture and movement of the limbs. Any marked difference between the two sides is abnormal. The normal position of the limbs is in flexion. Look for weakness or paralysis in the face and in the arms suggesting injury to the facial nerve or brachial plexus. Flaccid paralysis in both legs in a newborn infant is usually due to spina bifida with myelomeningocoele.

Primitive reflexes

Primitive reflexes are present in the normal newborn infant and disappear between 3 and 6 months of age. They are responses to specific stimuli and depend to some extent on the baby's state of wakefulness. The absence of one or more of these reflexes in the newborn period may indicate some abnormality of the brain or perhaps a local abnormality in the affected limb or neuromuscular pathway.

Moro reflex This is the most useful of the primitive reflexes. It is correctly called the 'startle' reflex and should be elicited with care and gentle handling. The baby's body is supported with one arm and hand and his head with the other hand. The hand holding the head is suddenly lowered a few centimetres allowing the baby's head to drop back (Fig. 16.13). In a positive response the baby abducts and extends his arms and finally flexes them. A diminished or absent response suggests some cerebral abnormality. A clearly unilateral response suggests some local abnormality such as a fracture or brachial plexus injury in the arm on the side which does not respond.

Other primitive reflexes are:

Rooting reflex In this reflex the baby turns his head towards the stimulus of a touch on the side of the face, searching for the nipple.

Palmar grasp reflex A finger is placed across the palmar surface of the baby's fingers, which flex and grip the examiner's.

Stepping reflex The baby is held upright with his feet resting on a firm surface. As one foot presses down on the surface, the other leg flexes at the hip and knee in a stepping movement. As this response is alternated from one leg to the other the baby makes a walking movement.

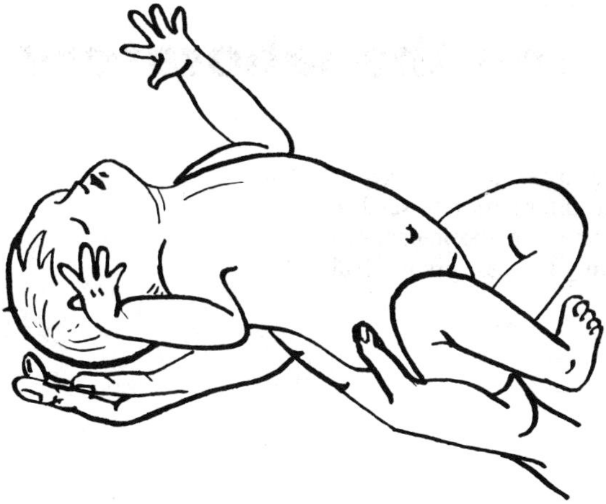

Fig. 16.13 Eliciting the Moro reflex.

17
Using the laboratory

Cooperation with laboratories requires mutual understanding between clinicians and laboratory workers. Pathology now embraces a series of specialized subjects and clinicians cannot be expected to be familiar with the detailed performance of all tests that they request. However they should know the following:

1 What *investigation* to request in given circumstances.
2 The discomfort and possible risk to the patient of an investigation.
3 What *information* the pathologist requires about the patient.
4 What *specimens* are required and how they should be obtained and transmitted to the laboratory.
5 The approximate cost in time and money of an investigation.
6 The possible risk of a specimen to the laboratory worker (infected material or Australia antigen-positive sera).
7 How to make the *best use* of the results received from the laboratory. In the case of complicated investigations, the clinician and the pathologist should agree a programme of investigation and discuss the results.

WHAT INVESTIGATION TO REQUEST

The result of any laboratory investigation is only one part of the information required to make a diagnosis. It may have as much or as little significance as any other physical finding. The plan of investigation has to be decided from the facts elicited by history taking and physical examination. However, the widespread use of automation in haematology and biochemistry means that tests are often performed in a 'package'. It is necessary to know what is offered in each package and to choose the appropriate one, rather than the single test. The availability of these routines should not lead to the abandonment of the eclectic approach that adds to the patient's comfort, the speed of diagnosis and the continued education of the doctor.

Certain investigations are often necessary to monitor the natural history of a disease and its treatment. For example the white blood cell count has to be followed serially in cases of leukaemia and the sedimentation rate in rheumatoid arthritis. There should therefore be a planned series of repeat tests, as is often necessary when following the resolution of a metabolic disorder. Tests should not be repeated without good reason and, if repeated, the interval between them should be logically decided.

WHAT INFORMATION TO SEND

A source of serious error can be failure to identify correctly the source of a specimen from a given patient. Therefore laboratories design their request forms with care and it is essential that all details required are filled in, accurately and legibly. Usually it is necessary to record the patient's surname and first name, address (or ward and bed number), the hospital serial number and the sex and date of birth of the patient. These details are all the more necessary in parts of the world where many family names are very similar.

Requests must also indicate the exact nature of the material sent, its source and the precise nature of the investigations required. The date on which the specimen is collected must be recorded. For many biochemical tests it is necessary to record the exact time at which the specimen is collected.

It is desirable that the patient's tentative diagnosis should be recorded together with any relevant clinical comment. A note of current antibiotic therapy is necessary with all requests for bacteriologial examinations. Similarly, any therapy that might influence biochemical investigations should be recorded.

COLLECTION OF SPECIMENS

It is essential that specimens reach the laboratory fresh and in the correct kind of container. Specimens are best taken by hand to the laboratory as soon as they are obtained, but they can, if necessary, be sent by post (letter post only), provided they are suitably packed and labelled 'Fragile, With Care' and 'Pathological Specimen'. Such specimens must be placed in a sealed inner container and then packed in a wooden or metal box containing sufficient absorbent material to soak up all the liquid contents if the inner container is broken. Local and international regulations about the transmission of pathological material must be strictly adhered to.

Suitable containers are best obtained from the laboratory that is going to make the investigations. All containers must be perfectly clean and preferably sterile. This is of course essential for bacteriological specimens. Containers for blood should be completely dry. All containers must have properly fitting lids or caps. It is usually essential that the correct container should be used for each particular investigation (e.g. particular anticoagulants are necessary for particular chemical or other tests on blood). It is also desirable that the correct amount of material specified for a particular container should be placed in that container, and in any case no more than the amount specified.

All syringes and needles must be sterile and should either be of the disposable type or be dry-sterilized in a laboratory.

Venepuncture

A piece of rubber tubing is used as a tourniquet and applied round the upper arm over the middle of the biceps, so as to impede the venous but not the arterial flow. The skin at the bend of the elbow is 'painted' with 0·5% chlorhexidine in 70% alcohol or simply 70% spirit (iodine is expensive and can give rise to severe skin reactions). The skin is rendered tense by the operator's left hand; the syringe with the needle attached is held in the right hand and almost parallel with the patient's arm; the patient is asked to 'make a fist' and then the needle with the bevel upwards is inserted into a prominent vein—the median basilic is usually convenient—and the needle is pointed in the direction of the blood flow. The required amount of blood is then drawn up into the syringe and the tourniquet is removed before the needle is withdrawn, as otherwise a haematoma may form. For some purposes it is necessary to remove the tourniquet as soon as the needle enters the vein, so that free-flowing blood is withdrawn. As soon as the needle is withdrawn a swab is placed on the puncture site and the patient is instructed to hold his forearm firmly flexed against his arm for a minute or so. Occasionally a vein in the forearm or wrist may prove more convenient than one at the elbow, but the procedure is then usually more painful. A vein which can be *felt* is generally easier to enter than one which can only be *seen*.

Blood obtained by venepuncture should be placed immediately in a container suitable for the purpose for which it is to be used. The needle should first be removed from the syringe, since forcing the blood through the needle may cause haemolysis. Appropriate containers for particular investigations should be obtained from the laboratory.

Heparin and sequestrene (EDTA) are the most generally useful anticoagulants. Sequestrene can be used for most haematological investigations and heparin for most simple chemical tests, with the exception of blood glucose, for which bottles containing sodium fluoride are necessary.

For blood group and serological investigations blood should be taken into a dry sterile bottle or tube. If the specimen has to be sent to the laboratory by post, it is best to wait till the blood has clotted. Some serum should then be removed with a sterile needle and syringe, and this serum is sent separately, together with the blood clot.

Lumbar puncture

See p. 344.

MAKING THE BEST USE OF RESULTS

It is merely stating the obvious to say that the interpretation of any laboratory test will depend on the relevance of the test to the presumptive diagnosis and the interpreter's knowledge of pathology, biochemistry and physiology. The task of a clinical laboratory is to put these disciplines to work in the solution of a diagnostic problem.

All tests are subject to errors of performance. Fortunately these are rare, but the clinician will help the pathologist if he tells him of any 'rogue' result that does not accord with other data. All results will depend on the precision of the method used and the variability of the quality measured amongst a healthy population.

In non-quantitative tests, as in cytology, there may be false positives and false negatives. The laboratory should be able to say with what frequency these may occur. For instance, in cases of bronchial carcinoma, malignant cells are often to be detected in the sputum; however, in a very small proportion of examinations, apparently malignant cells in the sputum will be reported when there is no bronchial carcinoma. The clinician can give some weight to such findings by considering the patient. If the patient is a middle-aged man who smokes heavily, the report of malignant cells would be likely to be a true positive as bronchial carcinoma is prevalent in such patients. Conversely, if the patient is a non-smoking girl, the positive sputum report would be likely to be false.

For quantitative tests, as in biochemistry and much of haematology, the precision of a test can be determined statistically and its performance monitored within the laboratory and by cooperation with other laboratories.

Precision is the measure of the repeatability of a determination. If the method is very precise the spread of results around the 'true' value will be small and vice versa. The precision of measurement has to be linked to the variations of the 'true' value as found in a population of, say, 1000 healthy people. The results of the measurement performed on this group of normals can be plotted as a gaussian curve on either side of the mean value. It is conventional to express this normal range as the mean value plus or minus two standard deviations. Within this range will fall 95% of all normal results. However, it has to be remembered that one in 20 of normal results will fall just outside the normal range. Therefore a value just outside the range of normal does not necessarily indicate abnormality. It should also be remembered that normal ranges have to be established for the sex and age of the groups studied and also for the method as performed in each laboratory.

Appendix

CENTIGRADE AND FAHRENHEIT SCALES

The Centigrade (Celsius) scale is preferred.
The following table shows the relationship of the Centigrade and Fahrenheit scales, as far as is likely to be required in clinical work.

Centigrade	Fahrenheit	Centigrade	Fahrenheit
110	230	36.5	97.7
100	212	36	96.8
95	203	35.5	95.9
90	194	35	95
85	185	34	93.2
80	176	33	91.4
75	167	32	89.6
70	158	31	87.8
65	149	30	86
60	140	25	77
55	131	20	68
50	122	15	59
45	113	10	50
44	111.2	5	41
43	109.4	0	32
42	107.6	–5	23
41	105.8	–10	14
40.5	104.9	–15	5
40	104	–20	–4
39.5	103.1		
39	102.2	0.54	1
38.5	101.3	1	1.8
38	100.4	2	3.6
37.5	99.5	2.5	4.5
37	98.6		

To convert Fahrenheit to Centigrade:

$$X°\text{F} - 32 \times \frac{5}{9} = Y°\text{C}$$

To convert Centigrade to Fahrenheit:

$$X°\text{C} \times \frac{9}{5} + 32 = Y°\text{F}$$

SI UNITS

In this book the Système International d'Unités has been used as far as possible. This system aims to derive all measurements from seven basic units and to express all measurements as decimal fractions or multiples of these. Of the seven basic units the four which appear in this book are:

Physical quantity	Name of SI unit	Symbol
length	metre	m
mass	kilogram	kg
time	second	s
amount of substance	mole	mol

and the prefixes indicating the decimal fractions and multiples are:

Fraction	Prefix	Symbol
10^{-1}	deci-	d
10^{-2}	centi-	c
10^{-3}	milli-	m
10^{-6}	micro-	μ
10^{-9}	nano-	n
10^{-12}	pico-	p
10^{-15}	femto-	f
Multiple	**Prefix**	**Symbol**
10	deca-	da
10^2	hecto-	h
10^3	kilo-	k
10^6	mega	M

The litre (1 = dm^3) is also recognized as the unit of volume.

It follows that with the adoption of SI, certain familiar terms no longer are used, as is the case with measures of volume. A cubic centimetre (cc, cm^3) is replaced by the millilitre (ml) and the cubic millimetre (cmm, mm^3) by the microlitre (μl). In linear measure the micron (μ) should no longer be used; the correct unit is the micrometre (μm). Blood, intrauterine and intra-ocular pressures are measured in millimetres of mercury (mmHg) and intrathecal pressures in centimetres of CSF (cm CSF). It is recommended that the medical calorie or kilocalorie should now be converted to the joule (1 kcal = 4186.8J).

Further information on SI units may be obtained from *The Use of SI Units*, Publication PD 5686 of the British Standards Institution, and useful information on the SI units commonly used in medicine and biology is available in *Units, Symbols and Abbreviations: A Guide for Biological and Medical Editors and Authors*, published by the Royal Society of Medicine.

SOME APPROXIMATE CONVERSION TABLES

1 fluid ounce (fl oz)	= 28 ml
1 gallon UK (gal)	= 4.5 litres
1 grain (do not abbreviate)	= 65 mg
1 inch (in)	=25.4 mm
1 foot (ft)	= 0.3 m
1 ounce (oz)	= 28 g
1 pound (lb)	= 0.45 kg
1 calorie (cal)	= 4.2 J
1 kilocalorie (medical calorie, Cal)	= 4.2 kJ

Index

Note: Page numbers of figures and tables are in italic type.

Current Medical Treatment
5th edition

Edited by **C.W.H. Havard**, Vice Dean, The Royal Free Hospital School of Medicine; Consultant Physician and Physician in Charge of the Endocrine Unit, Royal Free Hospital; Consultant Physician, and Honorary Director of the Clinical Pharmacology Unit, Royal Northern Hospital, London—with 29 distinguished contributors

Complete coverage—Clinical pharmacology is now an established medical discipline but there is, however, far more to the management of the sick patient than purely pharmacokinetics and pharmacodynamics. This book fills the need for a comprehensive work on medical treatment.

The distinguished team of contributors consists of physicians actively engaged in the practice of medicine and the teaching of medical students.

A practical book of reference for the medical student and the house officer, this work is also a valuable guide for the postgraduate and for the general practitioner.

Well-organized by body system, the format of the book is conventional and provides easy access to the vital facts.

This edition contains new chapters on parenteral nutrition and problems specific for the elderly. The editorial policy of purposeful renewal of the contributors has been continued to ensure constant and fundamental revision. Most of the text has been completely re-written and eleven chapters have new authors.

Drug-induced Disease—C.W.H. Havard & R.M. Pearson • Antimicrobial Therapy—A.E. Dormer • Diuretics—C.W.H. Havard • Infectious Diseases and Immunization—H.P. Lambert & M.H. Wansbrough-Jones • Diseases of the Blood—A.V. Hoffbrand & J.E. Pettit • Diseases of the Reticulo-endothelial Tissue and Leukaemia—J.S. Malpas & T.A. Lister • Bleeding Disorders and Thrombosis—A.S. Gallus • Diseases of the Heart and Circulation—T.R. Evans • Diseases of the Alimentary Tract—J.E. Lennard-Jones • Diseases of the Pancreas and Liver—R.E. Pounder & H.C. Thomas • Renal Diseases—Paul Sweny • Metabolic and Nutritional Diseases—Harry Keen • Diseases of the Endocrine Glands—C.W.H. Havard • Disorders of Connective Tissues and Joints—J.T. Scott • Respiratory Diseases and Tuberculosis—P.D.B. Davies • Diseases of the Skin—S.K. Goolamali & M.W. Greaves • Diseases of the Eye—J.H. Dobree • Tropical Diseases and Infestations—Anthony P. Hall • Sexually Transmitted Diseases—M.W. Adler • Diseases of Children—T.H. Hughes-Davies • Domestic and Industrial Poisoning—George Kazantzis • Intensive Care Nutrition—H.A. Lee • Problems Specific to the Elderly—Michael F. Green

Baillière Tindall   Fifth Edition   1983   0 7020 0989 X   544 pp   30 illus.   HB